Diagnostic Ultrasound
Head and Neck

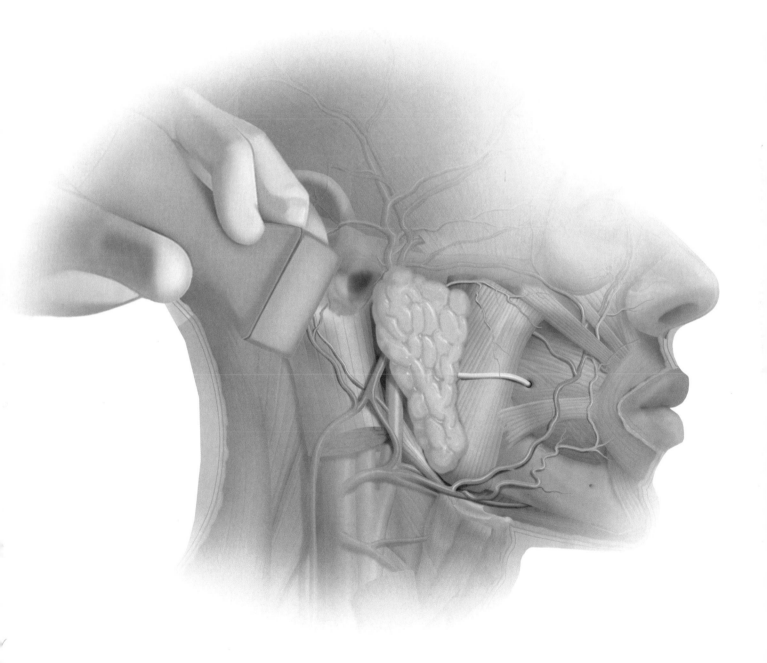

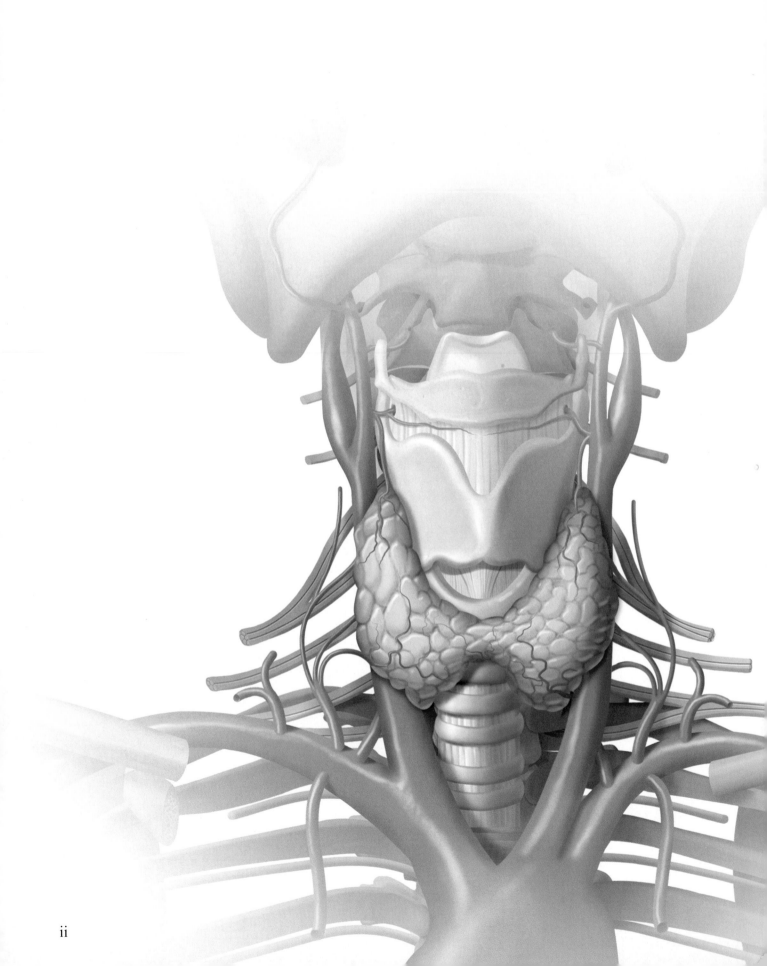

Diagnostic Ultrasound
Head and Neck

Anil T. Ahuja

MBBS (Bom), MD (Bom), FRCR, FHKCR, FHKAM (Radiology)

Professor of Imaging & Interventional Radiology
Chairman, Department of Imaging & Interventional Radiology
Prince of Wales Hospital
Faculty of Medicine
The Chinese University of Hong Kong
Hong Kong (SAR), China

AMIRSYS®

Names you know. Content you trust.®

First Edition

© 2014 Amirsys, Inc.

Compilation © 2014 Amirsys Publishing, Inc.

Printed in Canada by Friesens, Altona, Manitoba, Canada

ISBN: 978-1-937242-16-9

Notice and Disclaimer

Publisher Cataloging-in-Publication Data

Diagnostic ultrasound : head and neck / [edited by] Anil T. Ahuja.
    pages ; cm
    Head and neck
    Includes bibliographical references and index.
    ISBN 978-1-937242-16-9 (hardback)

1. Diagnostic ultrasonic imaging. 2. Head--Anatomy. 3. Neck--Anatomy. I. Ahuja, Anil. T.
II. Title: Head and neck.
[DNLM: 1. Head--ultrasonography--Atlases. 2. Neck--ultrasonography--Atlases.
3. Head--anatomy & histology--Atlases. 4. Neck--anatomy & histology--Atlases. WN 208]

RC78.7.U4 D515 2014
616.07543--dc23

To my late mum and dad, I owe it all to them. I have been blessed!

To Anita, no sister could have sacrificed more for the success of her brother. The rock in our lives.

To the three girls who make it all worthwhile: My precious wife, Reann, for her love, support, patience, and tolerance of my many imperfections; my lovely daughters, Sanjali and Tiana, for the sheer love, joy, happiness, and meaning they bring to our lives.

ATA

I dedicate my work on this book to the Head and Neck Imaging team in PWH. I could not have completed the task without the hard work and collaborative effort of each of the radiologists and technologists who helped me during this project.

To Anil, my mentor and friend, for his selfless sharing of knowledge and his leadership through this process and throughout the many years that I have known him.

I especially want to thank Dr. Ric Harnsberger and Dr. Donald Resnick for their mentoring, encouragement, and for serving as my inspiration.

Finally, to my mother and siblings, without whose love and support I certainly could not have accomplished this.

YYPL

To my beloved wife, Anna, lovely kids, Mike, Audrey, and Chloe, who bring happiness, hope, and courage to my life.

To my teacher of radiology, Anil, who instilled in me the love and passion for my specialty.

To ultrasound colleagues in my department, whose work has contributed so much to the progress in ultrasound.

KTW

Contributing Authors

Yolanda Y. P. Lee
MBChB, FRCR, FHKCR, FHKAM (Radiology)

Associate Consultant & Clinical Associate Professor (honorary)
Department of Imaging & Interventional Radiology
Prince of Wales Hospital
Faculty of Medicine
The Chinese University of Hong Kong
Hong Kong (SAR), China

K. T. Wong
MBChB, FRCR, FHKCR, FHKAM (Radiology)

Consultant & Clinical Associate Professor (honorary)
Department of Imaging & Interventional Radiology
Prince of Wales Hospital
Faculty of Medicine
The Chinese University of Hong Kong
Hong Kong (SAR), China

Carmen C. M. Cho
MBBS, FRCR, FHKCR, FHKAM (Radiology)

Associate Consultant & Clinical Assistant Professor (honorary)
Department of Imaging & Interventional Radiology
Prince of Wales Hospital
Faculty of Medicine
The Chinese University of Hong Kong
Hong Kong (SAR), China

Kunwar S. S. Bhatia

B Med Sci, BMBS, MRCS, DLO, FRCR

Assistant Professor
Department of Imaging & Interventional Radiology
Prince of Wales Hospital
Faculty of Medicine
The Chinese University of Hong Kong
Hong Kong (SAR), China

H. Y. Yuen

MBChB, FRCR, FHKCR, FHKAM (Radiology), MPH

Associate Consultant & Clinical Associate Professor (honorary)
Department of Imaging & Interventional Radiology
Prince of Wales Hospital
Faculty of Medicine
The Chinese University of Hong Kong
Hong Kong (SAR), China

Stella Sin Yee Ho

RDMS, RVT, PhD

Adjunct Associate Professor
Department of Imaging & Interventional Radiology
Prince of Wales Hospital
Faculty of Medicine
The Chinese University of Hong Kong
Hong Kong (SAR), China

Simon S. M. Ho

MBBS, FRCR

Clinical Associate Professor (honorary)
Department of Imaging & Interventional Radiology
Prince of Wales Hospital
Faculty of Medicine
The Chinese University of Hong Kong
Hong Kong (SAR), China

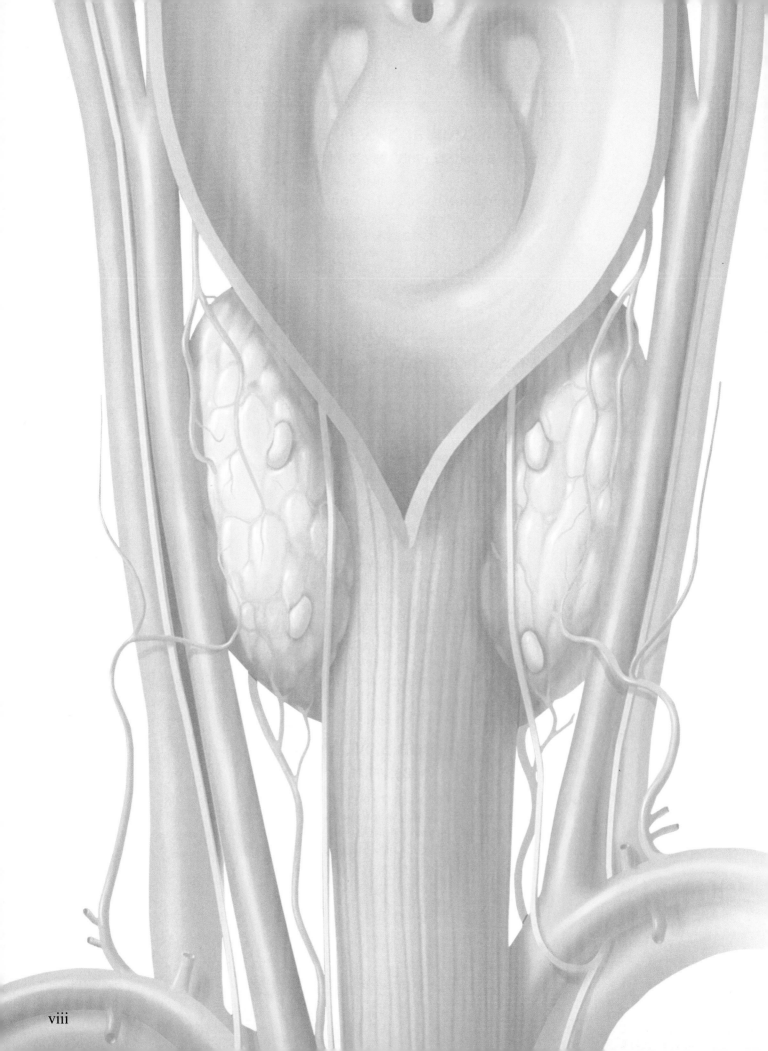

Preface

Ultrasound is a key imaging modality in the head and neck, both as a primary imaging tool and in other instances complementary to CT, MR, and nuclear medicine. Its role over the years has significantly expanded, and its practice is no longer restricted to imaging/radiology/ultrasound departments. Endocrinologists and head and neck surgeons use ultrasound extensively in their clinical practice as an initial localizing and diagnostic tool because it is more sensitive than palpation and accurately characterizes many lesions in head and neck. They also use it to safely guide confirmatory needle biopsy or therapy (radiofrequency ablation, ethanol injection, etc.) and for routine patient follow-up. This book was written to provide essential information to all practicing "sonologists" and to those who may be considering taking up head and neck ultrasound.

Diagnostic Ultrasound: Head and Neck is divided into three parts: Anatomy, diagnoses, and differential diagnosis. The first part, anatomy, covers relevant sonographic anatomy in the head and neck, with complementary images from CT and MR. The second part, diagnoses, the core content of the book, provides detailed sonographic descriptions of common head and neck lesions, key clinical information, and practical scanning tips for identifying the wide spectrum of diseases in this region. The third and final part provides differential diagnoses for common sonographic signs and appearances. Although the book focuses on ultrasound, readers will find images from other imaging modalities so as to highlight the importance of multimodality imaging in modern clinical practice.

This book is a compilation of the head and neck sections of three previous books published by Amirsys, namely *Diagnostic Imaging: Ultrasound*; *Diagnostic and Surgical Imaging Anatomy: Ultrasound*; and *Expertddx: Ultrasound*. The text and 400-plus images in the anatomy section remain relatively unchanged from the earlier book. The diagnoses section includes 20 diagnoses from the earlier books and 21 new diagnoses/chapters. This section also contains 1,000-plus images, almost all of which are new and accompanied by comprehensive annotation, including illustrative images of shearwave elastography and strain imaging. The key facts feature has been retained in this book and is ideal for quick review. The differential diagnosis section of this book features 250-plus images, more than half of which are new, and includes key references.

Any book of this nature involves hard work, but the opportunity to work with friends with similar interests makes it fun. It gives us all a platform to share our experience, images, and knowledge as well as learn from each other as well as test our levels of patience and tolerance. We remain indebted to all the authors, coauthors, sonographers, and medical editors, and to the Amirsys team who have gently cajoled and patiently guided us along the entire process, despite being in a different part of the world. Finally, we would like to thank Dr. Ric Harnsberger and Dr. Paula Woodward for their unflinching support over the years.

We hope our efforts in some small way help you in your routine clinical practice.

Anil T. Ahuja

MBBS (Bom), MD (Bom), FRCR, FHKCR, FHKAM (Radiology)

Professor of Imaging & Interventional Radiology
Chairman, Department of Imaging & Interventional Radiology
Prince of Wales Hospital
Faculty of Medicine
The Chinese University of Hong Kong
Hong Kong (SAR), China

Yolanda Y. P. Lee

MBChB, FRCR, FHKCR, FHKAM (Radiology)

Associate Consultant & Clinical Associate Professor (honorary)
Department of Imaging & Interventional Radiology
Prince of Wales Hospital
Faculty of Medicine
The Chinese University of Hong Kong
Hong Kong (SAR), China

K. T. Wong

MBChB, FRCR, FHKCR, FHKAM (Radiology)

Consultant & Clinical Associate Professor (honorary)
Department of Imaging & Interventional Radiology
Prince of Wales Hospital
Faculty of Medicine
The Chinese University of Hong Kong
Hong Kong (SAR), China

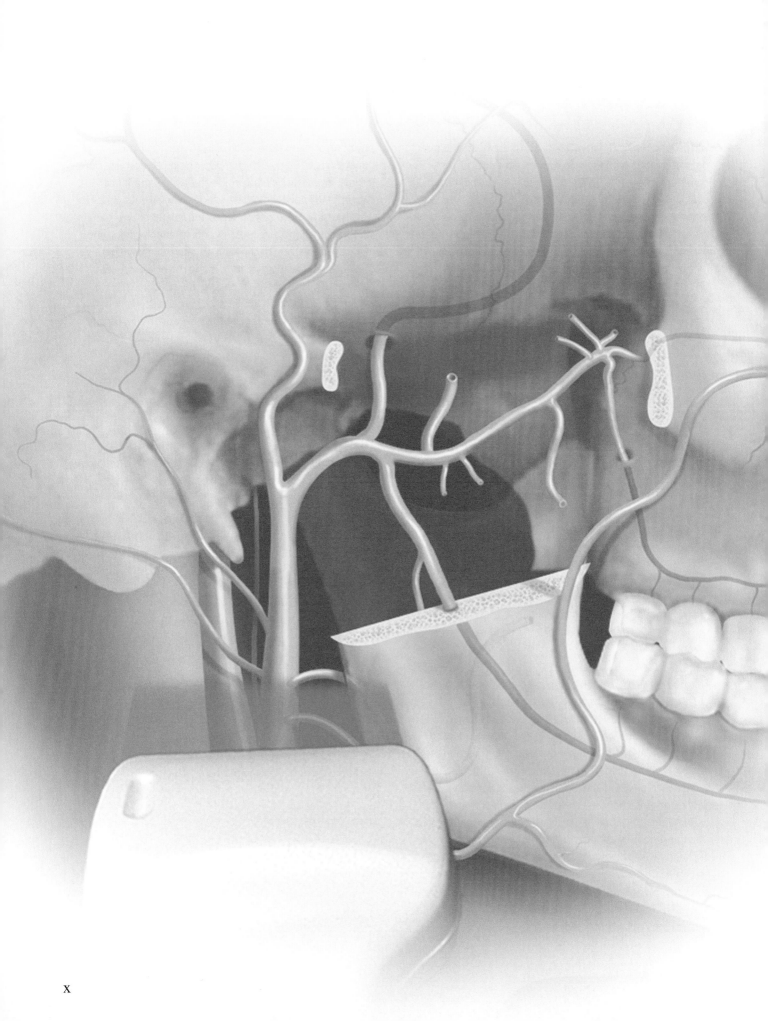

x

Acknowledgements

Text Editing
Dave L. Chance, MA, ELS
Angela M. Green Terry, BA
Sarah J. Connor, BA
Tricia L. Cannon, BA

Image Editing
Jeffrey J. Marmorstone, BS
Lisa A. M. Steadman, BS
Kevin Lo Hoi Nga

Medical Editing
Ryan Chi Hang Nung, MBChB(H.K.), FRCR
Jacqueline Ching Man Sitt, MBBS(H.K.), FRCR
Simon Sin Man Wong, MBBS(H.K.), FRCR
Janice Wong Li Yu, MBBS(H.K.), FRCR

Illustrations
Richard Coombs, MS
Lane R. Bennion, MS
Laura C. Sesto, MA

Art Direction and Design
Laura C. Sesto, MA
Tom M. Olson, BA

Lead Editor
Arthur G. Gelsinger, MA

Publishing Leads
Katherine L. Riser, MA
Rebecca L. Hutchinson, BA

AMIRSYS®

Names you know. Content you trust.®

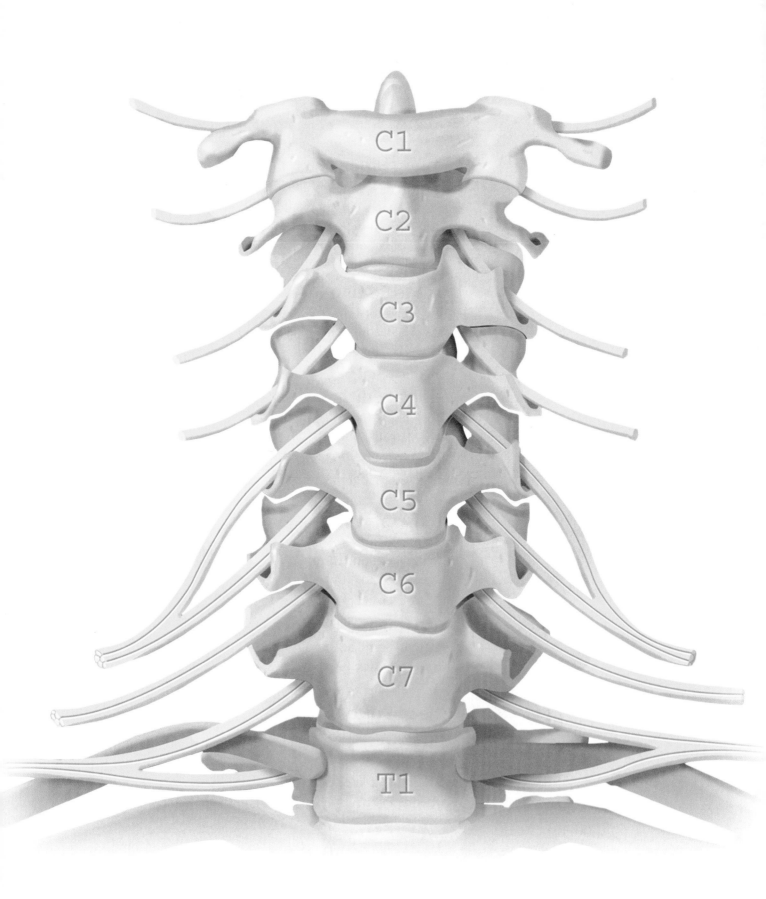

Sections

TABLE OF CONTENTS

PART II
Diagnoses

SECTION 1
Introduction and Overview

SECTION 2
Thyroid and Parathyroid

SECTION 3
Lymph Nodes

SECTION 6
Vascular

Diagnostic Ultrasound
Head and Neck

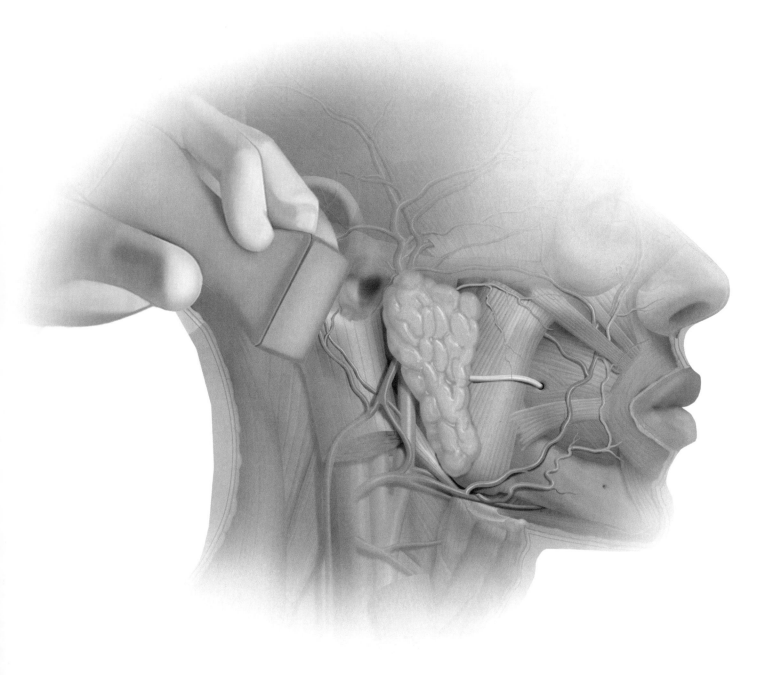

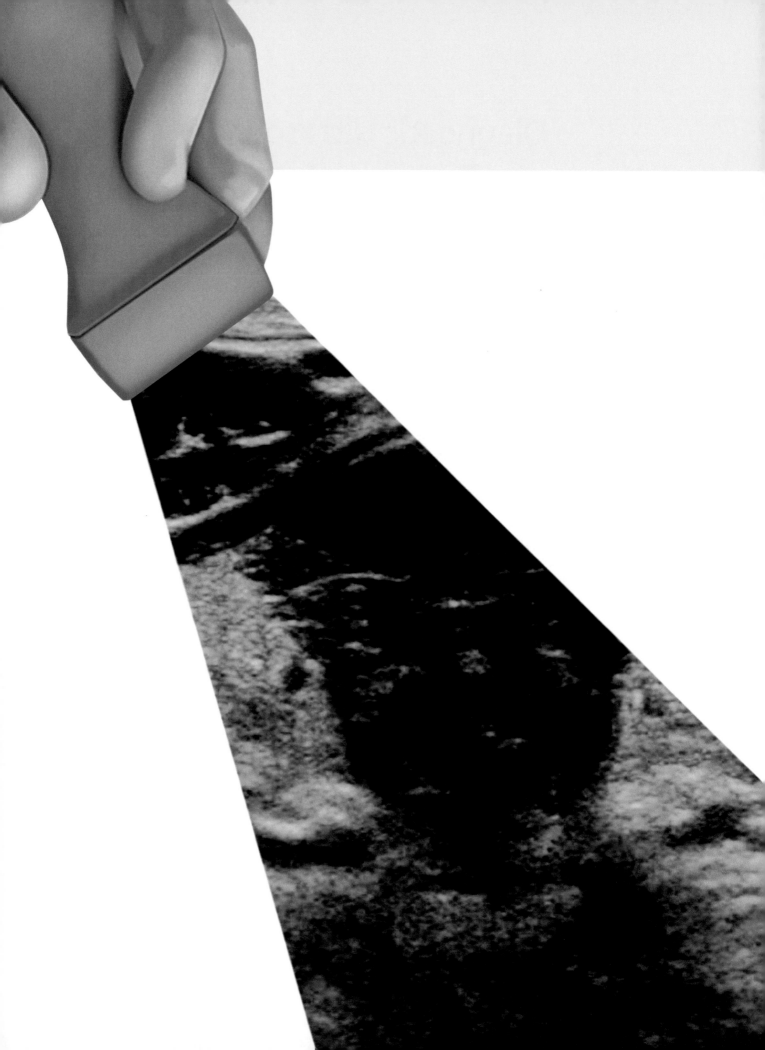

SECTION 1
Head and Neck

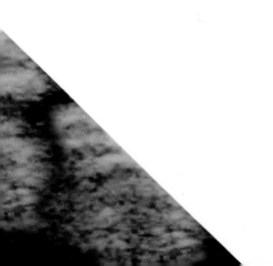

NECK

TERMINOLOGY

Abbreviations
- Suprahyoid neck (SHN)
- Infrahyoid neck (IHN)

Definitions
- SHN: Spaces from skull base to hyoid bone (excluding orbits, paranasal sinuses, and oral cavity) including parapharyngeal (PPS), pharyngeal mucosal (PMS), masticator (MS), parotid (PS), carotid (CS), buccal (BS), retropharyngeal (RPS), and perivertebral (PVS) spaces
- IHN: Spaces below hyoid bone to thoracic inlet, including visceral space (VS), posterior cervical space (PCS), anterior cervical space (ACS), CS, RPS, and PVS

IMAGING ANATOMY

Overview
- Fascial spaces of SHN and IHN are key for cross-sectional imaging
  - Concept is difficult to apply with ultrasound
- Ultrasound anatomy is based on division of neck into anterior and posterior triangles
  - Anterior triangle: Bounded anteriorly by midline and posteriorly by posterior margin of sternomastoid muscle
    - Further divided into suprahyoid and infrahyoid portions
    - Suprahyoid portion: Divided by anterior belly of digastric muscle into submental and submandibular triangles
    - Infrahyoid portion: Divided by superior belly of omohyoid muscle into muscular and carotid triangles
  - Posterior triangle: Bound anteriorly by posterior margin of sternomastoid muscle and posteriorly by anterior border of trapezius muscle
    - Apex formed by mastoid process, base of triangle formed by clavicle
    - Subdivided by posterior belly of omohyoid muscle into occipital triangle (superior) and supraclavicular triangle (inferior)
- Submental region
  - Key structures include anterior belly of digastric muscle, mylohyoid, genioglossus and geniohyoid muscles, sublingual glands, and lingual artery
- Submandibular region
  - Key structures include submandibular gland, mylohyoid muscle, hyoglossus muscle, anterior and posterior bellies of digastric muscle, facial vein, and anterior division of retromandibular vein (RMV)
- Parotid region
  - Key structures include parotid gland, masseter and buccinator muscles, RMV, and external carotid artery (ECA)
- Cervical region
  - Upper cervical region: Skull base to hyoid bone/carotid bifurcation
    - Key structures include internal jugular vein (IJV), carotid bifurcation, jugulodigastric node, and posterior belly of digastric muscle
  - Mid cervical region: Hyoid bone to cricoid cartilage
    - Key structures include IJV, common carotid artery (CCA), vagus nerve, and lymph nodes
  - Lower cervical region: Cricoid cartilage to clavicle
    - Key structures include IJV, CCA, superior belly of omohyoid, and lymph nodes
- Supraclavicular fossa
  - Key structures include trapezius, sternomastoid, omohyoid muscles, brachial plexus elements, and transverse cervical nodes
- Posterior triangle
  - Bordered anteriorly by sternomastoid muscle and posteriorly by trapezius muscle
  - Floor formed by scalene muscles, levator scapulae, and splenius capitis muscles
- Midline
  - Key structures include hyoid bone, strap muscles, thyroid, larynx, and tracheal rings

ANATOMY IMAGING ISSUES

Imaging Recommendations
- Use of high-resolution transducers is essential
- Color/power Doppler examination provides useful supplementary information to grayscale ultrasound
- US is very sensitive in identifying abnormalities (and in characterizing many head and neck soft tissue lesions)
  - Combination with FNAC provides specificity and increased diagnostic accuracy
- US + FNAC usually provides adequate information for patient management
- Cross-sectional imaging (CT, MR) may be required for
  - Large mass, when detailed anatomical extent is not fully examined by US
  - Deep-seated lesion with suboptimal US visualization and evaluation
  - Preoperative assessment of relevant adjacent structures (e.g., bone involvement)

Imaging Approaches
- Ultrasound imaging protocol
  - Start in submental region by scanning in transverse plane
  - Next, scan the submandibular region in transverse and longitudinal/oblique planes
  - Then scan parotid region in transverse and longitudinal planes
  - Now examine upper cervical, mid cervical, and lower cervical regions in transverse plane
  - Then examine supraclavicular fossa with transducer held transversely
  - Now scan posterior triangle transversely along a line drawn from mastoid process to ipsilateral acromion
  - Finally, scan midline and thyroid gland in both transverse and longitudinal planes
- This protocol is robust and can be tailored to suit individual clinical conditions
- Transverse scans quickly identify normal anatomy and detect abnormalities
- Any abnormality identified is further examined in longitudinal/oblique planes (grayscale and Doppler)
- In restless children, it may not be possible to follow the above protocol
  - It would therefore be best to evaluate primary area of interest 1st, before the child becomes uncooperative

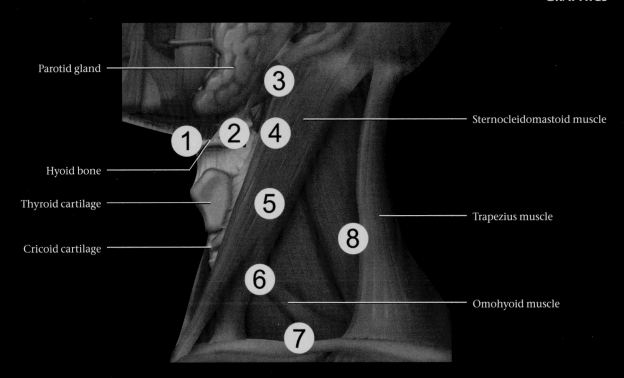

Parotid gland

Sternocleidomastoid muscle

Hyoid bone

Thyroid cartilage

Trapezius muscle

Cricoid cartilage

Omohyoid muscle

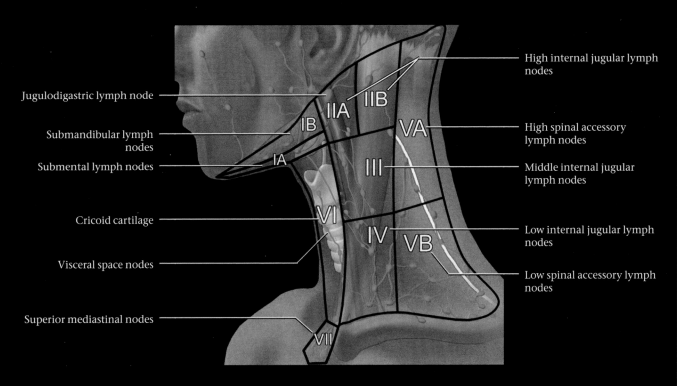

Jugulodigastric lymph node

High internal jugular lymph nodes

Submandibular lymph nodes

High spinal accessory lymph nodes

Submental lymph nodes

Middle internal jugular lymph nodes

Cricoid cartilage

Visceral space nodes

Low internal jugular lymph nodes

Low spinal accessory lymph nodes

Superior mediastinal nodes

(Top) Schematic diagram shows the protocol for ultrasound examination of the neck with 8 regions scanned in order: (1) submental region, (2) submandibular region, (3) parotid region, (4) upper cervical region, (5) mid cervical region, (6) lower cervical region, (7) supraclavicular fossa, and (8) posterior triangle. The above protocol is robust and helps to adequately evaluate the neck for common clinical conditions. Note that deep structures cannot be adequately assessed by ultrasound. *(Bottom)* Lateral oblique graphic of the neck shows the anatomic locations of the major nodal groups of the neck. Division of the internal jugular nodal chain into high, middle, and low regions is defined by the level of the hyoid bone and cricoid cartilage. Similarly, the spinal accessory nodal chain is divided into high & low regions by the level of the cricoid cartilage.

GRAPHICS

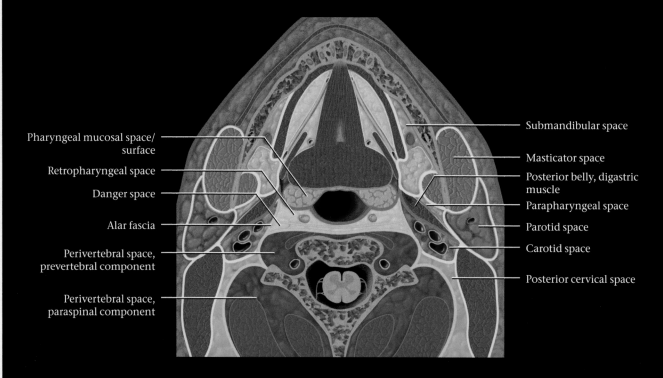

Pharyngeal mucosal space/ surface

Retropharyngeal space

Danger space

Alar fascia

Perivertebral space, prevertebral component

Perivertebral space, paraspinal component

Submandibular space

Masticator space

Posterior belly, digastric muscle

Parapharyngeal space

Parotid space

Carotid space

Posterior cervical space

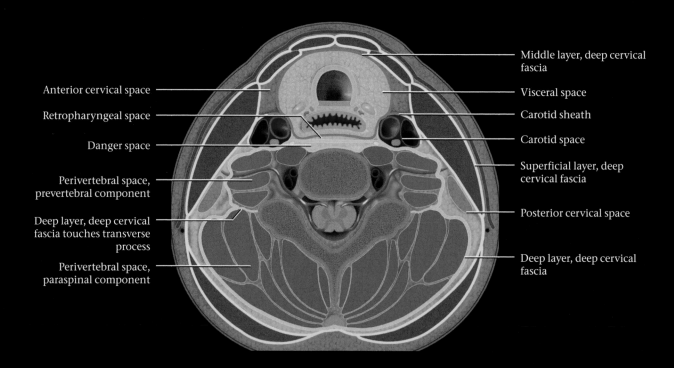

Anterior cervical space

Retropharyngeal space

Danger space

Perivertebral space, prevertebral component

Deep layer, deep cervical fascia touches transverse process

Perivertebral space, paraspinal component

Middle layer, deep cervical fascia

Visceral space

Carotid sheath

Carotid space

Superficial layer, deep cervical fascia

Posterior cervical space

Deep layer, deep cervical fascia

(Top) Axial graphic shows the suprahyoid neck spaces at the level of the oropharynx. The superficial (yellow line), middle (pink line), and deep (turquoise line) layers of deep cervical fascia (DCF) outline the suprahyoid neck spaces. Notice the lateral borders of the retropharyngeal & danger spaces are called the alar fascia and represent a slip of the deep layer of DCF. (Bottom) Axial graphic depicts the fascia and spaces of the infrahyoid neck. The 3 layers of DCF are present in the suprahyoid and infrahyoid neck. The carotid sheath is made up of all 3 layers of DCF (tricolor line around carotid space). Notice the deep layer completely circles the perivertebral space, diving in laterally to divide it into prevertebral and a paraspinal components. Although the spaces are not adequately demonstrated by US, it is important to be familiar with the concept in order to understand neck anatomy.

TRANSVERSE ULTRASOUND

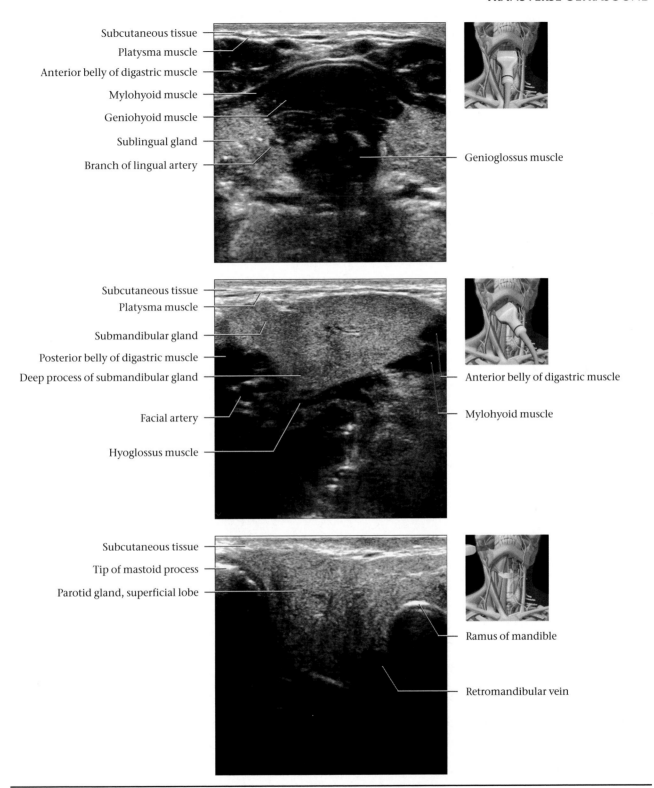

(Top) Standard transverse grayscale ultrasound image shows the submental region. The mylohyoid muscle is an important landmark for the division of the sublingual (deep to mylohyoid muscle) and submandibular (superficial to mylohyoid muscle) spaces. Part of the extrinsic muscles of the tongue, including the geniohyoid and genioglossus, are visualized. *(Middle)* Standard transverse grayscale ultrasound image shows the submandibular region. The submandibular gland is the key structure with its homogeneous echotexture. The gland sits astride the mylohyoid and posterior belly of the digastric muscles. *(Bottom)* Standard transverse grayscale ultrasound image shows the parotid region. Note that the deep lobe is obscured by shadowing from the mandible and cannot be evaluated. The retromandibular vein serves as a landmark for the intraparotid facial nerve.

NECK

TRANSVERSE ULTRASOUND

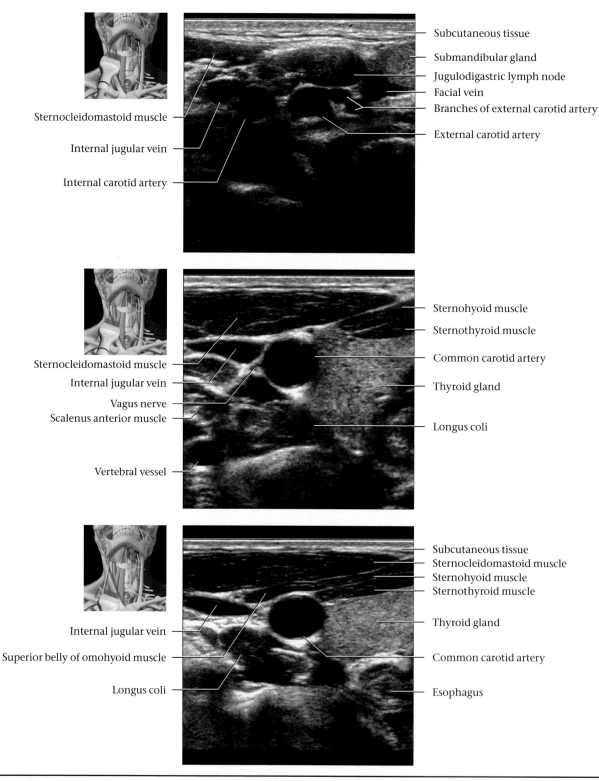

(Top: labels)
- Sternocleidomastoid muscle
- Internal jugular vein
- Internal carotid artery
- Subcutaneous tissue
- Submandibular gland
- Jugulodigastric lymph node
- Facial vein
- Branches of external carotid artery
- External carotid artery

(Middle: labels)
- Sternocleidomastoid muscle
- Internal jugular vein
- Vagus nerve
- Scalenus anterior muscle
- Vertebral vessel
- Sternohyoid muscle
- Sternothyroid muscle
- Common carotid artery
- Thyroid gland
- Longus coli

(Bottom: labels)
- Internal jugular vein
- Superior belly of omohyoid muscle
- Longus coli
- Subcutaneous tissue
- Sternocleidomastoid muscle
- Sternohyoid muscle
- Sternothyroid muscle
- Thyroid gland
- Common carotid artery
- Esophagus

(Top) Standard transverse grayscale ultrasound image shows the upper cervical level. Key structures include the internal jugular vein, the proximal internal and external carotid arteries, and the jugular chain lymph nodes. The jugulodigastric node is the most prominent and consistently seen on ultrasound. (Middle) Standard grayscale ultrasound image shows the mid cervical level. Note the vagus nerve is clearly seen on ultrasound. (Bottom) Standard grayscale ultrasound image shows the lower cervical level. The thyroid gland is related to the common carotid and internal jugular vein laterally. The anterior strap muscles (including the sternohyoid and sternothyroid muscles) and the superior belly of the omohyoid are clearly visualized.

TRANSVERSE ULTRASOUND

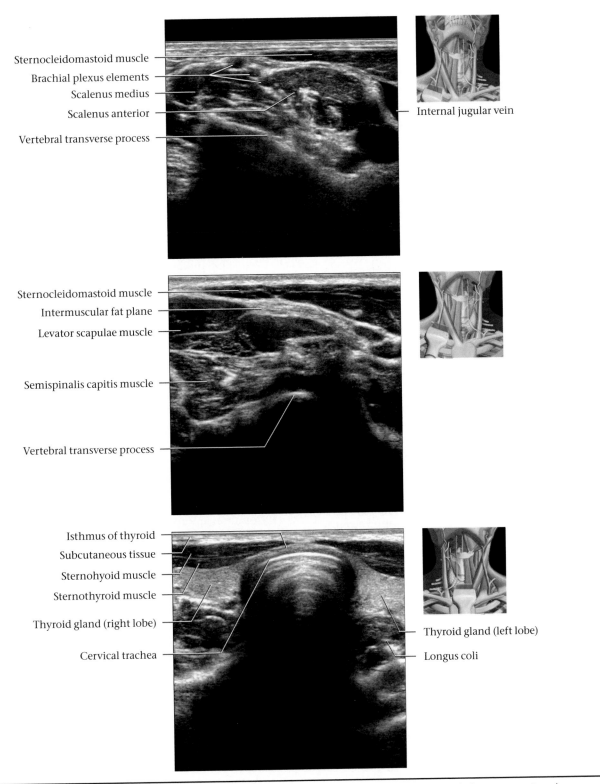

Sternocleidomastoid muscle
Brachial plexus elements
Scalenus medius
Scalenus anterior
Vertebral transverse process
Internal jugular vein

Sternocleidomastoid muscle
Intermuscular fat plane
Levator scapulae muscle
Semispinalis capitis muscle
Vertebral transverse process

Isthmus of thyroid
Subcutaneous tissue
Sternohyoid muscle
Sternothyroid muscle
Thyroid gland (right lobe)
Cervical trachea
Thyroid gland (left lobe)
Longus coli

(Top) Standard grayscale ultrasound image shows the supraclavicular fossa. Note that the trunks of the brachial plexus are consistently seen on high-resolution ultrasound at this site. *(Middle)* Standard transverse grayscale ultrasound image shows the posterior triangle. Note that the intermuscular fat plane is visible. The spinal accessory nerve and lymph nodes are important contents of the posterior triangle. *(Bottom)* Standard transverse grayscale ultrasound image shows the midline of the lower anterior neck. The isthmus of the thyroid gland, the trachea, and the longus coli are key structures to be identified.

SUBLINGUAL/SUBMENTAL REGION

TERMINOLOGY

Synonyms
- Sublingual space (SLS), submental triangle

Definitions
- Sublingual region (SLR): Paired nonfascial-lined spaces of oral cavity in deep oral tongue, above floor of mouth, superomedial to mylohyoid muscle

IMAGING ANATOMY

Overview
- Borders of submental triangle are readily defined on ultrasound
  - Floor is formed by mylohyoid muscle
  - Apex is limited anteriorly by symphysis menti
  - Base is bounded posteriorly by hyoid bone
  - Anterior belly of digastric muscle represents sides of triangle
- SLS is deep space of oral cavity superomedial to mylohyoid muscles
  - Contains key neurovascular structures of oral cavity
  - Includes glossopharyngeal nerve (CN9), hypoglossal nerve (CN12), lingual nerve (branch of V3), lingual artery and vein

Anatomy Relationships
- SLS relationships
  - SLS in deep oral tongue superomedial to mylohyoid muscle and lateral to genioglossus-geniohyoid muscles
  - Communication between sublingual spaces occurs in midline anteriorly as a narrow isthmus beneath frenulum
  - SLS communicates with submandibular space (SMS) and inferior parapharyngeal space (PPS) at posterior margin of mylohyoid muscle
    - There is no fascia dividing posterior SLS from adjacent SMS
    - Therefore, there is direct communication with SMS and PPS in this location

Internal Contents
- Major muscles forming borders of submental triangle
  - Anterior belly of digastric muscle
    - Marks lateral border of the submental triangle
  - Mylohyoid muscle
    - Muscle of the floor of mouth
    - Muscular sling between medial aspect of mandibular bodies
    - Anterior attachment to mandible inferior to origins of genial muscles
    - Separates SLS (deep to mylohyoid muscle plane) from SMS (superficial to mylohyoid muscle)
  - Genioglossus and geniohyoid muscles
    - Form root of tongue
    - Together with hyoglossus muscle, they make up major extrinsic muscles of tongue
- Posterior aspect of SLS is divided into medial and lateral compartments by hyoglossus muscle
- Lateral compartment contents
  - Hypoglossal nerve
    - Motor to intrinsic and extrinsic muscles of tongue

- Intrinsic muscles of tongue include inferior lingual, vertical, and transverse muscles
  - Lingual nerve: Branch of mandibular division of trigeminal nerve (CNV3) combined with chorda tympani branch of facial nerve
    - Lingual nerve branch of CNV3: Sensation to anterior 2/3 of oral tongue
    - Chorda tympani branch of facial nerve: Anterior 2/3 of tongue taste and parasympathetic secreto-motor fibers to submandibular ganglion/gland
  - Sublingual glands and ducts
    - Lie in anterior SLS bilaterally
    - ~ 5 small ducts open under oral tongue into oral cavity
    - With age, sublingual glands atrophy, becoming difficult to see on imaging
  - Submandibular glands and submandibular ducts
    - Submandibular gland deep margin extends into posterior opening of SLS
    - Submandibular duct runs anteriorly to papillae in anteromedial subfrenular mucosa
- Medial compartment contents
  - Glossopharyngeal nerve (CN9)
    - Provides sensation to posterior 1/3 of tongue
    - Carries taste input from posterior 1/3 of tongue
    - Located more cephalad in medial compartment compared to lingual artery and vein
  - Lingual artery and vein
    - Vascular supply to oral tongue
    - Seen running just lateral to genioglossus muscle

ANATOMY IMAGING ISSUES

Questions
- What defines a mass as primary to SLS?
  - Center of lesion is superomedial to mylohyoid muscle and lateral to genioglossus muscle
- Common lesions in submental region include
  - Congenital lesions: Epidermoid/dermoid cyst
  - Enlarged lymph node: Reactive, inflammatory or neoplastic (metastatic/lymphomatous nodes)
  - Inflammatory conditions: Ranula, abscess
  - Sublingual gland lesions: Sialadenitis, calculus, benign/malignant salivary gland tumor

Imaging Recommendations
- High-resolution ultrasound is ideal imaging tool for evaluating submental masses
- Major structures are best seen on transverse scans with patient's neck in slight hyperextension
- For more deep-seated lesions (e.g., deep to root of tongue), MR is necessary for better anatomical assessment
  - Ultrasound may help in directing a needle for guided biopsy of such lesions

RELATED REFERENCES

1. La'porte SJ et al: Imaging the floor of the mouth and the sublingual space. Radiographics. 31(5):1215-30, 2011
2. Ahuja AT et al: Practical Head & Neck Ultrasound. London: Greenwich Medical Media, 2000

SUBLINGUAL/SUBMENTAL REGION

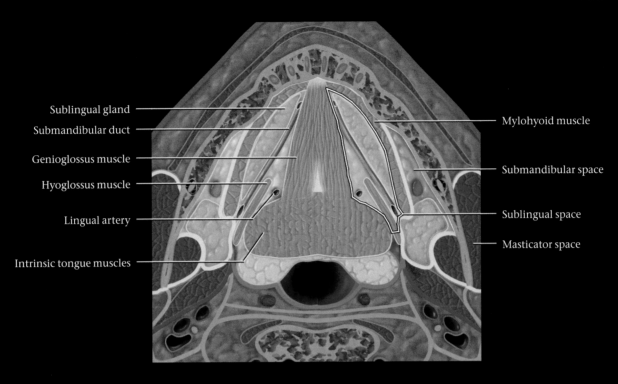

- Sublingual gland
- Submandibular duct
- Genioglossus muscle
- Hyoglossus muscle
- Lingual artery
- Intrinsic tongue muscles

- Mylohyoid muscle
- Submandibular space
- Sublingual space
- Masticator space

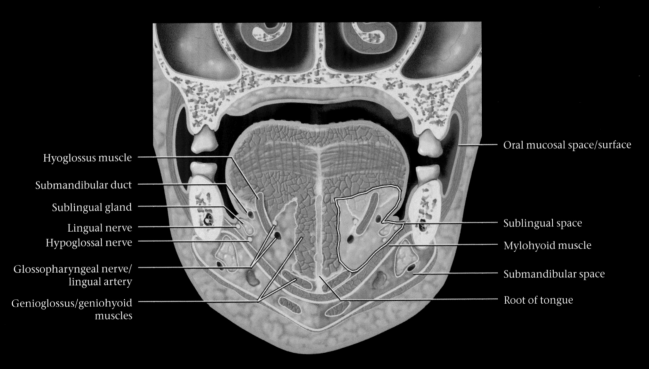

- Hyoglossus muscle
- Submandibular duct
- Sublingual gland
- Lingual nerve
- Hypoglossal nerve
- Glossopharyngeal nerve/ lingual artery
- Genioglossus/geniohyoid muscles

- Oral mucosal space/surface
- Sublingual space
- Mylohyoid muscle
- Submandibular space
- Root of tongue

(Top) Axial graphic through the body of the mandible shows the sublingual space (on patient's left, shaded in green) situated superomedial to the mylohyoid muscle and lateral to the genioglossus muscle. Notice the absence of fascia surrounding the sublingual space. The yellow line represents the superficial layer of deep cervical fascia. *(Bottom)* Coronal graphic through the oral cavity shows position of the mylohyoid muscle, which is the landmark in this area. The sublingual space (SLS) is shaded in green. The medial SLS compartment contains the glossopharyngeal nerve (CN9) and lingual artery/vein, and the lateral SLS compartment contains the submandibular duct, sublingual gland, lingual nerve, and hypoglossal nerve (CN12). The fascia-lined (yellow line) submandibular space is inferolateral to the mylohyoid muscle.

SUBLINGUAL/SUBMENTAL REGION

TRANSVERSE ULTRASOUND

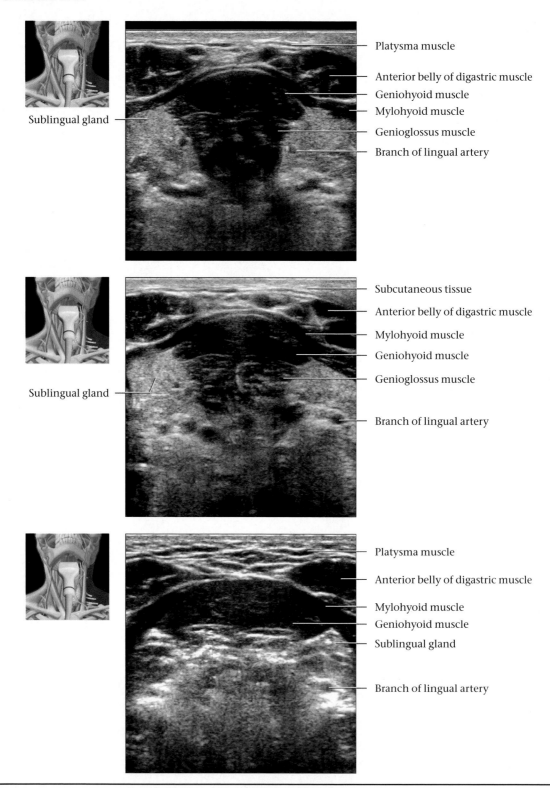

(Top) Platysma muscle — Anterior belly of digastric muscle — Geniohyoid muscle — Mylohyoid muscle — Genioglossus muscle — Branch of lingual artery — Sublingual gland

(Middle) Subcutaneous tissue — Anterior belly of digastric muscle — Mylohyoid muscle — Geniohyoid muscle — Genioglossus muscle — Branch of lingual artery — Sublingual gland

(Bottom) Platysma muscle — Anterior belly of digastric muscle — Mylohyoid muscle — Geniohyoid muscle — Sublingual gland — Branch of lingual artery

(Top) *More anterior transverse grayscale ultrasound of the submental and sublingual region is shown. The mylohyoid muscle is the landmark for division of sublingual space (deep to the mylohyoid plane) and submandibular space (superficial to the muscle plane). The sublingual gland appears as homogeneous, hyperechoic structures lateral to the geniohyoid/genioglossus muscle. Branches of lingual artery can be easily picked up on transverse plane. The submandibular duct sits alongside the lingual vessels, and a submandibular calculus may impact at this site.* *(**Middle**) More posterior transverse grayscale ultrasound allows the clear depiction of extrinsic muscles of the tongue at the root. (**Bottom**) Transverse grayscale ultrasound shows the submental region in a more posterior location.*

SUBLINGUAL/SUBMENTAL REGION

POWER DOPPLER ULTRASOUND AND CORONAL MR

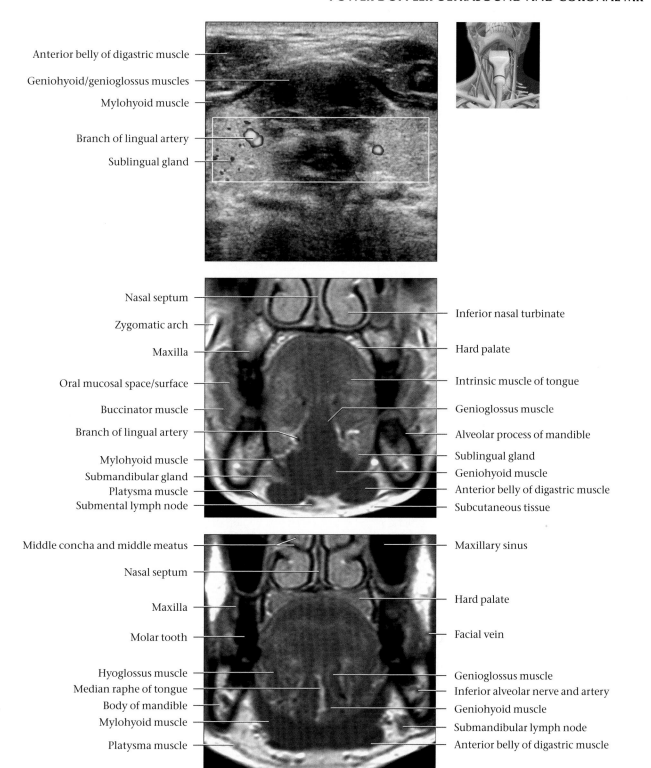

(Top) Power Doppler ultrasound of the submental region shows the presence of color flow within the branches of the lingual artery. The use of Doppler examination aids in differentiation from the dilated submandibular duct. **(Middle)** Correlative coronal T1WI MR shows the floor of the mouth and tongue. The mylohyoid muscle is the landmark separating the sublingual and submandibular spaces. **(Bottom)** Correlative coronal T1WI MR shows the floor of the mouth and tongue in a location more posterior to the previous image. For optimal use of ultrasound, the operator must also be familiar with the correlative anatomy on other imaging modalities.

SUBLINGUAL/SUBMENTAL REGION

LONGITUDINAL AND TRANSVERSE ULTRASOUND

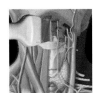
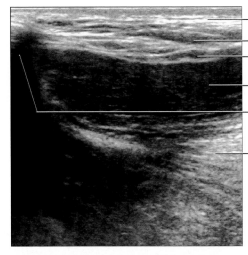

Subcutaneous tissue
Platysma muscle
Mylohyoid muscle
Geniohyoid muscle
Mandible
Genioglossus muscle

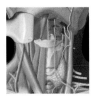
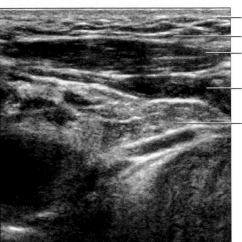

Subcutaneous tissue
Platysma muscle
Anterior belly of digastric muscle
Mylohyoid muscle
Sublingual gland

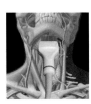
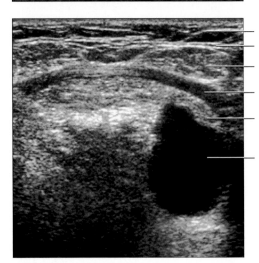

Subcutaneous tissue
Platysma muscle
Anterior belly of digastric muscle
Mylohyoid muscle
Sublingual space
Ranula

(Top) Longitudinal grayscale ultrasound of the submental region shows the relationship of the mylohyoid, geniohyoid, and genioglossus muscles. Note that scanning just off the midline will show more of the anterior belly of the digastric muscle rather than the mylohyoid muscle anteriorly. *(Middle)* Parasagittal longitudinal grayscale ultrasound shows the submental region. The sublingual gland is visualized within the sublingual space (deep to the mylohyoid muscle) underneath the anterior belly of the digastric and mylohyoid muscles. *(Bottom)* Transverse grayscale ultrasound shows a well-circumscribed, anechoic, cystic lesion in the left sublingual space (i.e., deep to the mylohyoid muscle plane). The appearance is suggestive of a ranula; relationship to the mylohyoid determines whether it is a simple or diving ranula.

SUBLINGUAL/SUBMENTAL REGION

SAGITTAL MR AND TRANSVERSE ULTRASOUND

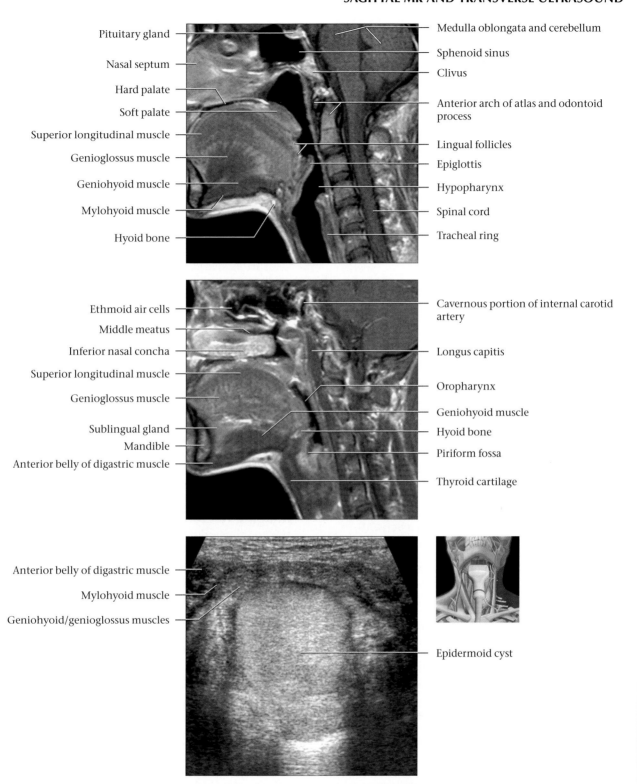

Pituitary gland — — Medulla oblongata and cerebellum

Nasal septum — — Sphenoid sinus

Hard palate — — Clivus

Soft palate — — Anterior arch of atlas and odontoid process

Superior longitudinal muscle — — Lingual follicles

Genioglossus muscle — — Epiglottis

Geniohyoid muscle — — Hypopharynx

Mylohyoid muscle — — Spinal cord

Hyoid bone — — Tracheal ring

Ethmoid air cells — — Cavernous portion of internal carotid artery

Middle meatus —

Inferior nasal concha — — Longus capitis

Superior longitudinal muscle — — Oropharynx

Genioglossus muscle —

Sublingual gland — — Geniohyoid muscle

Mandible — — Hyoid bone

Anterior belly of digastric muscle — — Piriform fossa

— Thyroid cartilage

Anterior belly of digastric muscle —

Mylohyoid muscle —

Geniohyoid/genioglossus muscles —

— Epidermoid cyst

(Top) Correlative sagittal T1WI MR shows the floor of the mouth close to the midline. Note the positions of the mylohyoid and geniohyoid muscles between the mandible anteriorly and hyoid bone posteriorly. (Middle) Sagittal T1WI MR shows the floor of the mouth in the paramedian plane. Note that the anterior belly of the digastric muscle is now seen as it extends anteromedially to insert on the inner cortex of the mandible. (Bottom) Transverse grayscale ultrasound of the submental region shows a well-circumscribed, homogeneous, hyperechoic, midline mass deep to the mylohyoid, geniohyoid, and genioglossus muscles. The appearances and anatomical location of the lesion are suggestive of an epidermoid cyst. Congenital lesions in the neck are site specific, and familiarity with the correlative anatomy is often the best clue to their diagnosis.

SUBMANDIBULAR REGION

TERMINOLOGY

Abbreviations
- Submandibular space (SMS)

Definitions
- Fascial-lined space inferolateral to mylohyoid muscle, containing submandibular gland, lymph nodes, and anterior belly of digastric muscles

IMAGING ANATOMY

Overview
- One of the distinct locations within the oral cavity that may be used to develop location-specific differential diagnoses
  - Other locations include oral mucosal space/surface, sublingual space, and root of tongue

Anatomy Relationships
- Inferolateral to mylohyoid muscle
- Deep to platysma muscle
- Cephalad to hyoid bone
- Communicates posteriorly with sublingual space and inferior parapharyngeal space at posterior margin of mylohyoid muscle
- Continues inferiorly into infrahyoid neck as anterior cervical space

Internal Contents
- Submandibular gland
  - 1 of 3 major salivary glands
  - Divided anatomically into superficial and deep lobes by the mylohyoid muscle
  - Superficial lobe is larger and in SMS itself
    - Superficial layer, deep cervical fascia (SL-DCF) forms submandibular gland capsule
    - Crossed by facial vein and cervical branches of facial nerve (marginal mandibular branch)
  - Smaller deep lobe, often called deep "process"
    - Tongue-like extension of gland that wraps around posterior aspect of mylohyoid muscle
    - Projects into posterior aspect of sublingual space
    - Submandibular duct projects off deep lobe into sublingual space
  - Submandibular gland innervation
    - Parasympathetic secretomotor supply from chorda tympani branch of facial nerve
    - Comes via lingual branch of CNV3
- Submental (level IA) and submandibular (level IB) nodal groups
  - Receive lymphatic drainage from anterior facial region
    - Including oral cavity, anterior sinonasal, and orbital areas
  - A few elliptical lymph nodes with preserved internal architecture is a constant normal finding
- Anterior belly of digastric muscle
  - Divides suprahyoid portion into submental and submandibular triangles
- Hyoglossus muscle
  - Deep to mylohyoid muscle; marks anterior margin of submandibular gland
  - Submandibular duct runs between hyoglossus muscle and mylohyoid muscle
- Facial vein and artery pass through SMS
  - Facial vein courses anteriorly and superiorly to submandibular gland
- Anterior division of retromandibular vein (RMV)
  - Outlines posterior border of submandibular gland
- Caudal loop of CN12
  - Passes through SMS before looping anteriorly and cephalad into tongue muscle
- Tail of parotid gland may "hang down" into posterior submandibular space

ANATOMY IMAGING ISSUES

Questions
- Major clinical-radiological question when mass is present in SMS: Is lesion nodal or submandibular gland in origin?
  - If "beaking" of submandibular gland tissue around lesion margin is present, and lesion is completely surrounded by glandular parenchyma, lesion origin is in submandibular gland
  - Fatty cleavage plane between mass and submandibular gland identifies lesion as nodal in origin
  - Internal architecture (e.g., presence of echogenic hilum) helps to identify lymph node
- Consider major differential diagnoses for mass in submandibular region
  - Congenital lesion: Epidermoid cyst, cystic hygroma
  - Inflammatory condition: Submandibular gland sialadenitis/abscess, diving ranula, chronic sclerosing siadenitis (Kuttner tumor), Sjögren syndrome
  - Lymph node enlargement: Reactive, inflammatory, or neoplastic (secondary or lymphomatous)
  - Benign salivary gland tumor, lipoma
  - Malignant salivary gland tumor

Imaging Recommendations
- Scan submandibular region in transverse and longitudinal/oblique planes, as these best demonstrate floor of submandibular region, hyoglossus, and mylohyoid muscles
- Always establish origin of mass (i.e., submandibular glandular or extraglandular mass), as this will help to narrow differential diagnosis
- Remember to evaluate glandular/extraglandular ductal dilatation and lymph nodes at this location

Imaging Pitfalls
- Distinction between submandibular glandular mass and enlarged lymph node can be difficult, especially if mass is large
- Lesions of parotid tail may appear in posterior submandibular region clinically
- Coronal MR helps to evaluate and localize large masses at this site

RELATED REFERENCES

1. Agarwal AK et al: Submandibular and sublingual spaces: diagnostic imaging and evaluation. Otolaryngol Clin North Am. 45(6):1311-23, 2012

GRAPHICS

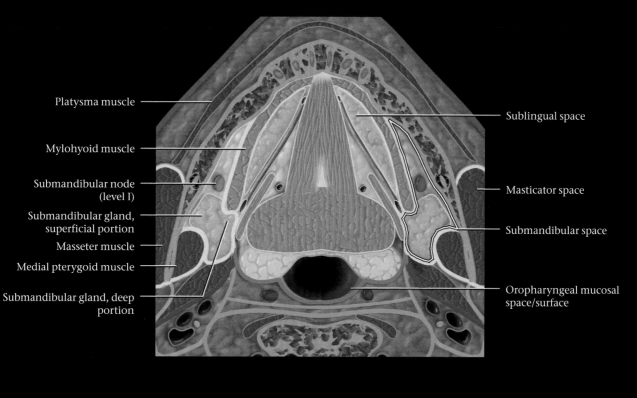

Platysma muscle

Mylohyoid muscle

Submandibular node (level I)

Submandibular gland, superficial portion

Masseter muscle

Medial pterygoid muscle

Submandibular gland, deep portion

Sublingual space

Masticator space

Submandibular space

Oropharyngeal mucosal space/surface

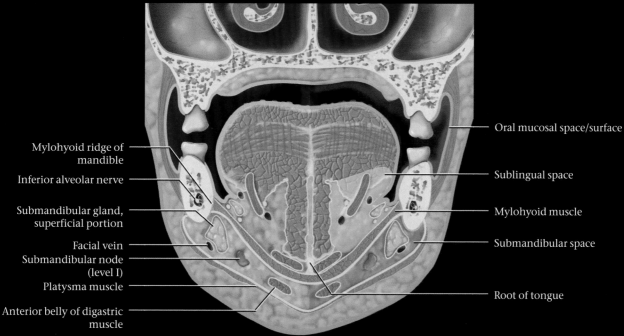

Mylohyoid ridge of mandible

Inferior alveolar nerve

Submandibular gland, superficial portion

Facial vein

Submandibular node (level I)

Platysma muscle

Anterior belly of digastric muscle

Oral mucosal space/surface

Sublingual space

Mylohyoid muscle

Submandibular space

Root of tongue

(Top) Axial graphic shows the oral cavity with emphasis on the submandibular space (SMS), shaded in light blue on the patient's left. The SMS is inferolateral to the mylohyoid muscle. Note that the principal structures of the SMS are the submandibular gland and lymph nodes. *(Bottom)* In this coronal graphic through the oral cavity, the SMS is shaded in light blue. The superficial layer of the deep cervical fascia (yellow line) is seen lining the vertical horseshoe-shaped SMS inferolateral to the mylohyoid muscle. The contents of the SMS are the anterior belly of the digastric muscle, submandibular nodes, submandibular gland, and facial vein. Note that the platysma muscle forms the superficial margin of the SMS.

SUBMANDIBULAR REGION

TRANSVERSE ULTRASOUND

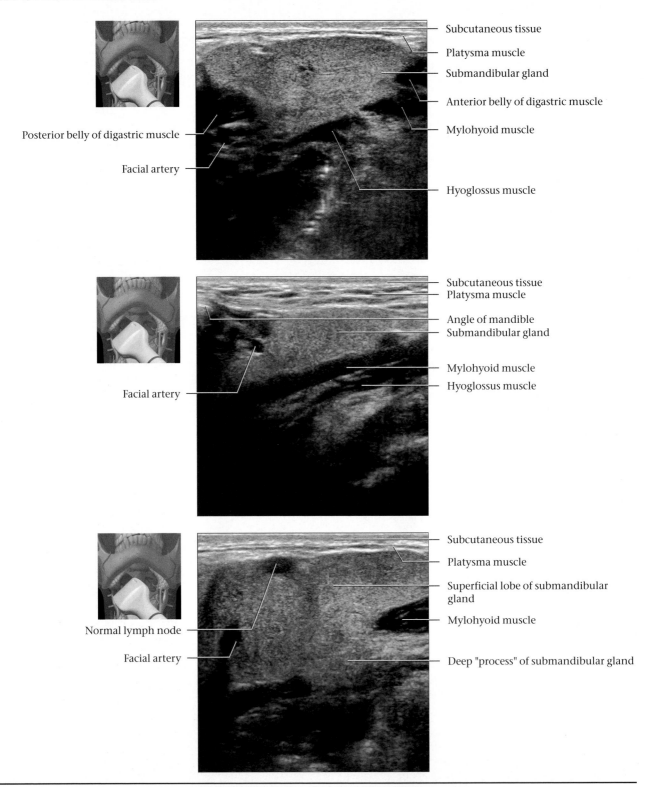

Posterior belly of digastric muscle

Facial artery

Subcutaneous tissue

Platysma muscle

Submandibular gland

Anterior belly of digastric muscle

Mylohyoid muscle

Hyoglossus muscle

Facial artery

Subcutaneous tissue

Platysma muscle

Angle of mandible

Submandibular gland

Mylohyoid muscle

Hyoglossus muscle

Normal lymph node

Facial artery

Subcutaneous tissue

Platysma muscle

Superficial lobe of submandibular gland

Mylohyoid muscle

Deep "process" of submandibular gland

(Top) Transverse grayscale ultrasound shows the submandibular region. The submandibular gland sits astride the posterior belly of the digastric and mylohyoid muscles. The hyoglossus muscle is seen deep to the submandibular gland. (Middle) Transverse grayscale ultrasound of the submandibular region (slightly more posterior scan) shows the consistent relationship of the submandibular gland superficial to the mylohyoid and hyoglossus muscles. The submandibular duct runs between these 2 muscles. (Bottom) Transverse grayscale ultrasound shows the submandibular gland. The gland is divided into superficial and deep lobes, demarcated by the free posterior edge of the mylohyoid muscle. Normal lymph nodes are a constant finding in this region.

SUBMANDIBULAR REGION

AXIAL MR AND POWER DOPPLER ULTRASOUND

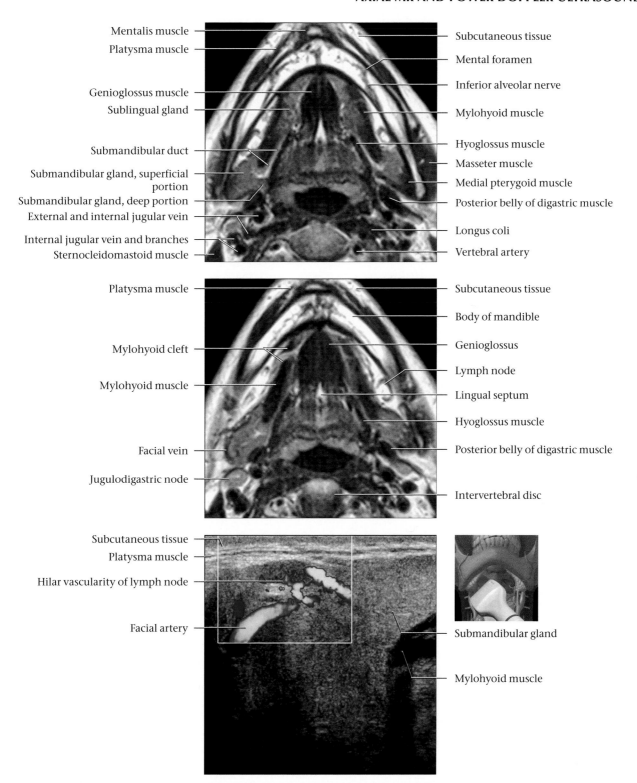

(Top) Axial T2WI MR shows the floor of the mouth. The SMS contains submandibular glands, fat, and lymph nodes. Note the high-signal submandibular ducts entering the posterior aspect of sublingual spaces bilaterally. **(Middle)** In a more inferior image, both submandibular glands are seen wrapping around the posterior margins of the mylohyoid muscles. The neurovascular pedicle to each side of the tongue is closely related to the hyoglossus muscle. **(Bottom)** Transverse power Doppler ultrasound of submandibular gland shows vascular flow within the facial artery. Note the presence of normal hilar vascularity within the lymph node.

SUBMANDIBULAR REGION

TRANSVERSE ULTRASOUND

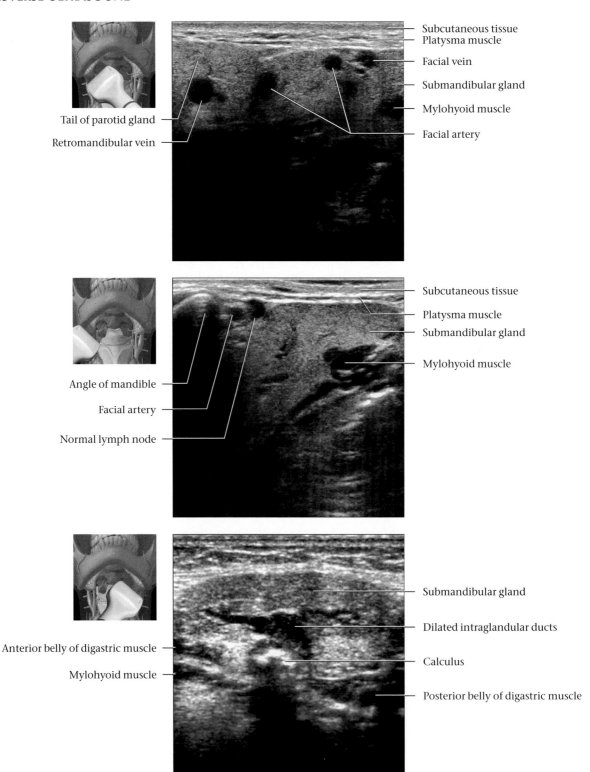

Subcutaneous tissue
Platysma muscle
Facial vein
Submandibular gland
Mylohyoid muscle
Facial artery

Tail of parotid gland
Retromandibular vein

Subcutaneous tissue
Platysma muscle
Submandibular gland
Mylohyoid muscle

Angle of mandible
Facial artery
Normal lymph node

Submandibular gland
Dilated intraglandular ducts
Calculus
Posterior belly of digastric muscle

Anterior belly of digastric muscle
Mylohyoid muscle

(Top) Transverse grayscale ultrasound shows the posterior submandibular region. Note the close proximity of the submandibular gland to the tail of the parotid gland. On ultrasound, it may be difficult to localize the origin of large lesions at this site. Displacement of vessels often provides the clue. (Middle) Longitudinal grayscale ultrasound shows the submandibular region. The submandibular gland is located inferior and posterior to the mandible and superficial to the mylohyoid muscle. (Bottom) Transverse grayscale ultrasound of the left submandibular gland shows a large obstructing calculus with intraglandular ductal dilatation. Note the glandular parenchyma appears heterogeneous and hypoechoic, compatible with sialadenitis secondary to obstruction.

SUBMANDIBULAR REGION

POWER DOPPLER ULTRASOUND AND PATHOLOGY

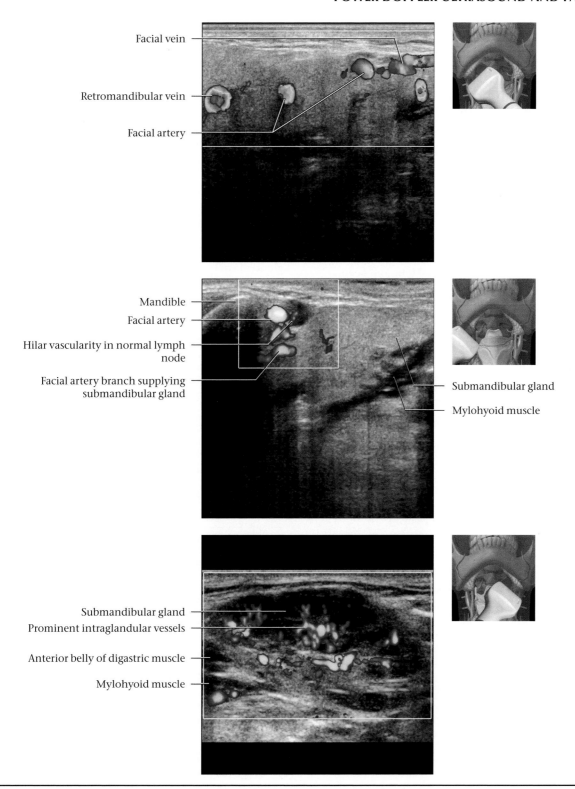

(Top) Transverse color Doppler ultrasound helps to identify and confirm important vascular landmarks in the posterior submandibular region, including the retromandibular vein and facial artery. (Middle) Longitudinal power Doppler ultrasound of the submandibular region shows the relationship of the facial artery to the superficial portion of the submandibular gland. The hilar vascularity of a normal lymph node and the vessels supplying the submandibular gland are seen. (Bottom) Transverse power Doppler ultrasound of the left submandibular gland shows an enlarged, heterogeneous submandibular gland with patchy hypoechoic "nodular" areas. Note, prominent intraglandular vessels running through "nodules" with no mass effect/displacement. No ductal dilatation or calculus is seen. These changes are also present in the contralateral gland (not shown), suggesting chronic sclerosing sialadenitis (Kuttner tumor).

PAROTID REGION

TERMINOLOGY

Abbreviations
- Parotid space (PS)

Definitions
- Paired lateral suprahyoid neck spaces enclosed by superficial layer of deep cervical fascia containing parotid glands, nodes, and extracranial facial nerve branches

IMAGING ANATOMY

Extent
- Extends from external auditory canal (EAC) and mastoid tip superiorly to below angle of mandible (parotid tail)

Internal Contents
- Parotid gland
  - Divided anatomically into superficial lobe and deep lobe by extracranial facial nerve
    - Superficial lobe: Constitutes ~ 2/3 of parotid glandular parenchyma
    - Deep lobe: Smaller component, projects into lateral parapharyngeal space (PPS)
- Extracranial facial nerve (CN7)
  - Exits stylomastoid foramen as single trunk; ramifies within PS lateral to retromandibular vein
  - Ramifying intraparotid facial nerve creates surgical plane between superficial and deep lobes
- External carotid artery (ECA)
  - Medial and smaller of the 2 vessels seen just behind mandibular ramus in PS
- Retromandibular vein (RMV)
  - Lateral and larger of the 2 vessels seen just behind mandibular ramus in parotid
  - Formed by union of superficial temporal vein and maxillary vein
  - Intraparotid facial nerve branches course just lateral to RMV
- Intraparotid lymph nodes
  - ~ 20 lymph nodes found in each parotid gland
  - Parotid nodes are 1st-order drainage for EAC, pinna, and surrounding scalp
- Parotid duct
  - Emerges from anterior PS, runs along surface of masseter muscle
  - Duct then arches through buccal space to pierce buccinator muscle at level of upper 2nd molar
- Accessory parotid glands
  - Project over surface of masseter muscle
  - Present in ~ 20% of normal anatomic dissections
- Masseter muscle
  - Muscle of mastication related to outer surface of mandibular ramus
  - Parotid duct runs anteriorly on its surface
- Buccinator muscle
  - Deep muscle of buccal space, extends anteriorly and just medially to anterior margin of masseter muscle
    - Parotid duct pierces to enter buccal mucosa at upper 2nd molar level

ANATOMY IMAGING ISSUES

Questions
- Is deep lobe of parotid gland involved?
  - For a parotid mass, it is important to determine location and extent of involvement in relation to extracranial facial nerve (i.e., superficial/deep lobe involvement)
    - Difference in surgical approach and risk of perioperative facial nerve injury
  - Intraparotid facial nerve is not visible with USG, CT, or MR, except proximally with high-resolution MR
  - On ultrasound, RMV is used as a marker for division of parotid gland into superficial and deep lobes (due to close proximity to CN7)

Imaging Approaches
- Scan in both transverse and longitudinal planes
  - Transverse scans define anatomic location of salivary gland masses in relation to ECA and RMV
  - Longitudinal scans help to better evaluate lesions in parotid tail and for Doppler examination
- USG cannot evaluate deep lobe mass or deep extension of superficial masses
  - Lower frequency transducer (e.g., 5 MHz) with gel block/standoff pad helps to evaluate large parotid mass with suspicious deep lobe extension
  - MR/CT is required for full anatomical delineation
  - US helps to direct needle for guided biopsy
- Always evaluate masseter muscle as its lesions clinically mimic parotid pathology
- Normal intraglandular ducts are seen as echogenic streaks within parotid parenchyma
  - When dilated, seen as 2 bright lines separated by fluid within
  - Extraglandular portion of duct is seen on US only if it is dilated

CLINICAL IMPLICATIONS

Clinical Importance
- Although US cannot visualize parotid deep lobe, it is still an ideal initial imaging modality to evaluate parotid masses, as most are located in superficial lobe
  - US characterizes common salivary masses and safely guides fine-needle aspiration cytology (FNAC)/biopsy for confirmation

EMBRYOLOGY

Embryologic Events
- Parotid space undergoes late encapsulation in embryogenesis

Practical Implications
- Late encapsulation results in intraparotid lymph nodes
- Warthin tumor arises within this lymphoid tissue (intraparotid > > periparotid > upper cervical)
- Parotid nodes are 1st-order drainage for malignancies of adjacent scalp, EAC, pinna, and deep face
- No such nodes in submandibular gland due to early encapsulation; therefore, no Warthin tumor or nodal metastases in submandibular gland (SMG)

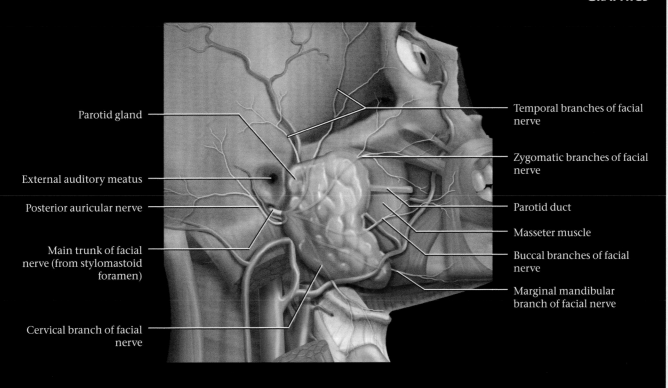

Parotid gland

External auditory meatus

Posterior auricular nerve

Main trunk of facial nerve (from stylomastoid foramen)

Cervical branch of facial nerve

Temporal branches of facial nerve

Zygomatic branches of facial nerve

Parotid duct

Masseter muscle

Buccal branches of facial nerve

Marginal mandibular branch of facial nerve

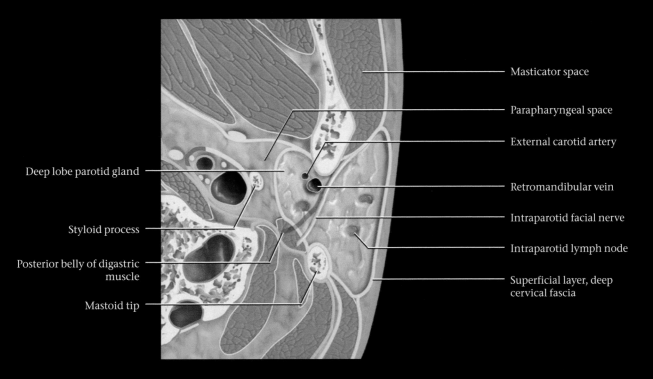

Deep lobe parotid gland

Styloid process

Posterior belly of digastric muscle

Mastoid tip

Masticator space

Parapharyngeal space

External carotid artery

Retromandibular vein

Intraparotid facial nerve

Intraparotid lymph node

Superficial layer, deep cervical fascia

(Top) Lateral schematic diagram shows the parotid region. The parotid gland is situated in front of the external auditory meatus and below the zygomatic arch. The parotid duct emerges from the anterior margin and passes superficial to the masseter muscle. The facial nerve, after emerging from the stylomastoid foramen, enters the parotid gland and divides into terminal branches to supply muscles of facial expression. *(Bottom)* Axial graphic shows the parotid space (PS) at the level of C1 vertebral body. The intraparotid course of the facial nerve extends from just medial to the mastoid tip to a position just lateral to the retromandibular vein, dividing the parotid gland into superficial and deep lobes.

PAROTID REGION

TRANSVERSE ULTRASOUND

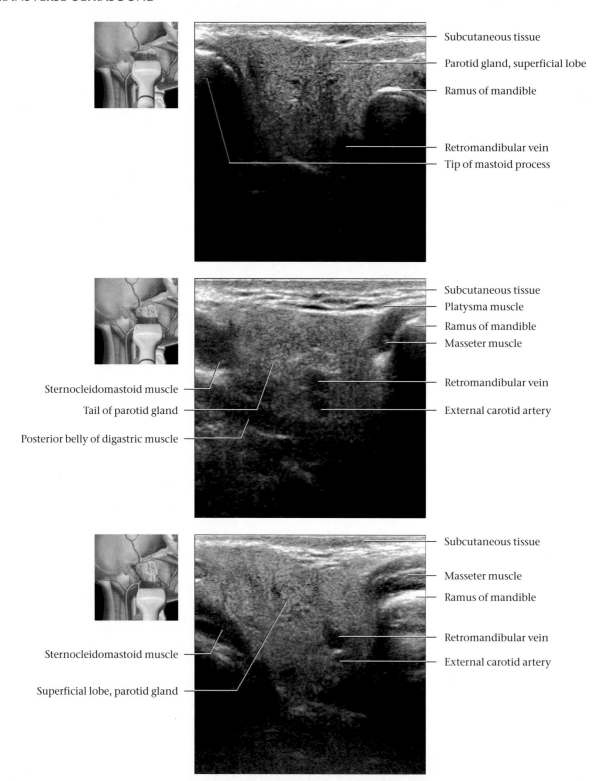

Subcutaneous tissue

Parotid gland, superficial lobe

Ramus of mandible

Retromandibular vein

Tip of mastoid process

Subcutaneous tissue

Platysma muscle

Ramus of mandible

Masseter muscle

Retromandibular vein

External carotid artery

Sternocleidomastoid muscle

Tail of parotid gland

Posterior belly of digastric muscle

Subcutaneous tissue

Masseter muscle

Ramus of mandible

Retromandibular vein

External carotid artery

Sternocleidomastoid muscle

Superficial lobe, parotid gland

(Top) Transverse grayscale ultrasound shows the parotid region. Note its relationship to the mastoid process and the mandibular ramus. The glandular parenchyma shows a homogeneous, hyperechoic pattern. The retromandibular vein is visualized as a round, anechoic structure within the parotid gland. (Middle) Transverse grayscale ultrasound shows the parotid tail region. The sternocleidomastoid muscle and the posterior belly of the digastric muscle are related to the posterior margin of the parotid tail. The retromandibular vein and external carotid artery serve as markers to infer the location of CN7. (Bottom) Transverse grayscale ultrasound shows the parotid gland. The retromandibular vein is usually larger and lateral to the external carotid artery within the parotid gland. Note that the deep lobe is obscured by shadowing from the mandibular ramus.

PAROTID REGION

AXIAL T1 MR & POWER DOPPLER ULTRASOUND

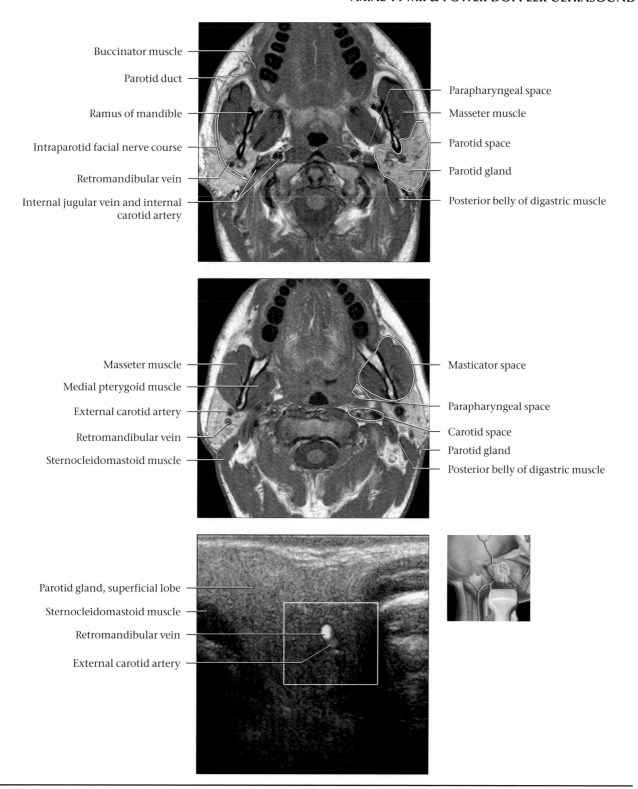

(Top) *Axial T1-weighted MR image at the oral pharyngeal level shows the parotid gland as a homogeneous T1-hyperintense structure posterolateral to the mandibular ramus and masseter muscle. Note the projected intraparotid facial nerve course drawn on the right.* **(Middle)** *Axial T1-weighted MR image shows a more inferior level of the parotid glands. The parotid space relates anteriorly to the masticator space, medially to the parapharyngeal space, and is separated medially by the posterior belly of digastric muscle from the carotid space.* **(Bottom)** *Power Doppler ultrasound helps to depict the retromandibular vein and external carotid artery, which are sometimes difficult to see in patients with bright fatty parotid glands. The RMV and ECA help to infer location of CN7.*

PAROTID REGION

LONGITUDINAL ULTRASOUND

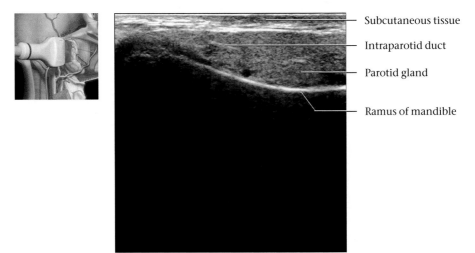

Subcutaneous tissue

Intraparotid duct

Parotid gland

Ramus of mandible

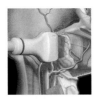
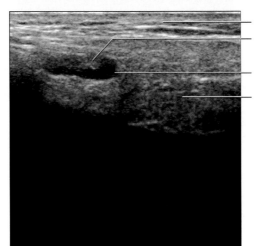

Subcutaneous tissue

Echogenic hilum in intraparotid lymph node

Intraparotid lymph node

Parotid gland

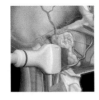
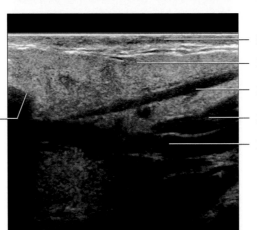

Subcutaneous tissue

Parotid gland, superficial lobe

Retromandibular vein

Posterior belly of digastric muscle

External carotid artery

Ramus of mandible

(Top) This is the 1st image in a series of longitudinal grayscale ultrasound scans of the parotid gland. The parotid gland is superficial to the ramus of the mandible. *(Middle)* Second image shows a normal intraparotid lymph node in the superficial lobe of the parotid gland. On high-resolution ultrasound, normal nodes are invariably seen in the parotid tail and in the pretragal parotid gland. The elliptical shape and normal internal architecture with echogenic hilum suggest its benign nature. *(Bottom)* Third image at the plane of the retromandibular vein is shown. Such anatomy is best seen in children and young adults where there is not much fat deposition in the gland.

CORONAL T1 MR & POWER DOPPLER ULTRASOUND

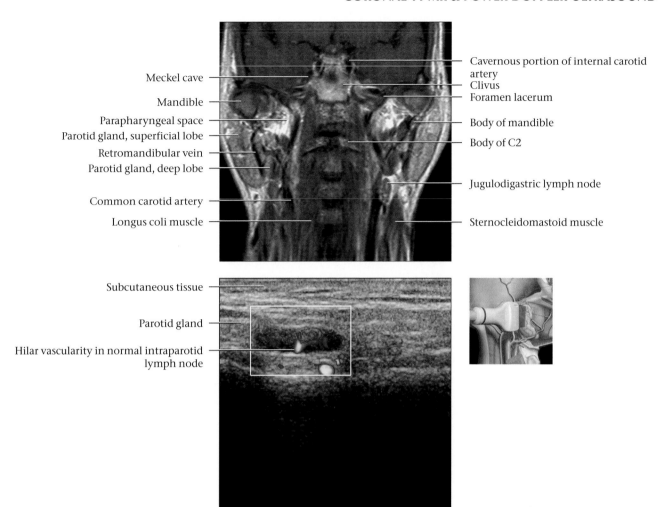

Meckel cave

Mandible

Parapharyngeal space
Parotid gland, superficial lobe
Retromandibular vein
Parotid gland, deep lobe

Common carotid artery

Longus coli muscle

Cavernous portion of internal carotid
artery
Clivus
Foramen lacerum

Body of mandible

Body of C2

Jugulodigastric lymph node

Sternocleidomastoid muscle

Subcutaneous tissue

Parotid gland

Hilar vascularity in normal intraparotid
lymph node

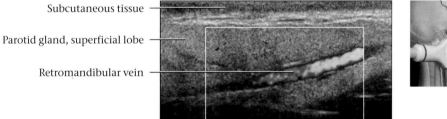

Subcutaneous tissue

Parotid gland, superficial lobe

Retromandibular vein

(Top) Coronal T1-weighted MR image shows the parotid glands. The retromandibular vein is seen as a signal-void tubular structure traversing the parotid gland vertically, helping to suggest the location of CN7. *(Middle)* Longitudinal power Doppler ultrasound of the parotid gland shows the presence of hilar vascularity within a normal intraparotid lymph node. On high resolution ultrasound, more nodes are seen in children compared to adults. *(Bottom)* Longitudinal power Doppler ultrasound of the parotid gland clearly delineates the retromandibular vein.

PAROTID REGION

TRANSVERSE ULTRASOUND

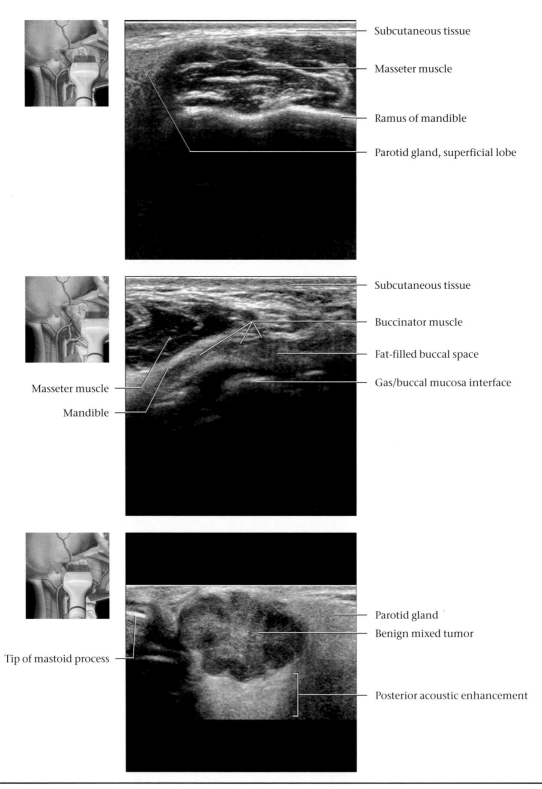

Subcutaneous tissue

Masseter muscle

Ramus of mandible

Parotid gland, superficial lobe

Subcutaneous tissue

Buccinator muscle

Fat-filled buccal space

Gas/buccal mucosa interface

Masseter muscle

Mandible

Parotid gland

Benign mixed tumor

Tip of mastoid process

Posterior acoustic enhancement

(Top) Transverse grayscale ultrasound of the anterior parotid region shows the masseter muscle superficial to the ramus of the mandible and closely related to the parotid gland. Note that masseter muscle lesions can mimic parotid pathology clinically. *(Middle)* Transverse grayscale ultrasound of the anterior parotid region/facial region shows the buccinator muscle as a thin, hypoechoic structure extending anteriorly and just medial to the anterior margin of the masseter muscle. The buccal space, which lies lateral to the buccinator muscle, is fat filled and contains the facial nerve, vein, artery, and the parotid duct. *(Bottom)* Transverse grayscale ultrasound of the right parotid gland shows a well-defined, solid, heterogeneous, hypoechoic mass with lobulated margin in the superficial lobe. Despite the solid nature of the tumor, there is intense posterior acoustic enhancement, often seen in benign mixed tumors. Pathology confirmed benign mixed tumor.

AXIAL T1 MR & TRANSVERSE ULTRASOUND

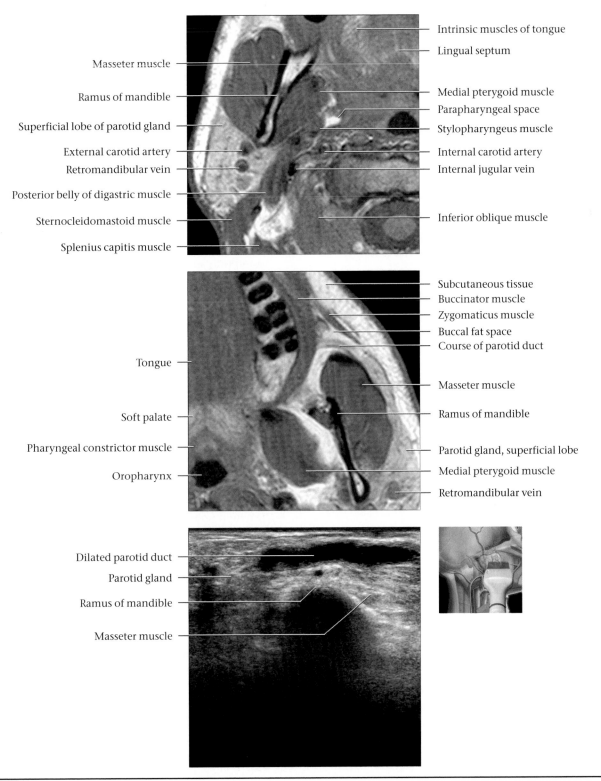

Masseter muscle

Ramus of mandible

Superficial lobe of parotid gland

External carotid artery

Retromandibular vein

Posterior belly of digastric muscle

Sternocleidomastoid muscle

Splenius capitis muscle

Intrinsic muscles of tongue

Lingual septum

Medial pterygoid muscle

Parapharyngeal space

Stylopharyngeus muscle

Internal carotid artery

Internal jugular vein

Inferior oblique muscle

Tongue

Soft palate

Pharyngeal constrictor muscle

Oropharynx

Subcutaneous tissue

Buccinator muscle

Zygomaticus muscle

Buccal fat space

Course of parotid duct

Masseter muscle

Ramus of mandible

Parotid gland, superficial lobe

Medial pterygoid muscle

Retromandibular vein

Dilated parotid duct

Parotid gland

Ramus of mandible

Masseter muscle

(Top) Axial T1WI MR of the right parotid region shows the relationship of the parotid gland to the masseter muscle and the ramus of the mandible, the parapharyngeal space and the posterior belly of the digastric muscle, and the upper sternocleidomastoid muscle. (Middle) Axial T1WI MR shows the anterior parotid region. The parotid duct courses anteromedially within the buccal fat space and pierces the buccinator muscle at the level of the upper 2nd molar into the buccal mucosa. (Bottom) Transverse grayscale ultrasound of the right parotid gland shows a grossly dilated parotid duct superficial to the ramus of the mandible and masseter muscles. The ductal dilatation is due to distal parotid ductal stricture close to the orificial opening. Note that the parotid gland itself is atrophic and heterogeneous, secondary to chronic infection.

UPPER CERVICAL LEVEL

TERMINOLOGY

Abbreviations
- Internal carotid artery (ICA)
- External carotid artery (ECA)
- Internal jugular vein (IJV)
- Jugulodigastric (JD) lymph node

Synonyms
- Carotid triangle
- Suprahyoid anterior triangle

Definitions
- Portion of anterior triangle adjacent to major vessels of carotid sheath
- Extends from skull base superiorly to hyoid bone inferiorly

IMAGING ANATOMY

Overview
- Cervical region is divided into upper, mid, and lower cervical levels in order to identify relevant groups of jugular cervical lymph nodes
- On ultrasound, upper cervical region is best scanned transversely from submandibular/parotid tail region to carotid bifurcation
- Major structures of upper cervical level: Cervical portion of ICA, ECA with origins of major branches, carotid bifurcation, IJV, posterior belly of digastric muscle, and JD lymph node

Internal Contents
- Cervical portion of ICA
  - 1 of 2 branches from common carotid artery
    - Runs lateral or posterolateral to ECA
    - Usually of larger caliber than ECA
    - Low-resistance arterial flow waveform on Doppler ultrasound
  - Supplies anterior part of brain, eye, and its appendages
  - Divided into bulbous, cervical, petrous, cavernous, and cerebral portions
  - Only first 2 portions lie extracranially and are accessible by ultrasound
  - No branch in extracranial portions
- ECA
  - Runs medial to cervical ICA
  - Smaller than ICA
  - High-resistance arterial flow waveform on Doppler ultrasound
  - Plays pivotal role in collateral circulation if arterial occlusion of ICA/vertebral artery
  - 1st branch: Superior thyroid artery
    - Readily detected by grayscale and Doppler examination
- Carotid bifurcation
  - ~ at level of hyoid bone (i.e., division between upper and midcervical levels)
  - Bulbous dilatation of proximal ICA beyond carotid bifurcation: Carotid bulb
  - Carotid body is located at carotid bifurcation
- IJV
  - Inferior continuation of sigmoid sinus from level of jugular foramen at skull base

- Right usually of larger caliber than left
- Lateral/posterolateral to internal carotid artery
- Acts as landmark for jugular cervical lymph nodes
- Posterior belly of digastric muscle
  - Key structure in separating parotid region superiorly from upper cervical level inferiorly
  - Runs anteroinferiorly from mastoid process to hyoid bone
  - Emerges deep to sternocleidomastoid muscle to abut tail of parotid gland
  - Major vessels run deep to muscle
    - From posterior to anterior: Internal jugular vein, internal carotid artery, and external carotid artery
- JD lymph node
  - Largest and most superior lymph node of deep jugular chain, also known as "sentinel" node of internal jugular chain
  - Resides close to carotid bifurcation/IJV
  - Orientated along line of digastric muscle
  - Commonly involved in head and neck cancer
- Vagus nerve
  - Descends from skull base within carotid sheath
  - Sandwiched between ICA medially and IJV
  - More difficult to see than in mid and lower cervical levels

ANATOMY IMAGING ISSUES

Questions
- What are common differential diagnoses for a mass in upper cervical level?
  - Enlarged lymph nodes: Reactive, inflammatory, and neoplasm (metastases/lymphoma)
  - Congenital lesion: 2nd branchial cleft cyst
  - Vascular lesion: IJV varix, IJV thrombosis
  - Neoplasm: Vagal schwannoma, carotid body tumor
- What are common sites?
  - JD lymph node is common site of nodal metastases from head and neck cancer
  - Common sites of primary include oral cavity (including tonsils and tongue), nasopharyngeal carcinoma
  - JD node also commonly involved in lymphoma
    - Multiple, often bilateral nodal involvement, pseudocystic/reticulated internal architecture on US

Imaging Recommendations
- Scan in transverse plane from submandibular region/parotid tail down to carotid bifurcation
  - Longitudinal scanning for more detailed assessment of internal architecture of lesion and evaluation of intralesional vascularity on Doppler
- Color flow imaging helps to identify major vessels and their anatomic relation to node/mass
  - Also provides flow information of cervical masses to characterize their nature
- US provides safe real-time guidance for fine-needle aspiration cytology (FNAC)/biopsy to further enhance diagnostic yield
  - FNAC/biopsy is not recommended for suspected carotid body tumor due to risk of uncontrolled bleeding

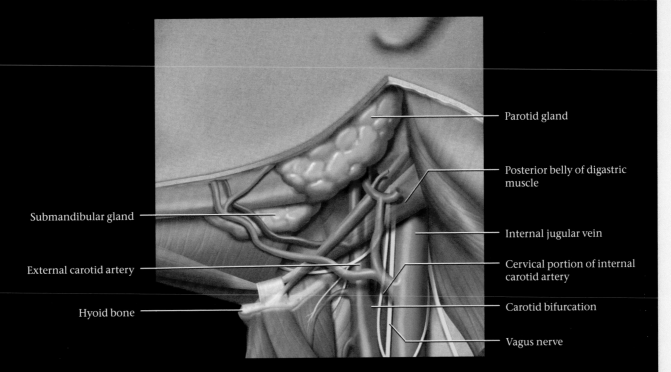

Parotid gland

Posterior belly of digastric muscle

Submandibular gland

Internal jugular vein

External carotid artery

Cervical portion of internal carotid artery

Hyoid bone

Carotid bifurcation

Vagus nerve

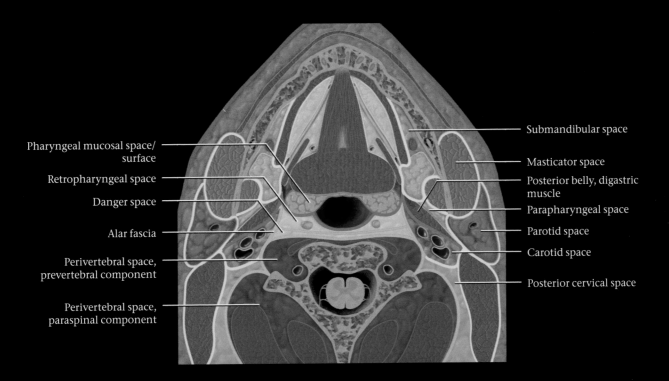

Pharyngeal mucosal space/ surface

Submandibular space

Masticator space

Retropharyngeal space

Posterior belly, digastric muscle

Danger space

Parapharyngeal space

Alar fascia

Parotid space

Perivertebral space, prevertebral component

Carotid space

Posterior cervical space

Perivertebral space, paraspinal component

(Top) Schematic diagram shows the key structures in the upper cervical level. The hyoid bone and the carotid bifurcation are 2 anatomical landmarks for the inferior margin of the upper cervical level. With high-resolution US, the jugulodigastric lymph node will be consistently seen at this site and should not be mistaken for pathology. Visualization of a similar node on the opposite side helps. *(Bottom)* Axial graphic shows the suprahyoid neck spaces at the level of the oropharynx. The superficial (yellow line), middle (pink line) and deep (turquoise line) layers of the deep cervical fascia outline the suprahyoid neck spaces. Ultrasound assessment of the upper cervical level involves scanning transversely along the major vessels of the carotid sheath (i.e., the internal carotid artery and internal jugular vein).

TRANSVERSE ULTRASOUND

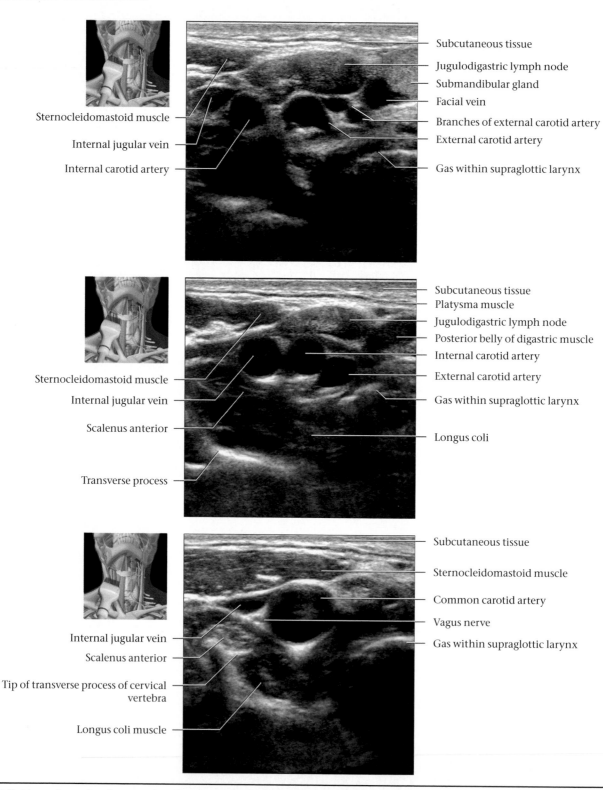

Sternocleidomastoid muscle

Internal jugular vein

Internal carotid artery

Subcutaneous tissue

Jugulodigastric lymph node

Submandibular gland

Facial vein

Branches of external carotid artery

External carotid artery

Gas within supraglottic larynx

Sternocleidomastoid muscle

Internal jugular vein

Scalenus anterior

Transverse process

Subcutaneous tissue

Platysma muscle

Jugulodigastric lymph node

Posterior belly of digastric muscle

Internal carotid artery

External carotid artery

Gas within supraglottic larynx

Longus coli

Internal jugular vein

Scalenus anterior

Tip of transverse process of cervical vertebra

Longus coli muscle

Subcutaneous tissue

Sternocleidomastoid muscle

Common carotid artery

Vagus nerve

Gas within supraglottic larynx

(Top) First image in a series of consecutive transverse grayscale ultrasound images of the upper cervical level clearly identifies key vascular landmarks, including the internal and external carotid arteries and the internal jugular vein. The uppermost and largest deep cervical lymph node (i.e., the jugulodigastric lymph node) is consistently seen on US in the upper cervical level anterior to the carotid arteries. It is usually elliptical, hypoechoic, and with echogenic hilum. *(Middle)* Second image shows the carotid bifurcation in the transverse plane. The external carotid artery is usually more medial and smaller than the internal carotid artery. *(Bottom)* Third image below the level of carotid bifurcation clearly shows the common carotid artery, internal jugular vein, and vagus nerve to be major structures within the carotid sheath.

UPPER CERVICAL LEVEL

AXIAL CECT

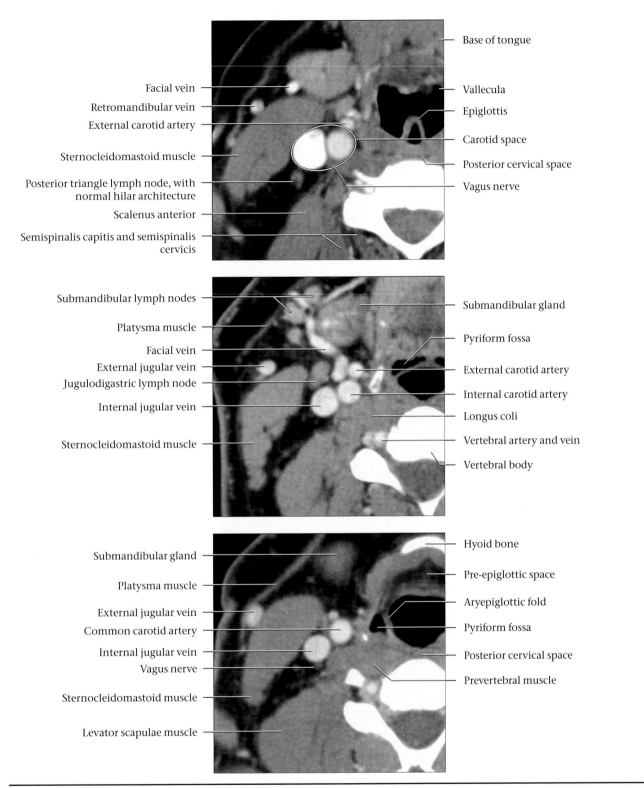

Labels (top image):
- Facial vein
- Retromandibular vein
- External carotid artery
- Sternocleidomastoid muscle
- Posterior triangle lymph node, with normal hilar architecture
- Scalenus anterior
- Semispinalis capitis and semispinalis cervicis
- Base of tongue
- Vallecula
- Epiglottis
- Carotid space
- Posterior cervical space
- Vagus nerve

Labels (middle image):
- Submandibular lymph nodes
- Platysma muscle
- Facial vein
- External jugular vein
- Jugulodigastric lymph node
- Internal jugular vein
- Sternocleidomastoid muscle
- Submandibular gland
- Pyriform fossa
- External carotid artery
- Internal carotid artery
- Longus coli
- Vertebral artery and vein
- Vertebral body

Labels (bottom image):
- Submandibular gland
- Platysma muscle
- External jugular vein
- Common carotid artery
- Internal jugular vein
- Vagus nerve
- Sternocleidomastoid muscle
- Levator scapulae muscle
- Hyoid bone
- Pre-epiglottic space
- Aryepiglottic fold
- Pyriform fossa
- Posterior cervical space
- Prevertebral muscle

(Top) At the level just above the hyoid bone, the carotid bifurcation can be seen. The vagus nerve is seen within the carotid sheath. *(Middle)* First in a series of axial CECT images shows the suprahyoid neck at the level of the free margin of epiglottis. The jugulodigastric lymph node is commonly seen; however, the internal architecture is better assessed on ultrasound than CECT. *(Bottom)* At the level of the hyoid bone, the carotid space now contains the common carotid artery, internal jugular vein, and vagus nerve only. The submandibular space is seen anteriorly, and is predominantly fat filled at this level. Familiarity with cross-sectional anatomy is key to optimal ultrasound examination of the neck, as lesions at this level are site specific.

UPPER CERVICAL LEVEL

TRANSVERSE ULTRASOUND

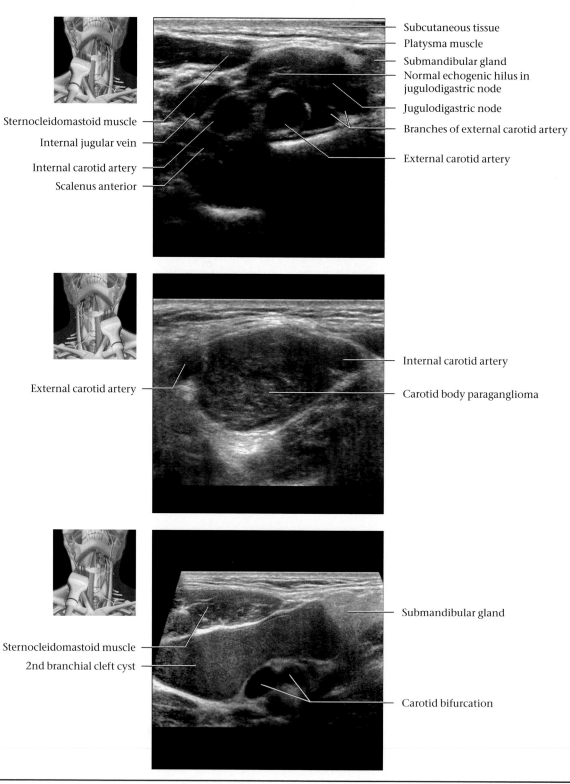

Subcutaneous tissue

Platysma muscle

Submandibular gland

Normal echogenic hilus in jugulodigastric node

Jugulodigastric node

Branches of external carotid artery

External carotid artery

Sternocleidomastoid muscle

Internal jugular vein

Internal carotid artery

Scalenus anterior

Internal carotid artery

Carotid body paraganglioma

External carotid artery

Submandibular gland

Sternocleidomastoid muscle

2nd branchial cleft cyst

Carotid bifurcation

(Top) Transverse grayscale ultrasound shows the upper cervical level. The normal jugulodigastric lymph node is elliptical in shape with preserved echogenic hilum. Its anatomical relationship with the major neck vessels is better appreciated on power Doppler ultrasound. (Middle) Transverse grayscale ultrasound of the left upper cervical level shows a large, heterogeneous, hypoechoic mass centered at the carotid bifurcation, splaying the internal and external carotid arteries. Appearances and location are strongly indicative of carotid body paraganglioma. (Bottom) Transverse grayscale ultrasound of the right upper cervical level shows a well-circumscribed cystic mass with a "pseudosolid" appearance along the medial edge of the sternomastoid muscle, posterior to the submandibular gland and superficial to major vessels within the carotid sheath. Location and appearances are suggestive of second branchial cleft cyst. This "pseudosolid" appearance is commonly seen in congenital neck cysts, including thyroglossal duct cysts.

POWER DOPPLER ULTRASOUND

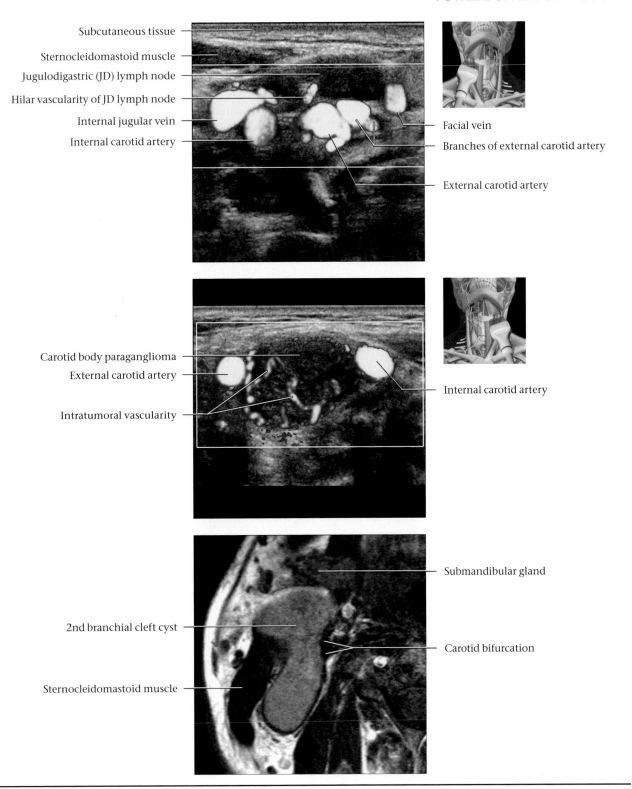

Subcutaneous tissue

Sternocleidomastoid muscle

Jugulodigastric (JD) lymph node

Hilar vascularity of JD lymph node

Internal jugular vein

Internal carotid artery

Facial vein

Branches of external carotid artery

External carotid artery

Carotid body paraganglioma

External carotid artery

Intratumoral vascularity

Internal carotid artery

Submandibular gland

2nd branchial cleft cyst

Carotid bifurcation

Sternocleidomastoid muscle

(Top) Transverse power Doppler ultrasound shows the upper cervical level. The major vessels, including the internal and external carotid arteries and the internal jugular vein, show color flow. Note the presence of normal hilar vascularity within the echogenic hilum of the jugulodigastric lymph node. *(Middle)* Transverse power Doppler ultrasound shows marked intratumoral vessels in carotid body paraganglioma. Note characteristic splaying of internal and external carotid arteries. *(Bottom)* Axial T1WI MR shows a lobulated right upper neck lesion with well-circumscribed margins located posterior to submandibular gland, along the medial edge of the sternocleidomastoid muscle and superficial to major arteries of the carotid sheath. Location of lesion is typical for 2nd branchial cleft cyst. Note T1-hyperintense signal within 2nd branchial cleft cyst due to proteinaceous intracystic content.

MIDCERVICAL LEVEL

TERMINOLOGY

Abbreviations
- Common carotid artery (CCA)
- Internal jugular vein (IJV)

Definitions
- Portion of anterior triangle adjacent to major vessels of carotid sheath
- Extends from hyoid bone superiorly to cricoid cartilage inferiorly

IMAGING ANATOMY

Overview
- Major lymphatic drainage of head and neck region is via deep jugular cervical lymph nodes, which are distributed along upper, mid, and lower cervical levels
- Key structures in midcervical level include CCA, IJV, vagus nerve, lymph nodes, omohyoid muscle, and esophagus

Internal Contents
- CCA
  - Arises from aortic arch directly on left from brachiocephalic trunk on right
  - Ascends neck within carotid sheath
    - Medial to IJV
    - Vagus nerve sandwiched between CCA and IJV
  - No named branches in midcervical level
  - Bifurcates into internal carotid artery (ICA) and external carotid artery (ECA) at level of hyoid bone
  - Low-resistance arterial flow pattern
- IJV
  - Inferior continuation of sigmoid sinus from jugular foramen at skull base
  - Major deep venous drainage from brain and neck
  - Descends within carotid sheath
    - Lateral to CCA at midcervical level
  - Joins subclavian vein to form brachiocephalic vein
  - During sonography, make sure IJV is compressible and has respiratory phasicity to rule out presence of thrombus
  - Occasionally presence of slow venous flow may mimic IJV thrombus
    - Real-time visualization of layering and a sharp linear interface help to distinguish it from thrombus
- Vagus nerve (CN10)
  - Extracranial segment starts superiorly from jugular foramen at skull base
  - Descends along posterolateral aspect of carotid artery within carotid sheath
    - Passes anterior to aortic arch on left and subclavian artery on right
  - Major autonomic nerve supply to visceral organs in thorax and abdomen
  - On transverse sonography, appears as round, hypoechoic structure with central echogenicity
    - Close relation to CCA, IJV are clues to its identification
    - On longitudinal scan, seen as long tubular hypoechoic structure with fibrillar pattern
- Lymph nodes

- Numerous lymph nodes are seen along deep jugular chain in midcervical level
- Receive lymphatic drainage from upper jugular chain and directly from adjacent structures including larynx, hypopharynx, and thyroid gland
  - Commonly involved in nodal metastases from common head and neck cancers
- Usually located anterior to vessels of carotid sheath
- Normal ultrasound appearances: Small, elliptical in shape, presence of echogenic hilus, preserved hilar vascularity on Doppler imaging
- Omohyoid muscle
  - Arises from anterior portion of body of hyoid bone
  - Runs obliquely to cross anterior to CCA and deep to sternocleidomastoid muscle
  - Intermediate tendon overlies IJV
    - Occasionally mistaken for a lymph node
  - Then runs obliquely across the inferior posterior triangle to attach to posterior aspect of lateral clavicle
- Cervical esophagus
  - Junction of cricopharyngeus muscle and proximal cervical esophagus is located in midcervical level
  - Lies posterior/posterolateral to trachea and medial to CCA
    - More commonly slightly off midline to the left
    - Asking patient to swallow during real-time sonography helps to accurately identify esophagus
  - On US, may be mistaken for parathyroid adenoma or paratracheal lymph node

ANATOMY IMAGING ISSUES

Imaging Approaches
- Scan in transverse plane along major vessels of carotid sheath (keep CCA and IJV in center of image)
  - From carotid bifurcation down to level of cricoid cartilage
- Longitudinal/oblique plane for better assessment of internal architecture and vascularity of any lesion detected on scanning in transverse plane
- Color flow imaging helps to identify major vessels and characterize lesions in this region
- USG also provides safe real-time guidance for fine-needle aspiration cytology (FNAC) or biopsy

CLINICAL IMPLICATIONS

Clinical Importance
- Common differential diagnoses for mass at midcervical level
  - Enlarged lymph nodes: Reactive, inflammatory, or neoplastic (metastases/lymphoma) disease
  - Inflammatory: Abscess
  - Congenital lesion: Lymphatic malformation, off-midline thyroglossal duct cyst
  - Neoplasm: Vagal schwannoma, esophageal lesion

RELATED REFERENCES

1. Ahuja AT et al. Imaging in head and neck cancer: A practical approach. London: Greenwich Medical Media, 2003

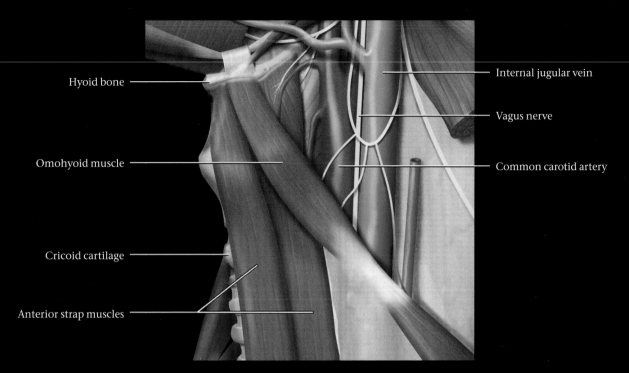

Hyoid bone

Omohyoid muscle

Cricoid cartilage

Anterior strap muscles

Internal jugular vein

Vagus nerve

Common carotid artery

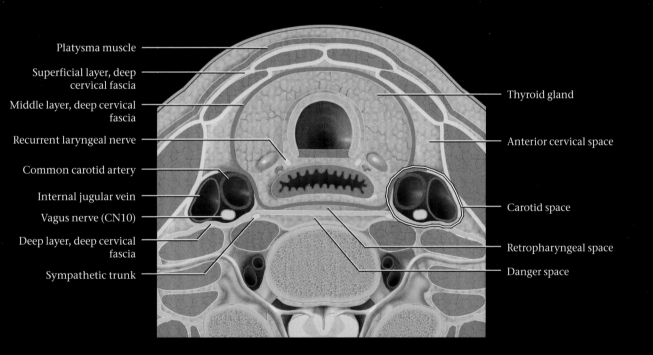

Platysma muscle

Superficial layer, deep cervical fascia

Middle layer, deep cervical fascia

Recurrent laryngeal nerve

Common carotid artery

Internal jugular vein

Vagus nerve (CN10)

Deep layer, deep cervical fascia

Sympathetic trunk

Thyroid gland

Anterior cervical space

Carotid space

Retropharyngeal space

Danger space

(Top) Schematic diagram shows the midcervical level, which contains key structures including the common carotid artery, the internal jugular vein, and the vagus nerve within the carotid sheath. The hyoid bone and the cricoid cartilage are the anatomical landmarks for the superior and inferior borders of the midcervical level, respectively. With high-resolution US, normal small jugular chain lymph nodes may be seen at this site and should not be mistaken for pathology. *(Bottom)* Axial graphic shows the middle cervical level in the infrahyoid neck. Note that the carotid sheath contains all 3 layers of the deep cervical fascia (tricolor line). In the infrahyoid neck, the carotid sheath is tenacious throughout its length. The infrahyoid carotid space contains the common carotid artery, the internal jugular vein, and the vagus cranial nerve.

MIDCERVICAL LEVEL

TRANSVERSE ULTRASOUND

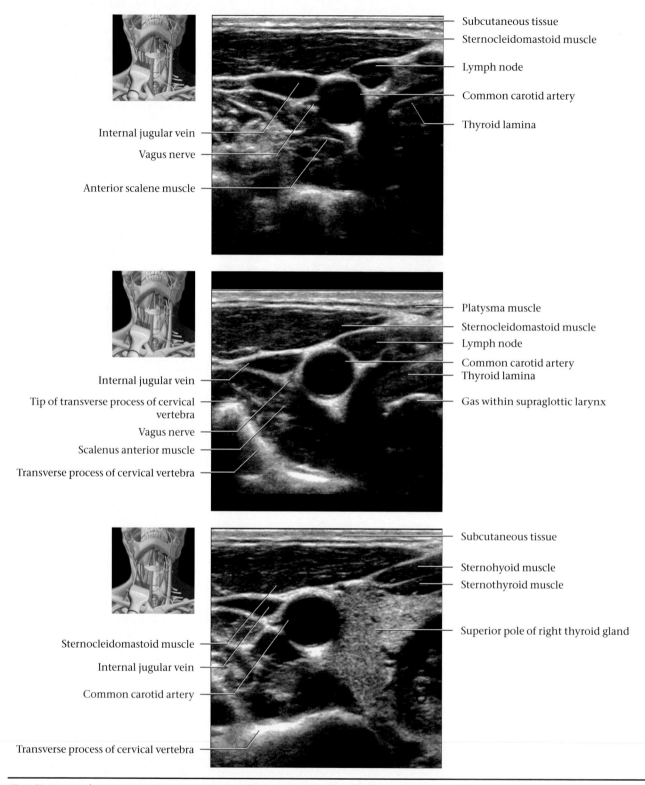

Subcutaneous tissue
Sternocleidomastoid muscle
Lymph node
Common carotid artery
Thyroid lamina

Internal jugular vein
Vagus nerve
Anterior scalene muscle

Platysma muscle
Sternocleidomastoid muscle
Lymph node
Common carotid artery
Thyroid lamina
Gas within supraglottic larynx

Internal jugular vein
Tip of transverse process of cervical vertebra
Vagus nerve
Scalenus anterior muscle
Transverse process of cervical vertebra

Subcutaneous tissue
Sternohyoid muscle
Sternothyroid muscle
Superior pole of right thyroid gland

Sternocleidomastoid muscle
Internal jugular vein
Common carotid artery
Transverse process of cervical vertebra

(Top) First image shows consecutive transverse grayscale ultrasound of midcervical level. Deep cervical lymph nodes are commonly found along and anterior to major vessels of the carotid sheath. These are commonly hypoechoic and elliptical with a normal echogenic hilum and hilar vascularity. (Middle) Second image shows midcervical level in transverse plane. At this level, the common carotid artery, internal jugular vein, and vagus nerve are the main structures within the carotid sheath. The vagus nerve is usually located between the CCA and the IJV, and appears as a small, round, hypoechoic nodule with a central echogenic dot. (Bottom) Third image shows the midcervical level. The cricoid cartilage may not be routinely seen on ultrasound, and visualization of the superior pole of the thyroid gland approximately coincides with this level.

AXIAL CECT

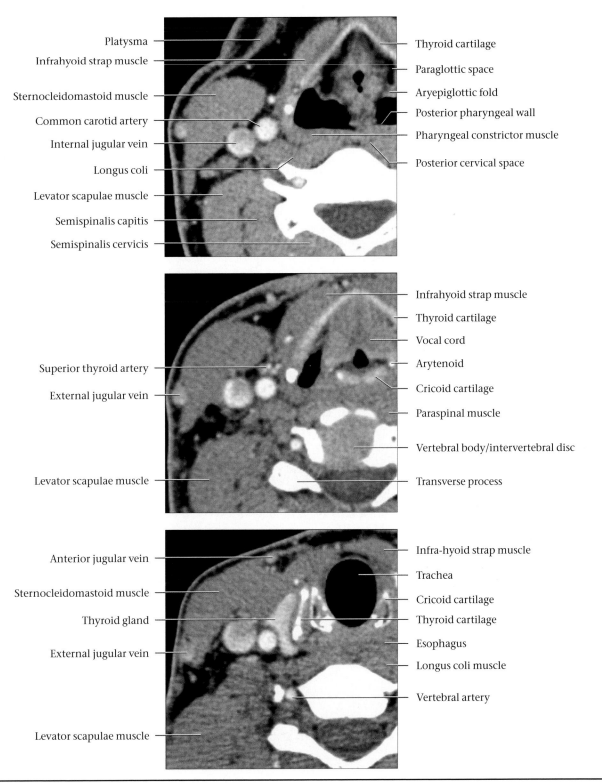

Platysma — Thyroid cartilage
Infrahyoid strap muscle — Paraglottic space
Sternocleidomastoid muscle — Aryepiglottic fold
Common carotid artery — Posterior pharyngeal wall
Internal jugular vein — Pharyngeal constrictor muscle
Longus coli — Posterior cervical space
Levator scapulae muscle —
Semispinalis capitis —
Semispinalis cervicis —

Superior thyroid artery — Infrahyoid strap muscle
External jugular vein — Thyroid cartilage
Vocal cord
Arytenoid
Cricoid cartilage
Paraspinal muscle
Levator scapulae muscle — Vertebral body/intervertebral disc
Transverse process

Anterior jugular vein — Infra-hyoid strap muscle
Sternocleidomastoid muscle — Trachea
Thyroid gland — Cricoid cartilage
External jugular vein — Thyroid cartilage
Esophagus
Longus coli muscle
Vertebral artery
Levator scapulae muscle —

(Top) CECT shows the upper thyroid cartilage level. Major structures of the midcervical level, including the common carotid artery, the internal jugular vein, and the sternocleidomastoid muscle are well demonstrated. Small lymph nodes are commonly seen adjacent to major vessels of the carotid sheath. (Middle) CECT shows the level of the lower thyroid lamina. Apart from the common carotid artery and the internal jugular vein, branches of the external carotid artery, such as the superior thyroid artery, can be demonstrated. (Bottom) CECT shows the level of the cricoid cartilage. The upper pole of the thyroid gland begins to be included in cross section. Note the presence of calcification/ossification in the thyroid lamina and cricoid cartilages, which is a normal age-related change.

MIDCERVICAL LEVEL

TRANSVERSE GRAYSCALE ULTRASOUND

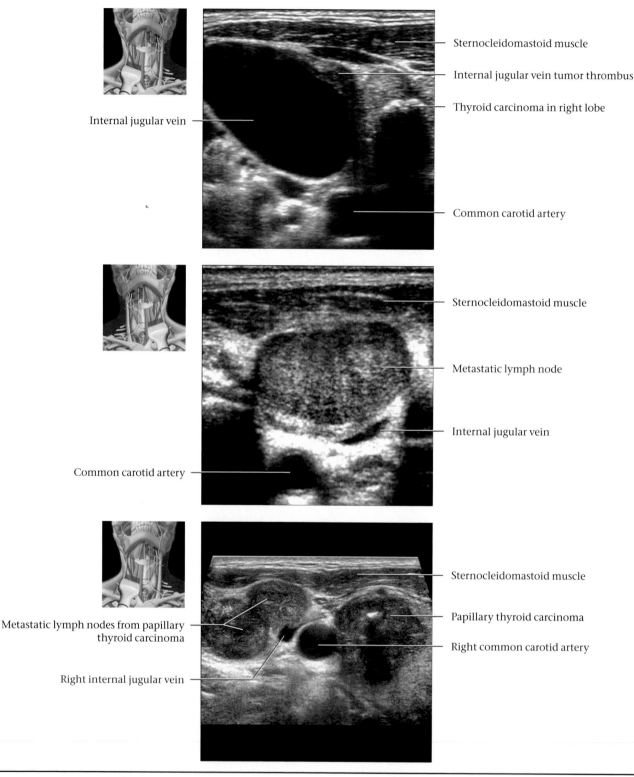

Internal jugular vein

Sternocleidomastoid muscle

Internal jugular vein tumor thrombus

Thyroid carcinoma in right lobe

Common carotid artery

Sternocleidomastoid muscle

Metastatic lymph node

Internal jugular vein

Common carotid artery

Metastatic lymph nodes from papillary thyroid carcinoma

Sternocleidomastoid muscle

Papillary thyroid carcinoma

Right common carotid artery

Right internal jugular vein

(Top) Transverse grayscale ultrasound of the right midcervical level shows an eccentric, hypoechoic thrombus in the anteromedial wall of the right internal jugular vein. Note the presence of an adjacent thyroid carcinoma in the right lobe. *(Middle)* Transverse grayscale ultrasound of the left midcervical level shows an enlarged, round, solid, hypoechoic, deep cervical lymph node with loss of echogenic hilum. The adjacent left internal jugular vein is compressed. Pathology showed metastatic squamous cell carcinoma. *(Bottom)* Transverse grayscale ultrasound of the right midcervical level shows multiple enlarged, round, solid, slightly hyperechoic lymph nodes with punctate calcification suggesting metastases from primary papillary thyroid carcinoma. Note thyroid papillary carcinoma seen as an ill-defined, solid, hypoechoic nodule with punctate and coarse calcification in the right lobe of the thyroid gland. The right internal jugular vein is compressed by enlarged lymph nodes but remains patent.

TRANSVERSE COLOR, DOPPLER, AND GRAYSCALE ULTRASOUND

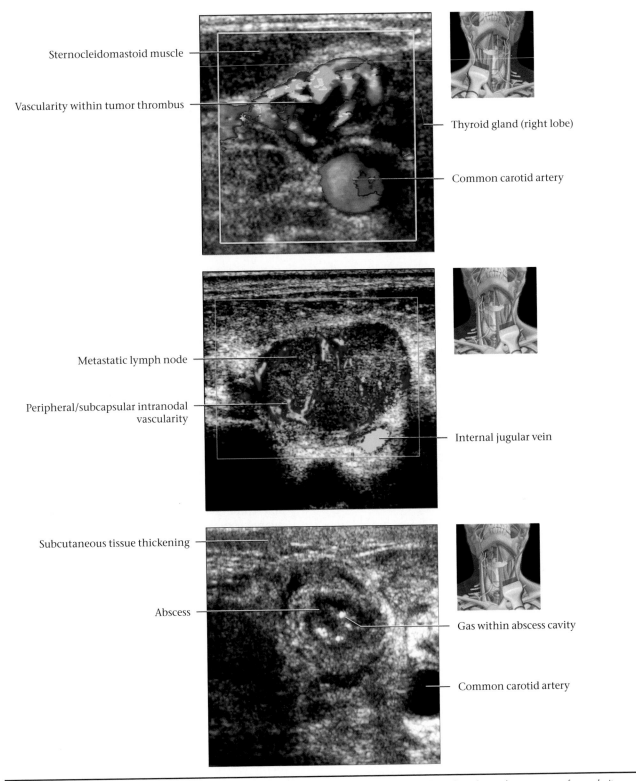

Sternocleidomastoid muscle

Vascularity within tumor thrombus

Thyroid gland (right lobe)

Common carotid artery

Metastatic lymph node

Peripheral/subcapsular intranodal vascularity

Internal jugular vein

Subcutaneous tissue thickening

Abscess

Gas within abscess cavity

Common carotid artery

(Top) *Transverse color Doppler ultrasound in a patient with occlusive internal jugular vein (IJV) thrombus shows the presence of vascularity within the IJV thrombus, suggesting it is a tumor thrombus rather than a bland venous thrombus.* *(Middle)* *Transverse power Doppler ultrasound shows the presence of peripheral/subcapsular intranodal vessels in a metastatic lymph node from head and neck squamous cell carcinoma. The vascularity is completely different from the hilar pattern of a normal cervical lymph node.* *(Bottom)* *Transverse grayscale ultrasound shows a neck abscess with fluid and gas within. The adjacent soft tissue is edematous and thickened. Note its close proximity to the common carotid artery, putting it at a risk of rupture.*

LOWER CERVICAL LEVEL AND SUPRACLAVICULAR FOSSA

TERMINOLOGY

Definitions

- Portion of lower anterior neck adjacent to carotid sheath, below level of cricoid cartilage and above level of clavicle

IMAGING ANATOMY

Overview

- Key structures in lower cervical level include common carotid artery (CCA), internal jugular vein (IJV), vagus nerve, subclavian artery, scalenus anterior muscle, and lymph nodes
- Important structures in supraclavicular fossa include trapezius muscle, sternocleidomastoid muscle, omohyoid muscle, brachial plexus elements, and transverse cervical chain lymph nodes

Internal Contents

- Subclavian artery
  - Arises from brachiocephalic trunk on right and aortic arch on left
  - Major arterial supply to upper limb
  - Contributes to arterial supply to neck structures and brain via vertebral artery
  - Junction of subclavian artery and CCA is readily identified on scanning in transverse plane in lower cervical level
    - Location marks root of neck
  - Origin of subclavian artery can be seen by angulating transducer inferiorly behind medial head of clavicle
- Scalenus anterior muscle
  - Runs inferiorly from transverse processes of cervical spine
  - Passes posterior to IJV to dip behind clavicle
  - Lies between 2nd part of subclavian artery posteriorly and subclavian vein anteriorly
  - Related posteriorly to scalenus medius muscle
    - Brachial plexus roots/rami lie between scalenus anterior muscle and scalenus medius muscle in supraclavicular fossa
    - Scanning inferiorly in transverse plane, brachial plexus roots/rami appear as small, round, hypoechoic structures emerging from behind lateral border of scalenus anterior muscle
- Brachial plexus (BP)
  - Formed from ventral rami of C5-T1 ± minor branches from C4, T2
  - Divided into roots/rami, trunks, division, cords, and terminal branches
    - Roots/rami: Originate from spinal cord levels C5-T1 enter posterior triangle by emerging between scalenus anterior and medius muscle
    - Trunks: Upper (C5-6), middle (C7), lower (C8-T1)
    - Divisions: Formed by each trunk, dividing into anterior and posterior branches in supraclavicular fossa
    - Cords: Lateral, medial, posterior cords descend behind clavicle to leave posterior triangle and enter axilla
    - Branches: In axilla
- Trapezius muscle
  - Anterior border marks posterior margin of posterior triangle and supraclavicular fossa and is easily recognized
  - Distal portion is attached to lateral clavicle
- Inferior belly of omohyoid muscle
  - Runs obliquely from intermediate tendon to traverse inferior portion of supraclavicular fossa
  - Divides occipital triangle superiorly from supraclavicular triangle inferiorly
- Transverse cervical chain lymph nodes
  - Seen adjacent to transverse cervical artery and vein, which arise from thyrocervical trunk and IJV
  - Related to and just superior to inferior belly of omohyoid muscle

ANATOMY IMAGING ISSUES

Imaging Approaches

- From midcervical level, proceed to scan in transverse plane along carotid sheath until medial head of clavicle (keep CCA and IJV in center of image)
- Then sweep laterally in transverse plane above mid/lateral portion of clavicle to assess supraclavicular fossa

Consider

- Enlarged lymph node is most common cause of mass in lower cervical level and supraclavicular fossa
  - Terminology
    - Omohyoid node: Deep cervical chain node just superior to omohyoid (where the omohyoid crosses IJV)
    - Virchow node: Signal node; lowest node of deep cervical chain nodes
    - Troisier node: Most medial node of transverse cervical chain nodes
  - Reactive nodes: Enlarged, cortical hypertrophy, preserved echogenic hilum and hilar vascularity
  - Tuberculous lymphadenitis: Matted, necrotic, enlarged nodes with soft tissue edema, and hypovascular/displaced hilar vascularity on power Doppler ultrasound
  - Metastatic nodes: Round, hypoechoic nodes with peripheral/subcapsular vascularity
  - Lymphomatous nodes: Large, heterogeneous, reticulated/pseudocystic appearance, increased peripheral and central vascularity, bilateral involvement
- Isolated metastatic lymph node in supraclavicular fossa is unusual from primary in head and neck region
  - Careful search for infraclavicular primary is indicated
  - Common primary from lung, breast, esophagus, and colorectal cancers
- Differential diagnoses
  - Brachial plexus schwannoma
  - Lipoma
  - Venous vascular malformation
  - Lymphatic malformation

RELATED REFERENCES

1. Ahuja AT et al. Imaging in Head and Neck Cancer: A Practical Approach. London: Greenwich Medical Media Limited, 2003

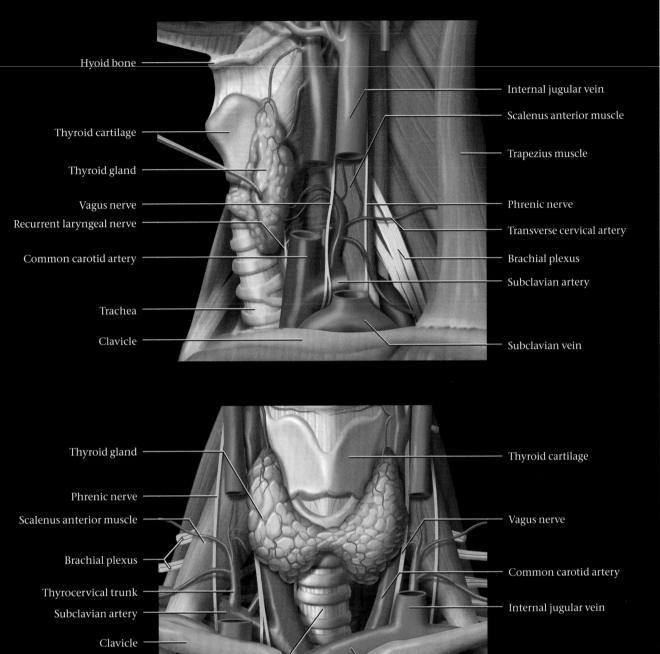

Hyoid bone

Thyroid cartilage

Thyroid gland

Vagus nerve

Recurrent laryngeal nerve

Common carotid artery

Trachea

Clavicle

Internal jugular vein

Scalenus anterior muscle

Trapezius muscle

Phrenic nerve

Transverse cervical artery

Brachial plexus

Subclavian artery

Subclavian vein

Thyroid gland

Phrenic nerve

Scalenus anterior muscle

Brachial plexus

Thyrocervical trunk

Subclavian artery

Clavicle

Trachea

Thyroid cartilage

Vagus nerve

Common carotid artery

Internal jugular vein

Left brachiocephalic vein

(Top) Graphic in lateral projection shows the anatomical relationship of major structures in the lower cervical level and supraclavicular fossa, including the common carotid artery, internal jugular vein, subclavian vessels, and brachial plexus. In assessing the supraclavicular fossa on ultrasound, adequate visualization is achieved by sweeping the transducer laterally in the transverse plane from the medial head of the clavicle. *(Bottom)* Graphic in frontal projection shows the lower cervical level and medial portion of the supraclavicular fossa. The major lymph nodes in these regions are mainly located close to the major vessels of the carotid sheath, including the Virchow node and the Troisier node. Presence of isolated malignant nodes at this site usually points to an infraclavicular primary. Proximity of these nodes to adjacent pulsatile vessels makes Doppler examination at this site suboptimal/difficult.

LOWER CERVICAL LEVEL AND SUPRACLAVICULAR FOSSA

TRANSVERSE ULTRASOUND

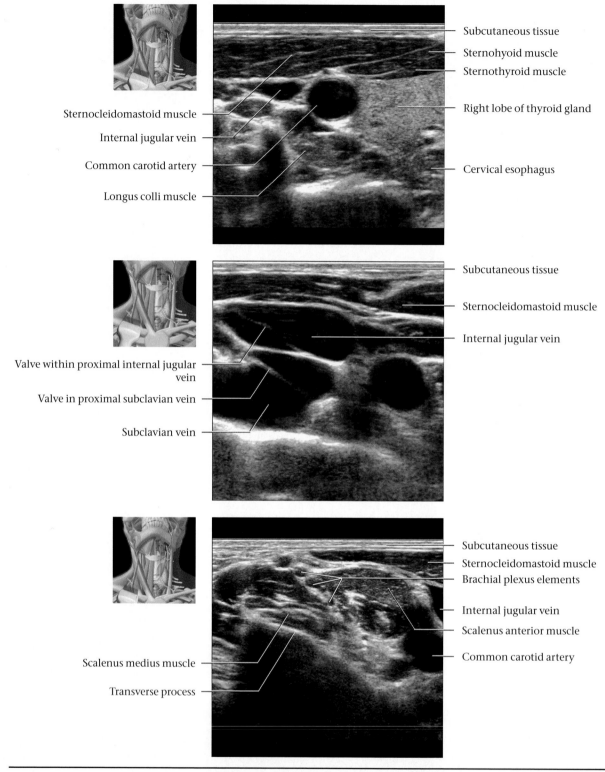

Subcutaneous tissue

Sternohyoid muscle

Sternothyroid muscle

Right lobe of thyroid gland

Cervical esophagus

Sternocleidomastoid muscle

Internal jugular vein

Common carotid artery

Longus colli muscle

Subcutaneous tissue

Sternocleidomastoid muscle

Internal jugular vein

Valve within proximal internal jugular vein

Valve in proximal subclavian vein

Subclavian vein

Subcutaneous tissue

Sternocleidomastoid muscle

Brachial plexus elements

Internal jugular vein

Scalenus anterior muscle

Common carotid artery

Scalenus medius muscle

Transverse process

(Top) First image in a series of transverse grayscale ultrasound images shows the lower cervical level. Major structures at this level include the common carotid artery, the internal jugular vein, the thyroid gland, and the overlying muscles of the anterior neck. *(Middle)* Second image shows the level of the medial supraclavicular fossa. Note the proximity of the proximal internal jugular vein to the subclavian vein at this site, which join to form the brachiocephalic vein. Supraclavicular lymph nodes are commonly found adjacent to these major vessels. *(Bottom)* Third image shows the lateral supraclavicular fossa. The scalenus anterior and medius muscles are clearly visualized with the trunks of the brachial plexus between them. US is often used to guide brachial plexus blocks. US also helps to exclude brachial plexus involvement by metastases at this site.

LOWER CERVICAL LEVEL AND SUPRACLAVICULAR FOSSA

AXIAL CECT AND POWER DOPPLER ULTRASOUND

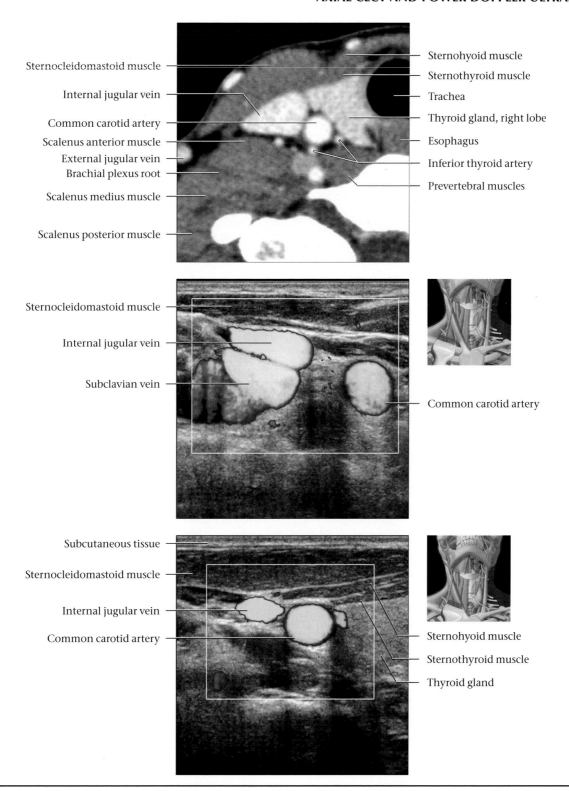

Sternocleidomastoid muscle

Internal jugular vein

Common carotid artery

Scalenus anterior muscle

External jugular vein

Brachial plexus root

Scalenus medius muscle

Scalenus posterior muscle

Sternohyoid muscle

Sternothyroid muscle

Trachea

Thyroid gland, right lobe

Esophagus

Inferior thyroid artery

Prevertebral muscles

Sternocleidomastoid muscle

Internal jugular vein

Subclavian vein

Common carotid artery

Subcutaneous tissue

Sternocleidomastoid muscle

Internal jugular vein

Common carotid artery

Sternohyoid muscle

Sternothyroid muscle

Thyroid gland

(Top) Axial CECT shows the lower cervical level. The relationship of the thyroid gland with the adjacent structures, including the carotid sheath, strap muscles, trachea, and esophagus is demonstrated. *(Middle)* Transverse power Doppler ultrasound in the supraclavicular fossa helps to delineate vascular structures in this region, including the confluence of the internal jugular vein and the subclavian vein. The proximal portion of the common carotid artery from the brachiocephalic trunk is also seen at this level. *(Bottom)* Transverse power Doppler US of the lower cervical level allows the clear depiction of the color-filled common carotid artery and internal jugular vein. Nodes are often seen at this site and are readily evaluated by US and biopsied/fine-needle aspirated under guidance.

LOWER CERVICAL LEVEL AND SUPRACLAVICULAR FOSSA

LONGITUDINAL ULTRASOUND AND PATHOLOGY

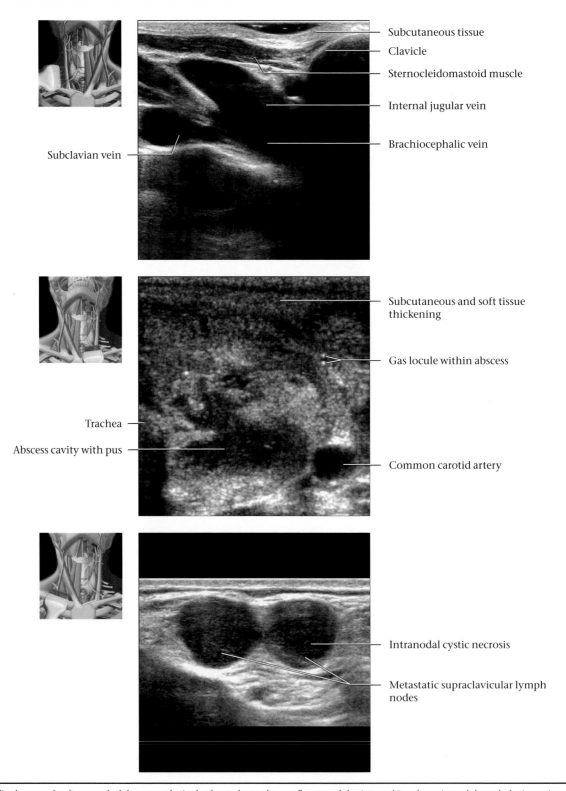

Subcutaneous tissue

Clavicle

Sternocleidomastoid muscle

Internal jugular vein

Brachiocephalic vein

Subclavian vein

Subcutaneous and soft tissue thickening

Gas locule within abscess

Trachea

Abscess cavity with pus

Common carotid artery

Intranodal cystic necrosis

Metastatic supraclavicular lymph nodes

(Top) Longitudinal grayscale ultrasound of the supraclavicular fossa shows the confluence of the internal jugular vein and the subclavian vein to form the brachiocephalic vein just above the medial portion of the clavicle. Nodes often nestle under these vessels, making biopsy access difficult. Pulsation from the vessels also makes Doppler evaluation of nodes at this level suboptimal. *(Middle)* Transverse grayscale ultrasound of the left lower cervical level shows abscess formation in the left lobe and perithyroidal soft tissue due to acute suppurative thyroiditis. Note the presence of pus and echogenic foci due to gas bubbles. *(Bottom)* Transverse grayscale ultrasound of the right supraclavicular fossa shows multiple enlarged, round, predominantly solid, hypoechoic lymph nodes with intranodal cystic necrosis and no adjacent soft tissue edema. Appearances are highly suspicious of metastatic lymph nodes. Isolated metastatic nodes at this site point to an infraclavicular primary, commonly from lung, breast, or esophagus.

CECT AND PATHOLOGY

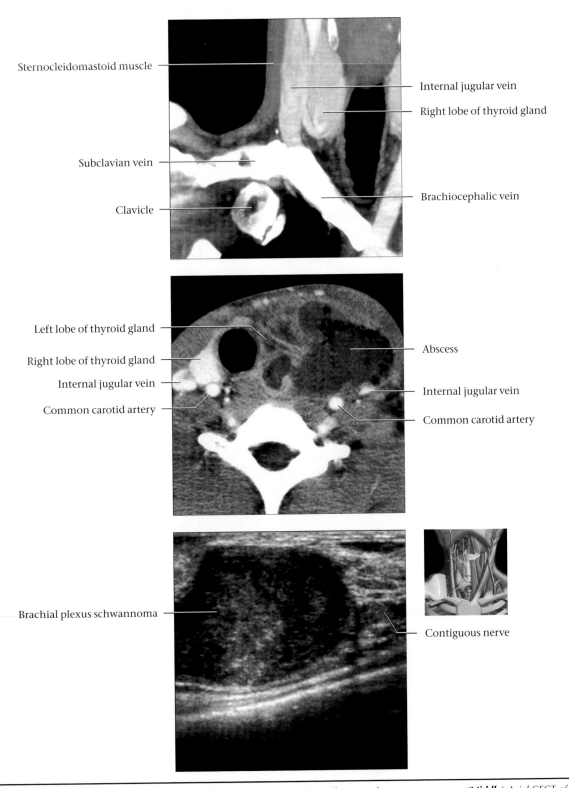

Sternocleidomastoid muscle

Internal jugular vein

Right lobe of thyroid gland

Subclavian vein

Brachiocephalic vein

Clavicle

Left lobe of thyroid gland

Abscess

Right lobe of thyroid gland

Internal jugular vein

Internal jugular vein

Common carotid artery

Common carotid artery

Brachial plexus schwannoma

Contiguous nerve

(Top) Coronal reformatted CECT of the lower neck and the supraclavicular fossa illustrates the venous anatomy. *(Middle)* Axial CECT of acute suppurative thyroiditis shows a large heterogeneous abscess with thick peripheral enhancement involving the left lobe of the thyroid gland and perithyroidal soft tissue. Note the presence of fluid and gas within the abscess cavity and marked subcutaneous thickening in left lower neck. *(Bottom)* Longitudinal grayscale ultrasound of the right supraclavicular fossa shows a solid, hypoechoic, lobulated mass contiguous with a thickened nerve. The appearances suggest a brachial plexus schwannoma. The continuation with a nerve is the clue to its diagnosis.

POSTERIOR TRIANGLE

TERMINOLOGY

Abbreviations
- Posterior cervical space (PCS)

Definitions
- Posterolateral fat-containing space in neck with complex fascial boundaries that extends from posterior mastoid tip to clavicle behind sternocleidomastoid muscle

IMAGING ANATOMY

Overview
- Posterolateral fat-filled space just deep and posterior to sternomastoid muscle
- Posterior border bound by anterior edge of trapezius muscle

Extent
- PCS extends from small superior component near mastoid tip to broader base at level of clavicle
- When viewed from side, appears as "tilting tent"

Anatomy Relationships
- Superficial space lies superficial to PCS
- Deep to PCS is perivertebral space
  - Anterior PCS is superficial to prevertebral component of perivertebral space
  - Posterior PCS is superficial to paraspinal component of perivertebral space

Internal Contents
- Fat is primary component of PCS
- Floor is formed by muscles running obliquely: Scalene muscles, levator scapulae, and splenius capitis muscles (from anterior to posterior)
  - Subdivided by inferior belly of omohyoid muscle into occipital and subclavian triangles
- Muscular floor is covered by superficial and deep layers of deep cervical fascia
- Spinal accessory nerve (CN11)
  - Arises from nerve cells in anterior gray column of upper 5 segments of spinal cord
  - Ascends alongside spinal cord and enter skull through foramen magnum
  - Unites with cranial root to exit through jugular foramen
  - Spinal portion then separates from cranial root
  - Motor supply to soft palate, pharynx, larynx, sternocleidomastoid, and trapezius muscles
- Spinal accessory lymph node chain
  - Level 5 spinal accessory nodes (SAN) further subdivide into A & B levels at hyoid bone
    - Level 5A: SAN above cricoid cartilage level
    - Level 5B: SAN below cricoid cartilage level
- Preaxillary brachial plexus
  - Segment of brachial plexus emerging from anterior and middle scalene gap passes through PCS
  - Leaves PCS with axillary artery into axillary fat
- Dorsal scapular nerve
  - Arises from brachial plexus (spinal nerves C4 & C5)
  - Motor innervation to rhomboid and levator scapulae muscles
- Transverse cervical artery and vein
  - Arises from thyrocervical trunk of subclavian artery and IJV respectively
  - Course in inferior posterior triangle and parallel to clavicle

ANATOMY IMAGING ISSUES

Imaging Approaches
- Scanning is usually undertaken in transverse plane
- From mastoid tip superiorly to acromion process inferiorly
  - Spinal accessory chain lymph nodes run from a point midway between mastoid process and angle of mandible to outer 1/3 of clavicle

Imaging Pitfalls
- On transverse scan, tips of transverse process of cervical vertebrae may be seen as echogenic structures with posterior acoustic shadowing
  - Do not mistake these for calcified lymph nodes
  - Longitudinal scan helps to clarify

Consider
- On US, normal-looking nodes are routinely found in posterior triangle of healthy individuals
- Most lesions in posterior triangle arise from spinal accessory chain lymph nodes
  - Reactive lymphadenopathy
    - Elliptical, preserved internal architecture and hilar vascularity
  - Infective lymphadenitis such as tuberculous lymphadenitis
    - Enlarged hypoechoic necrotic nodes with matting and soft tissue edema, avascular or displaced hilar vascularity
  - Metastatic lymph nodes
    - Primary from nasopharyngeal carcinoma and squamous cell carcinoma from other H&N sites
    - Enlarged, round, hypoechoic nodes with intranodal necrosis and peripheral vascularity
  - Lymphomatous nodes
    - Usually bilateral neck involvement
    - Enlarged, heterogeneous, reticulated/pseudocystic appearance, increased hilar and peripheral vascularity, hilar > > peripheral
- Other diseases that may occur in posterior triangle include
  - Congenital lesion: Lymphangioma, usually trans-spatial
  - Benign tumor: Lipoma, nerve sheath tumor

CLINICAL IMPLICATIONS

Clinical Importance
- CN11 runs in floor of posterior triangle
  - Accessory cranial neuropathy results when CN11 is injured
  - Most commonly injured during neck dissection for malignant squamous cell carcinoma (SCC) nodes
  - Less commonly injured by extranodal spread of SCC
- Spinal accessory nodes are main normal occupants of posterior cervical space

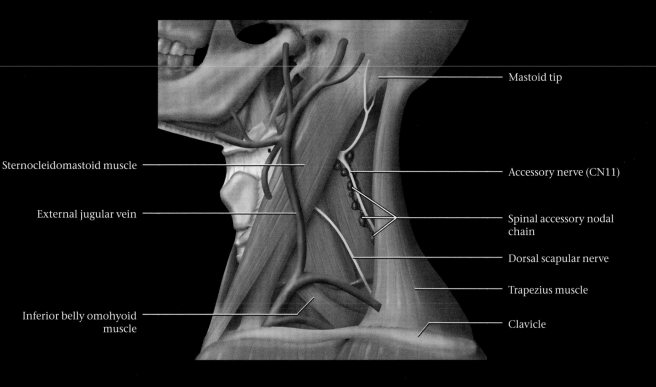

Mastoid tip

Sternocleidomastoid muscle

External jugular vein

Inferior belly omohyoid muscle

Accessory nerve (CN11)

Spinal accessory nodal chain

Dorsal scapular nerve

Trapezius muscle

Clavicle

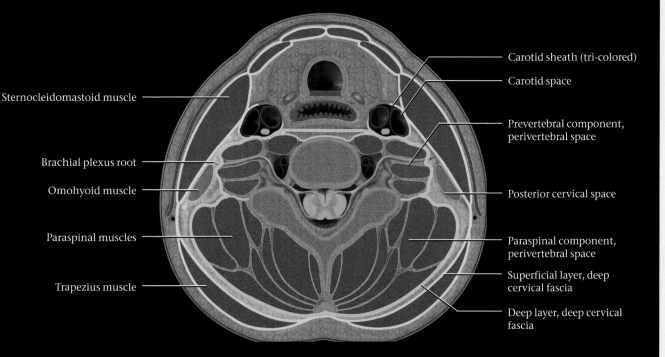

Sternocleidomastoid muscle

Brachial plexus root

Omohyoid muscle

Paraspinal muscles

Trapezius muscle

Carotid sheath (tri-colored)

Carotid space

Prevertebral component, perivertebral space

Posterior cervical space

Paraspinal component, perivertebral space

Superficial layer, deep cervical fascia

Deep layer, deep cervical fascia

(Top) Lateral graphic of the neck shows the posterior triangle as a "tilting tent" with its superior margin at the level of the mastoid tip and its inferior border at the clavicle. Note that it has 2 main nerves in its floor, the accessory nerve (CN11) and the dorsal scapular nerve. The spinal accessory nodal chain is its key occupant with regards to the kind of lesions found in the posterior triangle. *(Bottom)* Axial graphic through the thyroid bed of the infrahyoid neck depicts the posterior cervical space (PCS) with its complex fascial borders. The superficial layer of the deep cervical fascia is its superficial border while the deep layer of the deep cervical fascia is its deep border. Note the tri-color carotid sheath is its anteromedial border. The brachial plexus roots travel through the PCS on their way to the axillary apex.

POSTERIOR TRIANGLE

TRANSVERSE ULTRASOUND

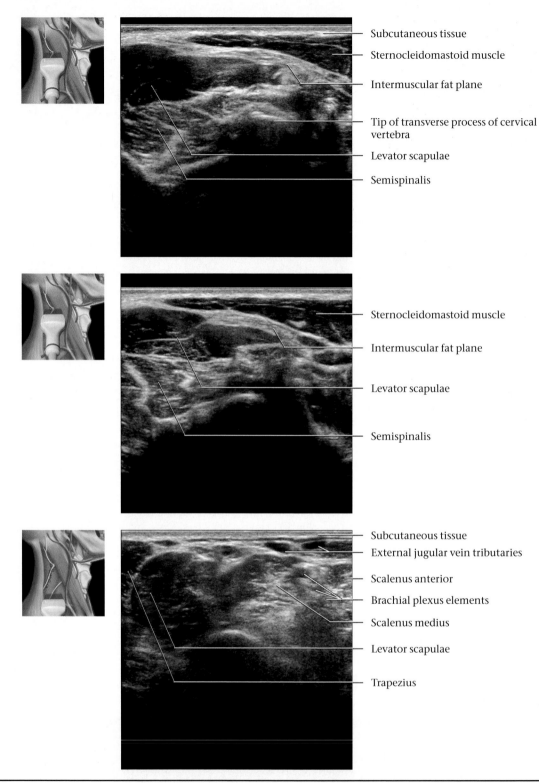

Subcutaneous tissue

Sternocleidomastoid muscle

Intermuscular fat plane

Tip of transverse process of cervical vertebra

Levator scapulae

Semispinalis

Sternocleidomastoid muscle

Intermuscular fat plane

Levator scapulae

Semispinalis

Subcutaneous tissue

External jugular vein tributaries

Scalenus anterior

Brachial plexus elements

Scalenus medius

Levator scapulae

Trapezius

(Top) First of 3 transverse grayscale ultrasound images shows the posterior triangle. The sternocleidomastoid muscle marks the anterior border of the posterior triangle. Muscles form the floor of the posterior triangle. Note the accessory nerve and nodes lie in the intermuscular fat plane. *(Middle)* Standard transverse grayscale ultrasound of the posterior triangle shows the intermuscular fat plane, which is best screened in this plane. Once pathology is detected further examination, particularly Doppler, is best done longitudinally. *(Bottom)* Lower level of the posterior triangle is shown. The trapezius muscle marks the posterior margin of the posterior triangle. The main bulk of the levator scapulae muscle forms the muscular floor.

AXIAL MR

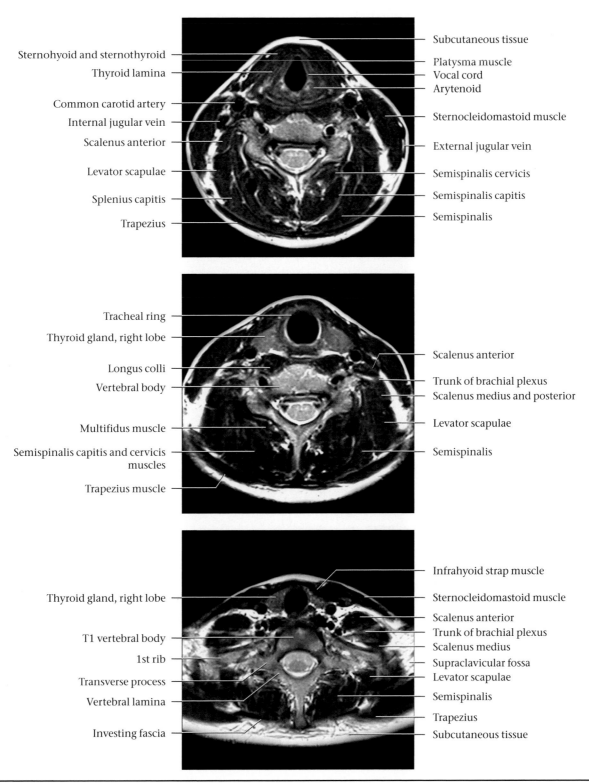

Sternohyoid and sternothyroid

Thyroid lamina

Common carotid artery

Internal jugular vein

Scalenus anterior

Levator scapulae

Splenius capitis

Trapezius

Subcutaneous tissue

Platysma muscle

Vocal cord

Arytenoid

Sternocleidomastoid muscle

External jugular vein

Semispinalis cervicis

Semispinalis capitis

Semispinalis

Tracheal ring

Thyroid gland, right lobe

Longus colli

Vertebral body

Multifidus muscle

Semispinalis capitis and cervicis muscles

Trapezius muscle

Scalenus anterior

Trunk of brachial plexus

Scalenus medius and posterior

Levator scapulae

Semispinalis

Thyroid gland, right lobe

T1 vertebral body

1st rib

Transverse process

Vertebral lamina

Investing fascia

Infrahyoid strap muscle

Sternocleidomastoid muscle

Scalenus anterior

Trunk of brachial plexus

Scalenus medius

Supraclavicular fossa

Levator scapulae

Semispinalis

Trapezius

Subcutaneous tissue

(Top) Axial PD MR of the neck at the level of the vocal cord shows the largely fat-filled posterior triangle with muscular floor. (Middle) Axial PD MR of the neck at the level of thyroid gland shows the scalenus medius muscle begins at the mid cervical level. The nerve roots and the trunk of the brachial plexus is seen emerging between the scalenus anterior and medius muscles. (Bottom) Axial PD MR of the lower posterior triangle shows the trunks of the brachial plexus between the scalenus anterior and the medius muscles, diverging posterior to the clavicle to axillary region. Note the content of the posterior triangle is predominantly fat with large muscles forming its boundaries.

POSTERIOR TRIANGLE

LONGITUDINAL AND TRANSVERSE US

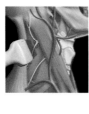 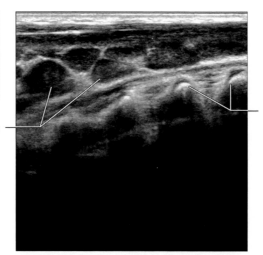

Reactive nodes

Tips of transverse process

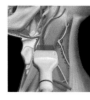 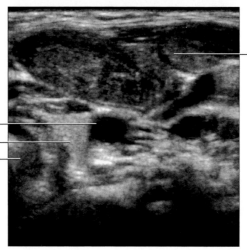

Sternocleidomastoid muscle pseudotumor

Common carotid artery

Left lobe of thyroid gland

Trachea

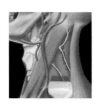 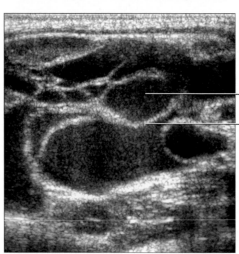

Lymphangioma

Internal septation

(Top) Longitudinal grayscale ultrasound of the posterior triangle shows a chain of reactive accessory nodes. Note their location in the intermuscular fat plane. Do not mistake the tips of the transverse processes with calcified nodes. (Middle) Transverse grayscale ultrasound in an infant with torticollis shows a heterogeneously enlarged left sternocleidomastoid muscle. The appearance is compatible with a sternocleidomastoid pseudotumor. (Bottom) Transverse grayscale ultrasound shows a large, multiseptated, cystic mass occupying the left posterior triangle in a child. The appearance is suggestive of a lymphatic malformation. These lesions are trans-spatial and frequently extend into other neck spaces.

POSTERIOR TRIANGLE

LONGITUDINAL US AND AXIAL MR

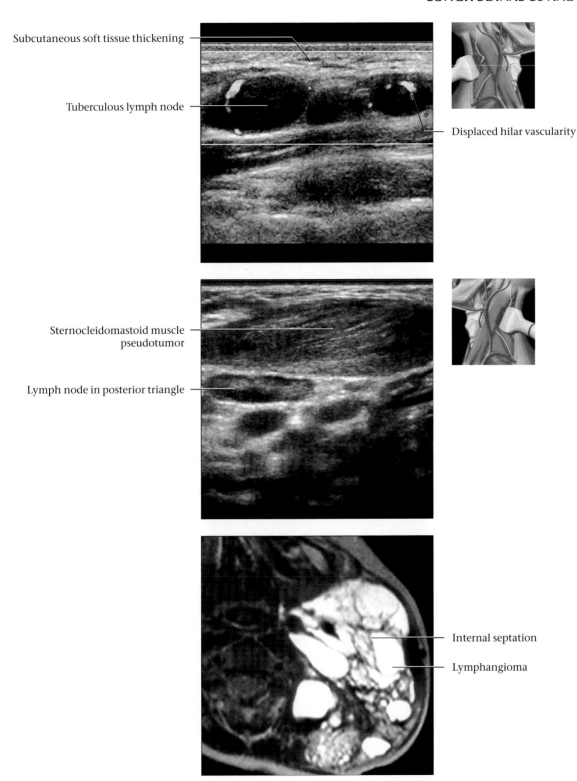

Subcutaneous soft tissue thickening

Tuberculous lymph node

Displaced hilar vascularity

Sternocleidomastoid muscle pseudotumor

Lymph node in posterior triangle

Internal septation

Lymphangioma

(Top) Longitudinal color Doppler ultrasound in the posterior triangle shows multiple, enlarged, hypoechoic lymph nodes with displaced hilar vascularity. Pathology showed tuberculous lymphadenitis. Once pathology is detected in transverse scans, it is better evaluated on a longitudinal scan, particularly if performing a Doppler examination. *(Middle)* Longitudinal grayscale ultrasound of the left posterior triangle shows the sternocleidomastoid muscle pseudotumor. Part of the normal muscular striations are preserved. *(Bottom)* Fat-suppressed T2WI MR of the neck shows the large lymphatic malformation occupying the left posterior triangle. Note the trans-spatial distribution of the lesion is better delineated by MR.

THYROID GLAND

IMAGING ANATOMY

Overview
- H- or U-shaped gland in anterior cervical neck formed from 2 elongated lateral lobes with superior and inferior poles connected by median isthmus
- 40% of people have pyramidal lobe ascending from isthmus area toward hyoid bone

Extent
- Extends from level of 5th cervical vertebra to 1st thoracic vertebra

Anatomy Relationships
- Thyroid gland lies anterior and lateral to trachea in visceral space of infrahyoid neck
- Posteromedially are tracheoesophageal grooves
  - Paratracheal lymph nodes, recurrent laryngeal nerve, parathyroid glands lie within the groove
- Posterolaterally are carotid spaces
  - Contains common carotid artery, internal jugular vein, vagus nerve
- Anteriorly are infrahyoid strap muscles
- Anterolaterally are sternocleidomastoid muscles

Internal Contents
- Thyroid gland
  - 2 lateral lobes (i.e., right and left lobes)
    - Measure ~ 4 cm in height
    - Each lobe has upper and lower poles
    - Lateral lobes are commonly asymmetric in size
  - Lateral lobes are joined by midline isthmus
  - On ultrasound, thyroid parenchymal echoes are fine, uniform, and hyperechoic compared to adjacent muscles
  - Echogenic thyroid capsule is clearly visualized and helps to differentiate thyroid lesions from extrathyroidal masses
- Arterial supply to thyroid gland
  - Superior thyroid arteries
    - 1st anterior branch of external carotid artery: Runs superficially on anterior border of lateral lobe, sending a branch deep into gland before curving toward isthmus where it anastomoses with contralateral artery
    - Proximal course closely associated with superior laryngeal nerve
  - Inferior thyroid arteries
    - Arise from thyrocervical trunk, a branch of subclavian artery
    - Ascend vertically, then curve medially to enter tracheoesophageal groove in plane posterior to carotid space
    - Most branches penetrate posterior aspect of lateral thyroid lobe
    - Closely associated with recurrent laryngeal nerve
  - Thyroidea ima occasionally present (3%)
    - Single vessel originating from aortic arch or innominate artery
    - Enters thyroid gland at inferior border of isthmus
- Venous drainage of thyroid gland
  - 3 pairs of veins arise from venous plexus on surface of thyroid gland
  - Superior and middle thyroid veins drain into internal jugular vein
  - Inferior thyroid veins drain into left brachiocephalic vein
- Lymphatic drainage of thyroid gland
  - Lymphatic drainage is extensive and multidirectional
  - Initial lymphatic drainage courses to periglandular nodes
    - Prelaryngeal, pretracheal (Delphian), and paratracheal nodes along recurrent laryngeal nerve
    - Paratracheal nodes drain along recurrent laryngeal nerve into mediastinum
    - Regional drainage occurs laterally into internal jugular chain (level 2-4) and spinal accessory chain (level 5), higher in neck along internal jugular vein

ANATOMY IMAGING ISSUES

Imaging Approaches
- Both longitudinal and transverse scans are required for comprehensive ultrasound assessment of thyroid gland
  - Transverse scan helps to locate thyroid nodules, their relationship to trachea, major vessels in carotid sheath, and to evaluate internal architecture and extrathyroid extension
  - Longitudinal scan helps to evaluate internal architecture, vascularity on Doppler, and extrathyroidal extension
- When evaluating thyroid nodule, examination is divided into
  - Ultrasound features of thyroid nodule
  - Assessment of adjacent structures (including trachea, esophagus, strap muscles, carotid artery, and internal jugular vein) and cervical lymph nodes

EMBRYOLOGY

Embryologic Events
- Thyroid gland originates from 1st and 2nd pharyngeal pouches (medial anlage)
- Originates as proliferation of endodermal epithelial cells on median surface of developing pharyngeal floor termed foramen cecum
- Bilobed thyroid gland descends anterior to pharyngeal gut along thyroglossal duct
- Inferior descent of thyroid gland anterior to hyoid bone and laryngeal cartilages

Practical Implications
- Thyroglossal duct cyst: Results from failure of involution of portion of thyroglossal duct
- Thyroid tissue remnants: From sequestration of thyroid tissue along thyroglossal duct
  - Seen anywhere along course of thyroglossal duct from foramen cecum to superior mediastinum
- Ectopic thyroid gland: From incomplete descent of thyroid into low neck
  - Seen anywhere along course from foramen cecum in tongue base to superior mediastinum
  - Most common location in neck is just deep to foramen cecum in tongue base (i.e., lingual thyroid)

RELATED REFERENCES

1. Sofferman RA et al. Ultrasound of the Thyroid and Parathyroid Glands. New York: Springer, 2012

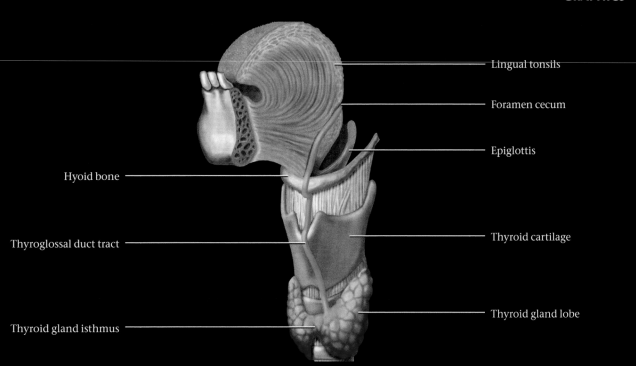

Lingual tonsils

Foramen cecum

Epiglottis

Hyoid bone

Thyroid cartilage

Thyroglossal duct tract

Thyroid gland lobe

Thyroid gland isthmus

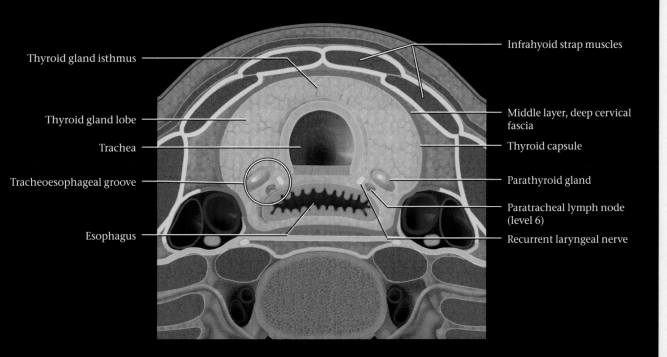

Thyroid gland isthmus

Infrahyoid strap muscles

Thyroid gland lobe

Middle layer, deep cervical fascia

Trachea

Thyroid capsule

Tracheoesophageal groove

Parathyroid gland

Paratracheal lymph node (level 6)

Esophagus

Recurrent laryngeal nerve

(Top) Sagittal oblique graphic displays the thyroglossal duct tract as it traverses the cervical neck from its origin at the foramen cecum to its termination in the anterior and lateral visceral space of the infrahyoid neck. The medial thyroid anlage arises from the paramedian aspect of the 1st and 2nd branchial pouches (foramen cecum area), then descends inferiorly through the tongue base, floor of mouth, and around and in front of the hyoid bone. *(Bottom)* Axial graphic at thyroid level depicts the thyroid lobes and isthmus in the anterior visceral space wrapping around the trachea. Note that there are 3 key structures found in the area of the tracheoesophageal groove, the recurrent laryngeal nerve, the paratracheal lymph node chain, and the parathyroid gland. The parathyroid glands may be inside or outside of the thyroid capsule.

THYROID GLAND

TRANSVERSE ULTRASOUND

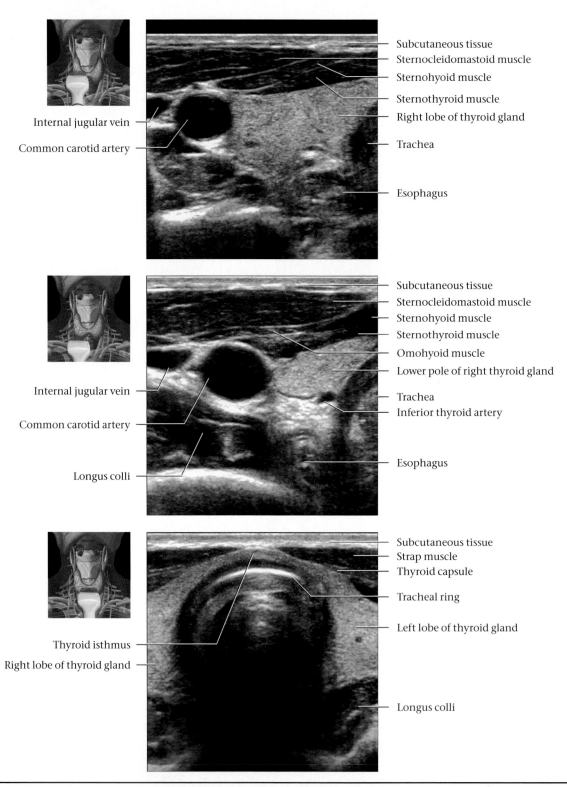

Internal jugular vein

Common carotid artery

Subcutaneous tissue
Sternocleidomastoid muscle
Sternohyoid muscle
Sternothyroid muscle
Right lobe of thyroid gland

Trachea

Esophagus

Internal jugular vein

Common carotid artery

Longus colli

Subcutaneous tissue
Sternocleidomastoid muscle
Sternohyoid muscle
Sternothyroid muscle
Omohyoid muscle
Lower pole of right thyroid gland

Trachea
Inferior thyroid artery

Esophagus

Thyroid isthmus
Right lobe of thyroid gland

Subcutaneous tissue
Strap muscle
Thyroid capsule

Tracheal ring

Left lobe of thyroid gland

Longus colli

(Top) Transverse grayscale ultrasound of the right lobe of the thyroid gland shows the homogeneous, hyperechoic echo pattern of the glandular parenchyma. Note its close anatomical relationship with the major vessels of the carotid sheath (internal jugular vein and common carotid artery) laterally, the trachea medially, and the cervical esophagus posteromedially. *(Middle)* Transverse grayscale ultrasound shows the level of the inferior pole of the thyroid gland. The inferior thyroid artery is a consistent finding related to and supplying the inferior pole. *(Bottom)* Midline transverse grayscale ultrasound shows the thyroid isthmus connecting the 2 lobes. The isthmus lies on the anterior surface of the trachea. In view of the intimate anatomical relationship between the thyroid gland and the trachea, a local tumor invasion to the trachea from malignant thyroid carcinoma is commonly seen, rendering surgical excision more extensive than total thyroidectomy.

THYROID GLAND

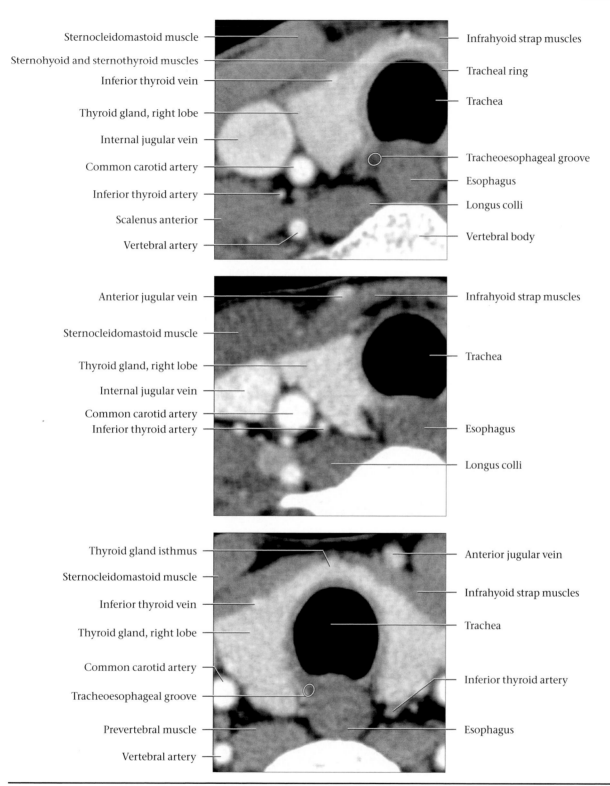

Top left labels:
Sternocleidomastoid muscle
Sternohyoid and sternothyroid muscles
Inferior thyroid vein
Thyroid gland, right lobe
Internal jugular vein
Common carotid artery
Inferior thyroid artery
Scalenus anterior
Vertebral artery

Top right labels:
Infrahyoid strap muscles
Tracheal ring
Trachea
Tracheoesophageal groove
Esophagus
Longus colli
Vertebral body

Middle left labels:
Anterior jugular vein
Sternocleidomastoid muscle
Thyroid gland, right lobe
Internal jugular vein
Common carotid artery
Inferior thyroid artery

Middle right labels:
Infrahyoid strap muscles
Trachea
Esophagus
Longus colli

Bottom left labels:
Thyroid gland isthmus
Sternocleidomastoid muscle
Inferior thyroid vein
Thyroid gland, right lobe
Common carotid artery
Tracheoesophageal groove
Prevertebral muscle
Vertebral artery

Bottom right labels:
Anterior jugular vein
Infrahyoid strap muscles
Trachea
Inferior thyroid artery
Esophagus

(Top) Correlative CECT image shows the right thyroid gland. The thyroid gland is seen as a triangular, homogeneously enhancing structure embracing the anterior aspect of the cervical trachea. The inferior thyroid artery seen on this CT is the main trunk, while that seen on the ultrasound image is a branch. *(Middle)* Axial CECT shows the lower pole of the thyroid gland. *(Bottom)* Axial CECT shows the neck at midline, indicating the tracheoesophageal groove. Remember that the recurrent laryngeal nerve, paratracheal nodes, and parathyroid glands may be seen on ultrasound in this location but they normally cannot be well demonstrated on routine CT images. Always evaluate extensions of the tumor into the trachea, tracheoesophageal groove, nodes, strap muscles, common carotid artery, and internal jugular vein.

THYROID GLAND

LONGITUDINAL ULTRASOUND

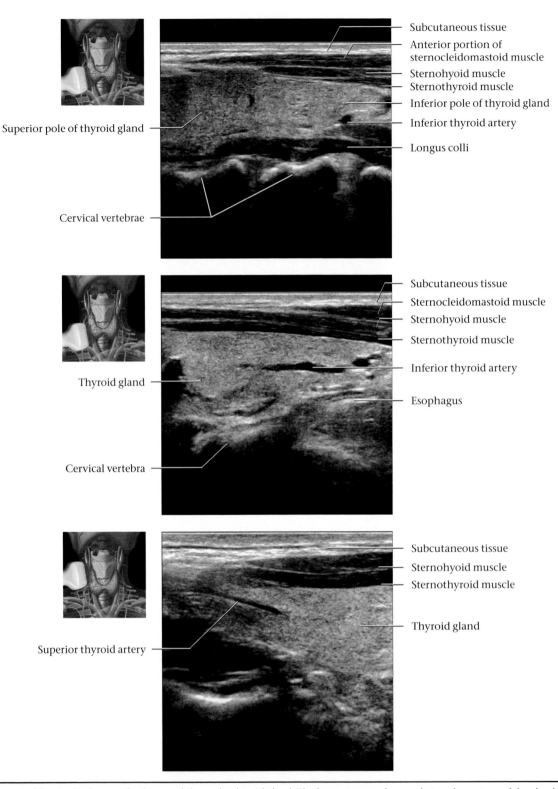

Subcutaneous tissue

Anterior portion of sternocleidomastoid muscle

Sternohyoid muscle

Sternothyroid muscle

Inferior pole of thyroid gland

Inferior thyroid artery

Longus colli

Superior pole of thyroid gland

Cervical vertebrae

Subcutaneous tissue

Sternocleidomastoid muscle

Sternohyoid muscle

Sternothyroid muscle

Inferior thyroid artery

Esophagus

Thyroid gland

Cervical vertebra

Subcutaneous tissue

Sternohyoid muscle

Sternothyroid muscle

Thyroid gland

Superior thyroid artery

*(Top) Parasagittal longitudinal grayscale ultrasound shows the thyroid gland. The homogeneous, hyperechoic echo pattern of the glandular parenchyma is better assessed on longitudinal scans. Part of the tortuous course of the inferior thyroid artery is constantly seen in relation to the lower pole. (**Middle**) Parasagittal longitudinal grayscale ultrasound shows the inferior thyroid artery coursing superiorly from the inferior pole within the glandular parenchyma. (**Bottom**) Parasagittal longitudinal grayscale ultrasound shows the superior thyroid artery, the 1st anterior branch of the external carotid artery, running inferiorly within and supplying the upper pole of the thyroid gland. Longitudinal scans best evaluate the glandular parenchyma and vascularity.*

THYROID GLAND

CORONAL REFORMATTED CECT AND VARIANT

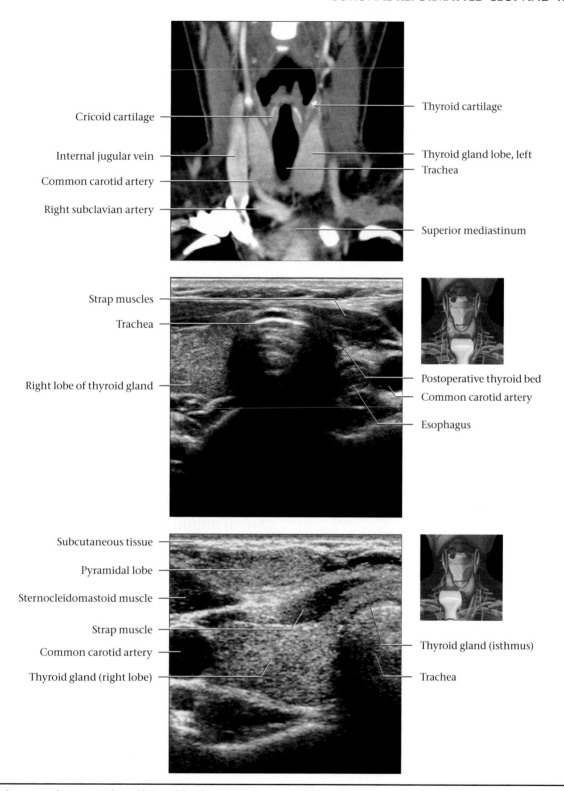

Cricoid cartilage

Internal jugular vein

Common carotid artery

Right subclavian artery

Thyroid cartilage

Thyroid gland lobe, left

Trachea

Superior mediastinum

Strap muscles

Trachea

Right lobe of thyroid gland

Postoperative thyroid bed

Common carotid artery

Esophagus

Subcutaneous tissue

Pyramidal lobe

Sternocleidomastoid muscle

Strap muscle

Common carotid artery

Thyroid gland (right lobe)

Thyroid gland (isthmus)

Trachea

(Top) In this image, the H- or U-shaped lobes of the thyroid gland are particularly well seen. Note the intimate relationship between the superomedial thyroid gland and the larynx. Remember that for thyroid malignancies the 1st-order nodes are the paratracheal nodes, which drain inferiorly into the superior mediastinum. (Middle) Transverse grayscale ultrasound in a patient with a previous history of a left thyroidectomy shows that the left thyroid bed is devoid of thyroid tissue and is occupied by the cervical portion of the esophagus and connective tissue. (Bottom) Transverse grayscale ultrasound shows the pyramidal lobe of the thyroid gland. The echo pattern is identical to the normal right thyroid lobe (i.e., homogeneous, hyperechoic) and is located anterior to the anterior strap muscle and connected to the isthmus.

PARATHYROID GLAND

TERMINOLOGY

Abbreviations
- Parathyroid gland (PTG)

Definitions
- Posterior visceral space (VS) endocrine glands that control calcium metabolism by producing parathormone

IMAGING ANATOMY

Anatomy Relationships
- PTG closely applied to posterior surface of thyroid lobes within visceral space
- Extracapsular (outside thyroid capsule) in most cases
- In vicinity of tracheoesophageal groove

Internal Contents
- Small lentiform glands posterior to thyroid glands in visceral space
- Normal measurements
  - ~ 6 mm in length, 3-4 mm transverse, and 1-2 mm in anteroposterior diameter
- In general, normal glands are not clearly visualized on US/CT/MR
  - Normal PTG may be seen by use of modern US machine and high-frequency transducer
  - Appear as small, well-circumscribed, hypoechoic nodules posterior to thyroid gland separated from echogenic thyroid capsule
- Normal number = 4
  - 2 superior and 2 inferior PTGs
  - May be as many as 12 total PTGs
- Normal positions of superior PTGs
  - Superior PTGs are more constant in position as compared with lower PTGs
  - Lie on posterior border of middle 1/3 of thyroid 75% of time
  - 25% found behind upper or lower 1/3 of thyroid
  - 7% found below inferior thyroidal artery
  - Rarely found behind pharynx or esophagus
- Normal positions of inferior PTGs
  - More variable in location
  - 50% of the inferior glands lie lateral to lower pole of thyroid gland
  - 15% lie within 1 cm of inferior thyroid poles
  - 35% position is variable residing anywhere from angle of mandible to lower anterior mediastinum
  - Intrathyroidal PTG are rare
- Arterial supply of PTGs
  - Superior PTG supplied by superior thyroid artery
  - Inferior PTG supplied by inferior thyroid artery

ANATOMY IMAGING ISSUES

Imaging Approaches
- Imaging for preoperative localization of parathyroid adenoma (PTA)
  - Ultrasonography
    - Best 1st examination for localizing most PTA
    - Use high-resolution linear array transducer (7.5-10 MHz)
    - Identifies 95% of PTA weighing > 1 gram

    - Easier to start scanning in transverse plane with patient's neck hyperextended
    - Start above thyroid at angle of mandible and move downward, scanning through thyroid to level of clavicle
    - Angulate transducer at clavicle to see any obvious lesion in mediastinum
    - On color flow imaging most PTAs demonstrate hypervascularity, mainly intraparenchymal and arterial, maybe blunt ending
    - Color flow imaging best done in longitudinal plane
  - Nuclear scintigraphy
    - Tc-99m sestamibi concentrates in PTA
    - Useful for detection of ectopic PTA (most common site below inferior thyroid pole)
  - Cross-sectional imaging (CT or MR)
    - Used for anatomic localization of ectopic PTA discovered with radionuclide exam

Imaging Pitfalls
- Parathyroid lesion may be confused with normal anatomical structures such as
  - Longus colli muscle, esophagus, blood vessels
  - Paratracheal lymph nodes (fine-needle aspiration [FNA] and internal vascularity help to identify)
  - Thyroid nodules in subcapsular location
- Detection of parathyroid lesion is limited in
  - Obese patients with short neck
  - Ectopic PTG (e.g., in mediastinum)
  - Postoperative neck, recurrent or persistent ↑ PTH

Consider
- Main indication for imaging of PTGs is localization of parathyroid adenoma causing hyperparathyroidism with hypercalcemia

CLINICAL IMPLICATIONS

Clinical Importance
- PTA is most common cause of primary hyperparathyroidism
- US localization facilitates minimally invasive parathyroidectomy
- US safely guides percutaneous injection of absolute alcohol in PTA

EMBRYOLOGY

Embryologic Events
- Superior PTGs develop from 4th branchial pouch along with primordium of thyroid gland
- Inferior PTGs develop from 3rd branchial pouch along with anlage of thymus
  - Descend variable distance with thymic anlage in thymopharyngeal duct tract
  - May descend into anterior mediastinum as far as pericardium

Practical Implications
- Abnormal PTG descent may cause inferior PTG to occupy "ectopic" sites
  - May be of critical importance when searching for parathyroid adenoma
    - In cases where surgical exploration for PTA is done without imaging, no PTA may be found if PTG is ectopic

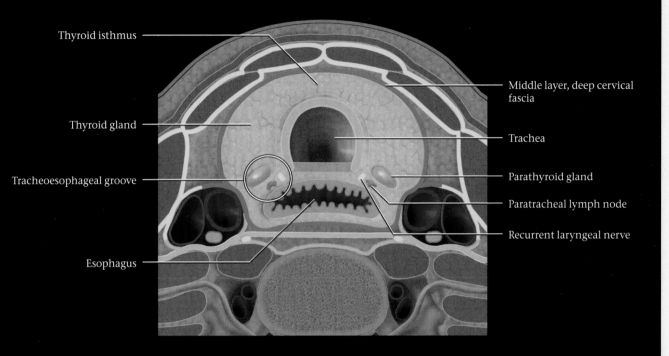

Thyroid isthmus

Middle layer, deep cervical fascia

Thyroid gland

Trachea

Tracheoesophageal groove

Parathyroid gland

Paratracheal lymph node

Recurrent laryngeal nerve

Esophagus

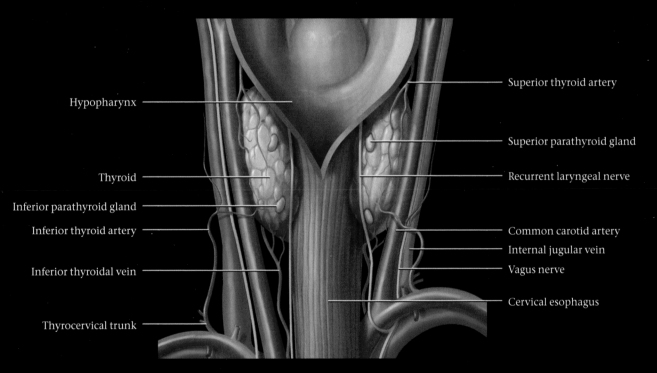

Hypopharynx

Superior thyroid artery

Superior parathyroid gland

Thyroid

Recurrent laryngeal nerve

Inferior parathyroid gland

Inferior thyroid artery

Common carotid artery

Internal jugular vein

Inferior thyroidal vein

Vagus nerve

Cervical esophagus

Thyrocervical trunk

(Top) Axial graphic at thyroid level depicts the superior parathyroid glands in the visceral space just posterior to the thyroid gland. Note that there are 3 key structures found in the area of the tracheoesophageal groove: The recurrent laryngeal nerve, the paratracheal lymph node chain, and the parathyroid gland. *(Bottom)* Coronal graphic illustrates the esophagus, parathyroid glands, and thyroid gland from behind. The drawing depicts the typical anatomic relationships of the paired superior and inferior parathyroid glands in the visceral space. Note the arterial supply to superior and inferior parathyroid glands from the superior and inferior thyroid arteries, respectively.

PARATHYROID GLAND

TRANSVERSE ULTRASOUND

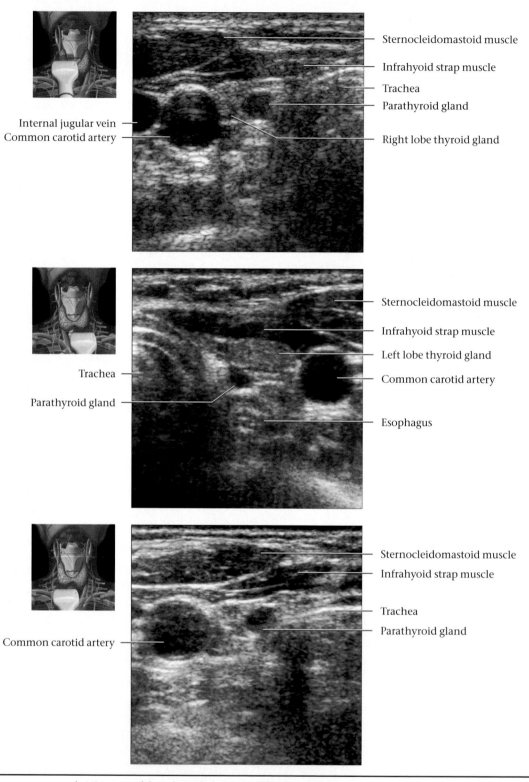

Sternocleidomastoid muscle

Infrahyoid strap muscle

Trachea

Parathyroid gland

Internal jugular vein

Common carotid artery

Right lobe thyroid gland

Sternocleidomastoid muscle

Infrahyoid strap muscle

Left lobe thyroid gland

Common carotid artery

Trachea

Parathyroid gland

Esophagus

Sternocleidomastoid muscle

Infrahyoid strap muscle

Trachea

Parathyroid gland

Common carotid artery

(Top) First of 3 transverse grayscale US images of the right neck shows a well-circumscribed, hypoechoic, right superior parathyroid gland medial to the common carotid artery and posterior to the superior right thyroid lobe. *(Middle)* US of the left neck at the level of the thyroid gland shows the left inferior parathyroid gland as a hypoechoic, ovoid lesion closely applied to the posterior left thyroid lobe. The esophagus is barely visible posterior to the parathyroid gland. *(Bottom)* US of the right neck demonstrates a right inferior parathyroid gland medial to the common carotid artery, lateral to the cervical trachea, and inferior to the right thyroid lobe. Note that it is not always possible to see normal parathyroid glands even with high-resolution ultrasound. Doppler will help in distinguishing it from paratracheal node.

PARATHYROID GLAND

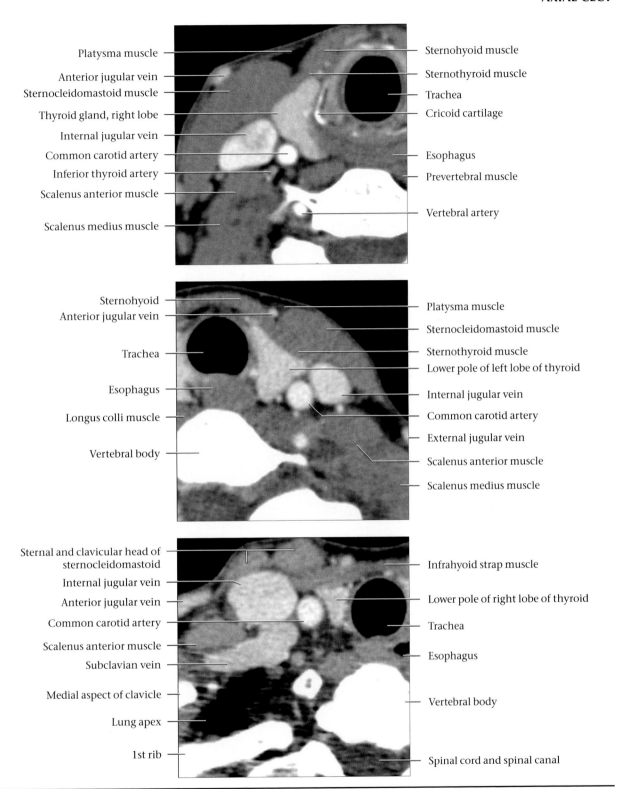

Platysma muscle — Sternohyoid muscle
Anterior jugular vein — Sternothyroid muscle
Sternocleidomastoid muscle — Trachea
Thyroid gland, right lobe — Cricoid cartilage
Internal jugular vein
Common carotid artery — Esophagus
Inferior thyroid artery — Prevertebral muscle
Scalenus anterior muscle
Scalenus medius muscle — Vertebral artery

Sternohyoid — Platysma muscle
Anterior jugular vein — Sternocleidomastoid muscle
Trachea — Sternothyroid muscle
— Lower pole of left lobe of thyroid
Esophagus — Internal jugular vein
Longus colli muscle — Common carotid artery
— External jugular vein
Vertebral body — Scalenus anterior muscle
— Scalenus medius muscle

Sternal and clavicular head of sternocleidomastoid — Infrahyoid strap muscle
Internal jugular vein
Anterior jugular vein — Lower pole of right lobe of thyroid
Common carotid artery — Trachea
Scalenus anterior muscle
Subclavian vein — Esophagus
Medial aspect of clavicle — Vertebral body
Lung apex
1st rib — Spinal cord and spinal canal

(Top) Axial CECT of the neck shows the level of the upper pole of the thyroid gland. A normal parathyroid gland is normally not seen. The anatomical location is commonly at the tracheoesophageal groove posterior to the thyroid gland. *(Middle)* Axial CECT of the neck shows the region of the lower pole of the thyroid's left lobe. *(Bottom)* Axial CECT shows the lower cervical level at the region of the lower pole of the right lobe of the thyroid gland. Note the normal parathyroid gland is not seen. Both CT and MR are used for anatomic localization of ectopic PTA discovered with radionuclide scan.

PARATHYROID GLAND

PATHOLOGY

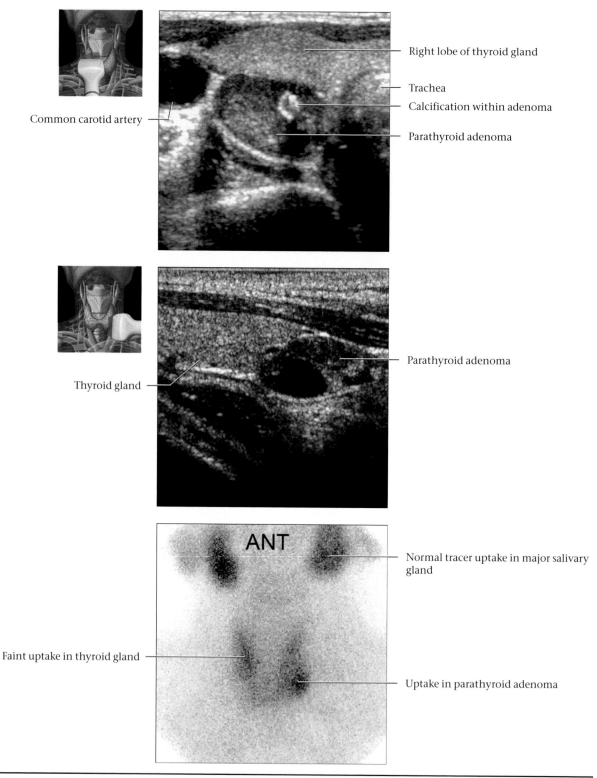

Right lobe of thyroid gland

Common carotid artery

Trachea

Calcification within adenoma

Parathyroid adenoma

Thyroid gland

Parathyroid adenoma

ANT

Normal tracer uptake in major salivary gland

Faint uptake in thyroid gland

Uptake in parathyroid adenoma

(Top) Transverse grayscale ultrasound shows a well-circumscribed, solid, round, hypoechoic PTA posterior to the upper pole of the right thyroid lobe. This patient had biochemical evidence of primary hyperparathyroidism. Note that the presence of calcification within adenoma is uncommon; it is more commonly seen with carcinoma. *(Middle)* Longitudinal grayscale ultrasound shows a well-circumscribed PTA inferoposterior to the lower pole of left lobe of the thyroid gland. The echotexture of the adenoma is heterogeneous. *(Bottom)* Planar sestamibi scintigraphy shows a solitary focus of increased tracer uptake superimposed on the lower pole of the left thyroid gland. The scintigraphic features are suggestive of solitary hyperfunctioning parathyroid adenoma.

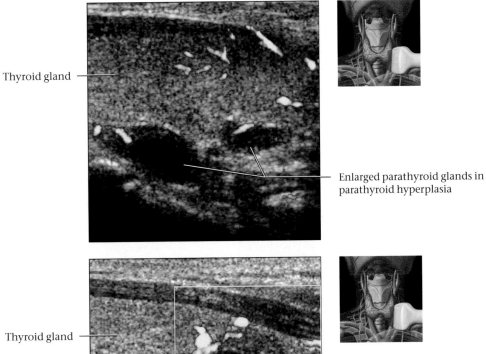

Thyroid gland

Enlarged parathyroid glands in parathyroid hyperplasia

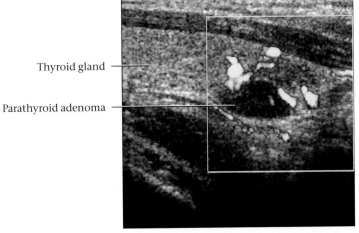

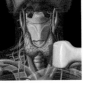

Thyroid gland

Parathyroid adenoma

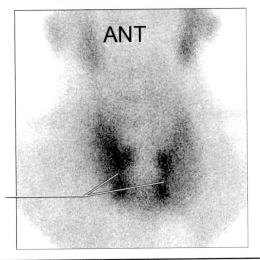

ANT

Multifocal/diffuse tracer uptake in parathyroid hyperplasia

(Top) *Power Doppler ultrasound at the level of the lower pole of the thyroid gland shows 2 enlarged, hypoechoic parathyroid glands with increased vascularity located posterior to the lower pole of thyroid gland. Multiplicity usually indicates parathyroid hyperplasia rather than double adenoma.* **(Middle)** *Longitudinal power Doppler ultrasound shows a parathyroid adenoma. Note the adenoma is slightly hypervascular in 90% of cases. Vascularity is best examined on longitudinal scans.* **(Bottom)** *Planar sestamibi scintigraphy reveals multifocal/diffuse tracer uptake superimposed on both sides of the thyroid gland. The scintigraphic features are compatible with parathyroid hyperplasia.*

LARYNX AND HYPOPHARYNX

TERMINOLOGY

Definitions
- Larynx: Cartilaginous skeleton bounded by ligaments and muscles at junction of upper and lower airway
- Hypopharynx: Caudal continuation of pharyngeal mucosal space, located between oropharynx and esophagus

IMAGING ANATOMY

Extent
- Larynx: Cranial margin at level of glossoepiglottic and pharyngoepiglottic folds with caudal margin defined by lower edge of cricoid
  - Superior connection: Oropharynx
  - Inferior connection: Trachea
- Hypopharynx: Extends from level of glossoepiglottic and pharyngoepiglottic folds superiorly to inferior border of cricoid cartilage (cricopharyngeus muscle)
  - Superior connection: Oropharynx
  - Inferior connection: Cervical esophagus

Internal Contents
- Laryngeal cartilages
  - Thyroid cartilage: Largest laryngeal cartilage
    - "Shields" larynx
    - 2 anterior laminae meet anteriorly at acute angle
    - Superior thyroid notch at anterosuperior aspect
    - Superior cornua are elongated and narrow, and they attach to thyrohyoid ligament
    - Inferior cornua are short and thick, articulating medially with sides of cricoid cartilage
  - Cricoid cartilage: Only complete ring in endolarynx
    - Provides structural integrity
    - 2 portions: Posterior lamina and anterior arch
    - Lower border of cricoid cartilage is junction between larynx above and trachea below
  - Arytenoid cartilage: Paired pyramidal cartilages that sit on the top posterior aspect of cricoid cartilage
    - Vocal and muscular processes are at level of true vocal cord (TVC)
    - Vocal processes: Anterior projections of arytenoids where posterior margins of TVC attach
  - Corniculate cartilage: Rests on top of superior process of arytenoid cartilage, within aryepiglottic (AE) fold
- Supraglottic larynx
  - Extends from tip of epiglottis above to laryngeal ventricle below
  - Contains vestibule, epiglottis, preepiglottic fat, AE folds, false vocal cord (FVC), paraglottic space, and arytenoid cartilages
  - Epiglottis: Leaf-shaped cartilage, larynx lid with free margin (suprahyoid), fixed portion (infrahyoid)
    - Petiole is "stem" of leaf that attaches epiglottis to thyroid lamina via thyroepiglottic ligament
    - Hyoepiglottic ligament attaches epiglottis to hyoid
    - Glossoepiglottic fold is midline mucous membrane covering hyoepiglottic ligament
  - Preepiglottic space: Fat-filled space between hyoid bone anteriorly and epiglottis posteriorly
  - AE folds: Projects from cephalad tip of arytenoid cartilages to inferolateral margin of epiglottis
    - Represents superolateral margin of supraglottis, dividing it from pyriform sinus (hypopharynx)
    - FVC: Mucosal surfaces of laryngeal vestibule of supraglottis
    - Paraglottic spaces: Paired fatty regions beneath FVC and TVC
      - Superiorly they merge into preepiglottic space, which terminates inferiorly at under surface of TVC
- Glottic larynx
  - TVC and anterior and posterior commissures
    - Composed of thyroarytenoid muscle (medial fibers are "vocalis muscle") covered by mucosa
    - Anterior commissure: Midline, anterior meeting point of TVC
- Subglottic larynx
  - Subglottis extends from under surface of TVC to inferior surface of cricoid cartilage
  - Mucosal surface of subglottic area is closely applied to cricoid cartilage
- Hypopharynx: Consists of 3 regions
  - Piriform sinus: Anterolateral recess of hypopharynx
    - Between inner surface of thyrohyoid membrane (above), thyroid cartilage (below), and AE folds (laterally)
    - Pyriform sinus apex (inferior tip) at level of TVC
    - Anteromedial margin of pyriform sinus is posterolateral wall of AE fold (marginal supraglottis)
  - Posterior hypopharyngeal wall: Inferior continuation of posterior oropharynx wall
  - Post cricoid region: Anterior wall of lower hypopharynx
    - Interface between hypopharynx and larynx
    - Extends from cricoarytenoid joints to lower edge of cricoid cartilage

ANATOMY IMAGING ISSUES

Imaging Recommendations
- Role of ultrasound (US) in laryngeal cancer is limited, particularly in era of MDCT and MR
- US may serve a supplementary role to clinical examination and CT/MR in assessing superficial extent of laryngeal tumor
- US combined with fine-needle aspiration cytology is useful for nodal staging of laryngeal tumor
- Although role of US in imaging of larynx is very limited, sonologist doing neck US should be familiar with its anatomy in order not to mistake its appearances for abnormalities

Imaging Sweet Spots
- Real-time US is well-suited to quickly evaluate vocal cord mobility in children presenting with hoarseness and stridor
- US also guides safe percutaneous vocal cord injection for patients with cord palsy, provided the degree of cartilaginous calcification does not obscure US visualization of vocal cord

Imaging Pitfalls
- Presence of motion and calcification/ossification within laryngeal cartilage (common in adult) restricts detailed sonographic assessment of internal laryngeal structures

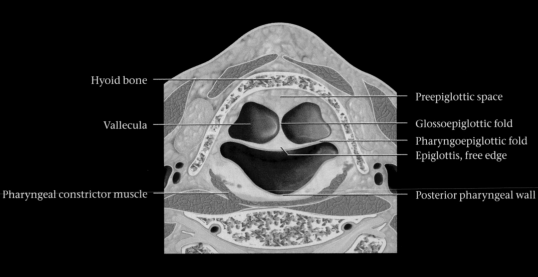

Hyoid bone — Preepiglottic space

Vallecula — Glossoepiglottic fold

Pharyngoepiglottic fold

Epiglottis, free edge

Pharyngeal constrictor muscle — Posterior pharyngeal wall

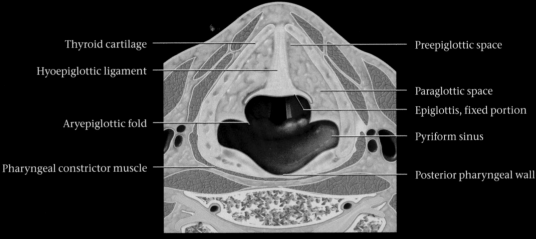

Thyroid cartilage — Preepiglottic space

Hyoepiglottic ligament

Paraglottic space

Epiglottis, fixed portion

Aryepiglottic fold — Pyriform sinus

Pharyngeal constrictor muscle — Posterior pharyngeal wall

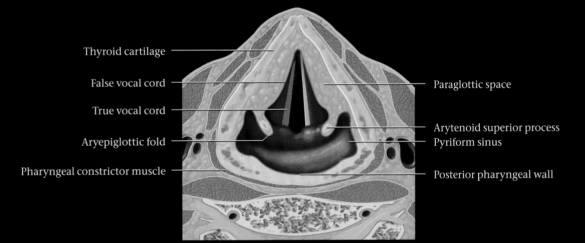

Thyroid cartilage

False vocal cord — Paraglottic space

True vocal cord

Aryepiglottic fold — Arytenoid superior process

Pyriform sinus

Pharyngeal constrictor muscle — Posterior pharyngeal wall

(Top) Axial graphic of the larynx and hypopharynx shows the roof of hypopharynx at the hyoid bone level and the high supraglottic structures. The free edge of the epiglottis is attached to the hyoid bone via the hyoepiglottic ligament, which is covered by the glossoepiglottic fold. (Middle) Graphic at the mid-supraglottic level shows the hyoepiglottic ligament dividing the lower preepiglottic space. No fascia separates the preepiglottic space from the paraglottic space. These 2 endolaryngeal spaces are submucosal in locations where tumors can hide from clinical detection. The aryepiglottic fold represents the junction between the larynx and hypopharynx. (Bottom) Graphic at the low supraglottic level shows false vocal cords formed by mucosal surfaces of laryngeal vestibule. The paraglottic space is beneath the false vocal cords, a common location for submucosal tumor spread.

LARYNX AND HYPOPHARYNX

GRAPHICS

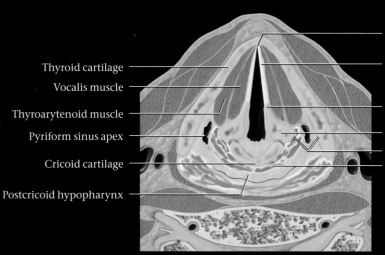

Anterior commissure

Thyroid cartilage

Vocal ligament

Vocalis muscle

Thyroarytenoid muscle

Vocal process, arytenoid cartilage

Pyriform sinus apex

Arytenoid cartilage

Cricoid cartilage

Thyroarytenoid gap

Posterior cricoarytenoid muscle

Postcricoid hypopharynx

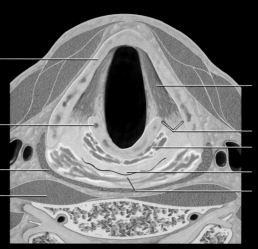

Thyroid cartilage

Undersurface of true vocal cord

Cricoid cartilage

Cricothyroid space

Posterior cricoarytenoid muscle

Pharyngeal constrictor muscle

Postcricoid hypopharynx

Longus capitis muscle

Posterior wall, hypopharynx

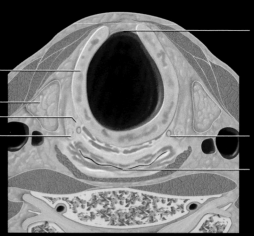

Cricothyroid membrane

Cricoid cartilage

Thyroid gland

Cricothyroid joint

Inferior cornu, thyroid cartilage

Recurrent laryngeal nerve

Cervical esophagus

(Top) Graphic at the glottic, true vocal cord level shows the thyroarytenoid muscle, which makes up the bulk of the true vocal cord. The medial fibers of the thyroarytenoid muscle are known as the vocalis muscle. Pyriform sinus apex is seen at the glottic level. *(Middle)* Graphic at the level of the undersurface of the true vocal cord shows the posterior lamina of the cricoid cartilage. Postcricoid hypopharynx represents the anterior wall of the lower hypopharynx and extends from the cricoarytenoid joints to the lower edge of the cricoid cartilage at the cricopharyngeus muscle. The posterior wall of the hypopharynx represents the inferior continuation of the posterior oropharyngeal wall and extends to the cervical esophagus. *(Bottom)* Graphic at the subglottic level shows the cricothyroid joint immediately adjacent to the recurrent laryngeal nerve, which is located in the tracheoesophageal groove.

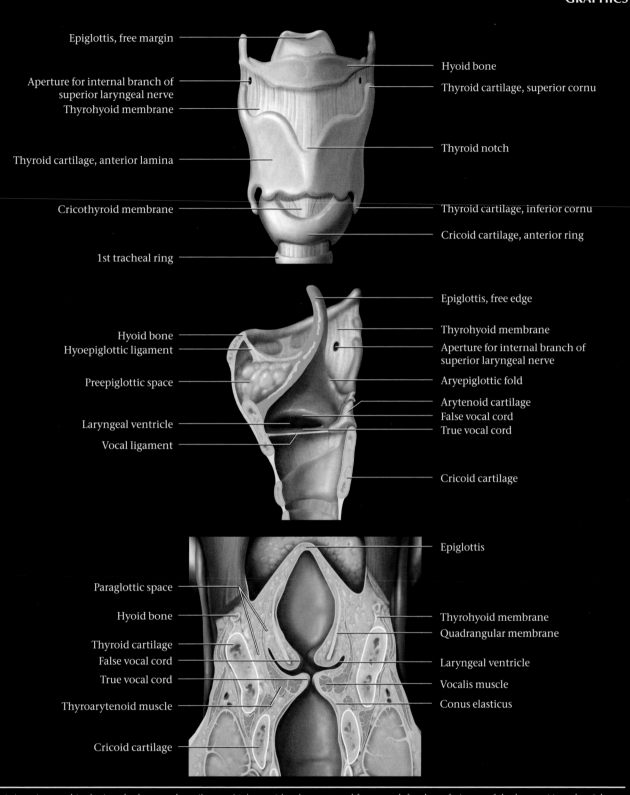

Epiglottis, free margin

Aperture for internal branch of superior laryngeal nerve

Thyrohyoid membrane

Thyroid cartilage, anterior lamina

Cricothyroid membrane

1st tracheal ring

Hyoid bone

Thyroid cartilage, superior cornu

Thyroid notch

Thyroid cartilage, inferior cornu

Cricoid cartilage, anterior ring

Hyoid bone
Hyoepiglottic ligament

Preepiglottic space

Laryngeal ventricle

Vocal ligament

Epiglottis, free edge

Thyrohyoid membrane

Aperture for internal branch of superior laryngeal nerve

Aryepiglottic fold

Arytenoid cartilage
False vocal cord
True vocal cord

Cricoid cartilage

Paraglottic space

Hyoid bone

Thyroid cartilage
False vocal cord
True vocal cord

Thyroarytenoid muscle

Cricoid cartilage

Epiglottis

Thyrohyoid membrane
Quadrangular membrane

Laryngeal ventricle

Vocalis muscle
Conus elasticus

(Top) Anterior graphic depicts the laryngeal cartilage, which provides the structural framework for the soft tissues of the larynx. Note that 2 large anterior laminae "shield" the larynx. The thyrohyoid membrane contains an aperture through which the internal branch of the superior laryngeal nerve and associated vessels course. **(Middle)** Sagittal graphic of the midline larynx shows the laryngeal ventricle air space, which separates false vocal cords above from true vocal cords below. **(Bottom)** Coronal graphic (posterior view) shows the false and true vocal cords separated by the laryngeal ventricle. The quadrangular membrane is a fibrous membrane that extends from the upper arytenoid and corniculate cartilages to the lateral epiglottis. The conus elasticus is a fibroelastic membrane that extends from the vocal ligament of the true vocal cord to the cricoid.

LARYNX AND HYPOPHARYNX

TRANSVERSE ULTRASOUND

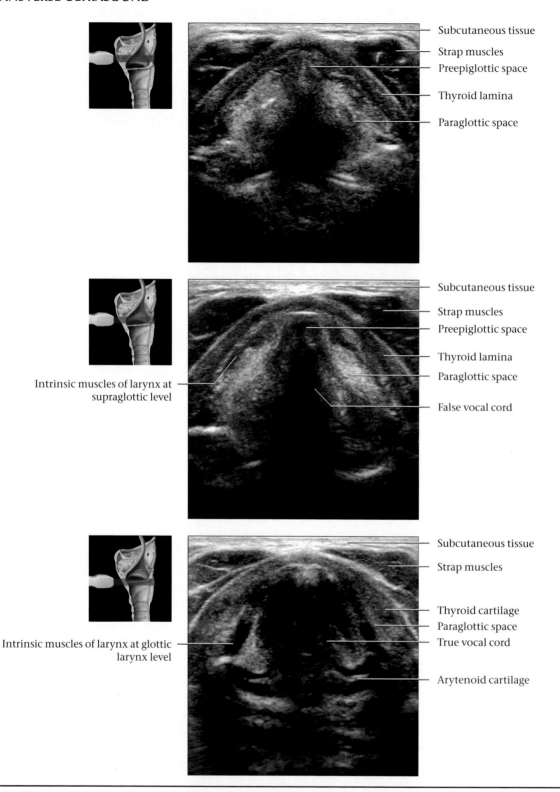

Subcutaneous tissue
Strap muscles
Preepiglottic space
Thyroid lamina
Paraglottic space

Intrinsic muscles of larynx at supraglottic level

Subcutaneous tissue
Strap muscles
Preepiglottic space
Thyroid lamina
Paraglottic space
False vocal cord

Intrinsic muscles of larynx at glottic larynx level

Subcutaneous tissue
Strap muscles

Thyroid cartilage
Paraglottic space
True vocal cord

Arytenoid cartilage

(Top) Axial grayscale ultrasound image of the larynx at the supraglottic larynx level shows that the thyroid laminae are the largest cartilaginous structure of the larynx and appear as thin, hypoechoic bands that join at the midline anteriorly. The hyperechoic, fat-filled paraglottic and preepiglottic spaces are important surgical landmarks for the staging of laryngeal carcinoma. *(Middle)* Transverse grayscale ultrasound of the larynx at the level of the false vocal cords shows abundant fat in the paraglottic spaces. The echo-poor intrinsic muscles of the larynx are embedded within the echogenic paraglottic fat. *(Bottom)* Transverse grayscale ultrasound of the larynx at the level of the true vocal cords shows that the arytenoid cartilage appears as echogenic foci posteriorly with attachments to the true vocal cords, which have distinct echo-poor appearances.

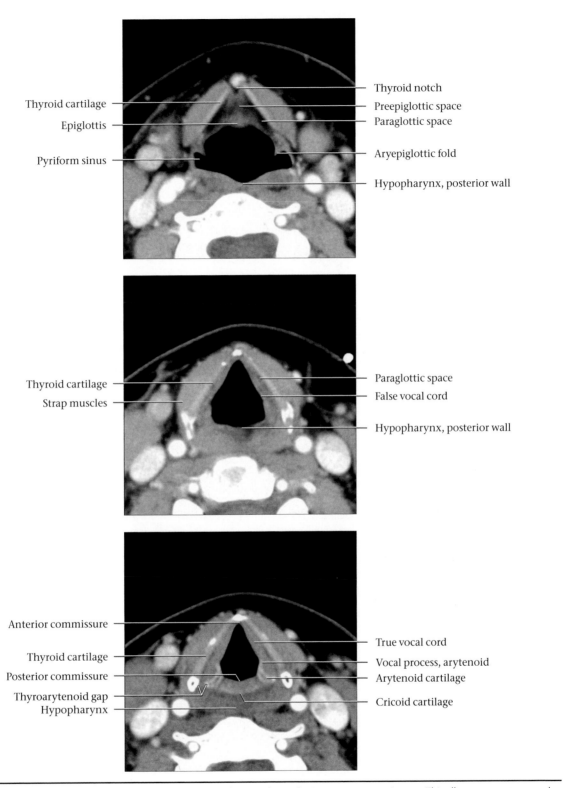

Thyroid cartilage
Epiglottis
Pyriform sinus

Thyroid notch
Preepiglottic space
Paraglottic space
Aryepiglottic fold
Hypopharynx, posterior wall

Thyroid cartilage
Strap muscles

Paraglottic space
False vocal cord
Hypopharynx, posterior wall

Anterior commissure
Thyroid cartilage
Posterior commissure
Thyroarytenoid gap
Hypopharynx

True vocal cord
Vocal process, arytenoid
Arytenoid cartilage
Cricoid cartilage

(Top) Axial CECT of the high supraglottic level shows that the preepiglottic and paraglottic spaces are continuous. This allows tumors to spread submucosally in these locations. The aryepiglottic fold, part of the larynx, represents a transition between the larynx and hypopharynx. *(Middle)* Axial CECT shows the low supraglottic level at the false vocal cord level. The paraglottic space represents the deep fatty space beneath the false vocal cords. Tumors that cross the laryngeal ventricle and involve false and true vocal cords are considered transglottic. *(Bottom)* Axial CECT at the glottic level shows the true vocal cords in abduction during quiet respiration. True vocal cord level is identified on CT when the arytenoid and cricoid cartilages are seen and muscle fills the inferior paraglottic space. The anterior and posterior commissures of the true vocal cords should be < 1 mm in normal patients. The postcricoid hypopharynx is typically collapsed.

LARYNX AND HYPOPHARYNX

LONGITUDINAL ULTRASOUND

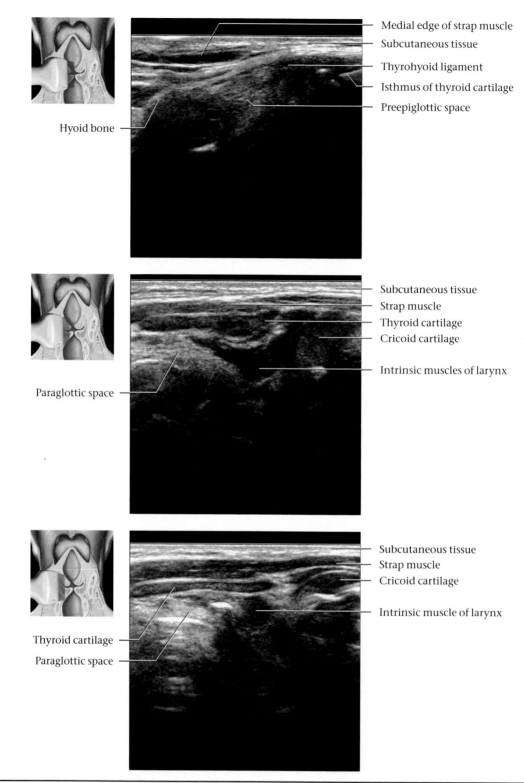

Hyoid bone

Medial edge of strap muscle
Subcutaneous tissue
Thyrohyoid ligament
Isthmus of thyroid cartilage
Preepiglottic space

Paraglottic space

Subcutaneous tissue
Strap muscle
Thyroid cartilage
Cricoid cartilage
Intrinsic muscles of larynx

Thyroid cartilage
Paraglottic space

Subcutaneous tissue
Strap muscle
Cricoid cartilage
Intrinsic muscle of larynx

(Top) Midline sagittal longitudinal grayscale ultrasound of the supraglottic larynx shows the fat-filled, echogenic, preepiglottic space underneath the thyrohyoid membrane. Tumor spread at this location is readily assessed by ultrasound. *(Middle)* Parasagittal longitudinal grayscale ultrasound of the larynx shows sonolucent thyroid and cricoid cartilages with no laryngeal calcification/ossification in a young adult. The paraglottic space is fat filled and appears echogenic. The intrinsic muscles of the larynx are embedded within the paraglottic space and are hypoechoic on ultrasound. *(Bottom)* Parasagittal longitudinal grayscale ultrasound shows the larynx further lateral than the previous image. Gas within the laryngeal lumen appears highly echogenic, casting posterior acoustic shadowing.

SAGITTAL AND CORONAL REFORMATTED NECT

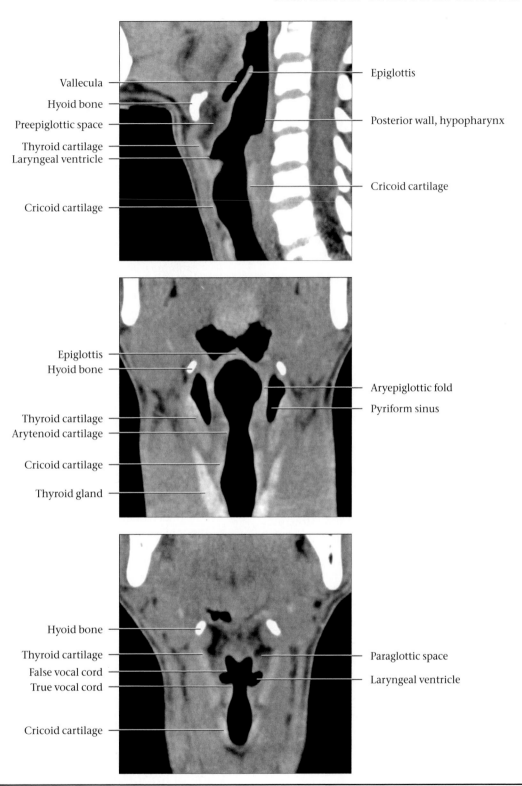

Vallecula — Epiglottis

Hyoid bone

Preepiglottic space — Posterior wall, hypopharynx

Thyroid cartilage
Laryngeal ventricle

Cricoid cartilage

Cricoid cartilage

Epiglottis
Hyoid bone

Thyroid cartilage — Aryepiglottic fold
Arytenoid cartilage — Pyriform sinus

Cricoid cartilage

Thyroid gland

Hyoid bone

Thyroid cartilage — Paraglottic space
False vocal cord — Laryngeal ventricle
True vocal cord

Cricoid cartilage

(Top) Parasagittal reformatted NECT shows the laryngeal ventricle air space that separates the false vocal cords above from the true vocal cords below. *(Middle)* In this coronal reformatted NECT, aryepiglottic folds are well seen as they extend from the lateral epiglottis to the arytenoid cartilage. The pyriform sinus is the most common location for tumors of the hypopharynx. *(Bottom)* In this coronal reformatted NECT, the laryngeal ventricle is visible as an air space between false vocal cords above and true vocal cords below. When a tumor crosses the laryngeal ventricle to involve the true and false cords, it is transglottic, which has important treatment implications. Coronal imaging is particularly useful for evaluation of transglottic disease. Note that ultrasound is unable to demonstrate such detailed anatomy, particularly of deeper structures.

CERVICAL TRACHEA AND ESOPHAGUS

TERMINOLOGY

Definitions
- Cervical trachea: Air-conveying flexible tube made of cartilage and fibromuscular membrane connecting larynx to lungs
- Cervical esophagus: Muscular food- and fluid-conveying tube connecting pharynx to stomach

IMAGING ANATOMY

Overview
- Trachea
  - 10-13 cm tube extending in midline from inferior larynx at ~ 6th cervical vertebral body to carina at upper margin of 5th thoracic vertebral body
- Esophagus
  - 25 cm tube extending in midline from inferior hypopharynx at ~ 6th cervical vertebral body to 11th thoracic vertebral body
  - Descends behind trachea and thyroid, lying in front of lower cervical vertebrae
    - Inclines slightly to the left in lower cervical neck and upper mediastinum, returning to midline at T5 vertebral body level

Anatomy Relationships
- Cervical trachea
  - Anterior: Infrahyoid strap muscles, isthmus of thyroid gland
  - Lateral: Lobes of thyroid gland
    - Tracheoesophageal groove structures: Recurrent laryngeal nerve, paratracheal nodes, parathyroid glands
  - Posterior: Cervical esophagus
- Cervical esophagus
  - Anterior: Cervical trachea
  - Anterolateral: Tracheoesophageal groove structures
  - Lateral: Common carotid artery, internal jugular vein, vagus nerve
  - Posterior: Retropharyngeal fascia/muscle

Internal Contents
- Cervical trachea
  - Tracheal cartilages
    - Each cartilage is imperfect ring of cartilage surrounding anterior 2/3 of trachea
    - Flat deficient posterior portion is completed with fibromuscular membrane
    - Cross-sectional shape of trachea is that of letter D, with flat posterior side
    - Smooth muscle fibers in posterior membrane (trachealis muscle) attach to free ends of tracheal cartilages and provide alteration in tracheal cross-sectional area
    - Hyaline cartilage calcifies with age
    - Minor salivary glands are sporadically distributed in tracheal mucosa
  - Blood supply: Inferior thyroid arteries and veins
  - Lymphatic drainage: Level VI pretracheal and paratracheal nodes
  - USG appearance
    - Hypoechoic tracheal ring composed of hyaline cartilage that is incomplete posteriorly
    - Ring-down artifacts from air in tracheal lumen
    - Midline behind thyroid isthmus
- Cervical esophagus
  - Begins at lower border of cricoid cartilage as continuation of hypopharynx
    - Upper limit is defined by cricopharyngeus muscle, which encircles it from front to back
  - Usually in slightly off-midline position to left in cervical portion
  - Long muscular tube consists of longitudinal and circular smooth muscles
  - Active peristalsis in antegrade (i.e., downward) direction
  - Blood supply: Inferior thyroid arteries and veins
  - Lymphatic drainage: Level VI paratracheal nodes
  - USG appearance
    - Circular configuration with alternating concentric echogenic/hypoechoic rings in transverse scan
    - Long tubular structure with alternating echogenic/hypoechoic layers representing mucosal, submucosal, muscular, and serosal layers on longitudinal scan
    - Presence of air in lumen; moves on swallowing

ANATOMY IMAGING ISSUES

Imaging Recommendations
- US is best done with patient's head slightly hyperextended
- Ask patient not to swallow during US
- Transverse and longitudinal scans are necessary for a comprehensive US examination
- Assess adjacent structures and regional neck nodes

Imaging Approaches
- Multislice CT is best imaging modality to assess local tumor extent of cervical esophageal/tracheal cancer
- Although more sensitive to cartilage invasion, MR may be degraded due to breathing artifacts
- Tumor extent
  - Thyroid cancer: Assessment of tumor invasion of trachea and esophagus; CT & MR are better than US
  - Esophageal cancer: Determine local tumor extent and invasion of adjacent structures (e.g., thyroid gland/trachea); CT is better than US

Imaging Pitfalls
- Tracheal ring calcification and intraluminal air render complete assessment of trachea difficult
- Intraluminal gas may obscure posterior esophageal wall
- Esophagus is a mobile tube and slips side to side in neck depending on direction head is turned
  - On US, esophagus may be on the right when head is turned to the left

CLINICAL IMPLICATIONS

Clinical Importance
- Recurrent laryngeal nerve is located in tracheoesophageal groove
  - Though the nerve itself is not usually visible on US, its expected course should be carefully examined by USG in patients with vocal cord palsy
- Primary tracheal tumors are rare
  - Often invaded/compressed/displaced by extrinsic mass (thyroid > > esophageal origin)

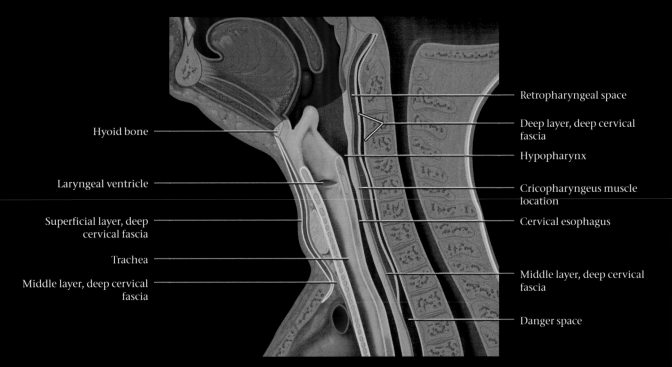

Retropharyngeal space

Deep layer, deep cervical fascia

Hypopharynx

Hyoid bone

Laryngeal ventricle

Cricopharyngeus muscle location

Superficial layer, deep cervical fascia

Cervical esophagus

Trachea

Middle layer, deep cervical fascia

Middle layer, deep cervical fascia

Danger space

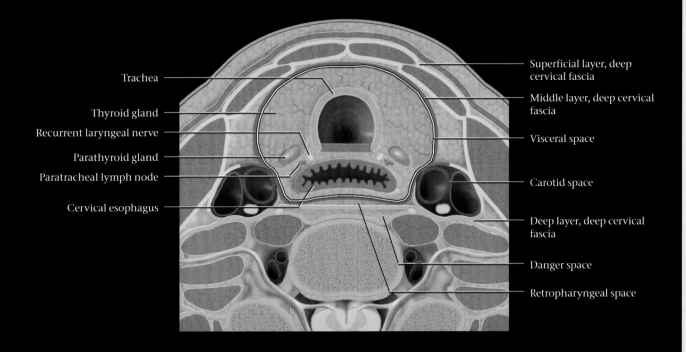

Trachea

Superficial layer, deep cervical fascia

Middle layer, deep cervical fascia

Thyroid gland

Recurrent laryngeal nerve

Visceral space

Parathyroid gland

Paratracheal lymph node

Carotid space

Cervical esophagus

Deep layer, deep cervical fascia

Danger space

Retropharyngeal space

(Top) Sagittal graphic shows the longitudinal relationships of the infrahyoid neck. Note that the middle layer of the deep cervical fascia (pink) encircles the trachea and esophagus as part of the visceral space. The trachea and esophagus are the inferior continuations of the airway and pharynx. *(Bottom)* Axial graphic shows the anteroposterior relationship of the trachea and esophagus in the lower neck. Note the middle layer of the deep cervical fascia surrounding the visceral space. Important components of the tracheoesophageal groove include the recurrent laryngeal nerve, paratracheal nodes, and parathyroid glands.

CERVICAL TRACHEA AND ESOPHAGUS

TRANSVERSE ULTRASOUND

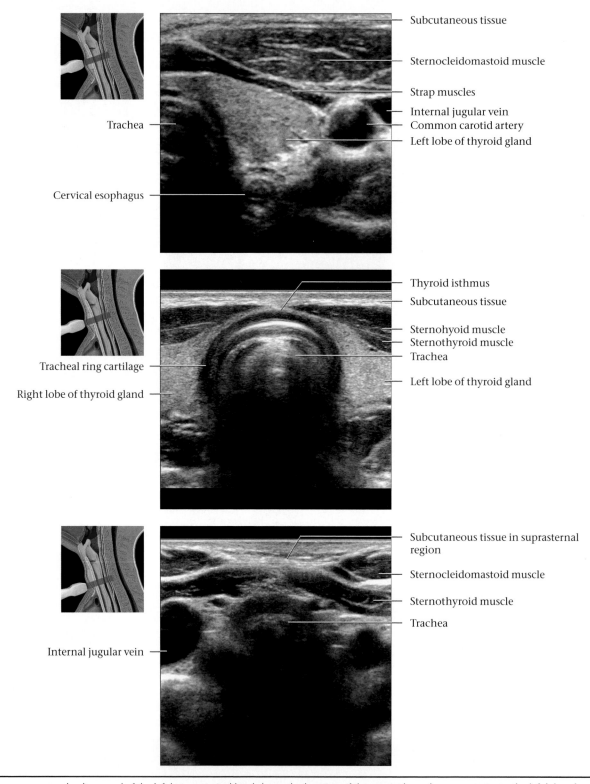

Subcutaneous tissue

Sternocleidomastoid muscle

Strap muscles

Internal jugular vein

Common carotid artery

Left lobe of thyroid gland

Trachea

Cervical esophagus

Thyroid isthmus

Subcutaneous tissue

Sternohyoid muscle

Sternothyroid muscle

Trachea

Left lobe of thyroid gland

Tracheal ring cartilage

Right lobe of thyroid gland

Subcutaneous tissue in suprasternal region

Sternocleidomastoid muscle

Sternothyroid muscle

Trachea

Internal jugular vein

(Top) Transverse grayscale ultrasound of the left lower cervical level shows the location of the cervical esophagus posterior to the left lobe of the thyroid gland and posterolateral to the trachea. The recurrent laryngeal nerve is located in the tracheoesophageal groove. The nerve is not visualized on USG. Note the circular configuration with alternating concentric echogenic/hypoechoic rings of the esophagus in cross section. (Middle) Transverse grayscale ultrasound of the midline anterior neck at the level of thyroid gland shows the trachea as a midline structure underneath the isthmus of the thyroid gland and related laterally to the thyroid lobes. Note the hypoechoic tracheal ring composed of hyaline cartilage that is incomplete posteriorly. (Bottom) Transverse grayscale ultrasound of the suprasternal region shows the lower cervical trachea underneath the insertion sites of the strap muscles.

CERVICAL TRACHEA AND ESOPHAGUS

AXIAL CECT

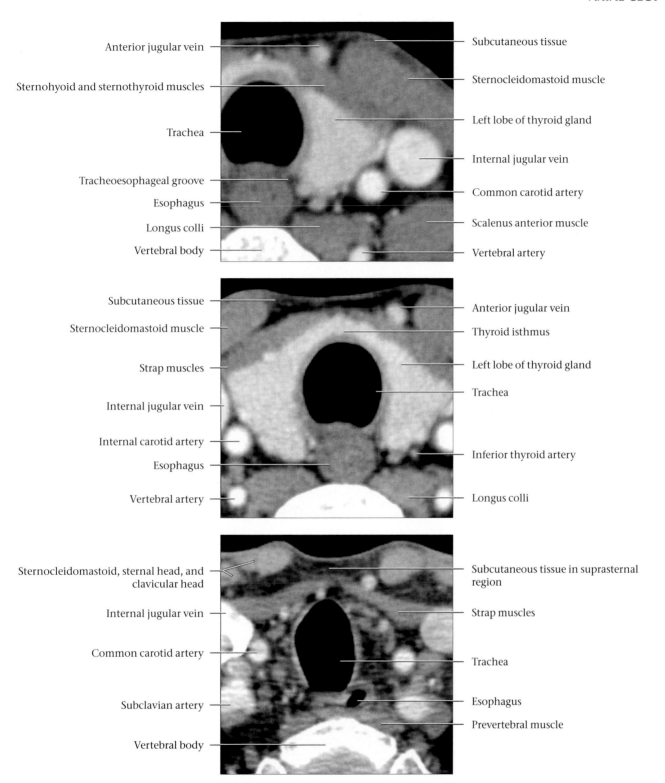

Anterior jugular vein

Sternohyoid and sternothyroid muscles

Trachea

Tracheoesophageal groove

Esophagus

Longus colli

Vertebral body

Subcutaneous tissue

Sternocleidomastoid muscle

Left lobe of thyroid gland

Internal jugular vein

Common carotid artery

Scalenus anterior muscle

Vertebral artery

Subcutaneous tissue

Sternocleidomastoid muscle

Strap muscles

Internal jugular vein

Internal carotid artery

Esophagus

Vertebral artery

Anterior jugular vein

Thyroid isthmus

Left lobe of thyroid gland

Trachea

Inferior thyroid artery

Longus colli

Sternocleidomastoid, sternal head, and clavicular head

Internal jugular vein

Common carotid artery

Subclavian artery

Vertebral body

Subcutaneous tissue in suprasternal region

Strap muscles

Trachea

Esophagus

Prevertebral muscle

(Top) Axial CECT image of the lower cervical level shows the close anatomical relationship of the trachea and the esophagus with adjacent structures, such as the thyroid gland. (Middle) Axial CECT of the lower cervical level shows the trachea surrounded by thyroid lobes and the isthmus and esophagus posterior to the trachea. (Bottom) Axial CECT at the level of the suprasternal region shows that the esophagus at this level is usually slightly off midline to the left in relation to the trachea. The esophagus and trachea are surrounded by mediastinal fat and related to the major vessels in the superior mediastinum. Although ultrasound is able to detect the spread of a thyroid tumor to the trachea and esophagus (and vice versa), CT and MR delineate the involvement much better.

CERVICAL TRACHEA AND ESOPHAGUS

LONGITUDINAL ULTRASOUND AND PATHOLOGY

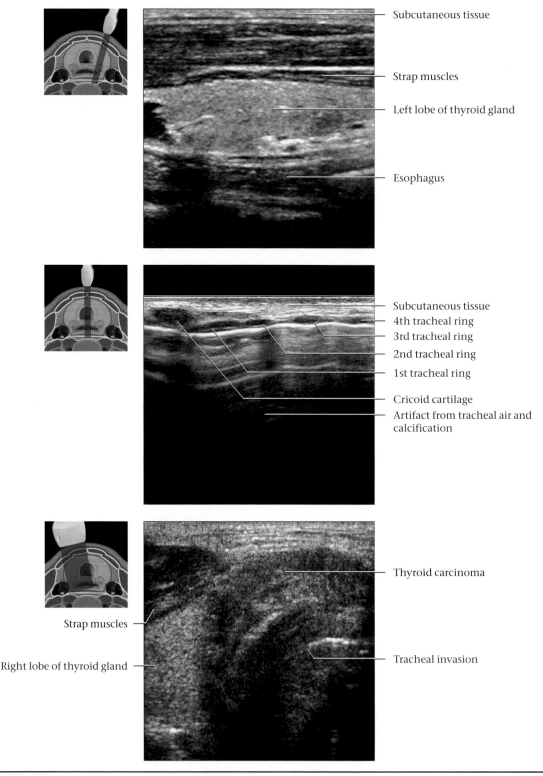

Subcutaneous tissue

Strap muscles

Left lobe of thyroid gland

Esophagus

Subcutaneous tissue
4th tracheal ring
3rd tracheal ring
2nd tracheal ring
1st tracheal ring
Cricoid cartilage
Artifact from tracheal air and calcification

Thyroid carcinoma

Strap muscles

Tracheal invasion

Right lobe of thyroid gland

(Top) Longitudinal grayscale ultrasound of the lower left neck at the thyroid gland level shows the cervical esophagus posterior to the left lobe of the thyroid gland. It is a long tubular structure with alternating echogenic/hypoechoic layers representing the mucosal, submucosal, muscular, and serosal layers. *(Middle)* Longitudinal grayscale ultrasound of the midline anterior neck shows the presence of hypoechoic tracheal rings along the cervical portion of the trachea. Note the hypoechoic, noncalcified, cricoid cartilage above the tracheal rings. *(Bottom)* Transverse grayscale ultrasound in a patient with thyroid carcinoma involving the isthmus and adjacent right lobe with local tumor invasion into trachea shows loss of definition of the hypoechoic tracheal ring, which is replaced by the tumor.

SAGITTAL REFORMATTED CECT AND PATHOLOGY

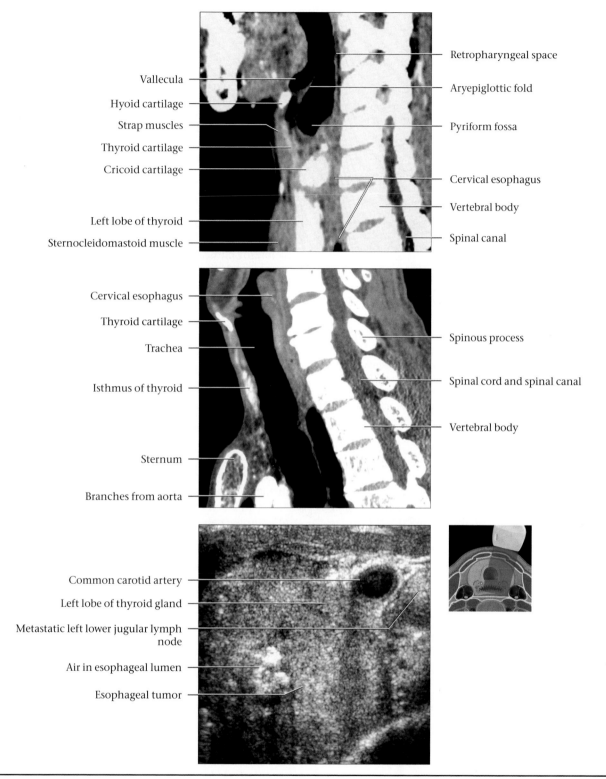

Vallecula

Hyoid cartilage

Strap muscles

Thyroid cartilage

Cricoid cartilage

Left lobe of thyroid

Sternocleidomastoid muscle

Retropharyngeal space

Aryepiglottic fold

Pyriform fossa

Cervical esophagus

Vertebral body

Spinal canal

Cervical esophagus

Thyroid cartilage

Trachea

Isthmus of thyroid

Sternum

Branches from aorta

Spinous process

Spinal cord and spinal canal

Vertebral body

Common carotid artery

Left lobe of thyroid gland

Metastatic left lower jugular lymph node

Air in esophageal lumen

Esophageal tumor

(Top) Oblique sagittal reformatted CECT image of the neck correlates with the image plane on ultrasound. The thyroid lobe is seen superficial to the esophagus. *(Middle)* Sagittal reformatted CECT of the neck in the midline shows the trachea anterior to the cervical esophagus, which is gas filled and inferior to the pharyngeal constrictor. *(Bottom)* Transverse grayscale ultrasound of the left lower cervical level shows a large heterogeneous mass posterior to and invading the lower pole of the left thyroid gland, compatible with known locally extensive esophageal carcinoma. Note the presence of left lower jugular lymph node metastases.

BRACHIAL PLEXUS

GROSS ANATOMY

Overview
- Brachial plexus (BP)
  - Major neural supply to upper limbs
  - Formed from ventral rami of C5-T1 ± minor branches from C4 &/or T2
  - Some proximal branches originate above BP proper
    - Dorsal scapular nerve, long thoracic nerve, nerves to scalene/longus colli muscles, and branch to phrenic nerve
    - Remaining minor and all major peripheral branches arise from BP proper
  - Divided into roots/rami, trunks, divisions, cords, and terminal branches
  - Roots/rami
    - Originate from spinal cord levels C5-T1
    - Enter posterior triangle by emerging between scalenus anterior and scalenus medius muscles
  - Trunks
    - Upper (C5-C6), middle (C7), lower (C8, T1)
    - Lower trunk lies behind 3rd part of subclavian artery
    - Minor nerves arise directly from trunks: Suprascapular nerve, nerve to subclavius muscle
  - Divisions
    - Formed by division of each trunk into anterior and posterior branches in supraclavicular triangle
    - Anterior divisions innervate anterior (flexor) muscles
    - Posterior divisions innervate posterior (extensor) muscles
    - No named minor nerves arise directly from divisions
  - Cords
    - Lateral cord (anterior divisions of superior and middle trunks) innervates anterior (flexor) muscles
    - Medial cord (anterior division of inferior trunk) innervates anterior (flexor) muscles
    - Posterior cord (posterior divisions of all 3 trunks) innervates posterior (extensor) muscles
    - Descend behind clavicle to leave posterior triangle and enter axilla
  - Terminal branches
    - Within axillary content
    - Musculocutaneous nerve (C5-C6) arises from lateral cord
    - Ulnar nerve (C8-T1) arises from medial cord
    - Axillary nerve (C5-C6), radial nerve (C5-T1), thoracodorsal nerve (C6-C8), and upper (C6-C7) and lower (C5-C6) subscapular nerves all arise from posterior cord

Anatomy Relationships
- Close anatomic proximity to subclavian artery and lymphatics
- Subclavian vein courses anterior to scalenus anterior, not in direct proximity to BP
- Nerves of BP enter axilla behind clavicle

IMAGING ANATOMY

Overview
- MR is the best modality for visualization of BP

- Surrounding perineural fat provides excellent visualization of nerves and allows them to be distinguished from adjacent soft tissues
- USG is alternative imaging technique to visualize small component of BP
  - Excellent spatial resolution provided by high-frequency transducer
  - Seen as long, tubular, hypoechoic structures against background of echogenic fat on longitudinal scan
  - Several small ovoid/round hypoechoic nodules in lower posterior triangle between scalenus anterior and scalenus medius muscles on transverse scan
  - Lack of flow distinguishes them from vascular structures

ANATOMY IMAGING ISSUES

Imaging Recommendations
- Knowledge of normal BP anatomy is critical for evaluating clinical abnormalities
- Nerve sheath tumor is one of the differential diagnoses for mass in lower posterior triangle/supraclavicular region
  - Demonstration of mass being contiguous with BP elements provides definitive diagnosis
- Sonographic appearances of nerve sheath tumor may overlap with abnormal lymph node
  - Identification of contiguous nerve obviates need for needle aspiration/biopsy, which may cause arm twitching
- USG is ideal for initial investigation of suspected BP schwannoma in neck
  - Also helps to evaluate BP involvement with metastatic nodes in lower posterior triangle/supraclavicular fossa

Imaging Approaches
- On US it may not be possible to definitively differentiate between rami, trunks, divisions, and cords
  - Therefore, often referred to as BP elements
- Roots/rami emerging from spine are better seen on longitudinal scans
- Roots/rami of BP (C5-T1) emerge into scalene triangle and are readily identified on transverse scans between scalenus anterior and medius
- Longitudinal scans help evaluation along their length
- Color/power Doppler distinguishes them from vessels

Imaging Pitfalls
- Infraclavicular portion of BP cannot be well demonstrated on USG

CLINICAL IMPLICATIONS

Clinical Importance
- Clinical symptoms and neurological signs help to localize lesions along BP
  - Erb-Duchenne palsy: Lesion in upper BP
  - Klumpke palsy: Lesion in lower BP
- BP nerve blocks are ideally done under ultrasound guidance
- Development of pain in BP schwannoma should raise suspicion of malignancy

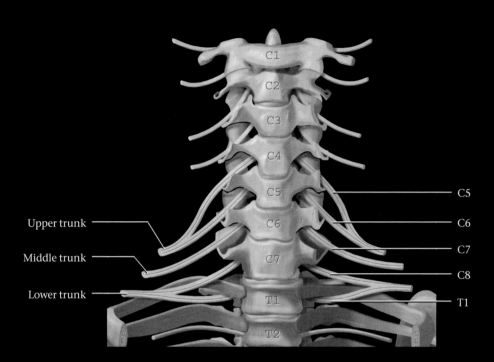

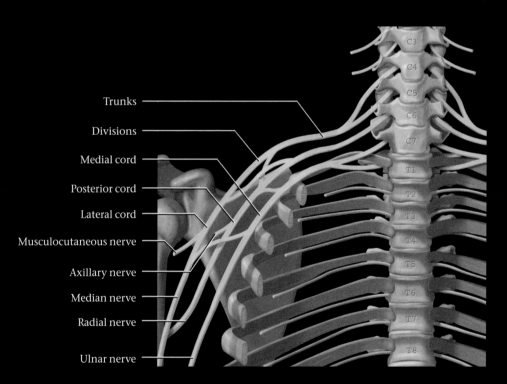

(Top) Coronal graphic of the cervical spine and supraclavicular brachial plexus demonstrates the cervical ventral primary rami combining to form the brachial plexus. The C1-C7 roots exit above the same numbered pedicle, C8 exits above the T1 pedicle, and more caudal roots exit below their corresponding numbered pedicles. The trunks are visualized on ultrasound in the lower posterior triangle and supraclavicular fossa. *(Bottom)* Coronal graphic of the brachial plexus demonstrates the more distal plexus elements extending into the axilla. The trunks recombine into posterior and anterior divisions that form the cords. The posterior cord forms the radial and axillary nerves. The medial cord forms the ulnar nerve, whereas the lateral cord forms the musculocutaneous nerve. The median nerve is formed from branches of both the lateral and the medial cords.

BRACHIAL PLEXUS

TRANSVERSE AND LONGITUDINAL ULTRASOUND

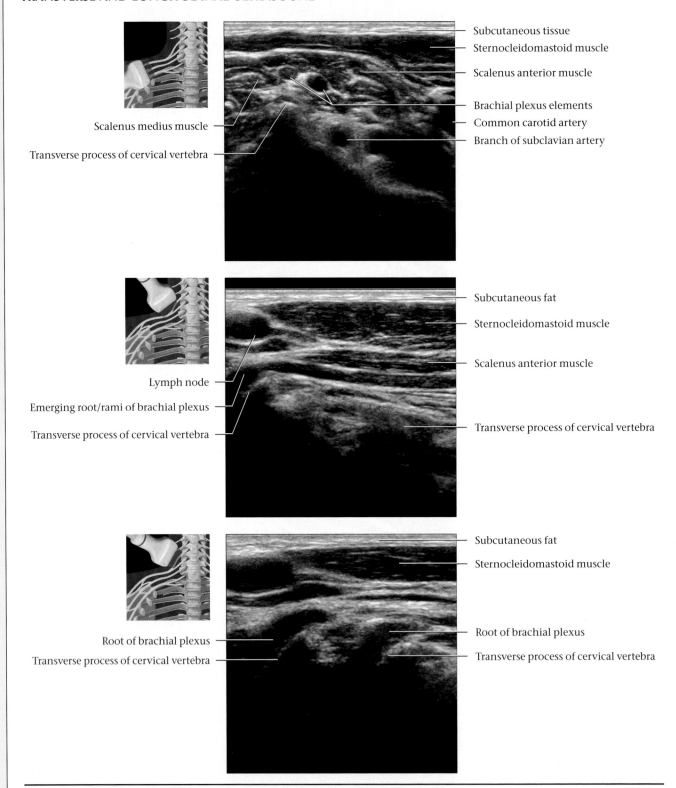

Subcutaneous tissue
Sternocleidomastoid muscle
Scalenus anterior muscle

Brachial plexus elements
Common carotid artery
Branch of subclavian artery

Scalenus medius muscle

Transverse process of cervical vertebra

Subcutaneous fat

Sternocleidomastoid muscle

Scalenus anterior muscle

Lymph node

Emerging root/rami of brachial plexus

Transverse process of cervical vertebra

Transverse process of cervical vertebra

Subcutaneous fat

Sternocleidomastoid muscle

Root of brachial plexus

Root of brachial plexus

Transverse process of cervical vertebra

Transverse process of cervical vertebra

(Top) Short-axis view grayscale ultrasound of the lower posterior triangle shows the elements of brachial plexus that appear as round, hypoechoic structures between the scalenus anterior and scalenus medius. *(Middle)* Longitudinal grayscale ultrasound of the posterior triangle of the neck shows the root and trunk of the brachial plexus, which appears as a thin, tubular, hypoechoic structure related superficially to the scalenus anterior muscle and deeply to the cervical vertebrae. *(Bottom)* Longitudinal grayscale ultrasound of the posterior triangle shows the emerging roots of the brachial plexus. Although USG identifies elements of the brachial plexus in the neck, MR delineates the entire anatomy better.

AXIAL AND CORONAL MR

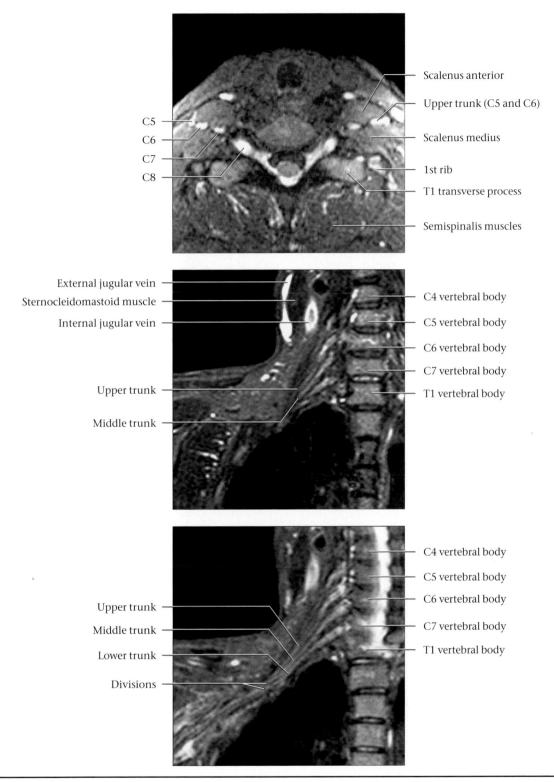

C5
C6
C7
C8

Scalenus anterior
Upper trunk (C5 and C6)
Scalenus medius
1st rib
T1 transverse process
Semispinalis muscles

External jugular vein
Sternocleidomastoid muscle
Internal jugular vein

C4 vertebral body
C5 vertebral body
C6 vertebral body
C7 vertebral body
T1 vertebral body

Upper trunk
Middle trunk

Upper trunk
Middle trunk
Lower trunk
Divisions

C4 vertebral body
C5 vertebral body
C6 vertebral body
C7 vertebral body
T1 vertebral body

(Top) Axial STIR MR at the C7-T1 level depicts the linear alignment of the C5-C8 ventral primary rami (VPR). C5 and C6 are in close proximity and form the left upper trunk. *(Middle)* Coronal T2WI MR of the brachial plexus shows the proximal cervical roots/VPR combining to form the upper and middle trunks of the brachial plexus. Normal nerve is slightly hyperintense to muscle on STIR and fat-saturated T2-weighted MR. *(Bottom)* Reformatted oblique coronal T2WI MR of the brachial plexus shows that the trunks and divisions of the brachial plexus continue from cervical nerve roots to the axilla.

BRACHIAL PLEXUS

PATHOLOGY

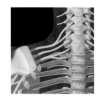
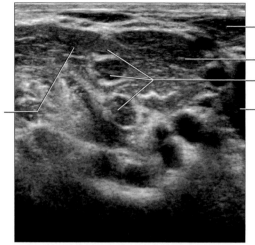
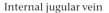

Sternocleidomastoid muscle

Scalenus anterior muscle

Thickened brachial plexus elements

Internal jugular vein

Scalenus medius muscle

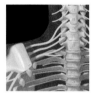
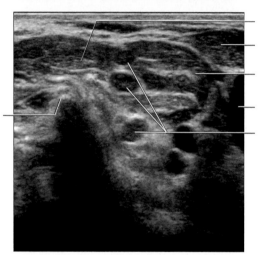

Scalenus medius muscle

Sternocleidomastoid muscle

Scalenus anterior muscle

Internal jugular vein

Thickened brachial plexus elements

Tip of transverse process of cervical vertebra

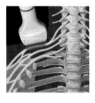
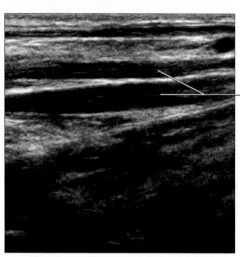

Thickened brachial plexus trunks

(Top) Transverse grayscale ultrasound of the right lower posterior triangle/supraclavicular fossa shows round, smooth, hypoechoic nodules between the scalenus anterior and medius muscles. The anatomical location suggests the possibility of thickened brachial plexus elements. *(Middle)* Transverse grayscale ultrasound at the lower level of the right posterior triangle/supraclavicular fossa shows the hypoechoic nodules persist and diverge. *(Bottom)* Longitudinal grayscale ultrasound of right posterior triangle/supraclavicular fossa confirms the elongated linear, hypoechoic, thickened elements of the brachial plexus. The patient had past history of neck irradiation for metastatic neck nodes, and the nerve thickening is likely secondary to post-radiation change.

PATHOLOGY

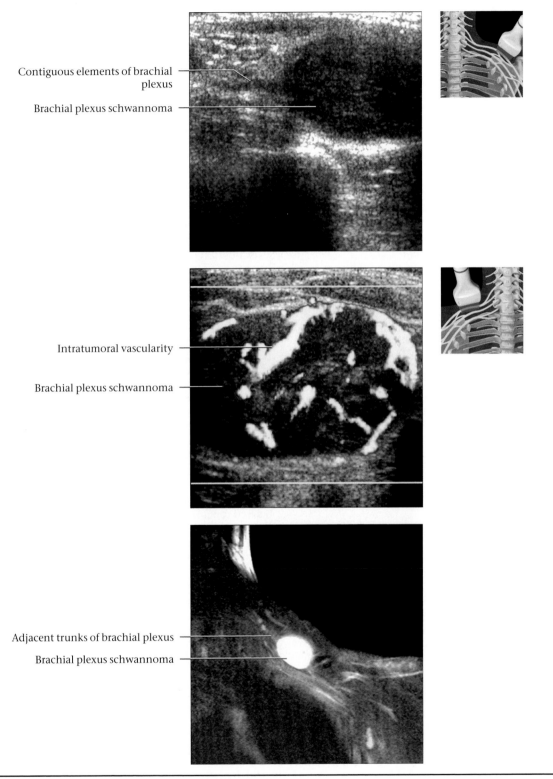

Contiguous elements of brachial plexus

Brachial plexus schwannoma

Intratumoral vascularity

Brachial plexus schwannoma

Adjacent trunks of brachial plexus

Brachial plexus schwannoma

(Top) Longitudinal grayscale ultrasound in the left supraclavicular fossa shows a round, solid, heterogeneous hypoechoic mass that continues with brachial plexus elements, suggesting a brachial plexus schwannoma. *(Middle)* Power Doppler ultrasound of a brachial plexus schwannoma demonstrates increased intralesional vascularity. *(Bottom)* Coronal fat-suppressed T2WI MR demonstrates a brachial plexus schwannoma with high signal intensity. The adjacent trunks of brachial plexus also appear mildly hyperintense on T2WI. The lesion is typically hypo-/isointense on T1WI and shows marked homogeneous enhancement after intravenous gadolinium (not shown).

VAGUS NERVE

TERMINOLOGY

Abbreviations
- Vagus nerve (CN10)

Synonyms
- 10th cranial nerve

IMAGING ANATOMY

Overview
- Mixed nerve (sensory, taste, motor, parasympathetic)
  - Parasympathetic nerve supplying regions of head and neck and thoracic and abdominal viscera
  - Additional CN10 components
    - Motor to soft palate (except tensor veli palatini muscle), pharyngeal constrictor muscles, larynx, and palatoglossus muscle of tongue
    - Visceral sensation from larynx, esophagus, trachea, and thoracic and abdominal viscera
    - Sensory nerve to external tympanic membrane, external auditory canal (EAC), and external ear
- 4 major segments: Intraaxial, cisternal, skull base, and extracranial
- Intraaxial segment
  - Vagal nuclei are in upper and middle medulla
    - Contain motor, sensory (including taste from epiglottis), and parasympathetic fibers
  - Fibers to and from these nuclei exit lateral medulla in postolivary sulcus inferior to glossopharyngeal nerve (CN9) and superior to bulbar portion of accessory nerve (CN11)
- Cisternal segment
  - Exits lateral medulla in postolivary sulcus between CN9 and bulbar portion of CN11
  - Travels anterolaterally through basal cistern together with CN9 and bulbar portion of CN11
- Skull base segment
  - Passes through posterior pars vascularis portion of jugular foramen (JF)
    - Accompanied by CN11 and jugular bulb
    - Superior vagal ganglion is found within JF
- Extracranial segment
  - Exits JF into nasopharyngeal carotid space
  - Inferior vagal ganglion lies just below skull base
  - Descends along posterolateral aspect of internal carotid artery (ICA) into thorax
    - Passes anterior to aortic arch on the left and subclavian artery on the right
  - Forms plexus around esophagus and major blood vessels to heart and lungs
  - Gastric nerves emerge from esophageal plexus and provide parasympathetic innervation to stomach
  - Innervation to intestines and visceral organs follows arterial blood supply to that organ
- Extracranial branches in head and neck
  - Auricular branch (Arnold nerve)
    - Sensation from external surface of tympanic membrane, EAC, and external ear
    - Passes through mastoid canaliculus extending from posterolateral JF to mastoid segment of facial nerve (CN7) canal
  - Pharyngeal branches
    - Pharyngeal plexus exits just below skull base
    - Sensory to epiglottis, trachea, and esophagus
    - Motor to soft palate and pharyngeal constrictor muscles
  - Superior laryngeal nerve
    - Motor to cricothyroid muscle
    - Sensory to mucosa of supraglottis
- Recurrent laryngeal nerve
  - On the right recurs at cervicothoracic junction, passing posteriorly around subclavian artery
  - On the left recurs in mediastinum, passing posteriorly under aorta at aortopulmonary window
  - Nerves recur in tracheoesophageal grooves
  - Motor to all laryngeal muscles except cricothyroid muscle
  - Sensory to mucosa of infraglottis

ANATOMY IMAGING ISSUES

Imaging Recommendations
- Extracranial segment is the only portion accessible for USG evaluation (upper, mid, lower cervical regions)
  - Lies between ICA/common carotid artery (CCA) and internal jugular vein (IJV) on transverse scans
  - Linear hypoechoic structure with central echogenic fibrillar pattern on longitudinal scan
  - On axial scans seen as round, hypoechoic structure with central echogenic focus
  - Best seen from level of carotid bifurcation down to lower cervical region
  - Color/power Doppler helps to distinguish it from small vessels in vicinity of major vessels of carotid sheath
- More easily visualized on USG in patients with previous radiotherapy
  - Appears diffusely thickened with smooth contour
- USG readily identifies CN10 schwannoma in upper, mid, or lower cervical region
  - Appears as round/ovoid solid hypoechoic mass
  - Related to ICA/CCA and IJV
    - No splaying of carotid bifurcation, which occurs in carotid body tumor
  - CN10 is contiguous with mass
  - Increased intranodular vascularity on power Doppler
  - USG features obviate the need for fine-needle aspiration/biopsy
- Recurrent laryngeal nerve cannot be confidently visualized on USG
  - In patient with vocal cord palsy, USG may help to detect abnormality in tracheoesophageal groove

Imaging Pitfalls
- USG cannot assess intrathoracic portion of CN10
  - CT is imaging modality of choice if CN10 lesion in mediastinum is suspected

CLINICAL IMPLICATIONS

Clinical Importance
- CN10 dysfunction
  - Proximal symptom complex (lesion between medulla and hyoid bone)
    - Multiple cranial nerves involved (CN9-CN12) with oropharyngeal and laryngeal dysfunction
  - Distal symptom complex (lesion below hyoid bone)
    - Isolated CN10 involvement with laryngeal dysfunction only

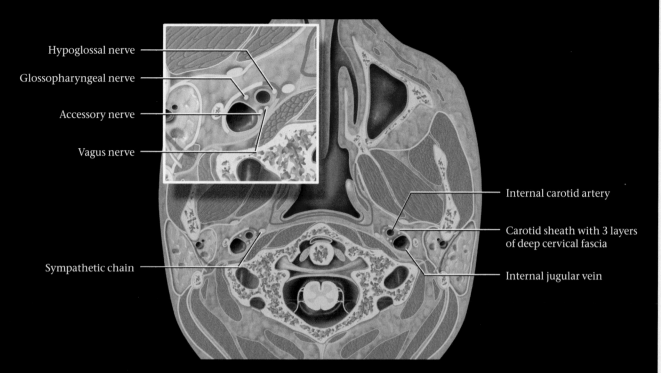

Hypoglossal nerve

Glossopharyngeal nerve

Accessory nerve

Vagus nerve

Internal carotid artery

Carotid sheath with 3 layers of deep cervical fascia

Sympathetic chain

Internal jugular vein

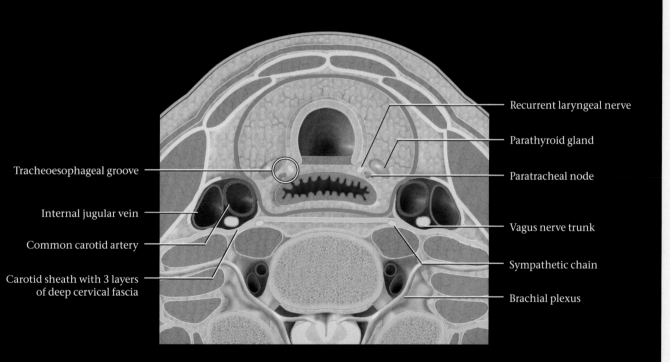

Recurrent laryngeal nerve

Parathyroid gland

Tracheoesophageal groove

Paratracheal node

Internal jugular vein

Common carotid artery

Vagus nerve trunk

Carotid sheath with 3 layers of deep cervical fascia

Sympathetic chain

Brachial plexus

(Top) Axial graphic of nasopharyngeal carotid spaces shows the extracranial vagus nerve situated posteriorly in the gap between the internal carotid artery and the internal jugular vein. Note that at this level the glossopharyngeal nerve (CN9), accessory nerve (CN11), and hypoglossal nerve (CN12) are all still within the carotid space. This site is not accessible on ultrasound. *(Bottom)* Axial graphic through the infrahyoid carotid spaces at the level of the thyroid gland demonstrates that the vagus trunk is the only remaining cranial nerve within the carotid space. It remains in the posterior gap between the common carotid artery and the internal jugular vein. Note the recurrent laryngeal nerve in the tracheoesophageal groove within the visceral space. Remember that the left recurrent laryngeal nerve turns cephalad in the aortopulmonary window in the mediastinum, whereas the right recurrent nerve turns at the cervicothoracic junction around the subclavian artery.

VAGUS NERVE

TRANSVERSE, POWER DOPPLER, AND LONGITUDINAL ULTRASOUND

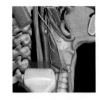
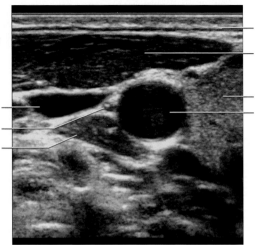

Subcutaneous tissue

Sternocleidomastoid muscle

Right lobe of thyroid gland
Common carotid artery

Internal jugular vein

Vagus nerve

Scalenus anterior

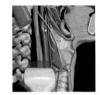
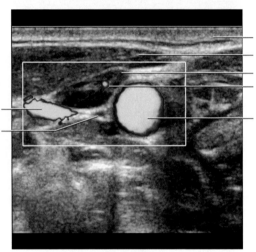

Subcutaneous tissue

Sternocleidomastoid muscle

Lymph node
Hilar vascularity in lymph node

Common carotid artery

Internal jugular vein

Vagus nerve

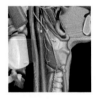
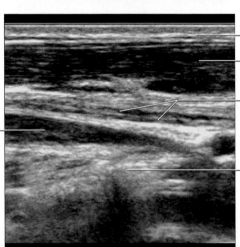

Subcutaneous tissue

Sternocleidomastoid muscle

Vagus nerve

Common carotid artery

Transverse process of cervical vertebra

(Top) Transverse grayscale ultrasound of the lower cervical level at the thyroid gland level shows the vagus nerve as a small, round, hypoechoic structure that exhibits central echogenicity within the carotid sheath and is located between the common carotid artery and the internal jugular vein. *(Middle)* Power Doppler ultrasound of the midcervical level in the transverse plane demonstrates the avascular nature of the vagus nerve adjacent to the common carotid artery and internal jugular vein. Note the presence of hilar vascularity in the adjacent normal deep cervical lymph node. *(Bottom)* Longitudinal grayscale ultrasound shows the vagus nerve, which appears as a long, thin, tubular, hypoechoic structure with a central echogenic fibrillary pattern within. On ultrasound, the vagus nerve is readily seen from the carotid bifurcation to the lower cervical region.

AXIAL AND CORONAL CECT

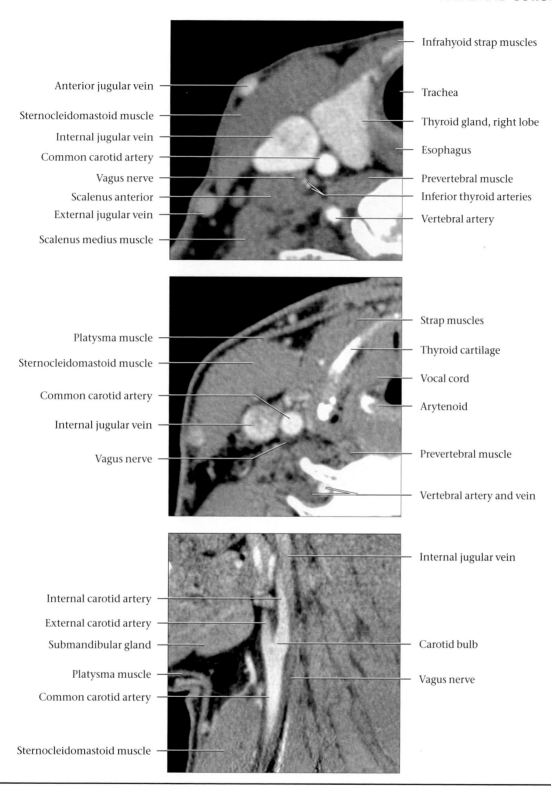

Anterior jugular vein

Sternocleidomastoid muscle

Internal jugular vein

Common carotid artery

Vagus nerve

Scalenus anterior

External jugular vein

Scalenus medius muscle

Infrahyoid strap muscles

Trachea

Thyroid gland, right lobe

Esophagus

Prevertebral muscle

Inferior thyroid arteries

Vertebral artery

Platysma muscle

Sternocleidomastoid muscle

Common carotid artery

Internal jugular vein

Vagus nerve

Strap muscles

Thyroid cartilage

Vocal cord

Arytenoid

Prevertebral muscle

Vertebral artery and vein

Internal jugular vein

Internal carotid artery

External carotid artery

Submandibular gland

Platysma muscle

Common carotid artery

Carotid bulb

Vagus nerve

Sternocleidomastoid muscle

(Top) *Axial CECT of the neck at the midcervical level shows the vagus nerve as an isodense dot in the posterior aspect of the carotid sheath. The inferior thyroid arteries are seen as contrast-enhanced dots in its proximity.* *(Middle)* *Axial CECT image of the neck in a different patient also shows the vagus nerve as an isodense dot in the posterior aspect of the carotid space.* *(Bottom)* *Oblique sagittal reformatted CECT image of the neck shows the course of the vagus nerve. It is closely related to the posterior aspect of the common carotid artery. Although CT demonstrates the vagus nerve in the neck, high-resolution ultrasound clearly evaluates its internal architecture.*

VAGUS NERVE

PATHOLOGY

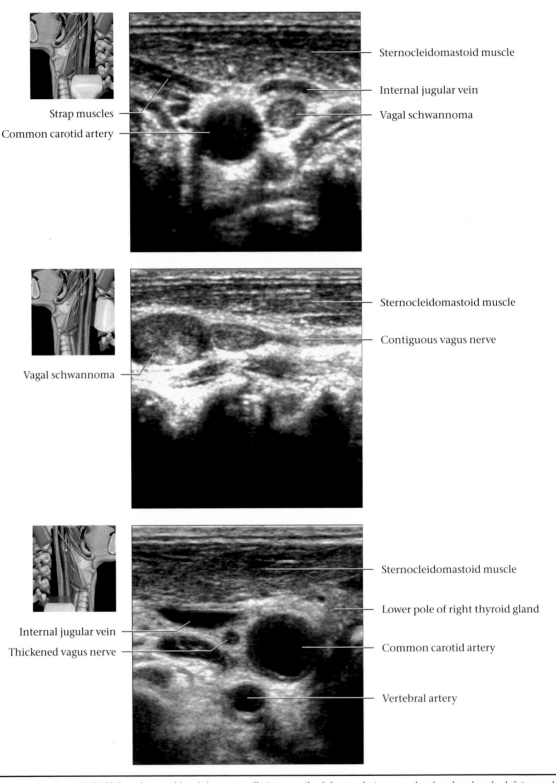

(Top) Transverse grayscale ultrasound of left midcervical level shows a well-circumscribed, hypoechoic mass closely related to the left internal jugular vein and common carotid artery. The anatomical location helps to identify the mass as originating from the vagus nerve. **(Middle)** Longitudinal grayscale ultrasound shows 2 well-circumscribed, oblong, solid, hypoechoic masses contiguous with the vagus nerve inferiorly. The appearances are of vagal schwannomas. **(Bottom)** Transverse grayscale ultrasound of the lower cervical level in a patient with previous neck irradiation for head and neck cancer shows that the vagus nerve is diffusely thickened with smooth contour as a result of post-irradiation change.

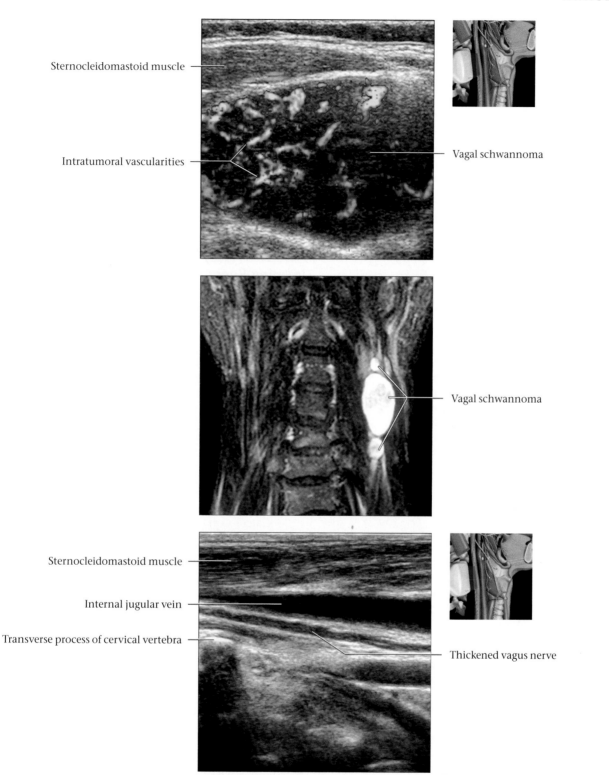

(Top) *Longitudinal power Doppler ultrasound of a vagal schwannoma reveals marked increased intratumoral vascularity. Ultrasound readily identifies a vagal nerve schwannoma and obviates the need for fine-needle aspiration cytology or biopsy.* **(Middle)** *Coronal fat-suppressed T2WI MR shows marked T2 hyperintensity of vagal schwannoma.* **(Bottom)** *Longitudinal grayscale ultrasound shows the diffusely thickened vagus nerve in relation to the internal jugular vein.*

CERVICAL CAROTID ARTERIES

TERMINOLOGY

Abbreviations
- Common (CCA), internal (ICA), and external (ECA) carotid arteries; vertebral artery (VA)

GROSS ANATOMY

Overview
- CCA terminates by dividing into ECA and ICA
- ECA is smaller of 2 terminal branches
  - Supplies most of head and neck (except eye, brain)
  - Has numerous anastomoses with ICA and VA (may become important source of collateral blood flow)
- ICA has no normal extracranial branches

IMAGING ANATOMY

Overview
- CCA
  - Right CCA originates from brachiocephalic trunk (BCT); left CCA originates from aortic arch (AA)
  - Courses superiorly in carotid space, anteromedial to internal jugular vein
  - Divides into ECA and ICA at ~ C3-C4 level
- Cervical ICA
  - 90% are posterolateral to ECA
  - Carotid bulb
    - Focal dilatation of ICA at its origin from CCA
    - Flow reversal occurs in carotid bulb
  - Ascending cervical segment
    - Courses superiorly within carotid space
    - Enters carotid canal of skull base (petrous temporal bone)
    - No named branch in neck
- ECA
  - Smaller and medial compared with ICA
  - Has 8 major branches in neck
  - Superior thyroid artery
    - 1st ECA branch (may arise from CCA bifurcation)
    - Arises anteriorly and courses inferiorly to apex of thyroid
    - Supplies superior thyroid and larynx
    - Anastomoses with inferior thyroid artery (branch of thyrocervical trunk)
  - Ascending pharyngeal artery
    - Arises from posterior ECA (or CCA bifurcation)
    - Courses superiorly between ECA and ICA
    - Visceral branches, muscular branches, and neuromeningeal branches
  - Lingual artery
    - 2nd anterior ECA branch
    - Loops anteroinferiorly, then superiorly to tongue
    - Major vascular supply to tongue, oral cavity, and submandibular gland
  - Facial artery
    - Originates just above lingual artery
    - Curves around mandible, then passes anterosuperiorly across cheek and is closely related to submandibular gland
    - Supplies face, palate, lip, and cheek
  - Occipital artery
    - Originates from posterior aspect of ECA
    - Courses posterosuperiorly between occiput and C1
    - Supplies scalp, upper cervical musculature, and posterior fossa meninges
  - Posterior auricular artery
    - Arises from posterior ECA above occipital artery
    - Courses superiorly to supply pinna, scalp, external auditory canal, and chorda tympani
  - Superficial temporal artery
    - Smaller of 2 terminal ECA branches
    - Runs superiorly behind mandibular condyle, across zygoma
    - Supplies scalp and gives off transverse facial artery
  - Internal maxillary artery
    - Larger of 2 terminal ECA branches
    - Arises within parotid gland, behind mandibular neck
    - Gives off middle meningeal artery (supplies cranial meninges)

ANATOMY IMAGING ISSUES

Imaging Recommendations
- Normal USG appearances of carotid arteries
  - CCA diameter: 6.3 ± 0.9 mm, smooth and thin intima, antegrade low-resistance arterial flow
  - ICA diameter: 4.8 ± 0.7 mm, smooth and thin intima, antegrade low-resistance flow
  - ECA diameter: 4.1 ± 0.6 mm, smooth and thin intima, antegrade high-resistance flow
- In assessing carotid arteries on USG, the following parameters should be examined
  - Intimal-medial thickness
    - Distance between leading edges of lumen-intima interface and media-adventitia interface at far edge
    - 0.5-1 mm in healthy adults
  - Presence of atherosclerotic plaques
    - Eccentric/concentric, noncircumferential/circumferential
    - Calcified plaque/soft plaque
  - Luminal diameter/area reduction
    - Should be measured on true cross-sectional view of affected artery
    - Color flow imaging helps to detect residual lumen in tight stenosis or in assessing indeterminate total occlusion
  - Spectral Doppler analysis
    - Arterial flow pattern: Low-resistance/high-resistance flow, antegrade/retrograde flow, special waveform (e.g., damped waveform, preocclusive "thump")
    - Peak systolic velocity (PSV) measurement
    - Systolic velocity ratio (SVR) measurement

Imaging Pitfalls
- Scanning technique must be meticulous to produce reliable Doppler ultrasound results
- Obliquity of imaging plane in relation to cross section of artery may wrongly estimate degree of stenosis

CLINICAL IMPLICATIONS

Clinical Importance
- Consider acute idiopathic carotidynia: Tender mass around distal carotid, near bifurcation
  - Vessel wall thickening, no luminal narrowing or velocity elevation

GRAPHIC & DIGITAL SUBTRACTION ANGIOGRAM

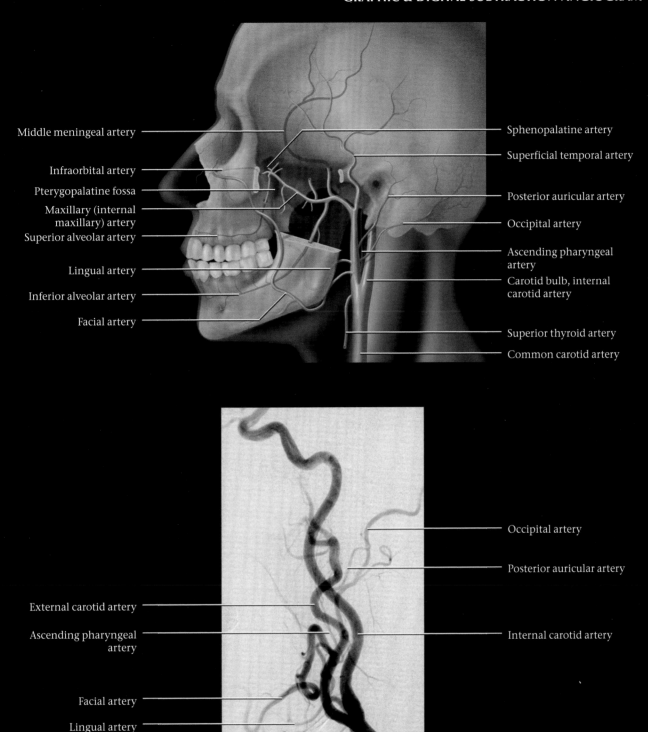

Middle meningeal artery

Infraorbital artery

Pterygopalatine fossa

Maxillary (internal maxillary) artery

Superior alveolar artery

Lingual artery

Inferior alveolar artery

Facial artery

Sphenopalatine artery

Superficial temporal artery

Posterior auricular artery

Occipital artery

Ascending pharyngeal artery

Carotid bulb, internal carotid artery

Superior thyroid artery

Common carotid artery

Occipital artery

Posterior auricular artery

External carotid artery

Ascending pharyngeal artery

Internal carotid artery

Facial artery

Lingual artery

Superior thyroid artery

(Top) Lateral graphic depicts the common carotid artery (CCA) and its 2 terminal branches, the external (ECA) and internal (ICA) carotid arteries. The scalp and the superficial facial structures are removed to show the deep ECA branches. The ECA terminates by dividing into the superficial temporal and internal maxillary arteries (IMA). Within the pterygopalatine fossa, the IMA divides into numerous deep branches. Its distal termination is the sphenopalatine artery, which passes medially into the nasal cavity. Numerous anastomoses between the ECA branches (e.g., between the facial and maxillary arteries) and between the ECA and the orbital and cavernous branches of the ICA provide potential sources for collateral blood flow. *(Bottom)* The early arterial phase of CCA angiogram is shown with bony structures subtracted. The major ECA branches are opacified.

CERVICAL CAROTID ARTERIES

COMMON CAROTID ARTERY

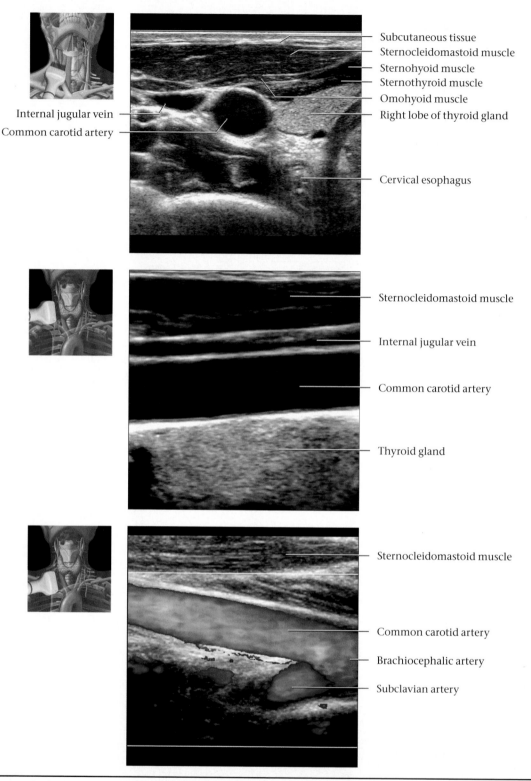

Internal jugular vein

Common carotid artery

Subcutaneous tissue

Sternocleidomastoid muscle

Sternohyoid muscle

Sternothyroid muscle

Omohyoid muscle

Right lobe of thyroid gland

Cervical esophagus

Sternocleidomastoid muscle

Internal jugular vein

Common carotid artery

Thyroid gland

Sternocleidomastoid muscle

Common carotid artery

Brachiocephalic artery

Subclavian artery

(Top) Transverse grayscale ultrasound shows the distal CCA at the level of the upper pole of the thyroid gland. Note that the wall in a normal individual is smooth with no intimal thickening or atherosclerotic plaque. The lumen is circular in cross section. There is no major named branch in the neck apart from the termination into ECA and ICA at the level of the hyoid bone. *(Middle)* Longitudinal grayscale ultrasound of the CCA shows the smooth outline of the intimal layer. *(Bottom)* Color Doppler ultrasound of the proximal CCA at the root of the neck in the longitudinal plane demonstrates the normal antegrade arterial flow in the cranial direction. Its origin along with the subclavian artery from the right brachiocephalic artery is also well demonstrated.

CERVICAL CAROTID ARTERIES

COMMON CAROTID ARTERY

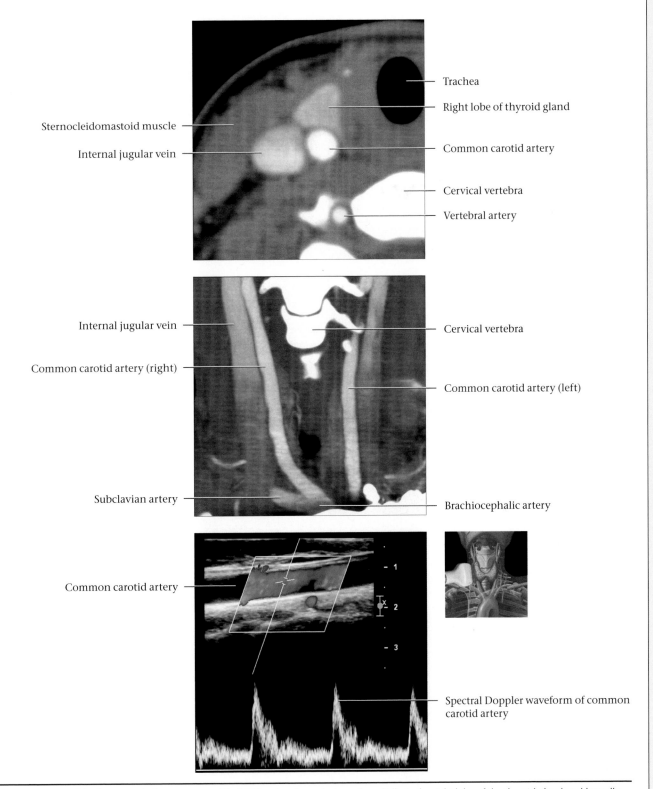

Sternocleidomastoid muscle

Internal jugular vein

Trachea

Right lobe of thyroid gland

Common carotid artery

Cervical vertebra

Vertebral artery

Internal jugular vein

Common carotid artery (right)

Cervical vertebra

Common carotid artery (left)

Subclavian artery

Brachiocephalic artery

Common carotid artery

Spectral Doppler waveform of common carotid artery

(Top) Axial CECT of the lower neck shows contrast-filled CCA related anteriorly and medially to the right lobe of the thyroid gland and laterally to the internal jugular vein. *(Middle)* Coronal reformatted CECT shows the normal contour and vertical course of the CCA. It originates from the brachiocephalic artery on the right at the root of the neck with the right subclavian artery. *(Bottom)* Spectral Doppler ultrasound of the CCA shows low-resistance arterial flow with a forward diastolic component. The scanning technique must be meticulous to produce a reliable Doppler assessment.

CAROTID BIFURCATION

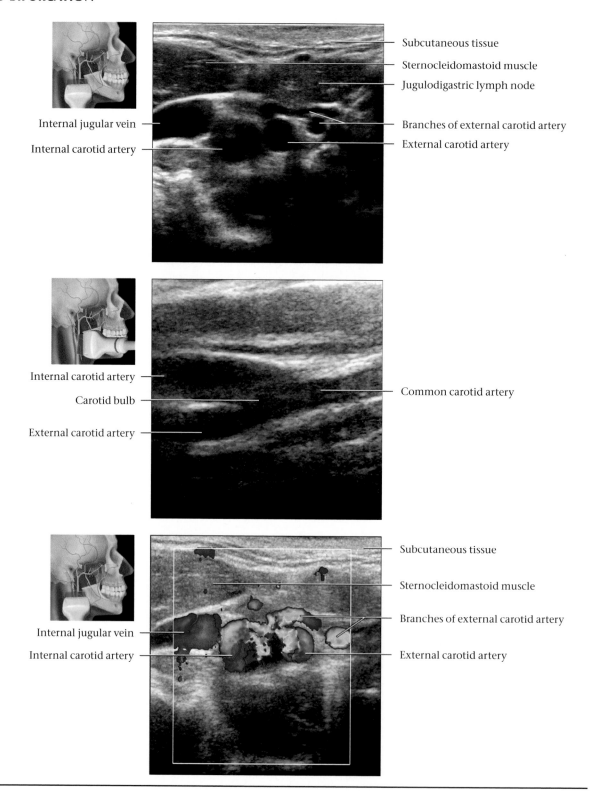

Subcutaneous tissue

Sternocleidomastoid muscle

Jugulodigastric lymph node

Internal jugular vein

Internal carotid artery

Branches of external carotid artery

External carotid artery

Internal carotid artery

Carotid bulb

External carotid artery

Common carotid artery

Subcutaneous tissue

Sternocleidomastoid muscle

Branches of external carotid artery

Internal jugular vein

Internal carotid artery

External carotid artery

(Top) Transverse grayscale ultrasound shows the upper cervical level at the carotid bifurcation. The CCA bifurcates into the ICA and ECA. The former is usually of larger caliber, laterally located, and has no branches in the neck. *(Middle)* Longitudinal grayscale ultrasound in coronal orientation demonstrates the carotid bifurcation. The proximal portion of the ICA is usually mildly dilated and is termed, "carotid bulb." At this site, the color/spectral Doppler study is more complex due to a disturbance of laminar flow and should not be misinterpreted as an abnormality. *(Bottom)* Color Doppler ultrasound of carotid bifurcation in a transverse plane demonstrates turbulent flow in the carotid bulb. Branches of ECA are easier to depict than on grayscale examination.

CERVICAL CAROTID ARTERIES

CAROTID BIFURCATION

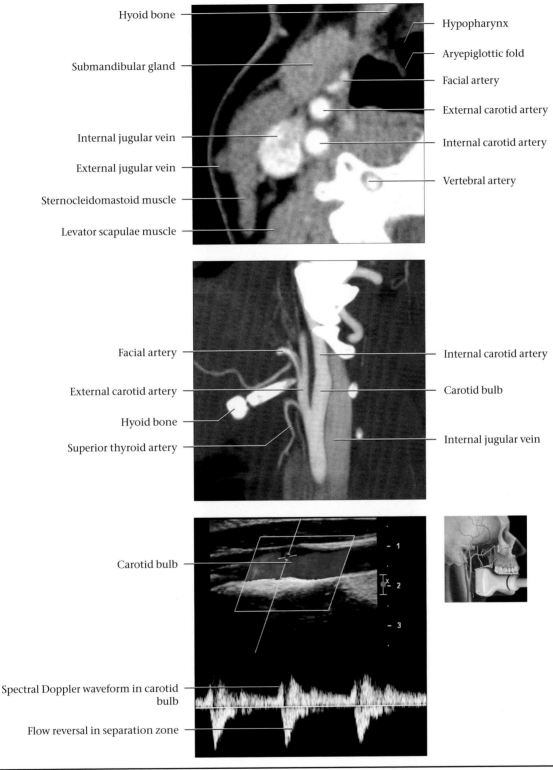

Hyoid bone

Submandibular gland

Internal jugular vein

External jugular vein

Sternocleidomastoid muscle

Levator scapulae muscle

Hypopharynx

Aryepiglottic fold

Facial artery

External carotid artery

Internal carotid artery

Vertebral artery

Facial artery

External carotid artery

Hyoid bone

Superior thyroid artery

Internal carotid artery

Carotid bulb

Internal jugular vein

Carotid bulb

Spectral Doppler waveform in carotid bulb

Flow reversal in separation zone

(Top) Axial CECT shows the upper neck just beyond the carotid bifurcation. The ICA is larger and more posterolateral in position than the ECA. *(Middle)* Maximum-intensity projection in the sagittal plane demonstrates carotid bifurcation into the ECA and ICA at the level of the hyoid bone. Note the branching nature of the ECA in contrast to the ICA. *(Bottom)* Spectral Doppler ultrasound shows the carotid bulb, which has a different flow pattern than the rest of the ICA. In early systole, blood flow is accelerated in a forward direction. As the peak systole is approached, a large separation zone with flow reversal develops. Flow separation should be seen in normal individuals, and its absence should raise the suspicion of plaque formation.

CERVICAL CAROTID ARTERIES

INTERNAL CAROTID ARTERY

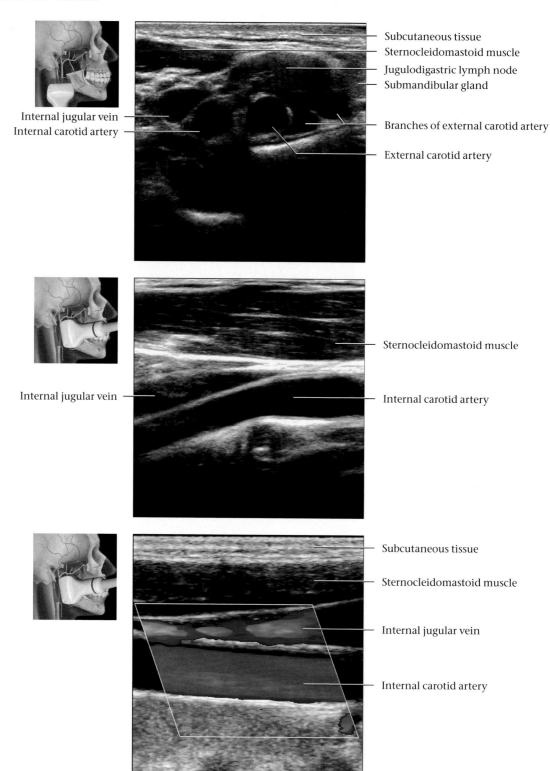

Subcutaneous tissue
Sternocleidomastoid muscle
Jugulodigastric lymph node
Submandibular gland

Internal jugular vein
Internal carotid artery

Branches of external carotid artery

External carotid artery

Sternocleidomastoid muscle

Internal jugular vein

Internal carotid artery

Subcutaneous tissue

Sternocleidomastoid muscle

Internal jugular vein

Internal carotid artery

(Top) Transverse grayscale ultrasound of the upper neck, just beyond the carotid bifurcation, shows the close anatomical relationship of the upper neck with the internal jugular vein, ECA, and jugulodigastric lymph node. *(Middle)* Longitudinal grayscale ultrasound shows the ICA. Note its smooth wall with no intimal thickening; it is free of atherosclerotic plaque in a normal individual. No branch is seen in the cervical region. *(Bottom)* Color Doppler ultrasound shows the ICA and the internal jugular vein in the longitudinal plane. Note that the normal antegrade flow is toward the cranial direction of the ICA and opposite the caudal direction of flow in the adjacent internal jugular vein.

INTERNAL CAROTID ARTERY

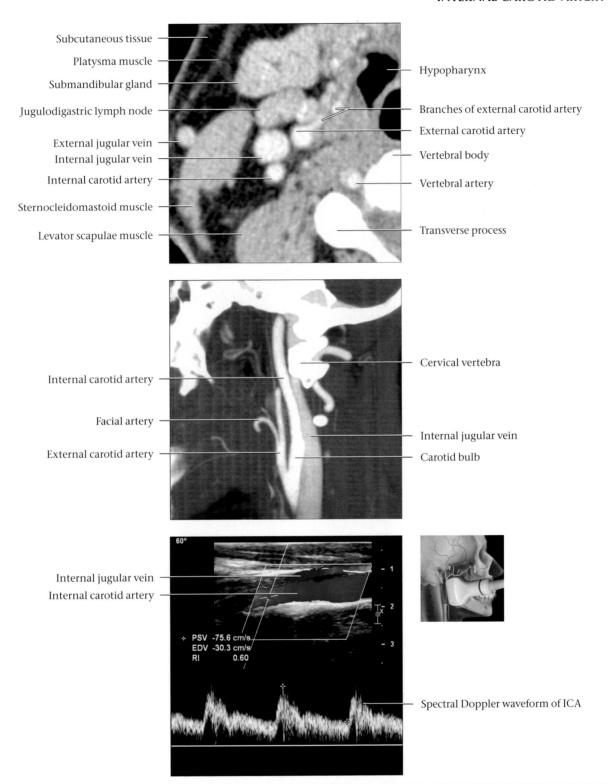

Subcutaneous tissue	Hypopharynx
Platysma muscle	
Submandibular gland	Branches of external carotid artery
Jugulodigastric lymph node	External carotid artery
External jugular vein	Vertebral body
Internal jugular vein	Vertebral artery
Internal carotid artery	
Sternocleidomastoid muscle	Transverse process
Levator scapulae muscle	

Internal carotid artery — Cervical vertebra

Facial artery

External carotid artery — Internal jugular vein — Carotid bulb

Internal jugular vein
Internal carotid artery

PSV -75.6 cm/s
EDV -30.3 cm/s
RI   0.60

Spectral Doppler waveform of ICA

(Top) Axial CECT of the upper neck shows the anatomical relation of the ICA with the internal jugular vein and branches of the ECA. *(Middle)* Maximum-intensity projection CECT in the sagittal plane shows the normal configuration and contour of the cervical portion of the ICA. Note the lack of an arterial branch from the cervical ICA in the neck in contrast to the ECA. Note the mild dilatation of the ICA at its origin (carotid bulb). *(Bottom)* Spectral Doppler ultrasound in the longitudinal plane shows the cervical portion of the ICA, which has a low-resistance flow pattern with antegrade flow in the diastolic phase. The waveform is different from that of the carotid bulb.

CERVICAL CAROTID ARTERIES

EXTERNAL CAROTID ARTERY

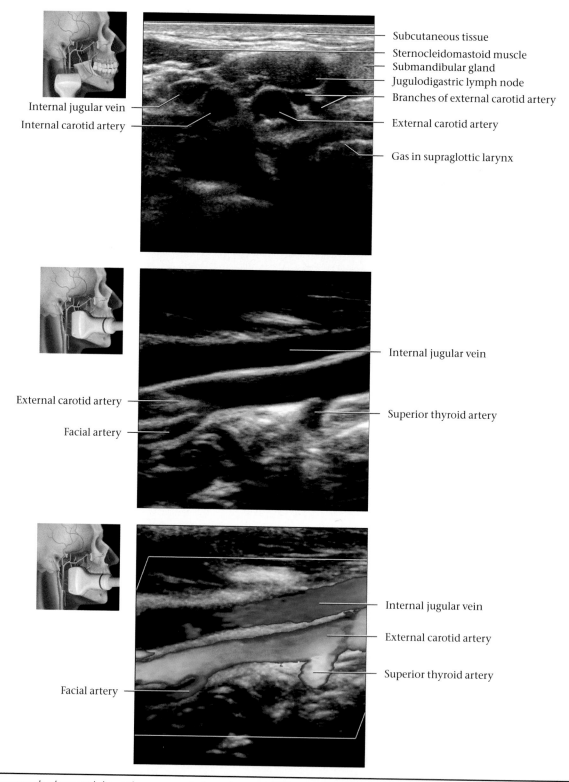

Internal jugular vein

Internal carotid artery

Subcutaneous tissue
Sternocleidomastoid muscle
Submandibular gland
Jugulodigastric lymph node
Branches of external carotid artery

External carotid artery

Gas in supraglottic larynx

External carotid artery

Facial artery

Internal jugular vein

Superior thyroid artery

Internal jugular vein

External carotid artery

Superior thyroid artery

Facial artery

(Top) Transverse grayscale ultrasound shows the upper neck above the carotid bifurcation. The position of the ECA medial to the ICA and internal jugular vein, posterior to the jugulodigastric lymph node, is well demonstrated. *(Middle)* Longitudinal grayscale ultrasound shows the ECA. Two anterior branches, the superior thyroid artery and the facial artery, are seen arising from the proximal portion of the ECA. They course inferiorly to the upper pole of the thyroid and superiorly to the facial region. *(Bottom)* Color Doppler ultrasound shows the ECA in the longitudinal plane. The antegrade flow in the cranial direction of the ECA is demonstrated. Note the opposite flow direction of the adjacent internal jugular vein.

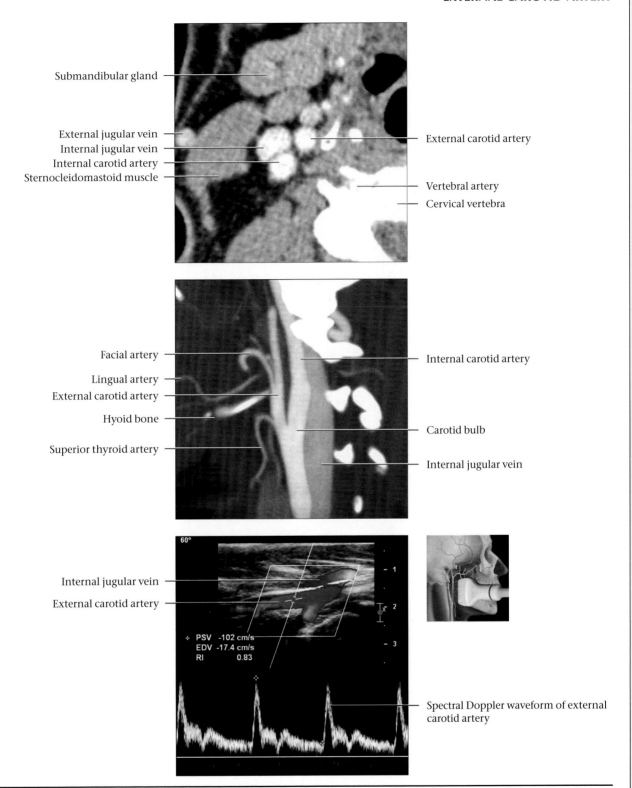

(Top) Axial CECT of the upper neck at the hyoid bone level shows the relationship of the ECA with the adjacent ICA and the internal jugular vein. (Middle) Maximum-intensity projection CECT in the sagittal plane shows the normal contour and configuration of the ECA. Note some of its major branches, including the superior thyroid artery, lingual artery, and facial artery, in its proximal portion. (Bottom) Spectral Doppler ultrasound of the ECA in longitudinal plane shows a high-resistance flow pattern with a low diastolic component. Contrarily, the CCA and ICA are of a low-resistance pattern with a high diastolic component.

CERVICAL CAROTID ARTERIES

GRAYSCALE AND DOPPLER ULTRASOUND

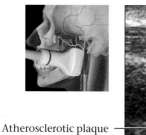
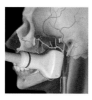
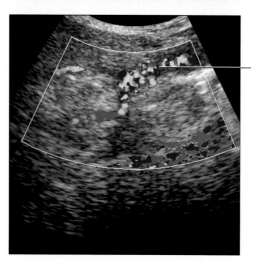
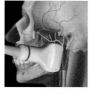
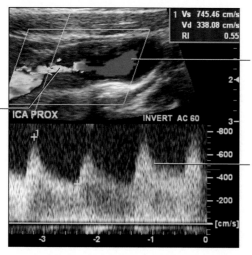

Sternocleidomastoid muscle

Internal jugular vein

Internal carotid artery

Atherosclerotic plaque

Stenotic segment, internal carotid artery

Internal carotid artery

Stenotic segment

Spectral waveform of stenotic internal carotid artery

(Top) Longitudinal grayscale ultrasound of the cervical portion of the ICA shows hypoechoic atherosclerotic plaque with marked luminal narrowing. *(Middle)* Longitudinal color Doppler ultrasound (same patient) helps to demonstrate the turbulent arterial flow through the severe stenotic segment in the proximal ICA. Color flow imaging is a useful tool to distinguish severe stenosis from complete occlusion. *(Bottom)* Spectral Doppler ultrasound of the proximal ICA demonstrates markedly elevated peak systolic and peak diastolic velocity, indicating severe stenosis.

GRAYSCALE AND DOPPLER ULTRASOUND

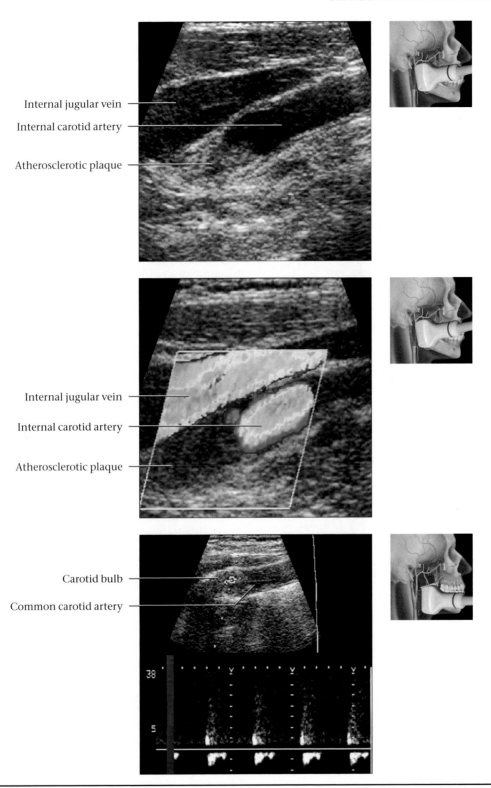

Internal jugular vein

Internal carotid artery

Atherosclerotic plaque

Internal jugular vein

Internal carotid artery

Atherosclerotic plaque

Carotid bulb

Common carotid artery

(Top) Longitudinal grayscale ultrasound of the cervical portion of the ICA shows a slightly hyperechoic atherosclerotic plaque causing complete arterial occlusion. *(Middle)* Color Doppler ultrasound (same patient) reveals an absence of arterial flow in the occluded segment of the ICA. *(Bottom)* Spectral Doppler ultrasound at the carotid bifurcation shows no detectable signal within the occluded segment and preocclusive "thump" proximal to the occluded segment. The carotid bulb was occluded on grayscale imaging (not shown).

VERTEBRAL ARTERIES

IMAGING ANATOMY

Overview
- Vertebral artery (VA): 4 segments
  - V1 segment (extraosseous segment)
    - Arises from 1st part of subclavian artery
    - Courses posterosuperiorly to enter C6 transverse foramen
    - Branches: Segmental cervical muscular, spinal branches
  - V2 segment (foraminal segment)
    - Ascends through C6-C3 transverse foramina
    - Turns superolaterally through inverted L-shaped transverse foramen of axis (C2)
    - Courses short distance superiorly through C1 transverse foramen
    - Branches: Anterior meningeal artery, unnamed muscular/spinal branches
  - V3 segment (extraspinal segment)
    - Exits top of atlas (C1) transverse foramen
    - Lies on top of C1 ring, curving posteromedially around atlantooccipital joint
    - As it passes around back of atlantooccipital joint, turns sharply anterosuperiorly to pierce dura at foramen magnum
    - Branches: Posterior meningeal artery
  - V4 segment (intradural/intracranial segment)
    - After VA enters skull through foramen magnum, courses superomedially behind clivus
    - Unites with contralateral VA at or near pontomedullary junction to form basilar artery
    - Branches: Anterior, posterior spinal arteries, perforating branches to medulla, posterior inferior cerebellar artery (PICA)
    - Arises from distal VA, curves around/over tonsil, gives off perforating medullary, choroid, tonsillar, cerebellar branches
- Basilar artery (BA)
  - Courses superiorly in prepontine cistern (in front of pons, behind clivus)
  - Bifurcates into its terminal branches, posterior cerebral arteries (PCAs), in interpeduncular or suprasellar cistern at or slightly above dorsum sellae
  - Branches: Pontine, midbrain perforating branches (numerous), anterior inferior cerebellar artery (AICA), superior cerebellar arteries (SCAs), PCAs (terminal branches)

Vascular Territory
- VA
  - Anterior spinal arteries (ASA): Upper cervical spinal cord, inferior medulla
  - Posterior spinal arteries (PSA): Dorsal spinal cord to conus medullaris
  - Penetrating branches: Olives, inferior cerebellar peduncle, part of medulla
  - PICA: Lateral medulla, choroid plexus of 4th ventricle, tonsil, inferior vermis/cerebellum
- BA
  - Pontine perforating branches: Central medulla, pons, midbrain
  - AICA: Internal auditory canal (IAC), CN7 and 8, anterolateral cerebellum
  - SCA: Superior vermis, superior cerebellar peduncle, dentate nucleus, brachium pontis, superomedial surface of cerebellum, upper vermis

Normal Variants, Anomalies
- Normal variants
  - VA: Variation in size from right to left, dominance common; origin from aortic arch in 5%
- Anomalies
  - VA/BA may be fenestrated or duplicated (may have increased prevalence of aneurysms)
  - Embryonic carotid-basilar anastomoses (e.g., persistent trigeminal artery)

ANATOMY IMAGING ISSUES

Imaging Recommendations
- V1 and V2 segments are amenable to USG examination
- Examination usually starts in V2 segment and proceeds downwards to V1 segment, then to its origin
- Examination of V2 segment
  - Transducer oriented longitudinally in midcervical region between trachea and sternocleidomastoid muscle
  - Angle transducer laterally from common carotid artery (CCA) and locate V2 segment posterior to acoustic shadowing of transverse processes
- Examination of V1 segment
  - Trace caudally from V2 to its origin
  - Left VA more difficult to visualize than right VA
  - Do not confuse with vertebral vein (VV) lying adjacent to VA, which can appear pulsatile
    - Color flow imaging helps to differentiate
- Normal waveform of vertebral artery on spectral Doppler analysis
  - Low resistance flow
  - Similar to that of CCA but with lower amplitude
  - PSV: 59 ± 17 cm/s; EDV: 19 ± 8 cm/s
  - Flow velocity asymmetry is common and related to caliber of VA

Imaging Pitfalls
- VA distal to V2 cannot be properly assessed by USG
  - Abnormalities in spectral Doppler waveform of VA at V1/V2 segment provide clue for disease beyond V2

EMBRYOLOGY

Embryologic Events
- Plexiform longitudinal anastomoses between cervical intersegmental arteries → VA precursors
- Paired plexiform dorsal longitudinal neural arteries (LNAs) develop, form precursors of BA
- Transient anastomoses between dorsal longitudinal neural arteries develop and ICAs appear (primitive trigeminal/hypoglossal arteries, etc.)
- Definitive VAs arise from 7th cervical intersegmental arteries, anastomose with LNAs
- LNAs fuse as temporary connections with ICAs regress → definitive BA, vertebrobasilar (VB) circulation formed

GRAPHICS AND VOLUME-RENDERED CTA

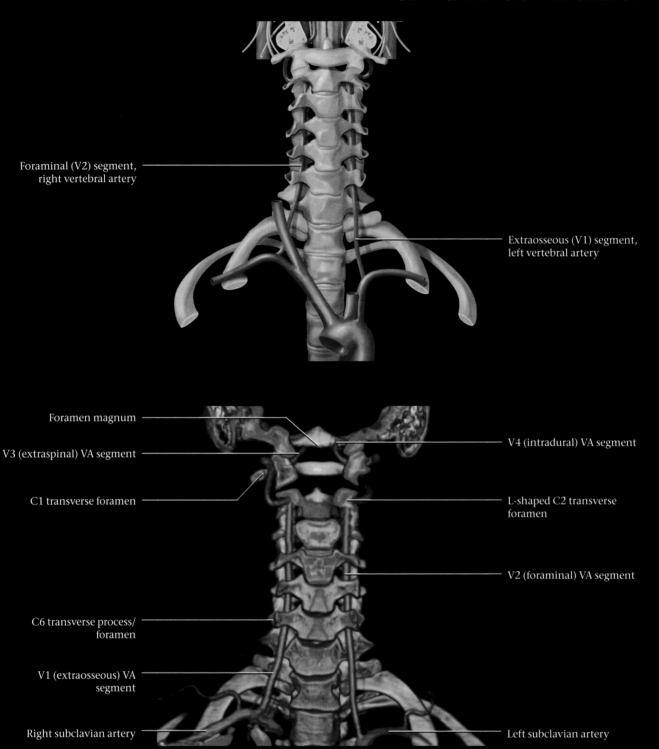

Foraminal (V2) segment, right vertebral artery

Extraosseous (V1) segment, left vertebral artery

Foramen magnum

V4 (intradural) VA segment

V3 (extraspinal) VA segment

C1 transverse foramen

L-shaped C2 transverse foramen

V2 (foraminal) VA segment

C6 transverse process/ foramen

V1 (extraosseous) VA segment

Right subclavian artery

Left subclavian artery

(Top) AP graphic shows 2 of the 3 extracranial segments of the vertebral arteries (VAs) and their relationship to the cervical spine. The extraosseous (V1) VA segments extend from the superior aspect of the subclavian arteries to the C6 transverse foramina. The V2 (foraminal) segment extends from C6 to the VA exit from the C1 transverse foramina. *(Bottom)* 3D-VRT CTA shows the extracranial VAs, which originate from the superior aspect of the subclavian arteries. The VAs typically enter the transverse foramina of C6 and ascend almost vertically to C2, where they make a 90° turn laterally in the L-shaped C2 transverse foramina before ascending vertically again to C1.

VERTEBRAL ARTERIES

TRANSVERSE, LONGITUDINAL GRAYSCALE AND COLOR DOPPLER

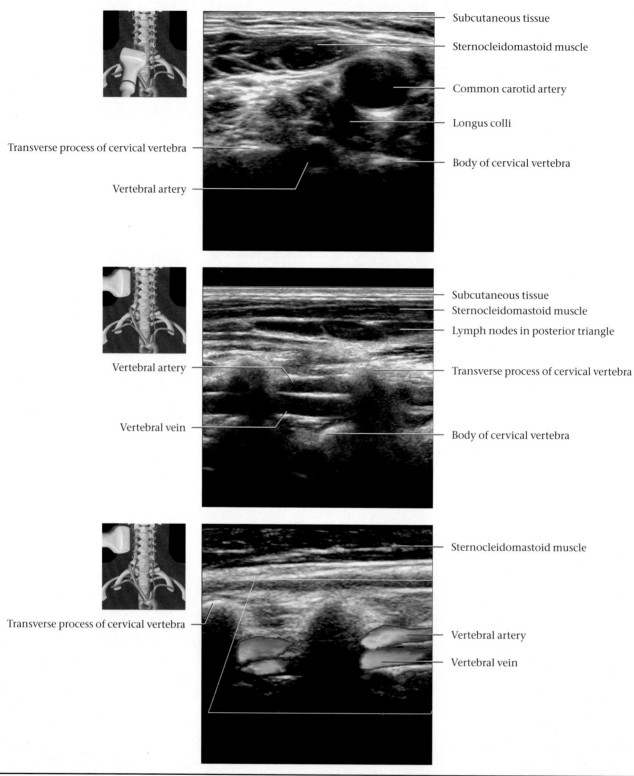

Subcutaneous tissue

Sternocleidomastoid muscle

Common carotid artery

Longus colli

Body of cervical vertebra

Transverse process of cervical vertebra

Vertebral artery

Subcutaneous tissue

Sternocleidomastoid muscle

Lymph nodes in posterior triangle

Vertebral artery

Transverse process of cervical vertebra

Vertebral vein

Body of cervical vertebra

Sternocleidomastoid muscle

Transverse process of cervical vertebra

Vertebral artery

Vertebral vein

(Top) Transverse grayscale ultrasound of the lower neck shows the proximal V1 segment of the vertebral artery, which arises from the 1st part of the subclavian artery and courses superiorly to enter the transverse foramina of the lower cervical vertebra. Note its posterior relationship to the longus colli at this level. *(Middle)* Longitudinal grayscale ultrasound of the posterior neck demonstrates the V2 segment of the vertebral artery within the transverse foramina of cervical vertebrae. Note the presence of dense posterior acoustic shadowing from the transverse processes, obscuring a clear view of the underlying vertebral vessels. *(Bottom)* Color Doppler ultrasound shows the V2 segment of the vertebral artery in the longitudinal plane. Note the opposite flow direction of the vertebral vein (i.e., craniocaudal direction) as compared with that of the vertebral artery (caudocranial direction).

VERTEBRAL ARTERIES

AXIAL AND CORONAL CECT, SPECTRAL DOPPLER

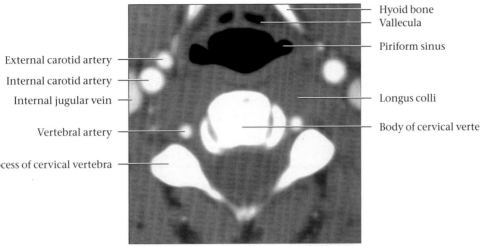

External carotid artery

Internal carotid artery

Internal jugular vein

Vertebral artery

Transverse process of cervical vertebra

Hyoid bone

Vallecula

Piriform sinus

Longus colli

Body of cervical vertebra

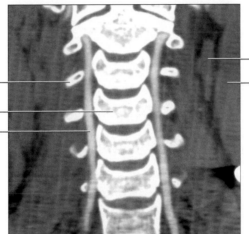

Transverse process of cervical vertebra

Body of cervical vertebra

Vertebral artery

Lymph nodes in posterior triangle

Sternocleidomastoid muscle

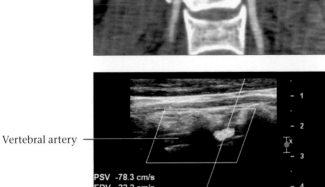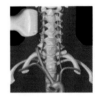

Vertebral artery

Spectral Doppler waveform of vertebral artery

PSV -78.3 cm/s
EDV -22.2 cm/s
RI   0.72

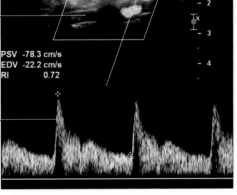

(Top) Axial CECT of the neck at the level of the hyoid bone shows the vertebral artery running in a caudocranial direction within the foramen transversarium of the cervical vertebrae. This portion is amenable for ultrasound examination. *(Middle)* Coronal reformatted CECT of the neck shows the vertical course of the vertebral arteries through the transverse foramina of C6 to C2 vertebrae. Note its close anatomical relationship with the transverse processes and bodies of the cervical vertebrae. *(Bottom)* Spectral Doppler ultrasound of the V2 segment of the vertebral artery is of low resistance, similar to that of the common carotid artery but with lower amplitude. Spectral analysis of the V2 segment provides a clue to stenosis/occlusion proximally and distally. For example, a high-resistance flow pattern without a diastolic flow component is often associated with a distal flow obstruction.

VERTEBRAL ARTERIES

GRAYSCALE AND DOPPLER ULTRASOUND

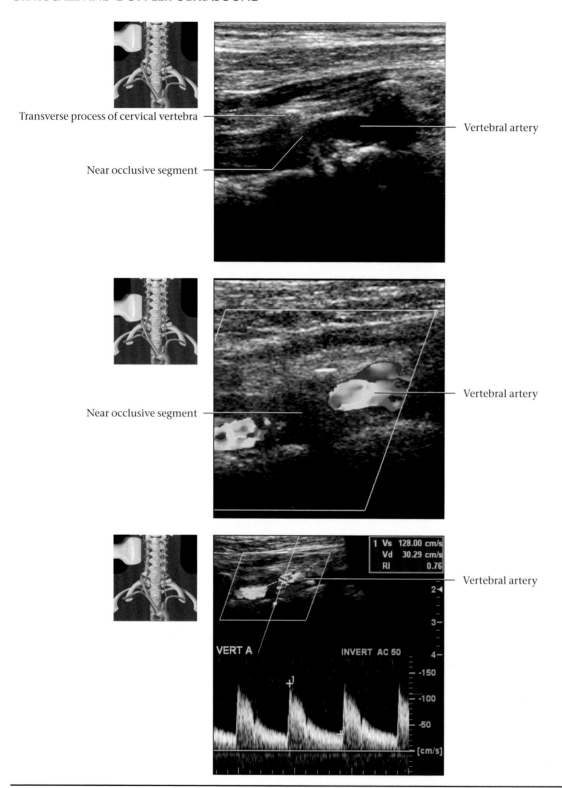

(Top) Longitudinal grayscale ultrasound of the V2 segment of the vertebral artery shows the presence of hypoechoic atherosclerotic plaque, causing near complete occlusion. *(Middle)* Color Doppler ultrasound of the vertebral artery (same patient) shows a lack of arterial color flow within the nearly occluded segment. *(Bottom)* Spectral Doppler ultrasound (same patient) shows a high-resistance flow pattern with elevated peak systolic and diastolic velocities.

GRAYSCALE AND DOPPLER ULTRASOUND

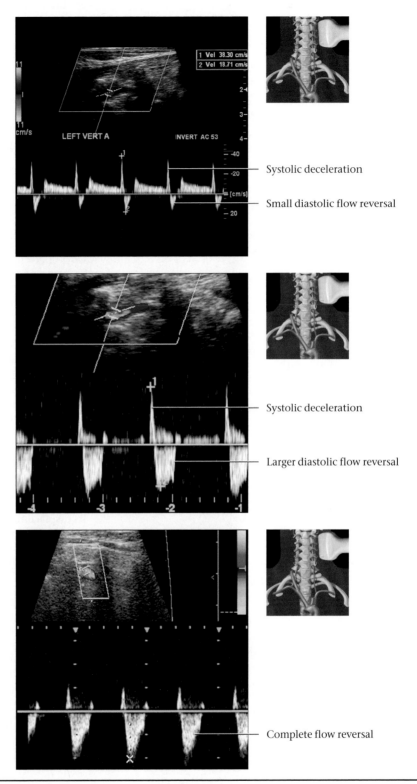

Systolic deceleration

Small diastolic flow reversal

Systolic deceleration

Larger diastolic flow reversal

Complete flow reversal

(Top) Spectral Doppler ultrasound shows a mild degree of subclavian steal syndrome. There is systolic deceleration of the vertebral flow in an antegrade direction with small diastolic flow reversal. *(Middle)* Spectral Doppler ultrasound shows a moderate degree of subclavian steal syndrome. The degree of systolic deceleration and diastolic flow reversal is more pronounced with alternating vertebral flow demonstrated. *(Bottom)* Spectral Doppler ultrasound shows severe subclavian steal syndrome. There is near complete reversal of flow in the vertebral artery with relative absent antegrade systolic flow. This pattern is commonly associated with the occurrence of vertebrobasilar symptoms.

NECK VEINS

TERMINOLOGY

Abbreviations
- Internal jugular vein (IJV)
- External jugular vein (EJV)
- Retromandibular vein (RMV)

GROSS ANATOMY

Overview
- Major extracranial venous system composed of facial veins, neck veins, scalp, skull (diploic), and orbital veins
- Facial veins
  - Facial vein
    - Begins at angle between eye, nose
    - Descends across masseter, curves around mandible
    - Joins IJV at hyoid level
    - Tributaries from orbit (supraorbital, superior ophthalmic veins), lips, jaw, facial muscles
  - Deep facial vein
    - Receives tributaries from deep face, connects facial vein with pterygoid plexus
  - Pterygoid plexus
    - Network of vascular channels in masticator space between temporalis/lateral pterygoid muscles
    - Connects cavernous sinuses and clival venous plexus to face/orbit tributaries
    - Drains into maxillary vein
  - RMV
    - Formed from union of maxillary and superficial temporal veins
    - Lies within parotid space
    - Passes between external carotid artery (ECA) and CN7 to empty into IJV
- Neck veins
  - EJV
    - From union of retromandibular and posterior auricular veins
    - Courses inferiorly on surface of sternocleidomastoid muscle
    - Drains into subclavian vein in supraclavicular fossa
    - Receives tributaries from scalp, ear, and face
    - Size, extent highly variable
  - IJV
    - Caudal continuation of sigmoid sinus from jugular foramen at skull base
    - Jugular bulb = dilatation at origin
    - Courses inferiorly in carotid space posterolateral to internal/common carotid arteries underneath sternocleidomastoid muscle
    - Unites with subclavian vein to form brachiocephalic vein
    - Size highly variable; significant side-to-side asymmetry common; right usually larger than left
  - Subclavian vein
    - Proximal continuation of axillary vein in thoracic inlet
    - EJV drains into subclavian vein
    - Subclavian vein joins IJV to form brachiocephalic vein
  - Vertebral venous plexus
    - Suboccipital venous plexus
    - Tributaries from basilar (clival) plexus, cervical musculature
    - Interconnects with sigmoid sinuses, cervical epidural venous plexus
    - Terminates in brachiocephalic vein

IMAGING ANATOMY

Overview
- Low pressure inside; easily compressible
  - Light probe pressure with good surface contact between transducer and skin to ensure optimal visualization
  - Use of Valsalva maneuver helps to distend major neck veins
- IJV
  - Largest vein of neck
  - Deep cervical chain lymph nodes commonly found along its course
  - Beware of thrombosis in patients with previous central venous catheterization or adjacent tumors
  - Always check for compressibility and phasicity on respiration
  - Presence of vascularity in IJV thrombosis is usually seen with a tumor thrombus rather than bland venous thrombus
- Subclavian vein
  - Accessible on USG by inferior tilting of transducer in supraclavicular fossa
  - Venous valves are present in most patients
  - Thrombosis/stenosis commonly seen in patients on chronic hemodialysis or with previous subclavian venous catheterization
- RMV
  - Serves as landmark on USG to infer position of intraparotid portion of facial nerve
  - Anterior division of RMV sandwiched between submandibular gland anteriorly and parotid tail posteriorly
    - Its displacement helps to determine origin of a mass in posterior submandibular region

ANATOMY IMAGING ISSUES

Imaging Pitfalls
- Neck veins are often overlooked, as most sonologists pay more attention to arteries than veins in neck
- Not all neck veins are readily assessed by ultrasound
  - Only large and superficial veins are clearly seen
- Asymmetric IJVs are common; 1 IJV may be many times the size of contralateral IJV
  - IJV venous varix: Extreme dilatation of IJV upon Valsalva maneuver with clinically palpable neck lump
- Slow flow within IJV may appear as low level hyperechoic intraluminal "mass"
  - May mimic IJV thrombus
  - Moving nature of echoes on real time ultrasound and sharp linear near-field interface help to distinguish artifacts from slow flow and IJV thrombus

CLINICAL IMPLICATIONS

Clinical Importance
- US safely guides needle for venous access
- Absence of respiratory phasicity is strong indicator of abnormality

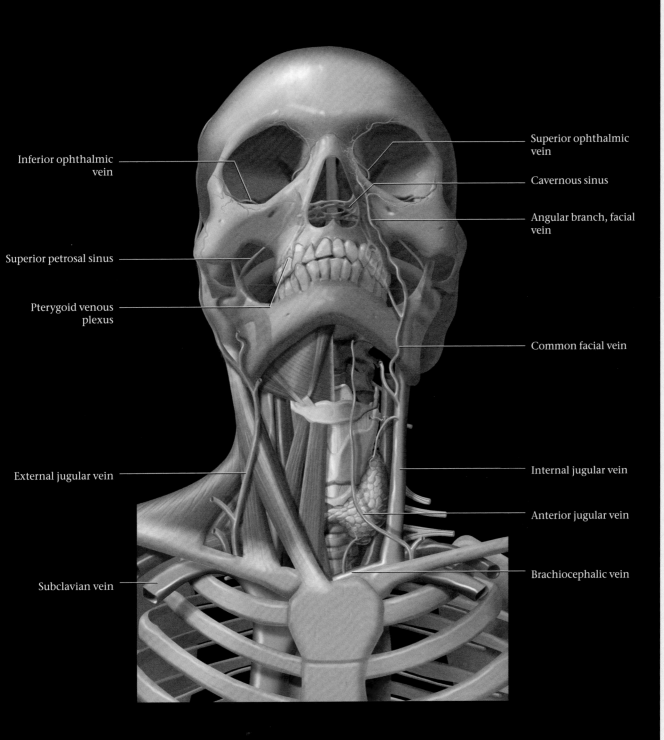

Inferior ophthalmic vein

Superior petrosal sinus

Pterygoid venous plexus

External jugular vein

Subclavian vein

Superior ophthalmic vein

Cavernous sinus

Angular branch, facial vein

Common facial vein

Internal jugular vein

Anterior jugular vein

Brachiocephalic vein

Anteroposterior view of the extracranial venous system depicts the major neck veins, their drainage into the mediastinum, and their numerous interconnections with the intracranial venous system. The pterygoid venous plexus receives tributaries from the cavernous sinus and provides an important potential source of collateral venous drainage if the transverse or sigmoid sinuses become occluded.

NECK VEINS

GRAYSCALE AND COLOR DOPPLER ULTRASOUND (IJV)

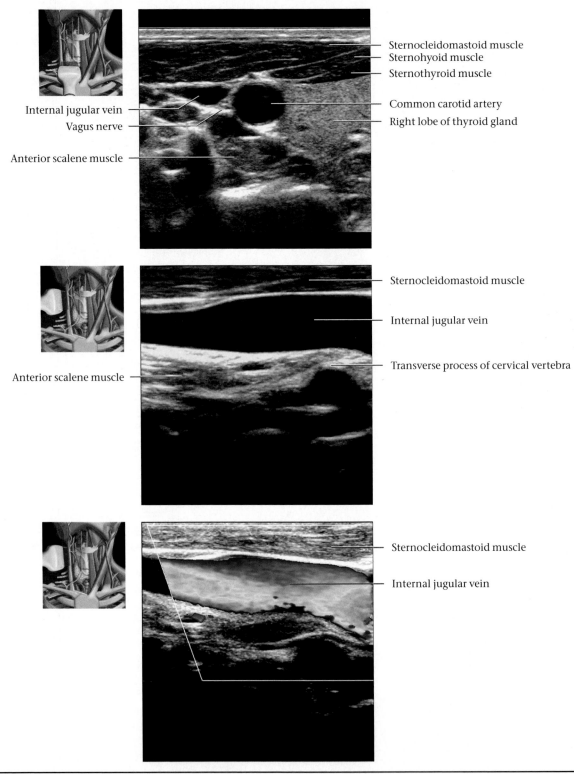

Internal jugular vein
Vagus nerve
Anterior scalene muscle

Sternocleidomastoid muscle
Sternohyoid muscle
Sternothyroid muscle
Common carotid artery
Right lobe of thyroid gland

Anterior scalene muscle

Sternocleidomastoid muscle
Internal jugular vein
Transverse process of cervical vertebra

Sternocleidomastoid muscle
Internal jugular vein

(Top) Transverse grayscale ultrasound of the lower cervical level shows the normal anatomical relationship between the internal jugular vein and the adjacent structures. It is underneath the sternocleidomastoid muscle and lateral to the common carotid artery and vagus nerve within the carotid sheath. *(Middle)* Longitudinal grayscale ultrasound shows the internal jugular vein in the midcervical level. The internal jugular vein appears as a tubular anechoic structure coursing in a vertical direction. It should be examined with light probe pressure and with compression to exclude a venous thrombosis. *(Bottom)* Corresponding color Doppler ultrasound in the longitudinal plane shows color flow filling the entire lumen of the internal jugular vein. The use of color Doppler helps to identify and evaluate the presence and nature of an IJV thrombus.

NECK VEINS

CECT AND SPECTRAL DOPPLER ULTRASOUND (IJV)

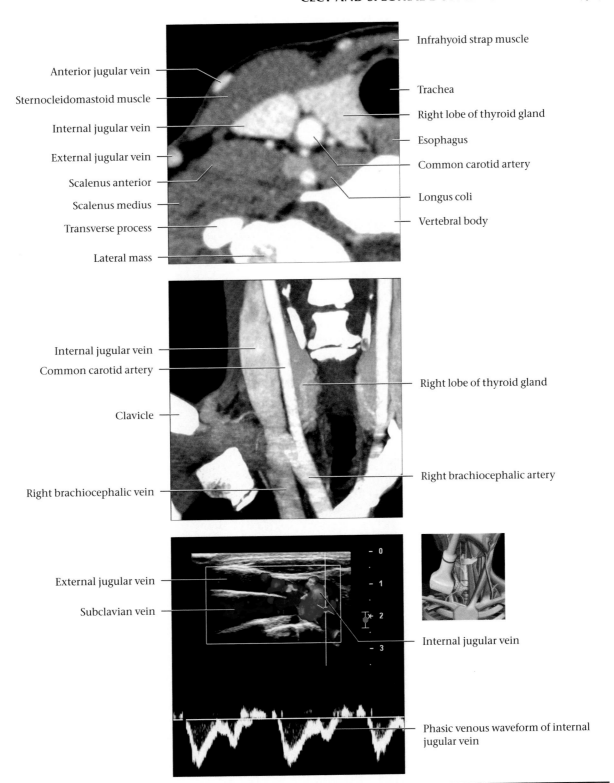

Anterior jugular vein

Sternocleidomastoid muscle

Internal jugular vein

External jugular vein

Scalenus anterior

Scalenus medius

Transverse process

Lateral mass

Infrahyoid strap muscle

Trachea

Right lobe of thyroid gland

Esophagus

Common carotid artery

Longus coli

Vertebral body

Internal jugular vein

Common carotid artery

Clavicle

Right brachiocephalic vein

Right lobe of thyroid gland

Right brachiocephalic artery

External jugular vein

Subclavian vein

Internal jugular vein

Phasic venous waveform of internal jugular vein

(Top) Axial CECT of the lower neck shows the internal jugular vein, which is usually larger than and lateral to the common carotid artery. The external jugular vein is in a subcutaneous location. *(Middle)* Coronal reformatted CECT of the lower neck shows the close anatomical relationship of the internal jugular vein and common carotid artery within the carotid sheath. The internal jugular vein continues inferiorly below the clavicle to join the subclavian vein to form the brachiocephalic vein. *(Bottom)* Transverse spectral Doppler ultrasound shows the internal jugular vein at the level of the supraclavicular fossa at the junction with the subclavian vein. The normal biphasic venous waveform, which varies with respiratory motion, can be easily demonstrated and helps to exclude the presence of obstructing venous thrombus.

GRAYSCALE AND COLOR DOPPLER ULTRASOUND (EJV)

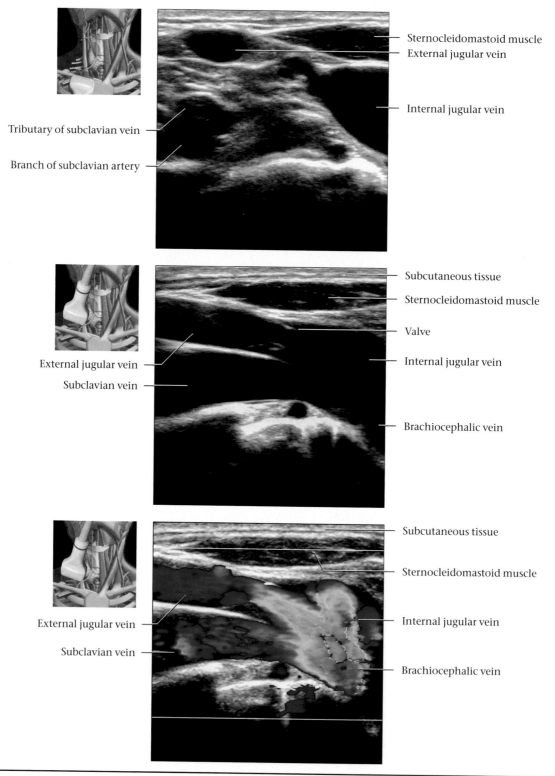

Sternocleidomastoid muscle
External jugular vein

Internal jugular vein

Tributary of subclavian vein

Branch of subclavian artery

Subcutaneous tissue

Sternocleidomastoid muscle

Valve

External jugular vein

Subclavian vein

Internal jugular vein

Brachiocephalic vein

Subcutaneous tissue

Sternocleidomastoid muscle

External jugular vein

Internal jugular vein

Subclavian vein

Brachiocephalic vein

(Top) Transverse grayscale ultrasound of right lower neck shows the location of the external jugular vein in relation to the sternocleidomastoid muscle. It appears as a distended, round, anechoic structure on Valsalva maneuver using light transducer pressure. *(Middle)* Transverse grayscale ultrasound shows the external jugular vein at the supraclavicular level, at the site of union with the subclavian vein, close to the terminal portion of the internal jugular vein. Valve leaflets are commonly seen within the major veins at the thoracic inlet level. *(Bottom)* Corresponding transverse color Doppler ultrasound at the supraclavicular level helps to depict the venous drainage of the external jugular vein to the subclavian vein. Note that the subclavian vein joins the internal jugular vein to form the brachiocephalic vein.

CECT AND SPECTRAL DOPPLER ULTRASOUND (EJV)

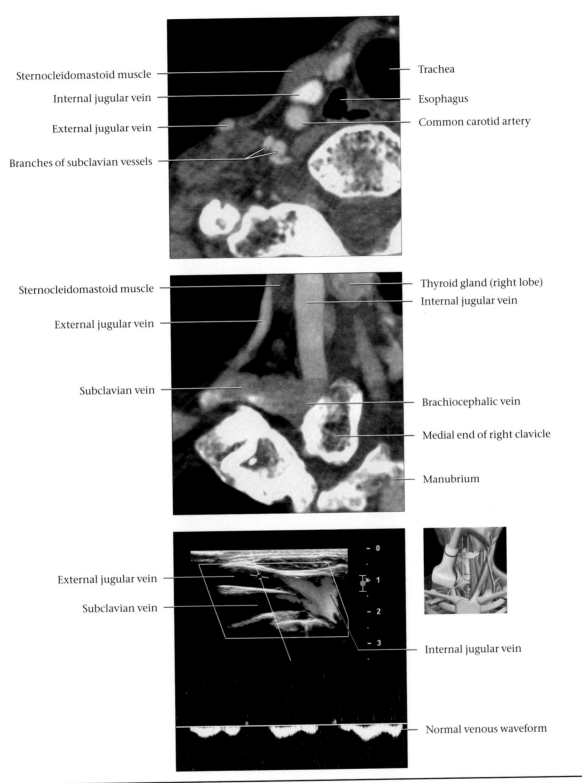

Sternocleidomastoid muscle

Internal jugular vein

External jugular vein

Branches of subclavian vessels

Trachea

Esophagus

Common carotid artery

Sternocleidomastoid muscle

External jugular vein

Subclavian vein

Thyroid gland (right lobe)

Internal jugular vein

Brachiocephalic vein

Medial end of right clavicle

Manubrium

External jugular vein

Subclavian vein

Internal jugular vein

Normal venous waveform

(Top) Axial CECT shows the right lower neck. Note the superficial anatomical location of the external jugular vein. Thus, light probe pressure is necessary for the assessment of the external jugular vein on ultrasound, because with increasing pressure, the vein will be compressed. *(Middle)* Coronal reformatted CECT shows the right lower neck. Note the drainage of the external jugular vein to the subclavian vein, which joins the IJV to form the brachiocephalic vein at the thoracic inlet level. *(Bottom)* Spectral Doppler ultrasound interrogating the terminal portion of the external jugular vein shows a normal, phasic, low-pressure venous waveform, which helps to confirm its patency.

NECK VEINS

LONGITUDINAL AND TRANSVERSE ULTRASOUND

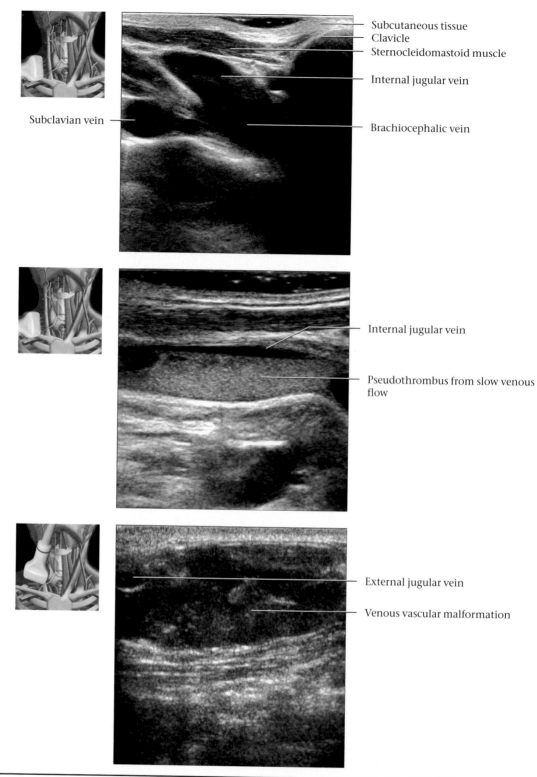

Subcutaneous tissue

Clavicle

Sternocleidomastoid muscle

Internal jugular vein

Subclavian vein

Brachiocephalic vein

Internal jugular vein

Pseudothrombus from slow venous flow

External jugular vein

Venous vascular malformation

(Top) Longitudinal grayscale ultrasound at the supraclavicular level shows the union of internal jugular vein and subclavian vein to form the brachiocephalic vein. The more distal portion of the brachiocephalic vein is obscured by the overlying clavicle, and is therefore, not assessed by ultrasound. *(Middle)* Longitudinal grayscale ultrasound of the right internal jugular vein shows a pseudothrombus phenomenon due to slow venous flow within the internal jugular vein. Note the layering with sharp linear border in the IJV lumen in the near field, which is the clue to distinguish it from venous thrombus. *(Bottom)* Transverse grayscale ultrasound of the right posterior triangle shows a well-defined hypoechoic mass with multiple internal sinusoidal spaces. The lesion is inseparable from the external jugular vein. Surgery confirmed a venous vascular malformation arising from the external jugular vein.

NECK VEINS

CECT, COLOR AND POWER DOPPLER ULTRASOUND

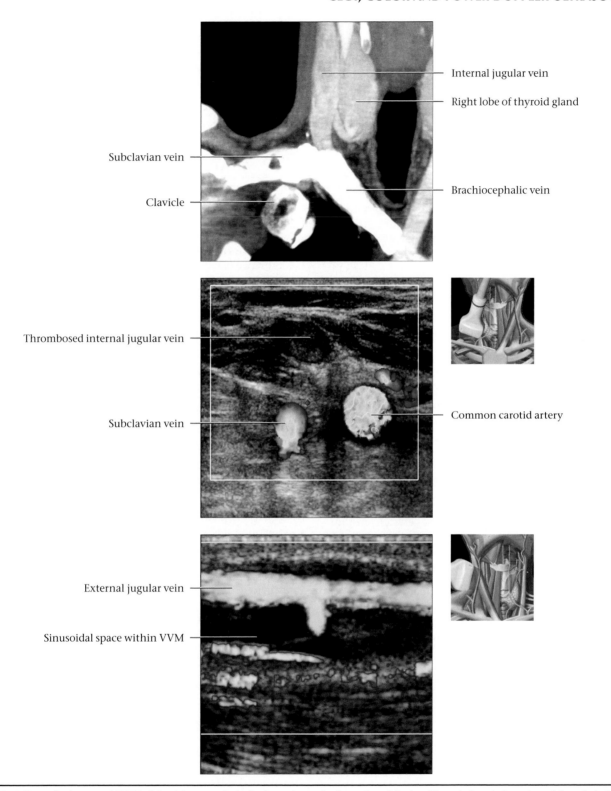

Internal jugular vein

Right lobe of thyroid gland

Subclavian vein

Brachiocephalic vein

Clavicle

Thrombosed internal jugular vein

Subclavian vein

Common carotid artery

External jugular vein

Sinusoidal space within VVM

(Top) Coronal reformatted CECT of the right supraclavicular fossa shows the formation of the brachiocephalic vein by union of the subclavian vein (dense contrast filling due to injection in ipsilateral antecubital fossa) and internal jugular vein. The brachiocephalic vein can be fully assessed on CECT as compared with ultrasound. *(Middle)* Transverse color Doppler ultrasound of the right supraclavicular level reveals intraluminal, hypoechoic, avascular echoes causing occlusion of the internal jugular vein. The appearances are of a bland venous thrombus due to prolonged central venous catheterization. *(Bottom)* Longitudinal power Doppler ultrasound shows the external jugular vein venous vascular malformation (VVM). Note the intimate relationship of the VVM and the external jugular vein. Sinusoidal spaces are usually not color filled due to very slow flow within.

CERVICAL LYMPH NODES

TERMINOLOGY

Synonyms

- Internal jugular chain (IJC): Deep cervical chain
- Spinal accessory chain (SAC): Posterior triangle chain
- Transverse cervical chain: Supraclavicular chain
- Anterior cervical chain: Prelaryngeal, pretracheal, paratracheal nodes
- Paratracheal node: Recurrent laryngeal node

Definitions

- Jugulodigastric node: "Sentinel" (highest) node, found at apex of IJC at angle of mandible
- Virchow node: "Signal" node, lowest node of deep cervical chain
- Troisier node: Most medial node of transverse cervical chain
- Omohyoid node: Deep cervical chain node superior to omohyoid as it crosses jugular vein
- Delphian node: Pretracheal node

IMAGING ANATOMY

Overview

- In normal adult neck there may be up to 300 lymph nodes
  - Small, oval/reniform shape
  - Internal structures: Capsule, cortex, medulla, hilum
- USG appearances of normal cervical lymph node
  - Small ovoid shape
  - Well-defined margin
  - Homogeneous hypoechoic cortex with echogenic hilus
  - Hilar vascularity on color/power Doppler examination
- Imaging-based nodal classification
  - Level I: Submental and submandibular nodes
    - Level IA: Submental nodes: Found between anterior bellies of digastric muscles
    - Level IB: Submandibular nodes: Found around submandibular glands in submandibular space
  - Level II: Upper IJC nodes: From posterior belly of digastric muscle to hyoid bone
    - Level IIA: Level II node anterior, medial, lateral or posterior to IJV; if posterior to IJV, node must be inseparable from IJV; contains jugulodigastric nodal group
    - Level IIB: Level II node posterior to IJV with fat plane visible between node and IJV
  - Level III: Mid IJC nodes
    - From hyoid bone to inferior margin of cricoid cartilage
  - Level IV: Lower IJC nodes
    - From inferior cricoid margin to clavicle
  - Level V: Nodes of posterior cervical space/spinal accessory chain
    - SAC nodes lie posterior to back margin of sternocleidomastoid muscle
    - Level VA: Upper SAC nodes from skull base to bottom of cricoid cartilage
    - Level VB: Lower SAC nodes from cricoid to clavicle
  - Level VI: Nodes of visceral space
    - Found from hyoid bone above to top of manubrium below
    - Midline group of cervical lymph nodes
    - Includes prelaryngeal, pretracheal, and paratracheal subgroups
  - Level VII: Superior mediastinal nodes
    - Between carotid arteries from top of manubrium above to innominate vein below
- Other nodal groups not included in standard imaging-based nodal classification
  - Parotid nodal group: Intraglandular or extraglandular
  - Retropharyngeal (RPS) nodal group: Medial RPS nodes and lateral RPS nodes (Rouviere node)
  - Facial nodal group

ANATOMY IMAGING ISSUES

Questions

- Useful USG features suspicious of malignancy
  - Shape: Round, long:short axis ratio < 2
  - Loss of echogenic hilus
  - Presence of intranodal necrosis (cystic/coagulation)
  - Presence of extracapsular spread: Ill-defined margin
  - Peripheral/subcapsular flow on color/power Doppler ultrasound
  - Increased intranodal intravascular resistance: Resistive index (RI) > 0.8, pulsatility index (PI) > 1.6
  - Internal architecture: Punctate calcifications in metastatic node from papillary thyroid carcinoma, reticulated/pseudocystic appearance of lymphomatous node
- No single finding is sensitive or specific enough; these signs should be used in combination
- FNAC helps to improve diagnostic accuracy
- Tuberculous nodes mimic metastatic nodes
  - Differentiating features: Intranodal necrosis, nodal matting, soft tissue edema and displaced hilar vascularity/avascularity, calcification (post treatment)

Imaging Approaches

- Nodal metastases from primary tumors are site specific; therefore, it is critical to understand usual patterns of lymphatic spread
- Equivocal nodes outside usual pattern are less suspicious
- Likely location of primary tumor can be suspected in patients presenting with nodal mass
- Nodal disease outside usual pattern may suggest aggressive tumor or prompt search for 2nd primary

Imaging Pitfalls

- Retropharyngeal (RPS) nodes and superior mediastinal nodes cannot be assessed by USG

CLINICAL IMPLICATIONS

Clinical Importance

- Presence of malignant SCCa nodes on staging are associated with 50% ↓ in long-term survival
  - If extranodal spread present, further 50% ↓
- Location of metastatic nodes in neck may help predict site of primary tumor
  - RPS and posterior triangle nodes seen in NPC, and lower cervical nodes in lung cancer
  - When Virchow node is found on imaging without upper neck nodes, primary is not in neck, and whole body imaging is warranted

GRAPHICS

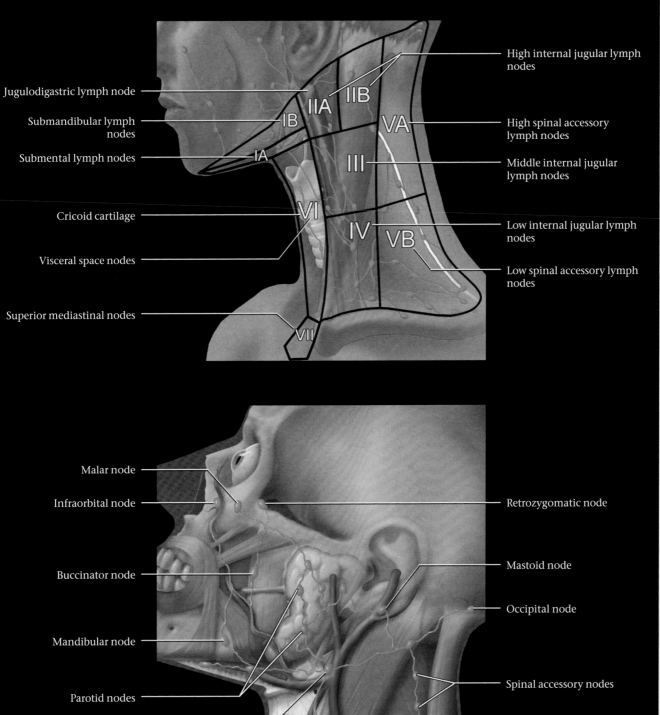

Jugulodigastric lymph node

Submandibular lymph nodes

Submental lymph nodes

Cricoid cartilage

Visceral space nodes

Superior mediastinal nodes

High internal jugular lymph nodes

High spinal accessory lymph nodes

Middle internal jugular lymph nodes

Low internal jugular lymph nodes

Low spinal accessory lymph nodes

Malar node

Infraorbital node

Buccinator node

Mandibular node

Parotid nodes

Jugulodigastric node

Retrozygomatic node

Mastoid node

Occipital node

Spinal accessory nodes

(Top) Lateral oblique graphic of the neck shows the anatomic locations for the major nodal groups of the neck. Division of the internal jugular nodal chain into high, middle, and low regions is defined by the level of the hyoid bone and cricoid cartilage. Similarly, the spinal accessory nodal chain is divided into high and low regions by the level of the cricoid cartilage. *(Bottom)* Lateral view shows facial nodes plus parotid nodes. None of these nodes bear level numbers but instead must be described by their anatomic location. Note that the internal jugular chain (IJC) is the final common pathway for all lymphatics of the upper aerodigestive tract and neck.

CERVICAL LYMPH NODES

TRANSVERSE AND LONGITUDINAL ULTRASOUND AND PATHOLOGY

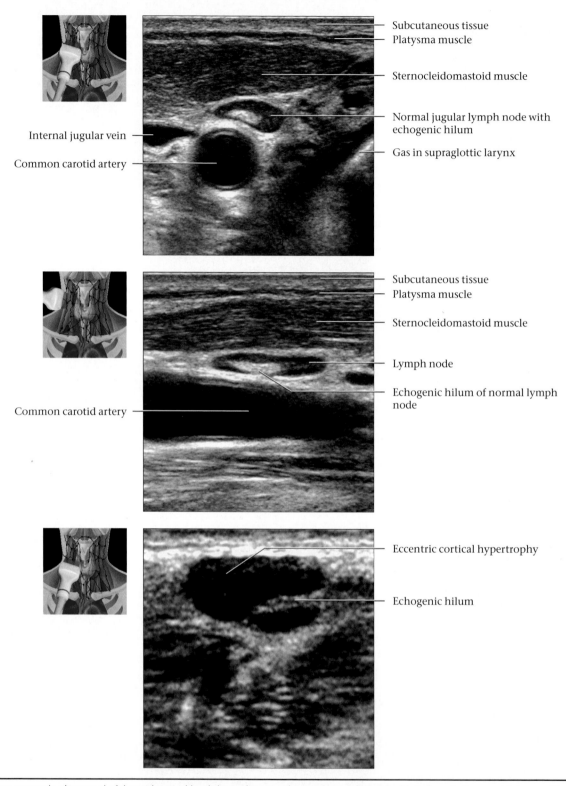

Subcutaneous tissue
Platysma muscle

Sternocleidomastoid muscle

Normal jugular lymph node with echogenic hilum

Gas in supraglottic larynx

Internal jugular vein

Common carotid artery

Subcutaneous tissue
Platysma muscle

Sternocleidomastoid muscle

Lymph node

Echogenic hilum of normal lymph node

Common carotid artery

Eccentric cortical hypertrophy

Echogenic hilum

(**Top**) Transverse grayscale ultrasound of the midcervical level shows the normal appearance of a cervical lymph node (i.e., ovoid shape with echogenic hilum). It is commonly found anterior to the carotid artery/internal jugular vein. (**Middle**) Longitudinal grayscale ultrasound of the midcervical level shows a normal elliptical hypoechoic lymph node with echogenic hilum anterior to the common carotid artery. (**Bottom**) Transverse grayscale ultrasound shows a reactive lymph node. It is mildly enlarged with cortical hypertrophy and preserved echogenic hilum. Note that with high-resolution ultrasound, the jugulodigastric node and other nodes in the jugular chain and accessory chain are invariably seen.

CERVICAL LYMPH NODES

POWER DOPPLER ULTRASOUND AND PATHOLOGY

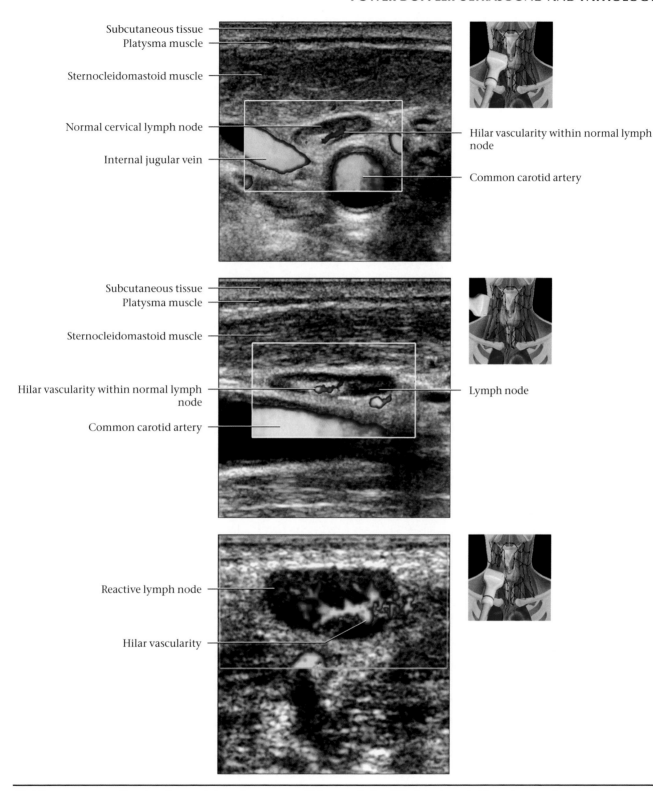

Subcutaneous tissue
Platysma muscle
Sternocleidomastoid muscle
Normal cervical lymph node
Internal jugular vein

Hilar vascularity within normal lymph node
Common carotid artery

Subcutaneous tissue
Platysma muscle
Sternocleidomastoid muscle
Hilar vascularity within normal lymph node
Common carotid artery

Lymph node

Reactive lymph node
Hilar vascularity

(Top) Transverse power Doppler ultrasound shows the presence of hilar vascularity within the echogenic hilum of a normal cervical lymph node. (Middle) Longitudinal power Doppler ultrasound shows hilar vascularity within the echogenic hilum of a normal cervical lymph node. The presence of echogenic hilum and hilar vascularity are good signs of cervical lymph node benignity. (Bottom) Transverse power Doppler ultrasound shows mild increase but preserved hilar vascularity in a reactive lymph node. Newer high-resolution transducers readily demonstrate nodal vascularity, both normal and abnormal.

CERVICAL LYMPH NODES

PATHOLOGY

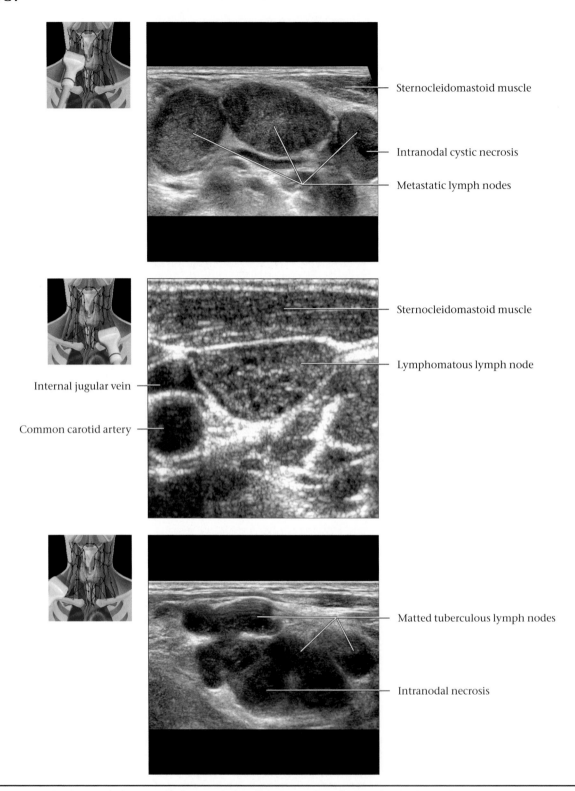

Sternocleidomastoid muscle

Intranodal cystic necrosis

Metastatic lymph nodes

Sternocleidomastoid muscle

Lymphomatous lymph node

Internal jugular vein

Common carotid artery

Matted tuberculous lymph nodes

Intranodal necrosis

(Top) Transverse grayscale ultrasound of upper neck shows multiple enlarged, round, predominantly solid, hypoechoic lymph nodes. Patient has known history of H&N cancer. Overall features are consistent with metastatic nodes. Presence of intranodal cystic necrosis, in patient with known primary malignancy, is indicative of the metastatic nature of lymph nodes. *(Middle)* Transverse grayscale ultrasound of a lymphomatous lymph node in mid deep jugular chain demonstrates the typical reticulated echo pattern. *(Bottom)* Transverse grayscale ultrasound shows multiple, matted, enlarged, heterogeneous, hypoechoic lymph nodes in the posterior triangle. Some of them demonstrate intranodal necrosis. A mild degree of edema is noted in the adjacent soft tissue. Features are compatible with tuberculous lymphadenitis.

CERVICAL LYMPH NODES

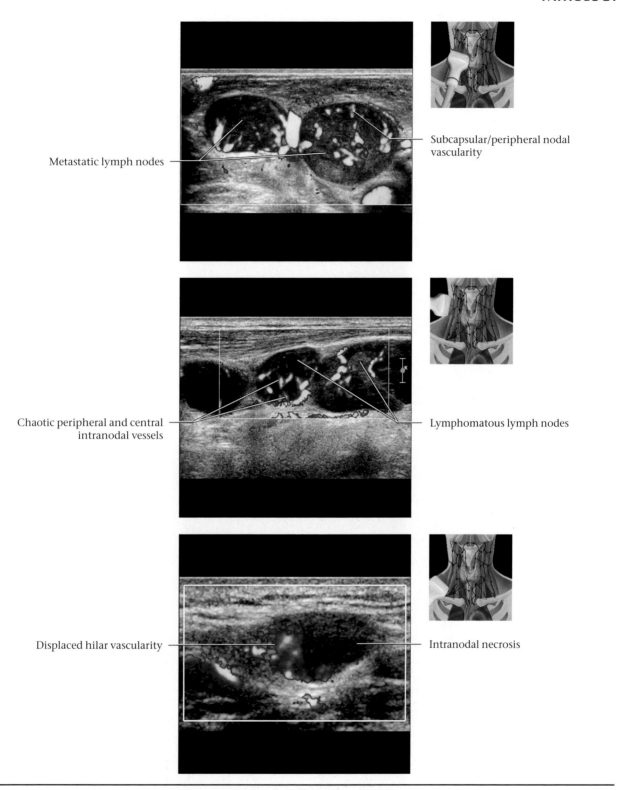

Metastatic lymph nodes

Subcapsular/peripheral nodal vascularity

Chaotic peripheral and central intranodal vessels

Lymphomatous lymph nodes

Displaced hilar vascularity

Intranodal necrosis

(Top) Transverse power Doppler ultrasound shows multiple subcapsular/peripheral intranodal vessels in multiple round, hypoechoic, solid lymph nodes at the upper cervical level. Pathology confirmed metastatic squamous cell carcinoma. *(Middle)* Longitudinal power Doppler ultrasound of multiple lymphomatous lymph nodes shows chaotic peripheral and central intranodal vessels. Note that hilar vascularity is more prominent than peripheral vascularity. *(Bottom)* Transverse power Doppler ultrasound shows a tuberculous lymph node in posterior triangle that is predominantly hypovascular with displaced hilar vascularity. The hypovascular portion corresponds to intranodal caseating necrosis.

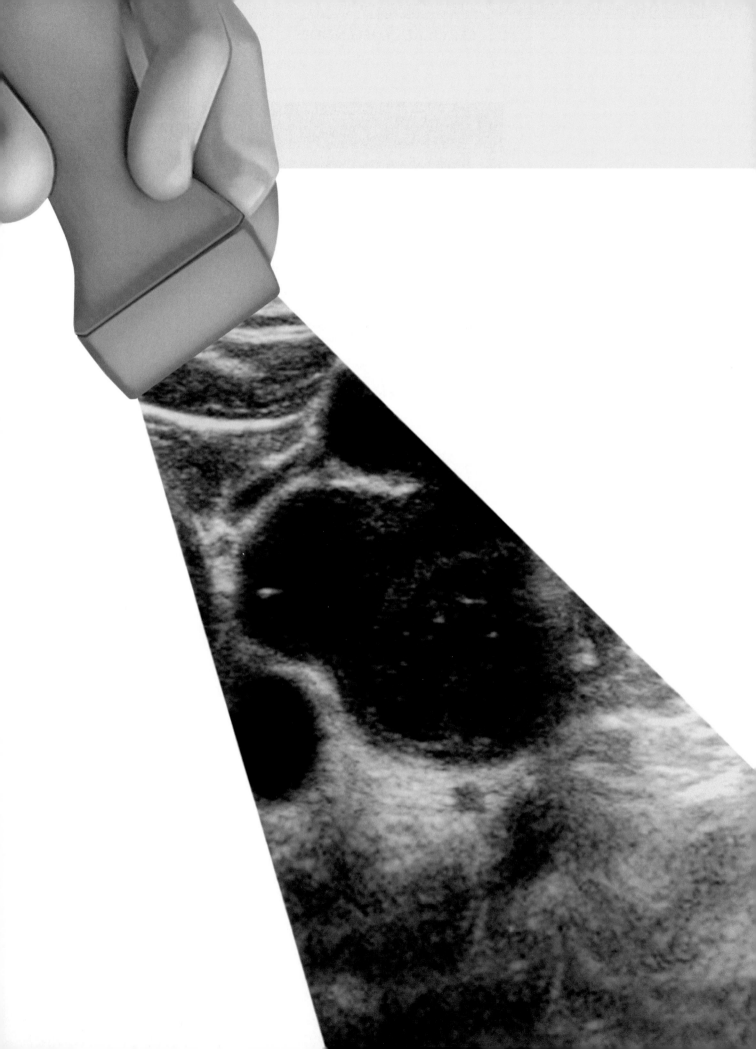

SECTION 1
Introduction and Overview

Introduction

Summary Thoughts: US in Head & Neck

In routine clinical practice, the major role of US in head & neck (H&N) is evaluating the thyroid gland and neck lymph nodes and differentiating them from miscellaneous lumps in the neck, salivary glands, and parathyroid gland. The superficial location of these structures makes them ideally suited to interrogation by high-resolution US, which is nonionizing in nature, readily available, and relatively inexpensive. Its high resolution makes it sensitive in detecting small abnormalities in H&N but at a cost of specificity. This is easily overcome by combining US with guided fine-needle aspiration cytology (FNAC), which increases the diagnostic accuracy. Therefore, in H&N, US is routinely combined with FNAC to identify lesions, characterize their nature, follow-up benign disease, and, in surveillance, detect potential complications and adverse sequelae. US portability has extended its use outside of radiology departments, and US is now extensively used by surgeons and endocrinologists in office-based settings to obtain relevant information quickly for patient management.

Does US with FNAC stand alone in assessment of H&N abnormalities? How does US complement CT, MR, and PET/CT, and vice versa? These are questions addressed daily in routine clinical practice by sonologists, radiologists, and clinicians practicing US. The use of imaging modalities is dependent on clinical indications and the organ being imaged. In H&N, the thyroid gland is by far the most common organ interrogated by US, and often, US is the only imaging modality required to adequately assess any abnormality. However, even in the thyroid, US does have limitations that are also applicable to other structures in the H&N, and these are inherent to US. For large lesions, US may be unable to evaluate their entire extent and involvement of adjacent structures. For others, US may be limited by deep location/multiplicity of lesions and attenuation of US by air and bone. For example, US may be unable to adequately assess extrathyroid extension of tumor and involvement of the trachea, esophagus, etc. for large thyroid tumors. In evaluating salivary glands, US cannot evaluate the deep lobe of the parotid gland, extrasalivary/parapharyngeal extent of tumor, or perineural involvement. For lymph nodes, in addition to not being able to assess many primary H&N cancers, US cannot evaluate retropharyngeal, oropharyngeal, or mediastinal lymphadenopathy that may be associated with H&N disease.

In addition to meticulous attention to technique and robust protocol, to perform high-quality diagnostic neck US, the sonologist must be familiar with

- Anatomy, known nodal draining sites of common H&N cancers, and location of head and neck masses, as these are site specific
- Limitations of US for evaluating extent of large masses, ectopic parathyroid, deep lobe of the parotid gland, and in the postoperative neck
- Guided biopsy/treatment techniques
- Use of CT, MR, and PET/CT, and imaging appearances of H&N abnormalities

Sonographic Evaluation of Lesions

Grayscale US

Evaluates size, shape, extent, margins, echogenicity, internal architecture (homogeneous/heterogeneous, ± cystic change, calcification), and location.

Size of a lesion alone is a poor predictor of its nature. Serial increase in size may be more useful in identifying malignant lesions in thyroid, salivary glands, and lymph nodes.

Malignant lymph nodes tend to be round in **shape** whereas benign nodes are usually elliptical. However, one must bear in mind that normal submandibular nodes may also be round in shape. Nerve sheath tumors may be fusiform, and malignant thyroid nodules taller than wide, but otherwise, shape has a limited role in predicting the nature of H&N lesions.

Margins are a good indicator of benignity/malignancy for thyroid and salivary gland lesions. Malignant lesions tend to be ill defined/infiltrative/spiculated whereas benign lesions are usually well defined; however, the opposite is the case for lymph nodes. Benign nodes tend to be ill defined as they excite periadenitis, thus blurring the borders of the node. The presence of ill-defined margins in an otherwise malignant node is a good indicator of extracapsular spread, a poor prognostic indicator.

Echogenicity of lesions may be compared to adjacent glandular parenchyma or other structures, usually muscle. In the thyroid gland, probability of malignancy ↓ as echogenicity of lesion ↑. Malignant nodes also tend to be hypoechoic except for metastatic nodes from thyroid papillary carcinoma, which are hyperechoic. Most salivary lesions are hypoechoic compared to adjacent salivary parenchyma, whereas neck lumps have variable echogenicity.

Internal echogenicity often helps to predict the nature of a lesion. Malignant lesions in thyroid and salivary glands tend to be heterogeneous, and metastatic nodes from SCCa, TB, and papillary thyroid cancers often show cystic change. Absence of hilar architecture is usually seen in malignant nodes but may be preserved in smaller nodes where the medullary sinuses are uninvolved by tumor cells. Punctate calcification is seen in thyroid papillary carcinoma and its metastatic nodes, whereas coarse calcification may be seen in benign multinodular thyroid, thyroid medullary cancer and its metastatic node and post-treatment TB nodes, and curvilinear calcification in venous vascular malformations (representing phleboliths).

Location of the lesion is also a good predictor of its nature, particularly as metastatic nodes in H&N have a known distribution (dependent on location of primary tumor) and neck masses are site-specific. Location of dermoid/epidermoid, thyroglossal duct cysts, branchial cysts, carotid paraganglioma, vagus/sympathetic schwannoma, ranula, etc. are anatomically/embryologically determined, and this aids in their identification.

Are there any grayscale features that are accurate predictors of the lesion's nature? In the thyroid, the presence of a solid, hypoechoic, ill-defined, heterogeneous, taller than wide nodule with fine echogenic calcification would be diagnostic of thyroid papillary carcinoma. On the other hand, spongiform appearance (aggregate of microcystic components in >

50% of nodule volume) and presence of "comet tail" artifact would be indicative of benign disease. Similarly, reticulated node and pseudocystic appearance of lymph node would suggest lymphoma and nodal matting, and soft tissue edema and intranodal necrosis will indicate TB. Continuation with vagus nerve and brachial plexus would identify vagal/brachial plexus schwannoma, and a striped/feathered appearance will confirm a lipoma. Presence of cystic septate spaces in a trans-spatial mass would indicate lymphatic malformation, and slow "to and fro" motion in a cystic septate nodule, ± curvilinear calcification, would suggest a VVM. Therefore, during real-time scanning, one is constantly mentally computing these signs to arrive at a specific diagnosis/differential diagnosis, and in many of the cases, FNAC then acts only as a confirmatory tool.

Doppler US ± Contrast

Assesses presence/absence of intralesional vascularity, distribution, intravascular resistance, flow velocities, and enhancement patterns and curves. In addition to distribution of vascularity, color flow Doppler also assesses flow velocity, direction, and intravascular resistance whereas power Doppler does not provide any information regarding flow direction. However, power Doppler is more sensitive in detecting presence/absence of flow and hence delineating its distribution, which is important in delineating benign from malignant lesions in thyroid and lymph nodes (limited for salivary lesions where the vascularity is variable). Therefore, power Doppler is preferred over color Doppler in evaluating intralesional vascularity in H&N.

Vascular distribution in thyroid gland: Most benign nodules have perinodular > intranodular vascularity, whereas malignant nodules have intranodular > perinodular vascularity. One must bear in mind, however, that a percentage of solid, nonhypervascular nodules may also be malignant. In nodules with follicular biopsy, assessment of intranodular vascularity is important, as follicular nodules with no/sparse intranodular flow have a 3% probability of cancer rather than 15-20% in unselected follicular nodules, whereas vascular follicular nodules have 50% probability of malignancy.

Vascular distribution in lymph nodes: With modern transducers, most (90%) nodes > 5 mm will demonstrate intranodular vascularity. Benign nodes tend to have hilar/central vascularity, whereas malignant nodes have peripheral vascularity (as angiogenesis induces vascular recruitment into periphery of nodes). Metastatic nodes may have a combination of hilar + peripheral vascularity (peripheral > hilar vascularity) in nodes where the medullary sinuses/hilar vessels are yet uninvolved. Lymphomatous nodes also have both hilar and peripheral vascularity (hilar > peripheral). Tuberculous nodes have areas of cystic necrosis/endarteritis, and these may appear avascular with hilar vessels being displaced by necrosis.

Vascularity in neck lumps and parathyroid: Parathyroid adenomas tend to show a single vessel within, which may ramify within the adenoma. VVMs often have very slow flow, which is better seen on grayscale rather than Doppler, and remaining common cystic H&N lesions other than pseudoaneurysms do not show significant vascularity. Carotid body paragangliomas show marked intralesional vascularity, whereas the presence of vascularity within nerve sheath tumors is variable.

Vascular resistance: Malignant lesions tend to have lower intravascular resistance, resistive index < 0.8 (1 for salivary lesions) and pulsatility index > 1.6 (2 for salivary lesions); however, its diagnostic accuracy may be limited, and estimating such parameters in tiny vessels is time consuming and difficult and is therefore not performed in routine clinical practice.

Elastography (Elasticity Imaging)

Evaluates firmness of tissues by measuring and displaying their displacements in response to a stimulus. Elasticity imaging (EI) can be performed using sonography, and tissue stimulation is achieved either by freehand compression, endogenous stimuli such as arterial pulsations, or focused pulses of US produced by a modified US transducer. US EI currently falls into 2 main types

- **Strain EI** calculates relative tissue strain, produces qualitative output as color-coded maps, and allows semiquantitative estimation of strain ratios for regions of interest defined by the operator. Firmer tissues displace less, hence display lower strain than soft tissues for a given stimulus
- **Shear wave elastography (SWE)** measures and maps the velocities of a specific type of tissue displacement (shear waves), which is increased in firmer tissues. From this data, tissue elasticity (elastic modulus) can be quantitatively estimated

Both EI methods can produce color-coded maps called elastograms in real time, which are usually overlaid as a partial transparency onto corresponding grayscale images during US examinations.

EI is currently undergoing intense scientific evaluation for tissue characterization in the body, although presently remains a research application in H&N. In general, malignant lesions tend to be firm, equating to lower strain or higher elastic modulus, whereas benign lesions are usually soft. Evidence from small studies is accumulating, which suggest high accuracies of EI in distinguishing papillary thyroid cancers from benign thyroid nodules and for discriminating metastatic from benign lymph nodes; however, its consistent reproducibility remains elusive. Its utility for other types of thyroid nodule, salivary masses, and neck lumps is less clear. Issues pertaining to standardization of EI technique, reproducibility, operator dependence, elastographic artifacts, and diagnostic performance, either in isolation &/or combined with conventional US, still need to be addressed in larger studies before EI can be used in routine practice.

No single sonographic feature is diagnostic. In routine clinical practice, a combination of features that includes grayscale and Doppler (± EI) helps in characterizing nature of abnormality.

Clinical Implications

Questions

The most common indication for H&N US is to evaluate thyroid gland, particularly multinodular thyroid (MNT). It is in the thyroid gland where US stands far superior to other modalities and is unquestionably the imaging modality of choice, particularly in evaluating thyroid nodules, and readily answers queries crucial to patient management.

Although prevalent in the community, the incidence of malignancy in MNT remains low; therefore, what is the role of US in MNT, particularly when the common thinking is that MNT confers

benignity? With the use of modern high-resolution transducers, one invariably detects multiple thyroid nodules, and presence of a solitary thyroid nodule is unusual. Therefore, on US, most cancers are detected against a background of MNT, and literature indicates that patients with multiple nodules have the same risk of cancer as those with single nodules. US identifies any suspicious nodule (solid, hypoechoic, ill-defined, taller than wide, punctate calcification, prominent intranodular vascularity) and guides confirmatory FNAC. In addition, US assesses local spread and metastatic adenopathy.

This raises the next question: **In absence of any suspicious nodule in MNT, does one need to biopsy, and if so, how is the nodule chosen?** In many centers, if there are no obvious suspicious nodules on US in a patient with MNT, no FNAC is done, and follow-up scans may be recommended. However, in extremely apprehensive patients, one may consider FNAC on a dominant nodule to reassure the patient. In others, large cystic nodules may be aspirated for cosmetic reasons.

If follow-up is recommended for FNAC proven benign nodules, when and how often should it be done? The recommendations for this are variable, but it is commonly agreed that follow-up scans may be done 6 months later (3-18 months), ± FNAC, and once a year thereafter. However, large nodules that have appeared suddenly or grown in size recently need to be followed up earlier, ± FNAC.

Does US have any role in evaluation of autoimmune thyroid disease (AITD)? Often, prior to US, the diagnosis of AITD is already made based on clinical signs, symptoms, and laboratory investigations. In some patients, however, these may overlap with other chronic illnesses, and diagnosis may not be that obvious. US helps in these instances. It helps to differentiate AITD from other conditions, such as subacute thyroiditis, and also distinguishes between Graves and Hashimoto thyroiditis (based on grayscale and Doppler features).

The real-time nature of US allows the sonologist to actively seek relevant imaging information that will help the clinician in managing nonthyroid abnormalities. It is therefore imperative for the sonologist to be familiar with anatomy, pathology, and imaging appearances and treatment aspects of H&N lesions. For example

- **Clinical features accurately suggest diagnosis of thyroglossal duct cyst (TDC), so why is US indicated?** In a patient with TDC, the sonologist confirms clinical diagnoses, establishes relation to hyoid bone, and identifies presence of normal thyroid or any features suspicious of malignancy in TDC. These are questions that need to be answered prior to treatment, and US readily provides the necessary information
- **How does US help to evaluate an upper neck mass?** US helps to confirm the nature of the mass and its anatomical location. A solid mass (on grayscale US) in the upper neck narrows the differential to common lesions at this site, which include enlarged node, schwannoma (vagus or sympathetic chain), or carotid body paraganglioma. Relation and vascular displacement help to distinguish between these. Vagus schwannoma separates IJV from CCA, whereas sympathetic schwannoma commonly displaces major vessels anteriorly, and carotid body paraganglioma straddles carotid bifurcation. Marked intratumoral vascularity with AV shunting would suggest paraganglioma, whereas schwannomas have scant vascularity susceptible to pressure, and abnormal nodes have characteristic vascularity that helps to separate reactive nodes from metastases and lymphoma
- Similarly, a cystic mass at the same site would raise other common diagnoses, such as 2nd branchial cleft cyst, cystic lymph nodes, lymphatic malformation, and venous vascular malformation. A combination of grayscale and Doppler features would help to distinguish between these diagnoses, and specific features should be sought, such as septa, slow swirling motion of debris within cystic portion, curvilinear/punctate calcification, and abnormal vascularity

What is the role of US in evaluating salivary glands? It is here that US has one of its major limitations, as it is unable to evaluate the deep lobe of the parotid gland, which is obscured from shadowing by the mandible and also due to its relatively deeper location in the neck. However, one must bear in mind that most parotid lesions occur in the superficial lobe, and most are benign. US clearly evaluates the superficial lobe, and its high resolution identifies any subtle focal or diffuse parenchymal abnormality. In addition, it accurately identifies focal parotid masses, characterizes their nature, and safely guides needle biopsy. It is also an invaluable tool for follow-up of lesions and for surveillance of any sinister change.

- US is ideal for submandibular and sublingual gland evaluation. It visualizes the entire gland, evaluates any parenchymal change (in patients with diffuse involvement) or calculus along the course of the duct (and intraglandular ± any complications). It characterizes focal masses, defines their extent and presence of adjacent abnormal nodes, and guides confirmatory biopsy. CT and MR are complementary tools where the entire extent of a large mass cannot be evaluated by US and for perineural spread of malignant masses

Is US useful in evaluating parathyroid adenoma? The commonly accepted gold standard for parathyroid localization is technetium sestamibi (± SPECT). However, it is often combined with other anatomical-based imaging modalities, such as CT, MR, and US. In our center, US is used as the initial imaging modality. When US and MIBI are concordant, focused parathyroidectomy is curative in the large majority of cases and may even obviate the need for intraoperative US or PTH estimation. In addition, US evaluates any concurrent pathology in the thyroid gland. US accurately identifies parathyroid adenoma in the vicinity of thyroid gland by its location, shape (flat, oval, arrowhead), and vascularity (prominent polar vessel ± ramification) and guides needle estimation of PTH when indicated. However, US has major limitations, as it does not evaluate ectopic adenoma and is limited in obese patients with short necks and following neck surgery. In such cases, MIBI + MR/CT is the likely approach, and parathyroid arteriography and venous sampling is considered when noninvasive imaging techniques are nondiagnostic.

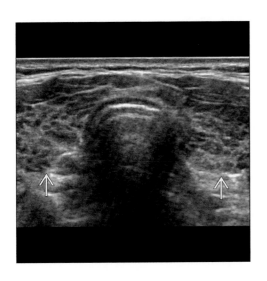

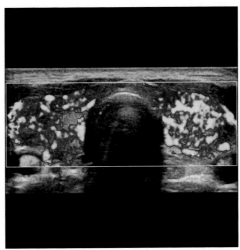

(Left) Transverse grayscale US in a patient with Hashimoto thyroiditis shows diffuse hypoechogenicity of the thyroid gland ➡ and small, hypoechoic, micronodular pattern (representing lymphocyte infiltration) and fibrous septa in thyroid parenchyma, clearly demonstrated by modern high-resolution transducers. *(Right)* Transverse power Doppler US shows diffuse hypervascularity ("thyroid inferno") in a patient with Graves disease, features not seen in toxic MNG and Hashimoto thyroiditis.

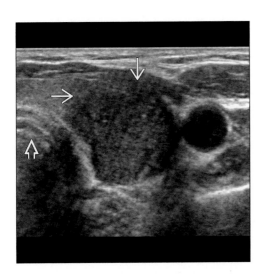

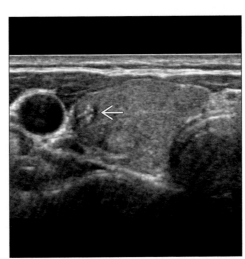

(Left) Transverse grayscale US shows an ill-defined (anteriorly and medially), solid, hypoechoic thyroid nodule ➡, suspicious for malignancy. In the thyroid gland, possibility of malignancy ↑ as echogenicity ↓. Note the trachea ➡. *(Right)* Transverse grayscale US shows a small, solid, hypoechoic thyroid nodule ➡ with fine echogenic foci, suspicious for papillary carcinoma. With ↑ use of modern high-frequency transducers, such suspicious nodules are increasingly seen as incidental lesions.

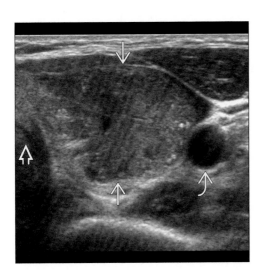

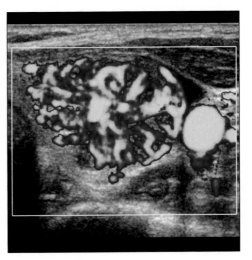

(Left) Transverse grayscale US shows an ill-defined, solid, hypoechoic nodule ➡ with fine echogenic foci in the left lobe of the thyroid gland. Note the trachea ➡ and common carotid artery ➡. *(Right)* Corresponding power Doppler US shows marked intranodular vascularity. Combination of grayscale (solid, hypoechoic, punctate echogenic foci) and Doppler features (hypervascularity) are highly suspicious of papillary thyroid cancer, and guided FNAC helps to confirm diagnosis.

(Left) Longitudinal grayscale US shows a noncalcified, homogeneous, iso-/hyperechoic thyroid nodule with hypoechoic halo ➡. Note that possibility of thyroid nodule being malignant ↓ as echogenicity ↑. *(Right)* Corresponding power Doppler US shows predominant perinodular/halo vascularity with sparse intranodular vessels. Hypoechoic, vascular halo around thyroid nodule = vascularity in compressed perinodular thyroid tissue and is often seen with benign thyroid nodules.

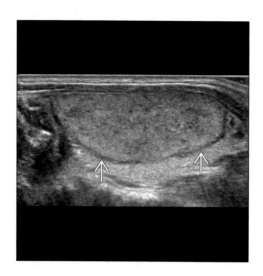
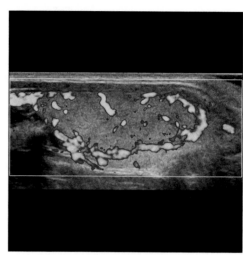

(Left) Longitudinal grayscale US shows a solid, hyperechoic (compared to adjacent muscle ➡) node with fine echogenic focus/calcification ➡. Hyperechogenicity and presence of fine intranodal calcification is diagnostic of metastases from thyroid papillary carcinoma. *(Right)* Corresponding power Doppler US shows marked, chaotic intranodal vascularity consistent with metastatic node. Reactive/benign nodes tend to demonstrate hilar vascularity.

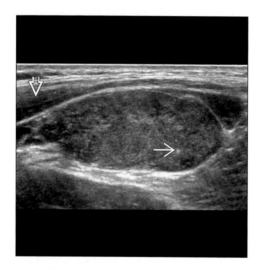
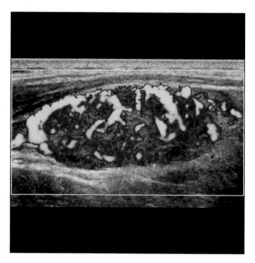

(Left) Longitudinal grayscale US shows solid, heterogeneous, hypoechoic nodes ➡. Note that with modern high-resolution transducers, one can see multiple hypoechoic areas within the node, giving it a reticulated appearance suggestive of lymphoma. *(Right)* Corresponding power Doppler US shows intranodal vascularity consistent with lymphoma (i.e., hilar > peripheral vascularity). Combination of grayscale and Doppler features helps to suggest nature of node and plan guided biopsy.

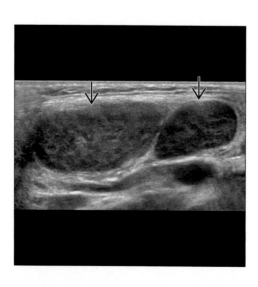
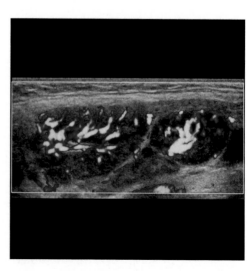

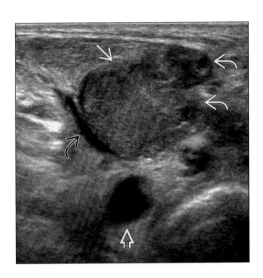

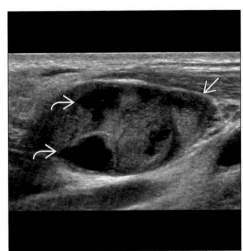

(Left) Transverse grayscale US shows malignant node indenting IJV ⊳ and anterior to CCA ⊳. Note that node ⊳ is characteristically hypoechoic in echogenicity; however, it shows ill-defined margins anteriorly ⊳, suggestive of extracapsular spread, a poor prognosticator in patients with metastatic SCCa. *(Right)* Longitudinal grayscale US shows a metastatic node ⊳ in a patient with known metastatic SCCa. Note multiple intranodal cystic areas ⊳ commonly seen in metastatic SCCa nodes.

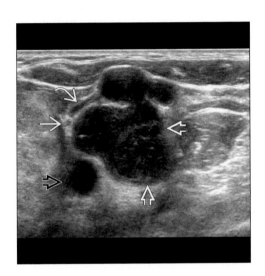

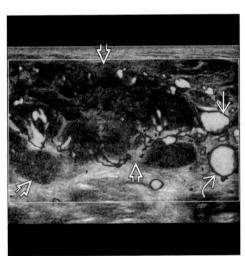

(Left) Transverse grayscale US shows a typical "collar stud" tuberculous abscess ⊳ in the neck. Note US clearly demonstrates its thick walls, necrotic nature, and anatomic relations to compressed IJV ⊳, CCA ⊳, and vagus nerve ⊳. *(Right)* Transverse power Doppler US shows a conglomerate of necrotic, matted nodes ⊳ in the right posterior triangle with intranodal and soft tissue vascularity, features typical of tuberculous lymphadenopathy. Note CCA ⊳ and IJV ⊳.

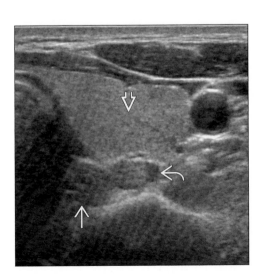

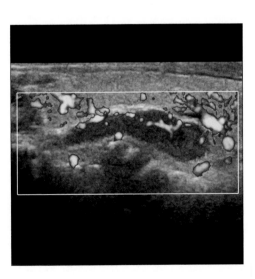

(Left) Transverse grayscale US in a patient with 1° hyperparathyroidism shows a well-defined, small parathyroid adenoma (PTA) ⊳ posterior to left thyroid gland ⊳ and juxtaesophageal ⊳ in location. US accurately identifies such adenomas, which are in the vicinity of thyroid gland, and any coexistent thyroid pathology. However, in postoperative neck and for ectopic parathyroid adenomas, US has limited role. *(Right)* Longitudinal power Doppler US shows arrowhead shape & central vascularity of PTA.

(Left) Transverse grayscale US in a patient with CN7 palsy shows solid, hypoechoic, malignant superficial parotid tumor ⮞ with ill-defined margins and extraglandular extension ➘. Note its posterior extension and proximity to the facial nerve ➡. Entire posterior extent of tumor cannot be defined by US. *(Right)* Power Doppler US shows markedly vascular superficial parotid tumor. Role of vascularity in differentiating benign from malignant lesions is limited for salivary masses.

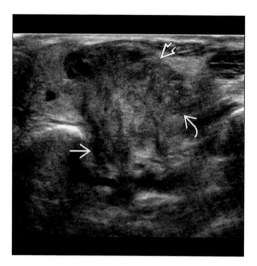
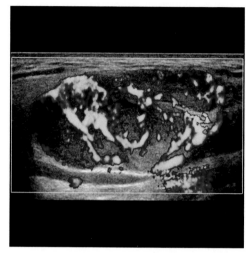

(Left) Color Doppler US of infant parotid shows diffuse, hypoechoic, parenchymal echopattern with marked ↑ in vascularity, typical for infantile hemangioma of parotid gland. US identifies lesion, obviates need for additional imaging/biopsy, and helps to reassure parents about benignity and resolution. *(Right)* Power Doppler US in a patient with malignant scalp lesion shows marked vascularity in small, metastatic intraparotid node. Embryologically, nodes are absent in submandibular gland.

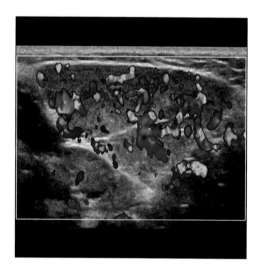
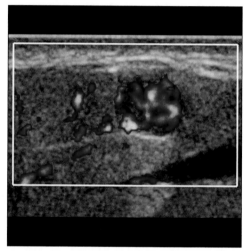

(Left) Grayscale US shows dilated submandibular duct ➡ with tiny obstructing calculus ➚ at its terminal end. US is ideal for evaluating submandibular calculi as it evaluates entire course of duct and identifies small calculus and associated parenchymal changes/ complications in gland. *(Right)* Transverse grayscale US of submandibular gland (SMG) shows characteristic cirrhotic SMG, typical of Kuttner tumor, which is often bilateral and symmetrical and may also involve parotid gland (SMG > parotid).

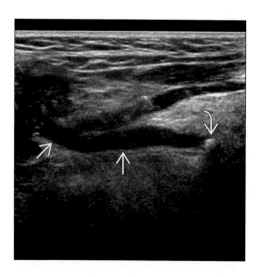
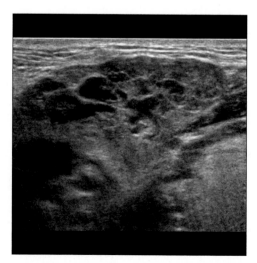

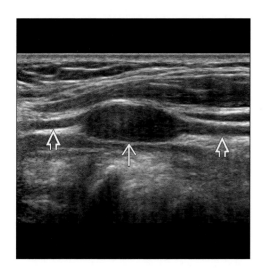

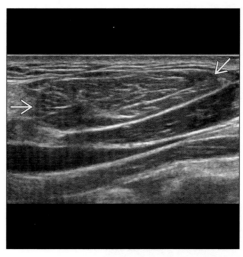

(Left) Longitudinal grayscale US shows a well-defined, noncalcified, solid, hypoechoic mass ⇨ in continuation with vagus nerve ⇨, indicating the vagus nerve sheath tumor. The ability of high-resolution US in identifying vagus nerve renders this diagnosis easy, obviating need for biopsy. *(Right)* Longitudinal grayscale US shows a well-defined mass ⇨ with multiple intralesional echogenic striations (feathered appearance) typical of lipoma, obviating need for biopsy.

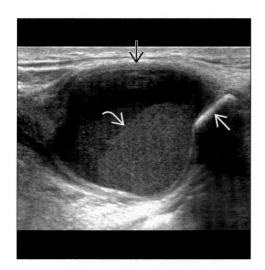

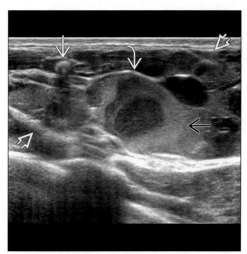

(Left) Longitudinal grayscale US shows suprahyoid TDC ⇨. Note its relation to hyoid bone ⇨, cystic nature, and avascular "solid" component ⇨ (on Doppler, not shown) indicating debris and not malignant change. US also identified normal thyroid tissue in thyroid bed. *(Right)* Longitudinal grayscale US shows a large VVM ⇨ with septa ⇨, fine echogenic debris ⇨ in vascular spaces, and echogenic focus/phlebolith ⇨. "To and fro" motion of debris is seen on grayscale US, indicating slow flow.

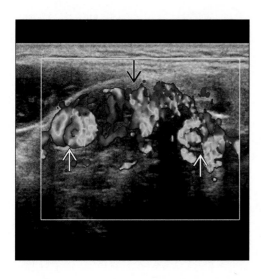

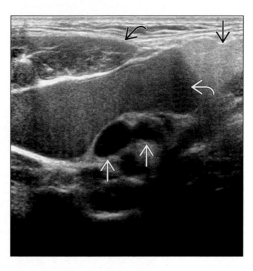

(Left) Transverse power Doppler US at level of carotid bifurcation ⇨ shows a large, markedly vascular mass ⇨ straddling bifurcation, appearances typical of carotid body tumor (CBT) with intralesional vascularity and AV shunting of blood. *(Right)* Transverse grayscale US a shows cystic mass ⇨ with fine debris anterior to carotid bifurcation ⇨, posterior to SMG ⇨, and under medial edge of sternomastoid muscle ⇨. Appearances and location are typical for 2nd BCC.

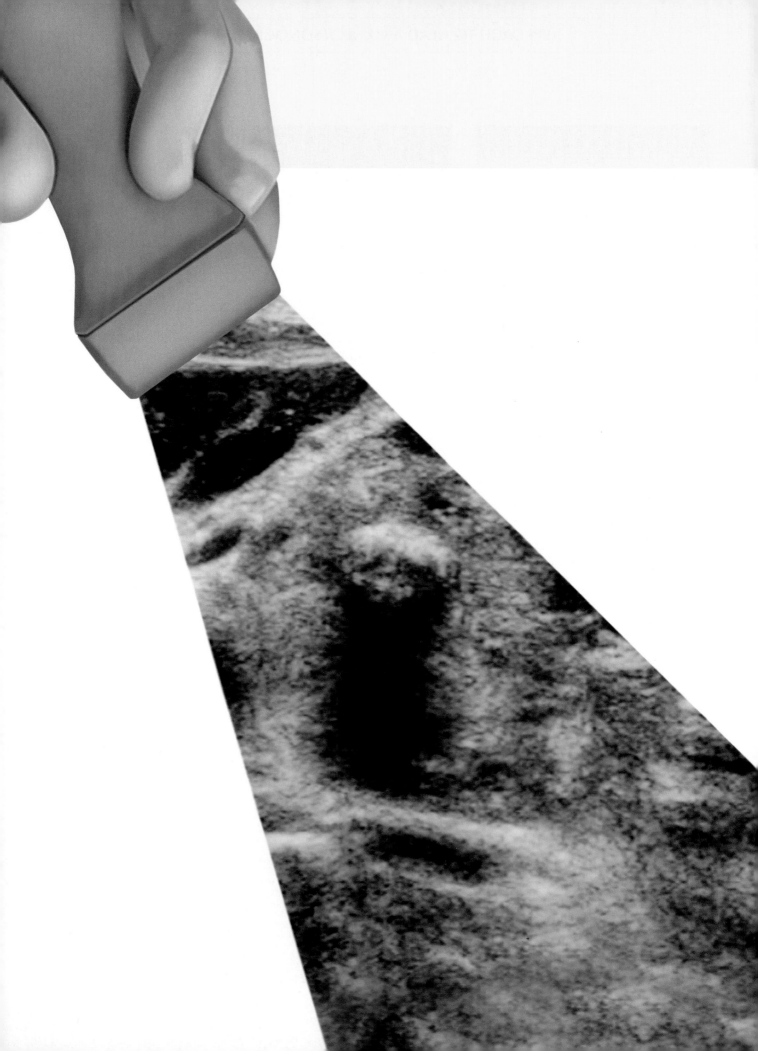

SECTION 2
Thyroid and Parathyroid

DIFFERENTIATED THYROID CARCINOMA

Key Facts

Imaging

- Sonographic features of **papillary carcinoma (PC)**
  - 10-20% are multifocal, 70% are solid, & 77-90% are hypoechoic
  - Punctate microcalcification is highly specific for PC, typically fine
  - Majority are ill-defined with irregular outlines
  - Large tumors invade strap muscles, esophagus, trachea, recurrent laryngeal nerve, neck vessels
  - Color Doppler: Chaotic vascularity within nodule, wall, & septa in nodules with cystic change
  - Nodes predominantly hyperechoic (80%) compared to muscles; 50% with punctate microcalcification
- US features suspicious of **follicular carcinoma (FC)**
  - Cannot differentiate benign follicular adenoma from FC on imaging or biopsy
  - Ill-defined solid tumor with hypoechoic, heterogeneous architecture

- Hypoechoic component to an iso-/hyperechoic solid mass; thick, irregular margins/capsule
- Obvious extrathyroid invasion into trachea, esophagus, strap muscles, & large vessels
- Color Doppler: Profuse, chaotic perinodular and intranodular vascularity; intranodular > perinodular

Top Differential Diagnoses

- Medullary carcinoma
- Follicular adenoma
- Anaplastic carcinoma

Diagnostic Checklist

- After evaluating thyroid gland, look for extracapsular spread, local invasion, & nodal metastasis
- PC is frequently detected against background multinodular goiter
- If staging CT is contemplated, do not give iodinated contrast; delay I-131 therapy up to 6 months

(Left) Transverse grayscale US shows a solid, ill-defined, hypoechoic nodule ➡ with punctate echogenic foci ➡ confined to the left lobe of the thyroid. Tumor hypoechogenicity is due to closely packed cell content & sparse colloid within. The carotid artery ➡ and trachea ➡ are also shown. (Right) Corresponding power Doppler US shows profuse, chaotic, intranodular vascularity. These features are typical of papillary carcinoma (PC) and readily confirmed by guided FNAC, which is safe despite marked intranodular vascularity.

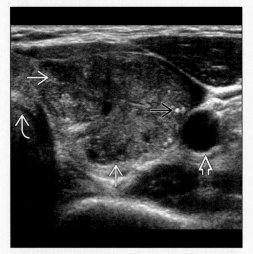
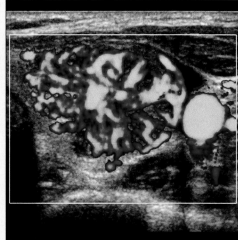

(Left) Transverse grayscale US shows a small, hypoechoic, ill-defined nodule ➡ in the right lobe of the thyroid. Note the adjacent solid, round node ➡ with absent hilus & echogenic focus ➡ within. Note typical nodal distribution. (Right) Corresponding power Doppler US shows marked abnormal intranodal vascularity consistent with a metastatic node. FNAC of the thyroid nodule and lymph node confirmed PC. Note the similarity in appearance between the primary tumor and the node on grayscale US.

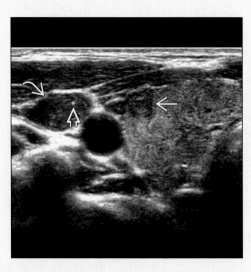
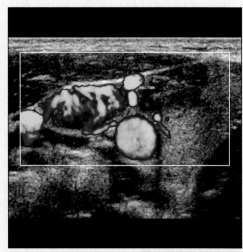

DIFFERENTIATED THYROID CARCINOMA

TERMINOLOGY

Definitions
- Thyroid malignancies with well-defined histologies; includes papillary carcinoma (PC) and follicular carcinoma (FC)

IMAGING

General Features
- Best diagnostic clue
  - Focal, intrathyroidal mass ± extracapsular invasion ± metastatic nodes ± distant metastases

Ultrasonographic Findings
- Grayscale US features of PC
  - 10-20% are multifocal, 70% are solid, and 77-90% are hypoechoic
    - Predominantly hypoechoic due to sparse colloid and closely packed cellular content
  - Punctate microcalcification is highly specific for PC; typically has fine calcification/echogenic foci ± posterior shadowing
  - Majority are ill-defined with irregular outlines, but 15-30% of tumors may show an incomplete halo
  - Tumor commonly spreads along rich lymphatic system in and adjacent to thyroid gland, accounting for multifocal tumors within thyroid and regional nodal spread
  - Large tumors may invade strap muscles, esophagus, trachea, recurrent laryngeal nerve, neck vessels
  - Color Doppler: Chaotic vascularity within nodule, wall, and septa in nodules with cystic change
- Grayscale US features of lymph node metastasis from PC
  - Distribution: Deep cervical, pre-/paratracheal, prelaryngeal, retropharyngeal, and mediastinal
  - Nodes predominantly hyperechoic (80%) compared with muscles; 50% with punctate microcalcification
  - Cystic necrosis (25%) with vascularity within solid portion and septa on color Doppler
  - US features of metastatic PC nodes often resemble primary thyroid tumor
- Grayscale US features of FC
  - Not possible to differentiate benign follicular adenoma from FC by imaging or biopsy
    - Differentiation made after surgery based on vascular and capsular invasion
    - Therefore, commonly lumped together as follicular lesions
  - Some cytologists may classify FCs into microfollicular or macrofollicular types
    - Microfollicular lesion may be FC 20-25%)
    - Macrofollicular lesions have a low risk of carcinoma
  - In most cases, FC develops from preexisting adenoma
  - US features suspicious for FC
    - Ill-defined solid tumor with hypoechoic, heterogeneous architecture
    - Hypoechoic component to an iso-/hyperechoic solid mass; thick irregular margins/capsule
    - Obvious extrathyroid invasion into trachea, esophagus, strap muscles, and large vessels
    - Color Doppler: Profuse, chaotic peri-/intranodular vascularity (intranodular > perinodular)

- Metastatic disease in bones, lungs, less commonly in lymph nodes; often present with metastases

Imaging Recommendations
- Best imaging tool
  - On US, solid, hypoechoic, punctate calcifications are specific for PC and correspond to psammoma bodies on microscopy
    - US identifies malignant nodules, guides fine-needle aspiration cytology (FNAC), and helps to follow-up/evaluate postsurgical thyroid bed
    - CT/MR used to stage large tumors as US may not define its entire extent and local infiltration
- Protocol advice
  - After evaluating thyroid gland, look for extracapsular spread, local invasion, and nodal metastasis
  - PC is frequently detected against background multinodular goiter
  - If staging CT is contemplated, do not give iodinated contrast; delay I-131 therapy up to 6 months

DIFFERENTIAL DIAGNOSIS

Medullary Carcinoma
- Mimics PC on US; coarse shadowing calcification and associated hypoechoic lymph nodes

Follicular Adenoma
- Solitary, well-defined, homogeneous, iso-/hyperechoic intrathyroidal mass with perinodular vascularity and no local invasion or adenopathy/metastases

Anaplastic Carcinoma
- Rapidly enlarging, invasive thyroid tumor that is hypoechoic, ill-defined, ± calcifications and profuse chaotic vascularity

Multinodular Goiter (MNG)
- Multiple nodules, heterogeneous, ± cystic change, ± coarse calcification and perinodular vascularity; always search for suspicious nodule against background MNG

PATHOLOGY

General Features
- Thyroid cancer
  - Differentiated thyroid carcinoma (DTCa): Papillary (80%) & follicular (10%); medullary carcinoma (5-10%); anaplastic carcinoma (1-2%)
- Patterns of spread
  - Local invasion with involvement of recurrent laryngeal nerves, trachea, esophagus
  - Nodal spread: Papillary (50%) > > follicular (10%) microscopic spread at presentation
  - Distant spread: Follicular (20%) > papillary (5-10%); typically spreads to lung, bone, & CNS
- Embryology anatomy
  - Nodal drainage from thyroid: Paratracheal, deep cervical, spinal accessory, retropharyngeal chains
  - DTCa accesses mediastinum via paratracheal chain

SELECTED REFERENCES

1. Wong KT et al: Ultrasound of thyroid cancer. Cancer Imaging. 5:157-66, 2005

(Left) Transverse grayscale US shows a focal, subtle, isoechoic right thyroid nodule ⇨ & diffuse, multiple, punctate, nonshadowing echogenic foci ⇨ in both lobes. The esophagus ⊡⇨ and trachea ⊡⇨ are also shown. *(Right)* Longitudinal US of the left lobe shows multiple echogenic foci ⇨ within the thyroid parenchyma. Surgery confirmed diffuse sclerosing variant of PC, which accounts for 0.7-5% of all PCs, commonly affects younger patients, and has ↑ incidence of nodal & lung metastases.

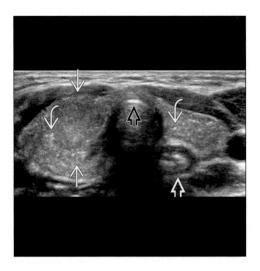
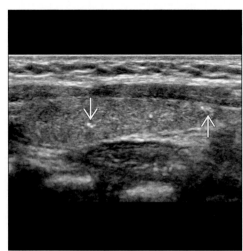

(Left) Longitudinal grayscale US shows a haloed ⇨, isoechoic nodule ⇨ with focal cystic change & septation confined to thyroid gland. Note the absence of echogenic foci within. *(Right)* Corresponding Doppler US shows halo vascularity ⇨ & prominent intranodular vascularity in the solid portion ⇨. Surgery confirmed minimally invasive FC, mimicking benign thyroid nodule. These patients have 3% fatality rate, rare metastases (8-10%), ± capsular penetration, and no vascular involvement.

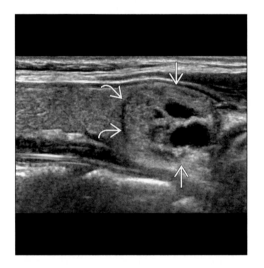
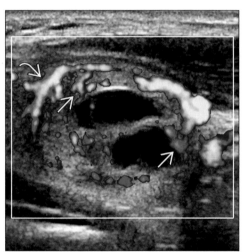

(Left) Longitudinal grayscale US shows a large, solid, hypoechoic, ill-defined thyroid mass ⇨. Note its infiltrative edges ⇨, suggesting malignant nature. *(Right)* Corresponding transverse grayscale US shows infiltrative edges and extrathyroid spread ⇨ of the left thyroid nodule. Note the thrombus in the distended middle thyroid vein ⊡⇨ (anterior to the common carotid artery ⊡⇨) extending into the internal jugular vein ⇨. Surgery confirmed FC. Tumor thrombus showed vascularity on Doppler.

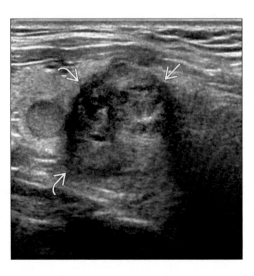
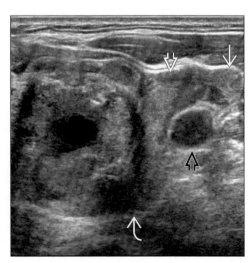

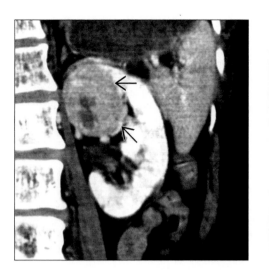

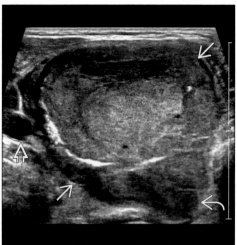

(Left) Coronal reformatted CECT shows well-defined left upper pole renal mass ➡. Other multiple bone & lung metastases were also present. Bone biopsy suggested follicular origin. (Right) Transverse grayscale US in the same patient shows solid, large, hypoechoic, noncalcified mass ➡ in right thyroid lobe with extrathyroid extension ➡. Note the close proximity of the carotid artery ➡ to the mass. Surgery confirmed thyroid FC, which often presents with hematogenous metastases, providing a clue to diagnosis.

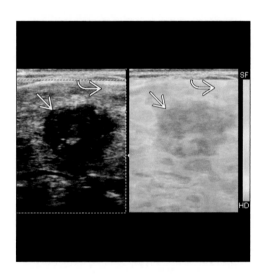

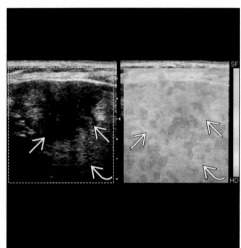

(Left) Longitudinal grayscale US & qualitative strain elastogram of PC ➡ are shown. Strain color scale ranges from purple (soft, elastic) to red (hard, inelastic). The tumor appears mostly red (inelastic) compared to normal thyroid ➡, which is mostly green (elastic), and is true positive for cancer on strain EI. (Right) Longitudinal US & qualitative strain elastogram show PC ➡ that is mostly green/yellow (elastic), similar to adjacent parenchyma ➡, and false-negative for cancer on strain EI.

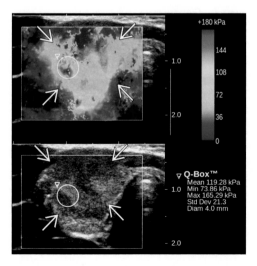

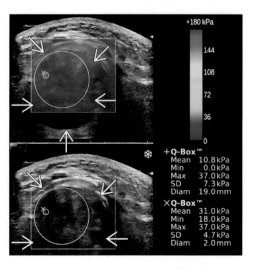

(Left) Transverse grayscale US & SWE show PC ➡. SWE scale ranges from blue (0 kPa, soft) to red (180 kPa, stiff). The tumor appears heterogeneous with large red areas. Circular ROI measures a maximum SWE of 165.3 kPa (very high). (Right) Transverse grayscale US & SWE show FC ➡ that is mostly blue (soft) with no high-stiffness areas. Circular ROI measures a maximum SWE of 37.0 kPa, which is low and overlaps with benign nodules. SWE cutoffs may be suboptimal for detecting FCs.

MEDULLARY THYROID CARCINOMA

Key Facts

Imaging

- Solitary or multiple or diffuse involvement of both lobes (especially familial type)
- Located predominantly in lateral upper 2/3 of gland in sporadic form
- Hypoechoic, solid tumor, frequently well defined but may have infiltrative borders
  - Echogenic foci in 80-90% representing amyloid deposition & associated calcification
  - Echogenic foci are usually dense & coarse with shadowing compared to papillary carcinoma
- Doppler: Chaotic intratumoral and intranodal vessels
- Ipsilateral lymph nodes along mid & low internal jugular chain, superior mediastinum
  - Hypoechoic ± coarse shadowing calcification
- ≤ 75% have lymphadenopathy at presentation
- On US, medullary thyroid carcinoma (MTC) is invariably mistaken for papillary carcinoma, which is much more common, and diagnosis made only after FNAC
- Sonographic clue to MTC rather than papillary carcinoma is multiplicity, presence of coarse shadowing tumoral calcification (punctate in papillary), and hypoechoic nodes (hyperechoic in papillary) ± coarse shadowing
- Evaluate adrenal & parathyroid gland if MTC is part of type 2 multiple endocrine neoplasia (MEN2)
- US identifies malignant nodule, guides needle for FNAC, and helps follow-up/evaluate postsurgical neck
- Consider familial syndromes with young patients or multifocal tumors

Top Differential Diagnoses

- Differentiated thyroid carcinoma
- Thyroid metastases
- Multinodular goiter (MNG)

(Left) Transverse grayscale US shows solid, hypoechoic medullary thyroid carcinoma (MTC) ➡ with central, dense, shadowing calcification ➡. Cancer risk in a solid nodule with dense central calcification is 2x higher than in a solid nodule without calcification. Note adjacent, smaller, similar nodule ➡. Multiplicity is seen in familial type of MTC. Note CCA ➡ and trachea ➡. (Right) Longitudinal grayscale US better demonstrates ill-defined edges ➡ of thyroid MTC. Calcification in MTC is associated with amyloid deposition.

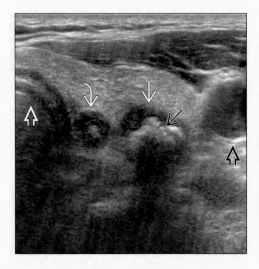
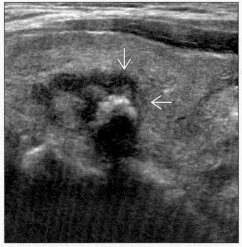

(Left) Transverse grayscale US shows postoperative MTC recurrence ➡ (solid & hypoechoic) low in right neck. Note CCA ➡, internal jugular vein ➡, and location of trachea ➡. (Right) Corresponding power Doppler US shows intratumoral vascularity. In postoperative patients, US is ideal initial imaging modality to detect neck recurrences and safely guide needle for FNAC confirmation. However, it is unable to evaluate mediastinal extent, distant disease, and local infiltration of large tumors.

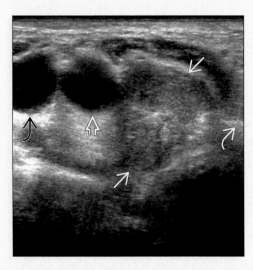
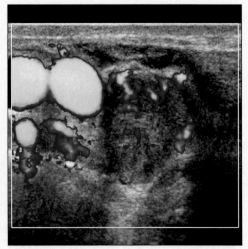

MEDULLARY THYROID CARCINOMA

TERMINOLOGY

Abbreviations
- Medullary thyroid carcinoma (MTC)

Definitions
- Rare neuroendocrine malignancy arising from thyroid parafollicular C cells that produce calcitonin

IMAGING

General Features
- Location
  - Within thyroid gland, lateral upper 2/3 of gland (site of maximum C-cell concentration)
- Morphology
  - Solid, usually well-circumscribed thyroid mass
  - More infiltrative type seen with familial forms
- Frequently multifocal; 2/3 of sporadic cases, almost all familial cases

Ultrasonographic Findings
- Grayscale ultrasound
  - Medullary thyroid carcinoma, primary tumor
    - Solitary or multiple or diffuse involvement of both lobes (especially familial type)
    - Located predominantly in lateral upper 2/3 of gland in sporadic form
    - Hypoechoic, solid tumor, frequently well defined but may have infiltrative borders
    - Echogenic foci in 80-90% representing amyloid deposition & associated calcification
    - Echogenic foci are usually dense & coarse with shadowing compared to papillary carcinoma
  - Lymph node metastases from medullary carcinoma
    - Ipsilateral lymph nodes along mid & low internal jugular chain, superior mediastinum
    - Lymph nodes predominantly hypoechoic ± coarse shadowing calcification
- Color Doppler
  - Chaotic intratumoral and intranodal vessels

Imaging Recommendations
- Best imaging tool
  - US is ideal initial tool for evaluation of thyroid nodule when combined with guided FNAC
    - Sonographically, MTC closely mimics papillary thyroid carcinoma, both primary tumor & metastatic node
    - On US, MTC is invariably mistaken for papillary carcinoma, which is much more common, and diagnosis made only after FNAC
    - Sonographic clue to MTC rather than papillary carcinoma is multiplicity, presence of coarse shadowing tumoral calcification (punctate in papillary), and hypoechoic nodes (hyperechoic in papillary) ± calcification with coarse shadowing
    - US identifies malignant nodule, guides needle for FNAC, and helps to follow-up/evaluate postsurgical thyroid bed and neck
    - Cross-sectional imaging is used to stage large tumors as US may not accurately define entire extent, local infiltration, & mediastinal nodes
- Protocol advice

- In addition to evaluating thyroid gland on US, look for extracapsular spread, local invasion, and nodal disease
- Evaluate adrenal and parathyroid gland if MTC is part of type 2 multiple endocrine neoplasia (MEN2)

DIFFERENTIAL DIAGNOSIS

Differentiated Thyroid Carcinoma
- Papillary carcinoma has punctate, fine calcifications
  - Nodes are hyperechoic, show cystic change, and punctate calcification

Thyroid Metastases
- Diffuse/focal enlargement of gland
- Well-defined, solid hypoechoic mass with abnormal vascularity
- Invariably associated with US evidence of disseminated disease in neck nodes, liver

Multinodular Goiter
- Diffusely enlarged gland with multiple nodules with coarse calcification, ± "comet tail" artifact

Follicular Adenoma
- Solitary, well-defined, noncalcified iso-/hyperechoic mass with homogeneous internal echogenicity and perinodular vascularity

CLINICAL ISSUES

Demographics
- Age
  - Sporadic form: Mean = 50 years
  - Familial form: Mean = 30 years
  - Can occur in children, especially with MEN2B
- Epidemiology
  - 5-10% all thyroid gland malignancies, ≤ 14% thyroid cancer deaths
  - 10% pediatric thyroid malignancies (MEN2)
  - Associated with MEN2 syndromes (autosomal dominant)
    - MEN2A: Multifocal MTC, pheochromocytoma, parathyroid hyperplasia, hyperparathyroidism
    - MEN2B: Multifocal MTC, pheochromocytoma, mucosal neuromas of lips, tongue, GI tract, conjunctiva; younger patients

Natural History & Prognosis
- Familial type almost always multifocal and bilateral
- 2/3 of sporadic cases are bilateral
- ≤ 75% have lymphadenopathy at presentation
- Distant metastases to lungs (miliary), liver, bones

DIAGNOSTIC CHECKLIST

Image Interpretation Pearls
- US appearance may mimic papillary thyroid carcinoma
- Consider familial syndromes in young patients or multifocal tumors

SELECTED REFERENCES

1. Sofferman RA et al: Ultrasound of the Thyroid and Parathyroid Glands. New York: Springer. 107-150, 2011

MEDULLARY THYROID CARCINOMA

(Left) Transverse grayscale US shows a solid, hypoechoic nodule ➡ with an ill-defined margin ➡ confined to the right thyroid lobe. Note CCA ⮞ and location of trachea ➡. *(Right)* Corresponding longitudinal grayscale US shows ill-defined edges ➡ and fine, nonshadowing echogenic foci ➡ within the thyroid nodule ➡. Note that sonographic appearances resemble thyroid papillary carcinoma. However, FNAC suggested MTC.

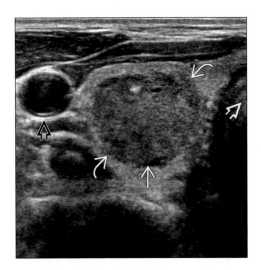
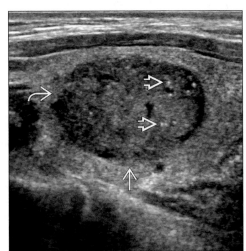

(Left) Transverse grayscale US through another plane (same patient) shows nonshadowing echogenic foci ➡ and additionally demonstrates cystic change ➡ in thyroid nodule ➡. Note CCA ⮞ and location of trachea ➡. *(Right)* Corresponding longitudinal grayscale US clearly demonstrates multiple nonshadowing echogenic foci ➡ and cystic change/septation ➡. On US, MTC is often mistaken for papillary thyroid carcinoma, which is far more common than MTC.

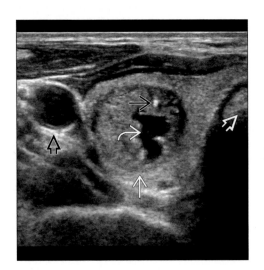
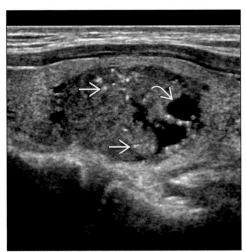

(Left) Transverse power Doppler US (same patient) shows marked chaotic intranodular vascularity in MTC. *(Right)* Transverse power Doppler US (through another plane) shows marked vascularity in the solid portion of MTC. Such profuse chaotic intranodular vascularity is highly suspicious for thyroid cancer. Compared with papillary cancer, MTC shows dense shadowing calcification (vs. punctate), hypoechoic nodes (vs. hyperechoic), and coarse shadowing nodal calcification (vs. punctate).

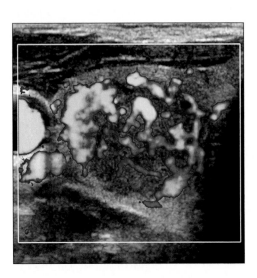
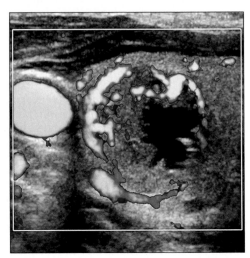

MEDULLARY THYROID CARCINOMA

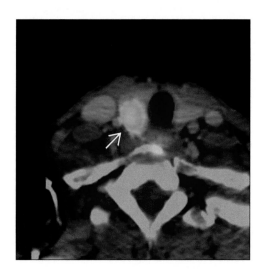
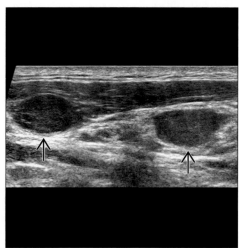

(Left) FDG PET/CT shows FDG-avid right thyroid MTC ➡. ATA guidelines suggest FDG-positive thyroid nodules undergo further evaluation including FNAC; risk of cancer in FDG-positive nodules is 33%, and such cancers may be aggressive. *(Right)* Longitudinal grayscale US shows metastatic nodes ➡ from thyroid MTC, which are usually hypoechoic (vs. hyperechoic in papillary carcinoma) and may have coarse shadowing calcification (vs. fine echogenic ± shadowing in papillary carcinoma).

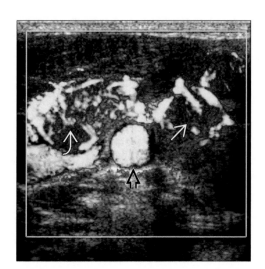
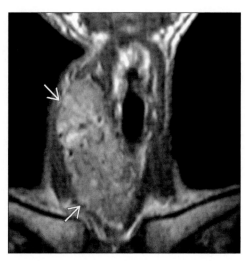

(Left) Power Doppler US shows abnormal chaotic vessels in thyroid MTC ➡ & the adjacent lymph node ➡. Note CCA ➡. Such prominent vessels should not prevent safe US-guided FNAC. *(Right)* Coronal T1WI MR shows the entire extent & infiltration of adjacent structures in a patient with a large thyroid MTC ➡. US readily identifies thyroid MTC, adjacent nodal spread, and safely guides FNAC for diagnosis, but cannot define extent & infiltration of large tumors; CT/MR are necessary.

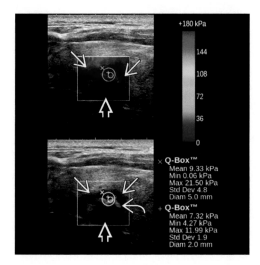
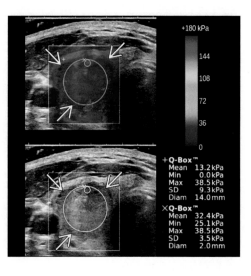

(Left) Longitudinal grayscale US & SWE show MTC ➡. SWE color scale ranges from blue (0 kPa, soft) to red (180 kPa, stiff). Hypoechoic MTC appears blue with maximum SWE of 21.5 kPa, which is low and overlaps with benign nodules. The deep aspect of the lesion ➡ is obscured by overlying tumor calcifications ➡ and lacks SWE signal. *(Right)* Transverse grayscale US & SWE show MTC ➡ appearing blue with a maximum SWE of 38.5kPa, which is low. SWE cutoffs may be inaccurate for detecting MTC.

ANAPLASTIC THYROID CARCINOMA

Key Facts

Imaging

- Invasive hypoechoic thyroid mass, ± focal calcification, ± necrosis against background of multinodular goiter (MNG) in elderly female, ± nodal or distant metastases
- Ill-defined hypoechoic tumor diffusely involving entire lobe or gland
- Background of MNG or DTCa
- Necrosis (78%), dense amorphous calcification (58%)
- Extracapsular spread with infiltration of trachea, esophagus, and perithyroid soft tissues & nerves
- Thrombus in internal jugular vein (IJV) and carotid artery (CA), causing expansion & occlusion of vessels
- Nodal or distant metastases in 80% of patients
- Color Doppler shows prominent, small, chaotic intratumoral vessels
- Necrotic tumor may be avascular/hypovascular (vascular infiltration/occlusion)

- Abnormal vascularity seen within metastatic nodes
- Vascularity seen in thrombus in vessels suggests tumor thrombus & not venous thrombus

Top Differential Diagnoses

- Differentiated thyroid carcinoma (DTCa)
- Non-Hodgkin lymphoma
- Thyroid metastases

Diagnostic Checklist

- Patients with ATCa are often old with poor general health & present with acute obstructive symptoms such as dyspnea, dysphagia, laryngeal nerve palsy
- US is ideal bedside imaging tool to evaluate ATCa, its gross extension, & nodal disease; readily combines with FNAC to confirm diagnosis
- US may be unable to evaluate exact infiltration into trachea, larynx, adjacent soft tissues, and mediastinal spread; CECT or MR may be necessary

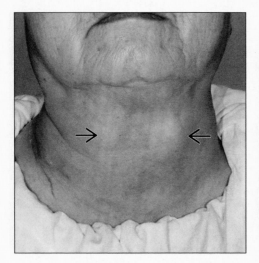
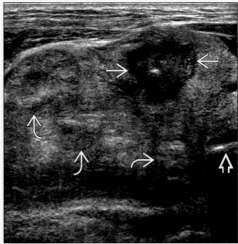

(Left) Elderly female patient with known multinodular goiter (MNG) presents with a rapidly enlarging mass in the thyroid region ➡, associated with hoarseness of voice and dysphagia. *(Right)* Transverse grayscale US shows thyroid enlargement and background multinodularity ➡. Note the markedly hypoechoic, heterogeneous, ill-defined thyroid nodule ➡ with infiltrating margins. Trachea ➡ is shown. Anaplastic thyroid carcinoma (ATCa) commonly occurs in elderly patients (7th decade, F > M) in the regions of endemic goiter.

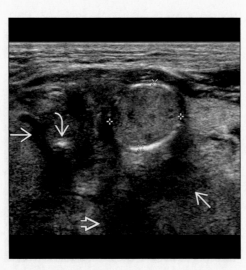
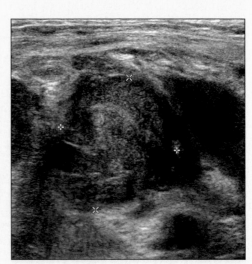

(Left) Grayscale US of the contralateral thyroid lobe shows a diffusely infiltrative tumor ➡ and focal area of amorphous ➡ and curvilinear calcification (calipers). Dense calcification reflects a longstanding goiter. Note extrathyroid spread posteriorly ➡. *(Right)* Transverse grayscale US (same patient) shows a solid, hypoechoic, ill-defined malignant lymph node (calipers) low in the neck. Nodal/distant metastases are seen in a majority of patients and intranodal cystic necrosis is seen in 50%.

ANAPLASTIC THYROID CARCINOMA

TERMINOLOGY

Abbreviations
- Anaplastic thyroid carcinoma (ATCa)

Definitions
- Lethal thyroid malignancy from thyroid-stimulating hormone transformation of either differentiated thyroid carcinoma or multinodular goiter (MNG)

IMAGING

General Features
- Best diagnostic clue
  - Invasive, hypoechoic thyroid mass, ± focal calcification, ± necrosis against background of MNG in elderly female, ± nodal or distant metastases
- Size
  - Typically > 5 cm at presentation
- Morphology
  - Primary tumor: Large, infiltrating thyroid mass
  - Primary tumor with MNG: Diffuse, heterogeneous thyromegaly with infiltrating margins

Ultrasonographic Findings
- Grayscale ultrasound
  - Ill-defined, hypoechoic tumor diffusely involving entire lobe or gland
  - Background of MNG or differentiated thyroid carcinoma (DTCa)
  - Necrosis (78%), dense amorphous calcification (58%)
    - Dense calcification reflects MNG calcification
  - Extracapsular spread with infiltration of trachea, esophagus, and perithyroid soft tissues and nerves
  - Thrombus in internal jugular vein (IJV) and carotid artery (CA) causing expansion and occlusion of vessels
  - Nodal or distant metastases in 80% of patients
    - Nodes are hypoechoic and necrotic in 50%
  - Color Doppler shows prominent, small, chaotic intratumoral vessels
    - Necrotic tumor may be avascular/hypovascular (vascular infiltration/occlusion)
    - Abnormal vascularity seen within metastatic nodes
    - Vascularity seen in thrombus in vessels suggests tumor thrombus, not venous thrombus

Imaging Recommendations
- Best imaging tool
  - Patients with ATCa are often elderly in poor general health and present with acute obstructive symptoms such as dyspnea, dysphagia, laryngeal nerve palsy
    - US is ideal bedside imaging tool to evaluate ATCa, its gross extension, and nodal disease; readily combines with FNAC to confirm diagnosis
    - US may be unable to evaluate exact infiltration into trachea, larynx, adjacent soft tissues, and mediastinal spread; CECT or MR may be necessary
    - CECT is preferable as patients' poor condition makes MR imaging suboptimal and CECT is faster
- Protocol advice
  - Check for background MNG/DTCa, extrathyroid and vascular infiltration of ATCa, and nodal and distant metastases in all patients

DIFFERENTIAL DIAGNOSIS

Non-Hodgkin Lymphoma
- Focal or diffuse, hypoechoic, ill-defined areas with abnormal vascularity, and background evidence of Hashimoto thyroiditis
- Associated solid, hypoechoic, reticulated lymphomatous nodes

DTCa
- Ill-defined, solid, hypoechoic, heterogeneous mass with abnormal vascularity ± punctate calcification ± adjacent nodal metastases ± vascular and extrathyroid infiltration

Thyroid Metastases
- Evidence of known primary and disseminated disease; solid, hypoechoic mass, ill/well defined, noncalcified, with abnormal vessels or diffuse hypoechoic enlarged thyroid and nodal metastasis

Medullary Carcinoma
- Solid, hypoechoic, ill-defined mass with coarse calcification and abnormal adjacent nodes

MNG
- Multiple, heterogeneous nodules ± dense calcification, cystic change, septa, "comet tail" artifact; no vascular or soft tissue infiltration and no nodal metastasis

CLINICAL ISSUES

Presentation
- Most common signs/symptoms
  - Rapidly growing, large, painful thyroid-area mass
  - 50% have associated symptoms from local invasion
    - Larynx or trachea: Dyspnea
    - 30% have recurrent laryngeal nerve palsy: Hoarseness
    - Esophagus: Dysphagia
  - Predisposing factors: Preexisting MNG, DTCa

Demographics
- Age
  - ATCa presents at later age than other thyroid malignancies, most typically 6th or 7th decade
- Epidemiology
  - Representing 1-2% of thyroid malignancy

Natural History & Prognosis
- Rapidly fatal, mean survival of 6 months after diagnosis

DIAGNOSTIC CHECKLIST

Consider
- Diagnosis based on clinical features, imaging, and biopsy
- Anaplastic carcinoma is always T4 tumor
- Intrathyroid disease = T4a = stage IVa
- Gross extrathyroid disease = T4b = stage IVb
- Metastatic disease = M1 = stage IVc

SELECTED REFERENCES

1. Wong KT et al: Ultrasound of thyroid cancer. Cancer Imaging. 5:157-66, 2005

ANAPLASTIC THYROID CARCINOMA

(Left) Transverse grayscale US shows large, solid, ill-defined ATCa ➡ diffusely involving both lobes of thyroid. Although US identifies the malignant nature of the mass and guides FNAC for diagnosis, it is unable to delineate the entire extent of large tumors, extrathyroid spread, infiltration of adjacent structures, and distant metastases. *(Right)* Corresponding axial CECT clearly demonstrates the entire extent of ATCa ➡, tracheal involvement, and airway displacement/slight narrowing ➡.

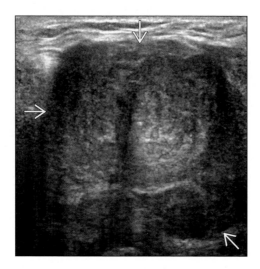
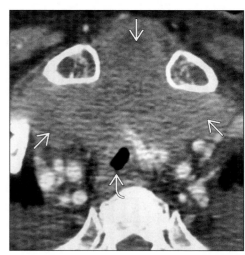

(Left) Clinical photograph shows an elderly male with ATCa who presented with recent, rapid enlargement of known thyroid mass associated with dysphagia, dyspnea, and hoarseness of voice. He was euthyroid and lung nodules were noted on chest x-ray. *(Right)* Axial CT in the same patient shows multiple lung metastases ➡. Nodal or distant metastases are present in the majority (~ 80%) of ATCa patients; extracapsular spread and vascular invasion occurs in 1/3 of patients.

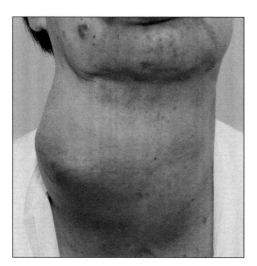
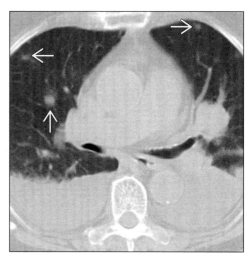

(Left) Corresponding transverse grayscale US shows a large, markedly hypoechoic, heterogeneous mass ➡ occupying most of the right thyroid lobe. Note posterior parts of the mass are not adequately assessed by US due to attenuation of the US. Note the right CCA ➡. *(Right)* Transverse grayscale US of the same patient shows a large thyroid tumor ➡ with intratumoral cystic necrosis ➡ and extrathyroid spread ➡. Guided FNAC confirmed the diagnosis of ATCa. Note the trachea ➡.

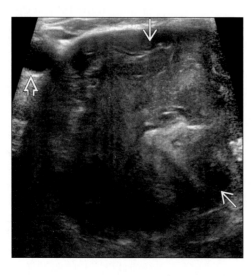
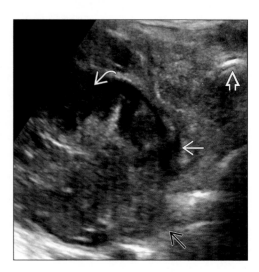

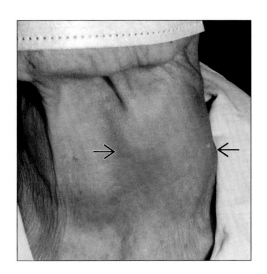

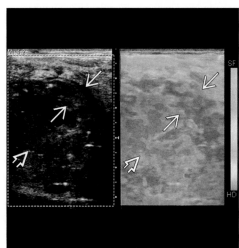

(Left) Clinical photo shows an elderly male presenting with a rapidly enlarging, painful mass in the thyroid region ➡. Clinical examination revealed a firm thyroid mass > 5 cm. *(Right)* Transverse grayscale US and qualitative strain elastogram show the thyroid with anaplastic thyroid carcinoma. Strain color scale (right) ranges from purple (soft) to red (hard). The solid margin of the tumor ➡ appears red (firm), whereas the more central, hypoechoic area ⇨, compatible with cystic necrosis, appears purple (soft).

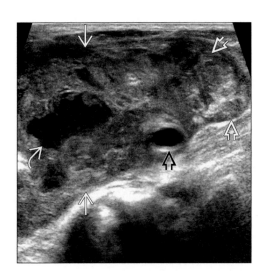

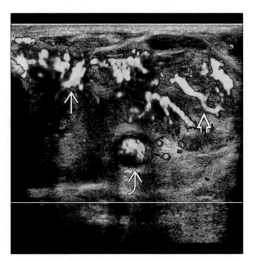

(Left) Transverse grayscale US shows a large, ill-defined thyroid mass ➡ with areas of cystic necrosis ➡, extracapsular spread, and adjacent malignant adenopathy ⇨. Note the CCA ⇨. *(Right)* Corresponding power Doppler US shows large vessels in thyroid tumor ➡ and chaotic vascularity in malignant lymph node ➡. Guided FNAC of thyroid mass confirmed diagnosis of ATCa. Necrotic ATCa may be hypovascular due to vascular infiltration and occlusion by tumor. Note the CCA ➡.

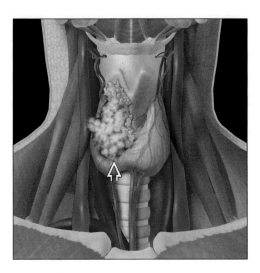

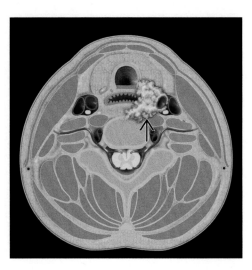

(Left) Coronal graphic shows a thyroid tumor ⇨ (T4a [stage IVa] disease). *(Right)* Axial graphic shows a thyroid tumor ➡ (T4b [stage IVb] disease). Note ATCa is always a T4 tumor. Intrathyroid disease is T4a (stage IVa), gross extrathyroid extension is T4b (stage IVb), metastatic disease is M1 (stage IVc). ATCa is rapidly fatal with a mean survival of 6 months after diagnosis. Demise is usually secondary to airway obstruction or complications of pulmonary metastases and treatment is usually palliative.

THYROID METASTASES

Key Facts

Imaging

- New-onset/rapidly enlarging hypoechoic, noncalcified thyroid nodule/mass in patient with known primary; lower pole > upper pole
- Common patterns
  - Noncalcified, well-circumscribed/ill-defined hypoechoic nodule
  - Diffuse heterogeneous hypoechoic thyroid ± goiter
  - Secondary involvement by direct extension from contagious structure (e.g., esophageal squamous cell carcinoma)
- Disorganized intralesional vascularity
- ± local invasion, cervical lymphadenopathy, other sites of distant metastasis, &/or rapid progression
- If US-guided FNA result is inconclusive, repeat biopsy + immunohistochemistry

Top Differential Diagnoses

- Thyroid adenoma

- Anaplastic thyroid carcinoma
- Differentiated thyroid carcinoma
- Thyroiditis
- Thyroid lymphoma

Pathology

- Source: Renal cell carcinoma (RCC) (48%) > lung, colorectal, breast > melanoma (4%) and sarcoma (4%)
- Immunohistochemical staining helps, especially when antibodies are selected based on known primary

Clinical Issues

- Uncommon, in 1.9-24% of patients with known 1°
- Poor prognosis due to concomitant disseminated metastasis and aggressive primary
- Prolonged disease-free survival reported after thyroidectomy in cases with slow-growing 1° (e.g., RCC, breast) and absence of extrathyroid metastases
- Long delay after diagnosis of primary possible

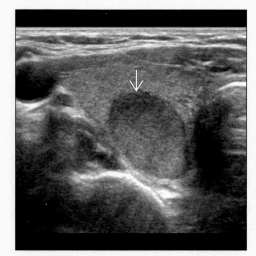
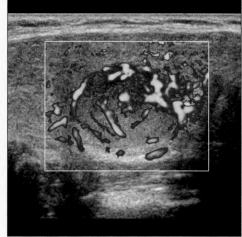

(Left) Transverse grayscale US shows a well-circumscribed, solid, homogeneously hypoechoic, noncalcified nodule ➡ in the lower pole of the right thyroid lobe, a common appearance of thyroid metastasis mimicking follicular lesion. *(Right)* Corresponding power Doppler US shows profuse, disorganized internal vascularity typical for thyroid metastasis but different from benign follicular adenoma (commonly perinodular or spoke wheel). US-guided FNA confirmed metastasis from endometrial carcinoma.

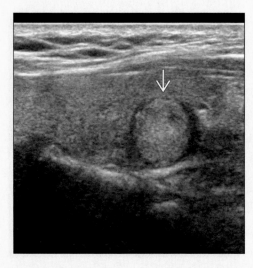
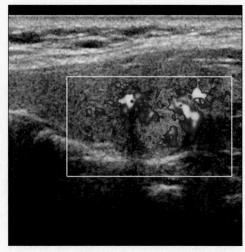

(Left) Longitudinal grayscale US shows a nodule ➡ in the lower pole of the thyroid in a patient with known carcinoma of the breast. It is well circumscribed, homogeneous, and isoechoic (similar to follicular adenoma). *(Right)* Corresponding longitudinal power Doppler US shows disorganized intranodular vascularity. In a patient with known primary, such a nodule should raise suspicion of thyroid metastases. In this case, FNA cytology (FNAC) confirmed metastasis from primary carcinoma of the breast.

THYROID METASTASES

TERMINOLOGY

Definitions
- Metastasis to thyroid gland from nonthyroid primary

IMAGING

General Features
- New-onset/rapidly enlarging hypoechoic, noncalcified thyroid nodule/mass in patient with known primary
- Location: Lower pole > upper pole

Ultrasonographic Findings
- Grayscale ultrasound
  - Common patterns
    - Well-circumscribed nodule (common)
      - Solitary or multifocal
      - Noncalcified, solid, homogeneous, hypoechoic/isoechoic, ± cystic change
    - Ill-defined mass
      - Heterogeneously hypoechoic mass, more often in lower pole, ± extension beyond thyroid capsule
      - Predominantly cystic mass with thick, irregular septa that appear similar to primary
    - Diffuse thyroid involvement
      - Diffuse heterogeneous, hypoechoic thyroid parenchyma ± diffuse enlargement of gland
    - Secondary involvement by direct extension from contagious structure (esophageal squamous cell carcinoma [SCCa], metastatic cervical nodes)
  - Local invasion possible
    - Through thyroid capsule, to strap muscles, encasing carotid arteries, etc.
    - Reported tendency of thyroid metastasis from renal cell carcinoma (RCC) to invade internal jugular vein
  - Rapid progression on follow-up scan
  - Lymphadenopathy related to known primary (supraclavicular from infraclavicular primary) or related to thyroid metastasis (central > lateral cervical)
  - Other sites of metastasis
    - Skin/muscle deposits; lung, brain, bone
- Power Doppler
  - Disorganized intratumoral vascularity

Imaging Recommendations
- Best imaging tool: Ultrasound with guided FNA

DIFFERENTIAL DIAGNOSIS

Thyroid Adenoma
- Typically solitary, oval-shaped, haloed
- Perinodular > intranodular vascularity

Anaplastic Thyroid Carcinoma
- Rapid clinical course; difficult to differentiate from thyroid metastasis in elderly patient with known primary

Differentiated Thyroid Carcinoma
- Punctate calcification in papillary carcinoma ± associated typical metastatic nodes

Thyroiditis
- Middle-aged female ± longstanding thyroid dysfunction

Thyroid Lymphoma
- Background Hashimoto thyroiditis
- ± systemic lymphoma

PATHOLOGY

Microscopic Features
- Source: RCC (48%) > lung, colorectal, breast > melanoma (4%) and sarcoma (4%); originates from primary that tends to spread hematologically
- FNA: > 70% correct diagnosis, > 20% misdiagnosed
  - Misdiagnosis ↑ in SCCa esophagus, cervix, RCC, and malignant melanoma
- Immunohistochemistry helps to exclude thyroid primary (except in certain cases of anaplastic thyroid cancer) and when antibodies are selected based on known primary

CLINICAL ISSUES

Presentation
- Enlarging thyroid nodule, goiter, dysphagia, dysphonia ± cough ± dramatic lower neck swelling and respiratory compromise
- 25% found incidentally on imaging or physical exam
- Euthyroid (88%) > hypo-/hyperthyroid (transient)
- Metachronous (80%) > synchronous (20%)
  - May be found 4.5 months to 21 years before diagnosis of primary
    - Metastases from lung primary is diagnosed earliest
- Extrathyroid metastases are present in 60% of patients with thyroid metastases

Demographics
- M:F = 1:1.4
- Occurs in 1.9-24% of patients with known primary

Natural History & Prognosis
- Poor prognosis due to concomitant disseminated metastasis and aggressive primary
- Prolonged disease-free survival reported after thyroidectomy in cases with slow-growing primary (e.g., RCC, breast) and absence of extrathyroid metastases

DIAGNOSTIC CHECKLIST

Image Interpretation Pearls
- Long delay after diagnosis of primary possible
- If ultrasound-guided FNA result is inconclusive, repeat biopsy + immunohistochemistry

SELECTED REFERENCES
1. Chung AY et al: Metastases to the thyroid: a review of the literature from the last decade. Thyroid. 22(3):258-68, 2012
2. Kim TY et al: Metastasis to the thyroid diagnosed by fine-needle aspiration biopsy. Clin Endocrinol (Oxf). 62(2):236-41, 2005
3. Pickhardt PJ et al: Sonography of delayed thyroid metastasis from renal cell carcinoma with jugular vein extension. AJR Am J Roentgenol. 181(1):272-4, 2003
4. Ahuja AT et al: Role of ultrasonography in thyroid metastases. Clin Radiol. 49(9):627-9, 1994

(Left) Longitudinal grayscale US shows an ill-defined, heterogeneously hypoechoic, noncalcified mass ➡ in the lower pole of the right thyroid lobe with possible extrathyroid extension ➡.
(Right) Corresponding longitudinal power Doppler shows profuse, disorganized intratumoral vascularity ➡. Appearances are highly suspicious for metastases in this patient with nasopharyngeal carcinoma, confirmed on FNAC. Note the indistinct border of the posterior thyroid capsule ➡ indicating local invasion.

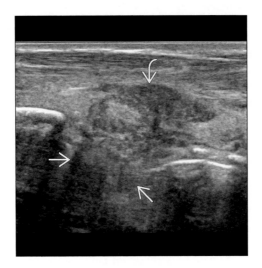
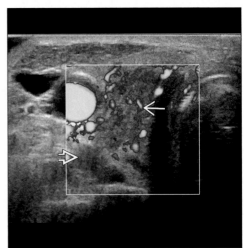

(Left) Transverse grayscale US in a patient with uterine leiomyosarcoma shows enlargement of the left thyroid lobe due to a large, solid, heterogeneous, noncalcified hypoechoic mass ➡. Note bulging of the thyroid capsule ➡ without definite infiltration of strap muscles ➡. Trachea ➡ and esophagus ➡ are displaced.
(Right) Corresponding axial CECT shows heterogeneous hypoenhancement of the thyroid mass ➡ and displaced trachea ➡ and esophagus ➡. FNAC confirmed thyroid metastases.

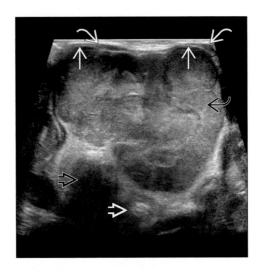
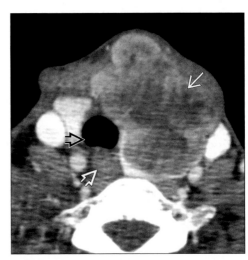

(Left) Transverse grayscale US of the left thyroid lobe in a patient with carcinoma of the lung shows a diffusely heterogeneous and hypoechoic thyroid gland ➡ with rounded contour.
(Right) Corresponding transverse grayscale US shows diffuse infiltration of the right thyroid lobe ➡ with a focal, solid, hypoechoic nodule ➡ within, and multiple abnormal nodes in the right posterior triangle ➡. US features suggest diffuse thyroid metastases, later confirmed by US-guided FNA.

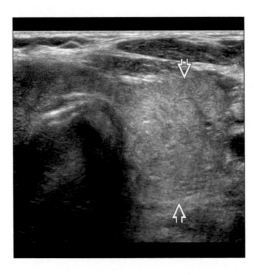
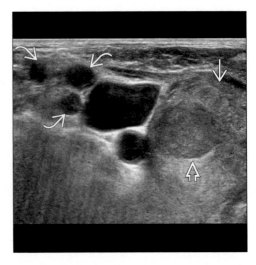

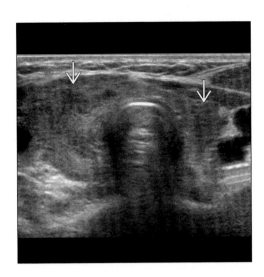

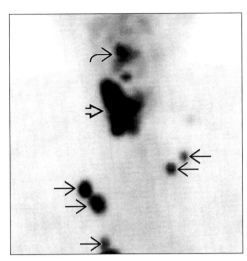

(Left) Transverse grayscale US shows a diffusely heterogeneous, hypoechoic thyroid parenchymal echo pattern bilaterally ➡️ (right > left lobe) in a patient with nasopharyngeal carcinoma. In view of patient's history, US features are highly suspicious of thyroid metastases. (Right) Corresponding anterior FDG PET/CT shows intense FDG uptake in the nasopharynx ➡️, thyroid ➡️, and lung ➡️, confirmed to be disseminated metastases. Diffuse uptake in right > left lobe of thyroid correlates with US findings.

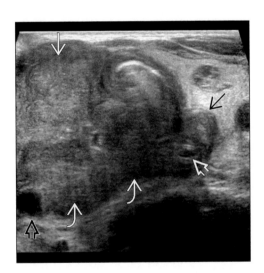

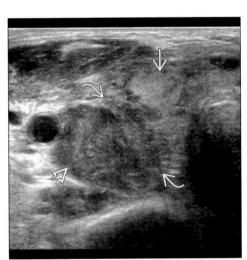

(Left) Transverse grayscale US shows a diffusely enlarged, hypoechoic right thyroid lobe ➡️ due to infiltration by a tumor ➡️ arising from the esophagus ➡️. Note the nasogastric tube ➡️ and encasement of the right common carotid artery ➡️. (Right) Transverse grayscale US in another patient shows direct invasion of the right thyroid lobe ➡️ by a metastatic lymph node ➡️ from carcinoma of the lung. Note the loss of echogenic thyroid capsule ➡️ and diffuse hypoechoic echo pattern of right thyroid lobe.

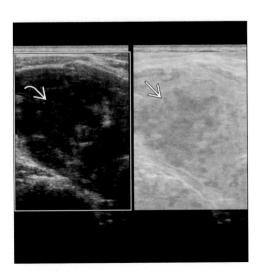

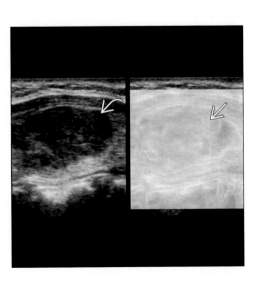

(Left) Transverse strain elastography shows stiff ➡️ (red) metastatic malignant melanoma involving the right thyroid lobe. Corresponding grayscale US shows an ill-defined hypoechoic mass ➡️ in the right thyroid lobe. (Right) Longitudinal strain elastography shows thyroid metastasis ➡️ that appears soft (green). The stiffness of a metastatic thyroid nodule may be variable. Note that it is solid, hypoechoic, and noncalcified ➡️ on accompanying grayscale US.

THYROID NON-HODGKIN LYMPHOMA

Key Facts

Imaging

- Rapidly enlarging, solid, noncalcified thyroid mass in patient with history of Hashimoto thyroiditis (HT)
- Background evidence of previous HT: Echogenic fibrous streaks in lobulated, hypoechoic gland
- Focal lymphomatous mass/nodule
  - Pseudocystic appearance with posterior enhancement
  - Well defined, solid, hypoechoic, heterogeneous, noncalcified, solitary/multiple, unilateral/bilateral
- Diffuse involvement
  - Hypoechoic, rounded gland with heterogeneous echo pattern
  - Simple thyroid enlargement, minimal change in echo pattern (often missed)
  - Presence of adjacent lymphomatous nodes and background HT may be only clue to diagnosis

- Lymphadenopathy: Reticulated or pseudocystic echo pattern
- Usually multiple nodes ± bilateral involvement
- Nodes are invariably solid; necrosis is not a feature
- Color Doppler: Thyroid nodules are nonspecific or hypovascular or have chaotic intranodular vessels
  - Nodes: Central > peripheral vascularity

Top Differential Diagnoses

- Anaplastic thyroid carcinoma, differentiated thyroid carcinoma, metastases to thyroid, multinodular goiter

Diagnostic Checklist

- Rapidly enlarging thyroid mass in elderly patient is usually due to thyroid non-Hodgkin lymphoma (NHL) or anaplastic carcinoma
- Absence of calcification, invasion, and necrosis is suggestive of NHL but not specific

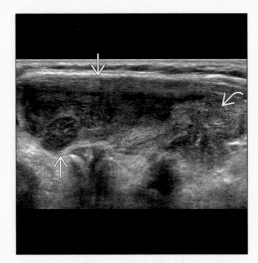
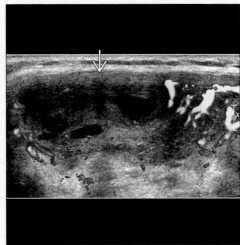

(Left) Longitudinal grayscale US shows an ill-defined, noncalcified, heterogeneous nodule ➡ with cystic areas in the upper pole of the thyroid. Note background evidence of Hashimoto thyroiditis (HT) in thyroid parenchyma ➡. *(Right)* Power Doppler US (same patient) shows no significant vascularity in the nodule ➡, which shows cystic change. In a patient with HT, any rapidly enlarging thyroid mass should raise suspicion of non-Hodgkin lymphoma (NHL). In this case, guided biopsy confirmed thyroid NHL.

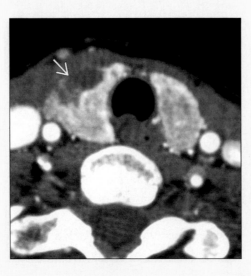
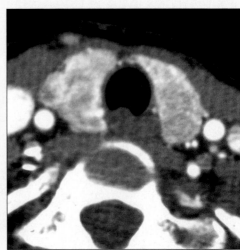

(Left) Axial CECT (same patient) shows heterogeneous thyroid parenchymal enhancement with a focal nodule ➡ in the right lobe. Lymphomatous thyroid nodules are usually solid and noncalcified, and the cystic necrosis/hemorrhage seen in this case is uncommon. *(Right)* Axial CECT through the thyroid gland (same patient) shows diffuse, patchy, heterogeneous enhancement of the thyroid gland, not the normal intense, homogeneous enhancement. This is reflective of background HT.

THYROID NON-HODGKIN LYMPHOMA

TERMINOLOGY

Abbreviations
- Thyroid non-Hodgkin lymphoma (NHL)

Definitions
- Primary thyroid NHL: Extranodal, extralymphatic lymphoma arising from thyroid gland

IMAGING

General Features
- Best diagnostic clue
  - Rapidly enlarging, solid, noncalcified thyroid mass in patient with history of Hashimoto thyroiditis (HT)
- Size
  - Often large (5-10 cm)
- Morphology
  - Diffuse, homogeneous thyromegaly if chronic lymphocytic thyroiditis is present
    - ± lymphomatous neck nodes
  - Primary tumor
    - Rapidly enlarging, homogeneous, solid mass
    - Single mass (80%), multiple masses, or diffusely infiltrated thyroid gland
    - Tendency to compress normal thyroid and surrounding structures without invasion
    - Necrosis, calcification, & hemorrhage are relatively uncommon (vs. anaplastic thyroid carcinoma)
  - Lymphadenopathy
    - When present, cervical nodes are usually multiple, bilateral, and solid/reticulated

Ultrasonographic Findings
- Color Doppler
  - Thyroid nodules: Nonspecific, hypovascular or have chaotic intranodular vessels
  - Nodes: Central > peripheral vascularity
- Background evidence of previous HT: Echogenic fibrous streaks in lobulated, hypoechoic gland
- Focal lymphomatous mass/nodule: Pseudocystic appearance with posterior enhancement
  - Well defined, solid, hypoechoic, heterogeneous, noncalcified, solitary/multiple, unilateral/bilateral
- Diffuse involvement: Hypoechoic, rounded gland with heterogeneous echo pattern
  - Simple thyroid enlargement, minimal change in echo pattern (often missed)
  - Presence of adjacent lymphomatous nodes and background HT may be the only clue to diagnosis
- Lymphadenopathy: Reticulated or pseudocystic echo pattern
  - Usually multiple nodes ± bilateral involvement
  - Nodes are invariably solid; necrosis is not a feature
  - Nodes cause mass effect on adjacent vessels but do not infiltrate carotid or jugular vein

Imaging Recommendations
- Best imaging tool
  - Thyroid NHL is often detected/suspected on routine serial follow-up US of HT
  - Development of focal hypoechoic nodules or ill-defined hypoechoic areas in patients with HT is suspicious for NHL
  - Presence of lymphomatous nodes on US during examination of patient with HT should raise suspicion of thyroid NHL
  - US-guided biopsy of thyroid ± neck nodes helps to confirm diagnosis
  - CECT of neck, chest, abdomen, and pelvis is required for staging when diagnosis is known
- Protocol advice
  - Lymphomatous nodules and nodes were previously described to have pseudosolid appearance: Anechoic with posterior enhancement but solid on biopsy
  - With modern transducers, such appearance is rare, and internal solid nature is clearly identified
    - Lymphomatous nodes have reticulated appearance on modern high-resolution transducers

DIFFERENTIAL DIAGNOSIS

Anaplastic Thyroid Carcinoma
- Rapidly enlarging, invasive thyroid mass in elderly patient against background of multinodular goiter
- Calcification, necrosis, and heterogeneous tumor with vascular and soft tissue extension and necrotic nodes

Differentiated Thyroid Carcinoma
- Unilateral, ill-defined, solid, hypoechoic mass with abnormal vascularity ± punctate calcification and adjacent characteristic adenopathy
- Large, invasive tumor may be indistinguishable from anaplastic carcinoma or lymphoma

Metastases to Thyroid
- May mimic thyroid lymphoma, but invariably there is evidence of disseminated disease and known primary
- Focal, solid, solitary/multiple, well-defined nodules with hypervascularity or diffuse thyroid enlargement with adjacent characteristic adenopathy

Multinodular Goiter
- Multiple, hypoechoic, heterogeneous, cystic/septated nodules with perinodular vascularity, coarse calcification, ± "comet tail" artifact
- Rapid increase in size: Spontaneous hemorrhage

CLINICAL ISSUES

Presentation
- Most common signs/symptoms
  - Rapidly enlarging thyroid mass, frequently with associated neck adenopathy in patient with HT
    - Low-grade NHL has slower growth rate

DIAGNOSTIC CHECKLIST

Image Interpretation Pearls
- Rapidly enlarging thyroid mass in elderly patient is usually due to thyroid NHL or anaplastic carcinoma
- Absence of calcification, invasion, and necrosis is suggestive of NHL but not specific

SELECTED REFERENCES

1. Sofferman RA et al: Ultrasound of the Thyroid and Parathyroid Glands. 1st ed. New York: Springer. 107-150, 2012

THYROID NON-HODGKIN LYMPHOMA

(Left) Axial grayscale US of the left lobe of the thyroid (same patient) shows hypoechoic, heterogeneous, parenchymal echogenicity with fine fibrotic streaks ➡️, which is the typical grayscale appearance of HT. Note the trachea ⏩ and common carotid artery ➡️. *(Right)* Longitudinal power Doppler US (same patient) shows prominent thyroid parenchymal vascularity in HT, reflecting thyroid-stimulating hormone (TSH) effect on thyroid gland.

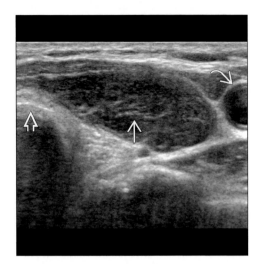
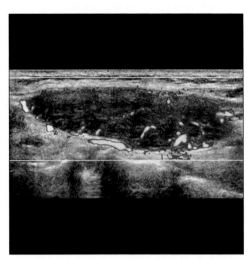

(Left) Axial T1WI C+ MR (same patient) shows focal lower signal ➡️ than the surrounding thyroid parenchyma, corresponding to a lymphomatous nodule (with cystic change) seen on US and CT. *(Right)* Axial T2WI MR (same patient) shows similar lymphomatous ➡️ involvement in the right lobe of the thyroid. MR clearly defines the extent of thyroid involvement and helps in disease staging. NHL confined to the thyroid is staged as IE; presence of regional nodes changes the stage to IIE.

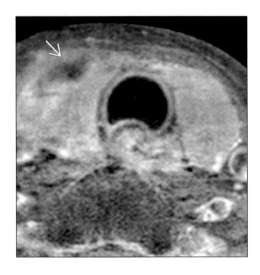
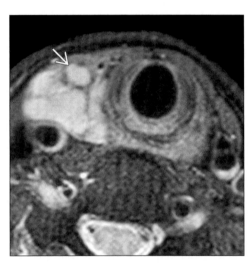

(Left) Transverse grayscale US and qualitative strain elastogram shows diffuse thyroid NHL ⏩. Strain color scale ranges from purple (elastic, soft) to red (inelastic, hard). It appears mostly inelastic, but strain EI may be misleading here as there is no normal thyroid for reference. *(Right)* Transverse grayscale US and SWE shows diffuse thyroid NHL ⏩. SWE color scale ranges from blue (0 kPa, soft) to red (180 kPa, stiff). It has maximum SWE of 30.5 kPa, which is only slightly higher than that of normal thyroid.

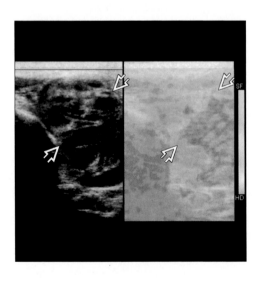
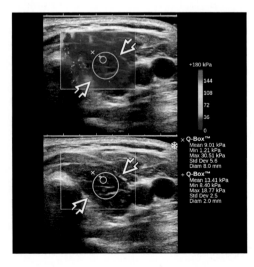

THYROID NON-HODGKIN LYMPHOMA

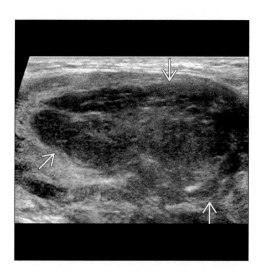

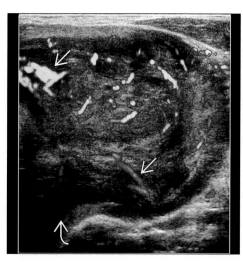

(Left) Longitudinal grayscale US in a patient with HT presenting with rapidly enlarging thyroid mass raising suspicion of thyroid NHL shows that most of left thyroid lobe is occupied by a large, solid, hypoechoic, noncalcified, heterogeneous mass ➡. *(Right)* Axial power Doppler US (same patient) shows scattered large vessels ➡ within the thyroid mass. US-guided biopsy confirmed thyroid NHL. Note suspicious extraglandular extension of the tumor posteriorly ➡. No abnormal neck nodes were identified on imaging.

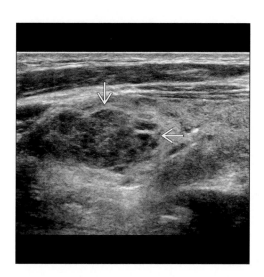

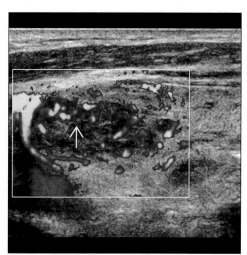

(Left) Longitudinal grayscale US of the contralateral lobe (same patient) also shows an ill-defined, solid, noncalcified, hypoechoic tumor ➡. *(Right)* Power Doppler US (same patient) shows marked intratumoral vascularity ➡. Note that 80% of thyroid NHLs are seen as solitary thyroid masses, whereas the rest present as multiple masses or diffuse infiltration. Thyroid lymphoma is most often diffuse large B-cell lymphoma. Others include B-cell mucosa-associated lymphoid tissue (MALT) and follicular lymphoma.

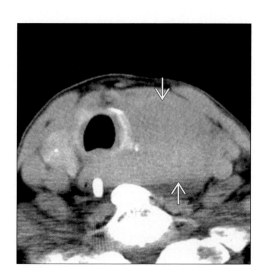

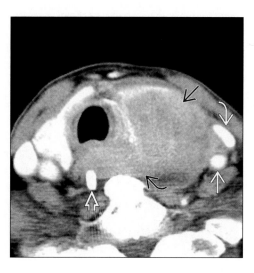

(Left) Axial NECT (same patient) shows a homogeneous, solid, noncalcified left thyroid mass ➡. *(Right)* Axial NECT (same patient) shows no obvious enhancement of the thyroid NHL mass ➡. Note its extraglandular extension ➡ posteriorly, displacement of the esophagus to the right (nasogastric tube in esophagus ➡), and mass effect but no infiltration of the left common carotid artery ➡ and internal jugular vein ➡.

MULTINODULAR GOITER

Key Facts

Imaging

- Multiplicity of nodules, bilateral diffuse involvement
- Despite being unencapsulated, nodules are sharply defined and haloed ± conglomeration
- Solid nodules are often isoechoic with small proportion being hypoechoic (5%)
- Heterogeneous internal echo pattern with internal debris, septa, solid/cystic portions
- Dense shadowing calcification (curvilinear, dysmorphic, coarse) ± multiple
- Nodules with "comet tail" artifact, highly suggestive of colloid nodule (mimics microcalcification)
- Cystic component due to degeneration, hemorrhage, or colloid within nodule
- Background thyroid parenchymal echoes are coarse & heterogeneous (fine bright echoes in normal gland)
- Color Doppler: Peripheral > intranodular vascularity

- Color Doppler: Septa and intranodular solid portions are avascular (organizing blood, clot)

Top Differential Diagnoses

- Papillary carcinoma
- Follicular carcinoma
- Anaplastic thyroid carcinoma
- Medullary carcinoma

Diagnostic Checklist

- Role of US in MNG: Detect any suspicious nodule, guide biopsy, and identify any retrosternal extension
- Look for papillary carcinoma in MNG: solid, ill-defined, hypoechoic nodule, punctate microcalcification and chaotic intranodular vessels
- Evaluate neck for metastatic nodes: Solid/cystic, hyperechoic, punctate microcalcification, abnormal vascularity, pre-/paratracheal & deep cervical chain

(Left) Transverse grayscale US shows multiple solid, haloed, hyperechoic (compared to adjacent muscle) nodules ➡️ *in an enlarged left lobe of thyroid. Note the trachea* ⬅️ *and left common carotid artery (CCA)* ➡️. *(Right) Corresponding longitudinal grayscale US shows multiple solid, hyperdense nodules* ➡️ *of variable sizes in thyroid. Note the absence of suspicious features such as hypoechogenicity, punctate calcification, and taller than wide shape, which may necessitate guided FNAC to rule out malignancy.*

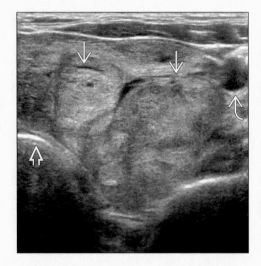
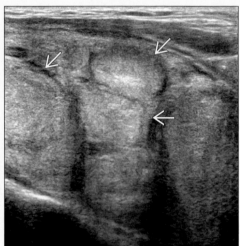

(Left) Longitudinal grayscale US shows a haloed, noncalcified, heterogeneous thyroid nodule ➡️ *with focal cystic change* ➡️ *and fine septation. (Right) Corresponding power Doppler US shows predominantly perinodular vascularity, vascular halo* ➡️, *and intranodular vascularity. Halo represents compressed thyroid tissue & its vascularity. Thick avascular halo represents fibrous capsule around neoplastic mass. Presence/absence of halo is not a good indicator of the nodule's nature (benign vs. malignant).*

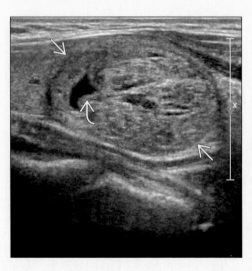
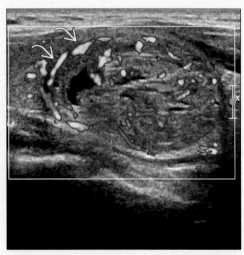

MULTINODULAR GOITER

TERMINOLOGY

Definitions
- Diffuse, multinodular enlargement of thyroid gland in response to chronic TSH stimulation
- Plunging/substernal/retrosternal goiter: Inferior extension of multinodular goiter (MNG) into mediastinum

IMAGING

General Features
- Best diagnostic clue
  - Well-marginated, diffuse enlargement of thyroid gland with a heterogeneous, nodular appearance
  - Calcifications, fibrosis, cystic change, and hemorrhage produce heterogeneous imaging appearance
- Location
  - Visceral space, thyroid bed
    - Substernal extension occurs in 37% of patients
- Size
  - May be very large (> 15 cm)
- Morphology
  - Well-defined, diffuse thyroid enlargement in visceral space of infrahyoid neck
    - Carotid spaces displaced away from midline; trachea compressed between enlarged thyroid lobes

Ultrasonographic Findings
- Grayscale ultrasound
  - Multiple nodules, bilateral diffuse involvement
  - Solid nodules are often isoechoic with small proportion being hypoechoic (5%)
  - Despite being unencapsulated, nodules are sharply defined and haloed ± conglomeration
    - Halo composed of vessels and compressed thyroid
  - Heterogeneous internal echo pattern with internal debris, septa, solid/cystic portions
    - Solid portion within often represents blood clot
  - Dense shadowing calcification (curvilinear, dysmorphic, coarse) ± multiple
  - Nodules with "comet tail" artifact, highly suggestive of colloid nodule (mimics microcalcification)
  - Cystic component due to degeneration, hemorrhage, or colloid within nodule
  - Background thyroid parenchymal echoes are coarse and heterogeneous (fine bright echoes in normal gland)
  - Color Doppler: Peripheral > intranodular vascularity
  - Color Doppler: Septa and intranodular solid portions are avascular (organizing blood, clot)

Imaging Recommendations
- Best imaging tool
  - US is ideal imaging modality as it evaluates thyroid nodules and adjacent mass effect, and identifies any suspicious nodule (± guided biopsy)
  - US is ideal for follow-up on apprehensive patients who are otherwise asymptomatic
  - Risk of malignancy in MNG is 1-5%; most common cancer is papillary thyroid cancer
    - Anaplastic carcinoma is usually seen against a background of multinodularity and is less common than papillary carcinoma
  - Look for papillary carcinoma in MNG: Search for solid, ill-defined, hypoechoic nodule, punctate microcalcification, and chaotic intranodular vessels
    - Evaluate neck for metastatic nodes: Solid/cystic, hyperechoic, punctate microcalcification, abnormal vascularity, pre-/paratracheal, deep cervical chain
  - US guides needle biopsy of suspicious nodules
  - US is unable to evaluate large goiters, particularly their infraclavicular/mediastinal extent, severity of airway compression; CT/MR are better
- Protocol advice
  - Main role of US in MNG is to identify presence of any suspicious nodule and guide biopsy
  - Evaluate neck for suspicious/metastatic nodes and for any retrosternal extension

DIFFERENTIAL DIAGNOSIS

Papillary Carcinoma
- Ill-defined, solid, hypoechoic nodule with punctate microcalcification and chaotic intranodular vessels
- Abnormal nodes: Solid/cystic, hyperechoic, punctate microcalcification, abnormal vessels

Follicular Carcinoma
- Ill- or well-defined, hypoechoic, solid nodule with abnormal vascularity, no calcification ± distant metastases
- Unilateral with normal thyroid tissue seen; other small heterogeneous nodules to suggest MNG may be seen

Anaplastic Thyroid Carcinoma
- Rapidly enlarging, heterogeneous, ill-defined, coarse calcification, invasive tumor originating from thyroid
- Esophagus, trachea, carotid space may be invaded

Medullary Carcinoma
- Ill-defined/well-defined, hypoechoic, solid nodule with abnormal vascularity and coarse shadowing calcification
- Abnormal nodes: Solid, hypoechoic, coarse shadowing focus, abnormal vessels, characteristic distribution

PATHOLOGY

General Features
- Associated abnormalities
  - Risk of cancer in MNG (5%)
    - Risk factors for malignancy: Radiation exposure, family history of thyroid carcinoma, rapid growth
- 95% MNG benign; 5% malignant
  - Incidence of malignancy in MNG ~ to a single nodule
  - Papillary carcinoma and anaplastic carcinoma may be seen with MNG
- MNG most common cause of asymmetric thyroid enlargement; 3-5% of general population affected in developed countries
- Substernal extension in 37%, majority anterior mediastinum, rarely posterior mediastinum

SELECTED REFERENCES

1. Sofferman RA et al. Ultrasound of the Thyroid and Parathyroid Glands. 1st ed. New York: Springer. 61-106, 2012

MULTINODULAR GOITER

(Left) Transverse grayscale US shows the characteristic spongiform/puff pastry/honeycomb appearance (aggregation of microcystic components in > 50% of nodule volume) of thyroid nodule ➡. Note the right CCA ⬈ and trachea ⬊. *(Right)* Corresponding longitudinal grayscale US shows a spongiform thyroid nodule ➡. Spongiform appearance is highly specific for hyperplastic nodule, has high negative predictive value for malignancy, and may obviate need for confirmatory FNAC.

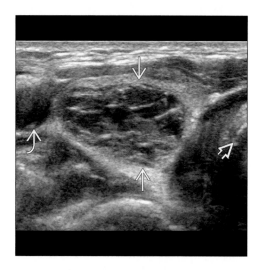
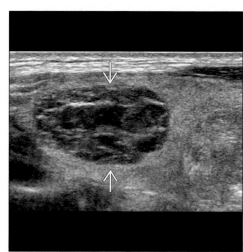

(Left) Transverse grayscale US shows multiple heterogeneous thyroid nodules, some with cystic change ➡ and dense shadowing calcification ➡. This appearance is commonly seen in MNG. Note trachea ⬊ and right CCA ⬈. *(Right)* Corresponding longitudinal grayscale US shows multiple solid nodules ➡ scattered within thyroid parenchyma. In MNG, the aim of US is to detect malignant nodules, as the risk of cancer in patients with multiple nodules is the same as in patients with solitary nodule.

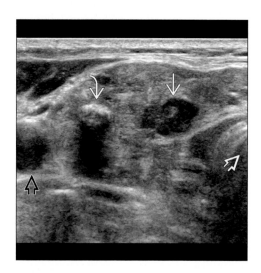
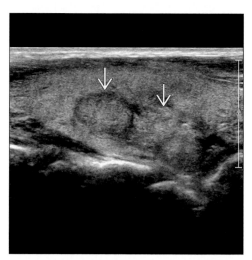

(Left) Transverse grayscale US shows diffuse enlargement of the thyroid, which is studded with multiple solid, hyperechoic nodules ➡. Note posterior parts of thyroid are not clearly seen due to sound attenuation in deeper parts. The trachea ⬊ is shown. *(Right)* Axial CECT clearly defines thyroid enlargement, its extent, & its relationship to adjacent structures. US cannot define the extent of large tumors, extrathyroid infiltration, mediastinal extension, airway compression, and malignancy when thyroid volume is high.

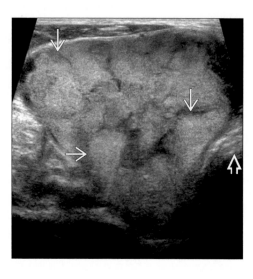
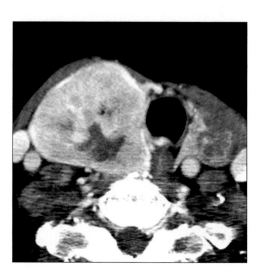

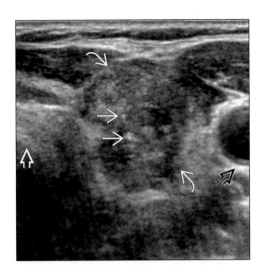

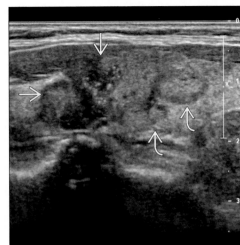

(Left) Transverse grayscale US shows a solid, ill-defined, hypoechoic thyroid nodule ➡ with punctate microcalcification ➡, typical features of papillary carcinoma. Note the trachea ➡ and left CCA ➡. *(Right)* Corresponding longitudinal grayscale US shows papillary carcinoma ➡. Note evidence of background multinodularity ➡. The primary role of US in MNG is to detect thyroid malignancy, guide FNAC (for increased accuracy), and evaluate the neck for associated metastatic lymph nodes.

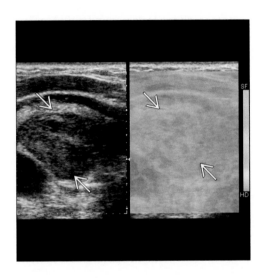

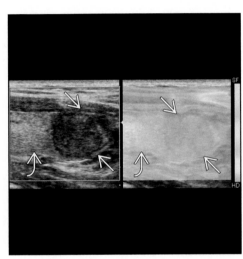

(Left) Transverse grayscale US and qualitative strain elastogram show a hyperplastic thyroid nodule ➡. Strain color scale ranges from purple (elastic/soft) to red (inelastic/hard). The nodule is mostly green & purple, indicating an elastic lesion. *(Right)* Longitudinal grayscale US and qualitative strain elastogram show a hyperplastic thyroid nodule ➡. It is mostly green (elastic) and appears more elastic than the adjacent parenchyma ➡. Both nodules are true-positive for benign nodule on strain EI.

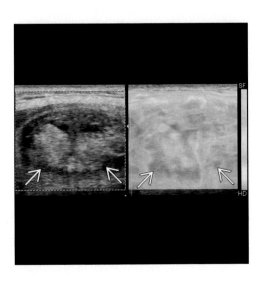

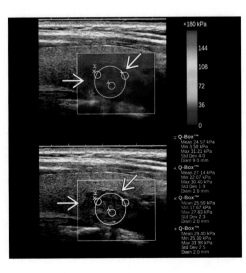

(Left) Longitudinal grayscale US and qualitative strain elastogram show a hyperplastic thyroid nodule ➡. It is mostly red (inelastic) and is false-positive for cancer on strain EI. *(Right)* Longitudinal grayscale US & SWE shows a hyperplastic nodule ➡. SWE color scale ranges from blue (0 kPa, soft) to red (180 kPa, stiff). The nodule appears blue, similar to the adjacent thyroid parenchyma, with maximum stiffness of 34.0 kPa, which suggests a soft nodule. This is true-positive for benign nodule on SWE.

THYROID ADENOMA

Key Facts

Terminology

- True adenoma: Benign neoplasm of thyroid glandular epithelium with fibrous encapsulation
- Adenomatous nodule: Focal adenomatous hyperplasia with incomplete capsule; cold nodule

Imaging

- Solid, homogeneous, noncalcified, well-defined, haloed, isoechoic or hyperechoic; hypoechoic is less common and has ↑ risk of malignancy
- Hürthle cell neoplasms have similar imaging characteristics to follicular nodule (FN)
- In general, differentiation between follicular adenoma and follicular carcinoma cannot be made by ultrasound, FNA, or core needle biopsy
- Defined by invasive features (nodular capsule or vascular penetration) at histology

- US features that raise suspicion of malignant FN: Ill-defined, hypoechoic component in otherwise iso-/hyperechoic nodule, thick irregular capsule
- Rarely, definite sonographic sign of malignant FN may be seen: Invasion beyond thyroid capsule &/or regional or distant metastasis, vascular thrombosis
- Absence of internal flow or predominantly peripheral flow indicates low probability of thyroid FN malignancy; predominant internal flow is associated with malignancy
- FA is usually slow growing; rapid enlargement occurs with spontaneous hemorrhage
- Adenomatous hyperplasia likely to have degenerative changes

Top Differential Diagnoses

- Multinodular goiter
- Thyroid differentiated carcinoma
- Medullary thyroid carcinoma

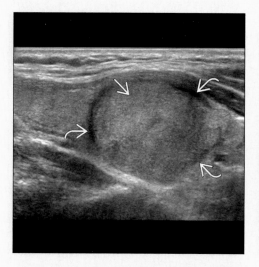
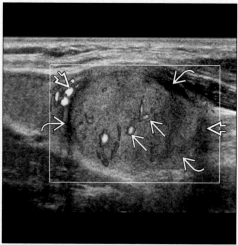

(Left) Longitudinal grayscale US shows typical appearance of follicular adenoma (FA) ➡: Well-defined, oval, solid, noncalcified, homogeneous, and isoechoic with a well-defined hypoechoic halo ➡. (Right) Corresponding longitudinal power Doppler US shows perinodular halo is avascular, likely representing a fibrous capsule ➡. Scattered, mixed perinodular ➡ and intranodular ➡ vascularity is seen. FNA showed a benign follicular lesion. Predominant intranodular flow is associated with malignancy.

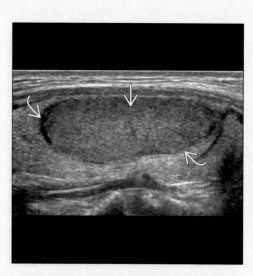
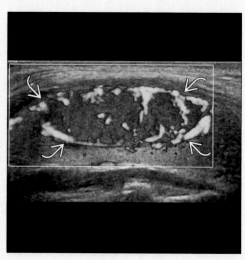

(Left) Longitudinal grayscale US shows a homogeneously hypoechoic follicular lesion ➡. FA can occasionally be hypoechoic, but such nodules have an increased risk of malignancy. Note the thin rim of a complete, hypoechoic halo ➡. (Right) Corresponding longitudinal power Doppler ultrasound shows predominantly perinodular vascularity ➡. The hypoechoic halo seen on grayscale predominantly represents compressed thyroid and perinodular vessels. A fibrous capsule around an adenoma is often avascular.

THYROID ADENOMA

TERMINOLOGY

Definitions
- True adenoma: Benign neoplasm of thyroid glandular epithelium with fibrous encapsulation
  - Follicular adenoma (FA) and Hürthle cell adenoma (HCA)
- Adenomatous nodule: Focal adenomatous hyperplasia with incomplete capsule; cold nodule

IMAGING

General Features
- Best diagnostic clue
  - Thyroid adenoma: Well-defined nodule compresses adjacent gland
  - Adenomatous nodule: Less distinct lesion contours, often multiple
  - Adenomatous nodules are more common than adenomas

Ultrasonographic Findings
- Grayscale ultrasound
  - Solid and homogeneous in 70%
  - Well-defined hypoechoic halo in 80% = compressed thyroid tissue &/or fibrous capsule
  - Isoechoic or hyperechoic to adjacent thyroid parenchyma
    - Hypoechoic appearance is less common and has higher risk of being malignant
  - Calcification and cystic change are rare
  - Hürthle cell neoplasms are rare and share similar imaging characteristics with follicular nodule (FN), usually diagnosed after FNA/biopsy/excision
  - In general, differentiation between FA and follicular carcinoma (FC) cannot be made by ultrasound, FNA, or core needle biopsy
    - Defined by invasive features (nodular capsule or vascular penetration) at microscopic level → histological diagnosis
    - FNA showing FN has 10-20% chance of malignancy
    - US features that raise suspicion of malignant FN: Ill-defined border, hypoechoic component in an otherwise iso-/hyperechoic nodule, thick irregular capsule
    - Rarely, definite sonographic sign of malignant FN may be seen: Invasion beyond thyroid capsule &/or regional or distant metastasis, vascular thrombosis
- Power Doppler
  - Typical vascular pattern
    - Type II vascularity = perinodular > intranodular
    - "Spoke-wheel" appearance = peripheral blood vessels extending toward center of lesion
  - Absence of internal flow or predominantly peripheral flow indicates low probability of thyroid FN malignancy; predominant internal flow is associated with malignancy

Nuclear Medicine Findings
- F18-FDG PET: Can be FDG avid
- Tc-99m pertechnetate or I-123
  - Hot nodule: Often autonomous adenoma, < 1% malignant
  - Cold nodule: 20% malignant

DIFFERENTIAL DIAGNOSIS

Multinodular Goiter
- Hyperplastic response of entire thyroid gland to stimulus as opposed to neoplastic nature of FA
- Multiple isoechoic, solid/heterogeneous, partially haloed nodules in diffusely enlarged thyroid gland ± spongiform appearance

Thyroid Differentiated Carcinoma
- Hypoechoic, ill-defined, heterogeneous nodule with punctate calcification, of taller than wide shape and abnormal vascularity ± associated typical metastatic nodes

Medullary Thyroid Carcinoma
- Hypoechoic, solid, ill defined, central dense calcification, abnormal vascularity, ± associated metastatic nodes

Lymphocytic Thyroiditis
- Mimics FA on grayscale US, mixed intra-/perinodular and disorganized vascularity, eggshell calcification possible, ~ 5% of all biopsied nodules

PATHOLOGY

General Features
- Results from genetic mutation or other genetic abnormality in precursor cell
- FA is defined as benign tumor with uniform, follicular cell differentiation encapsulated by fibrous capsule
- ± hemorrhage, fibrosis, calcification, and cystic change

Staging, Grading, & Classification
- Classified according to cellular architecture and relative amount of cellularity and colloid
  - Simple (normofollicular), fetal (microfollicular), colloid (macrofollicular), and embryonal (atypical); Hürthle cell lesion (oncocytic) is usually considered subtype of FA

Microscopic Features
- Differentiation between benign follicular adenoma and carcinoma generally depends on histopathology; FNA can suggest diagnosis of FN but cannot determine malignant capsular or vascular invasion
- 3 types of FNA results possible (by Bethesda system)
  - Benign follicular nodule: Macrofollicular subtype, essentially benign
  - FN or suspicious for FN: Hyperplastic proliferation (35%) and FA or FC (15-30%) → lobectomy for diagnosis
  - Hürthle cell lesion: 15-45% turn out to be malignant Hürthle cell carcinoma, require lobectomy for diagnosis

SELECTED REFERENCES

1. Glastonbury CG: Thyroid Adenoma. In Harnsberger HR et al: Diagnostic Imaging: Head & Neck. 2nd ed. Salt Lake City: Amirsys, Inc. 2011
2. Iared W et al: Use of color Doppler ultrasonography for the prediction of malignancy in follicular thyroid neoplasms: systematic review and meta-analysis. J Ultrasound Med. 29(3):419-25, 2010

THYROID ADENOMA

(Left) Transverse power Doppler US of the left lobe of the thyroid shows a "spoke-wheel" appearance often seen in a benign follicular neoplasm. The term "spoke-wheel" appearance describes peripheral vascularity ➡ with branches extending toward the center of the lesion ➡. *(Right)* Corresponding longitudinal power Doppler US also shows a vascular pattern ➡ reminiscent of a "spoke-wheel" pattern. Note the perinodular vessels extending toward the center of the nodule.

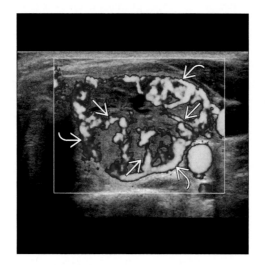
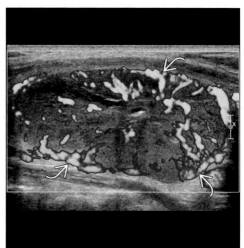

(Left) Transverse grayscale US of the left thyroid lobe shows FA with cystic change ➡, which is uncommon and represents hemorrhage/necrosis/cyst formation within the FA. Note that the nodule is otherwise iso-/hyperechoic with a thin rim of perilesional hypoechoic halo ➡, typical for a follicular nodule (FN). *(Right)* Corresponding transverse power Doppler US shows predominant peripheral vascularity ➡ with few intranodular vessels in a solid portion of the nodule with cystic areas ➡ being avascular.

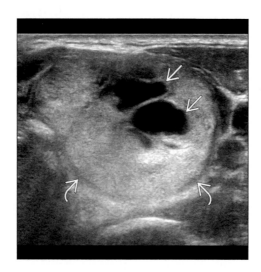
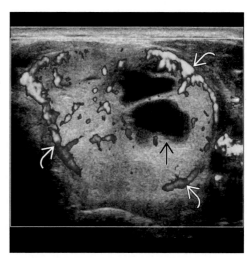

(Left) Transverse grayscale US shows a Hürthle cell lesion ➡, which is sonographically indistinguishable from a follicular lesion. Diagnosis is usually made after FNA/biopsy/hemithyroidectomy. *(Right)* Longitudinal grayscale US shows a histologically proven benign FA ➡ that was was incidentally found on F18-FDG PET due to FDG avidity (SUV max 10). A benign FA may be hypermetabolic; however, malignancy should be excluded in all hypermetabolic thyroid nodules due to ↑ risk.

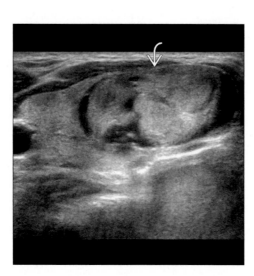
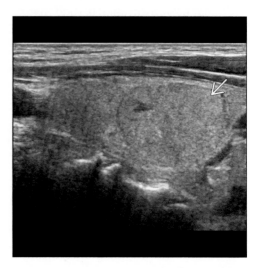

THYROID ADENOMA

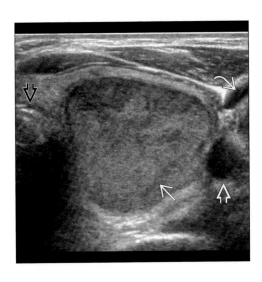 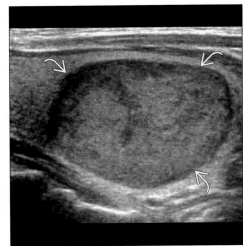

(Left) Transverse grayscale US shows the left lobe of the thyroid in a patient with recent-onset thyrotoxicosis and goiter. Note the solid, homogeneously hypoechoic, noncalcified, haloed nodule ➡ within the lower pole of the thyroid gland. Also note the trachea ➡, CCA ➡, and IJV ➡. *(Right)* Corresponding longitudinal grayscale US shows a complete perinodular hypoechoic halo ➡. Sonographic appearances are highly suggestive of a follicular lesion.

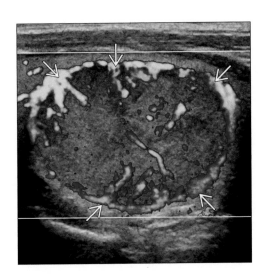 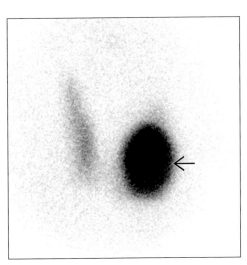

(Left) Longitudinal power Doppler US (same patient) demonstrates predominant perinodular vascularity ➡, often seen in FA. The overall appearances most likely represent an autonomous FA in the context of recent-onset thyrotoxicosis. *(Right)* Corresponding anterior Tc-99m pertechnetate thyroid scan of the same patient shows a hot nodule ➡, confirming toxic thyroid adenoma. When a follicular nodule is toxic/hot, it is likely to be benign adenoma.

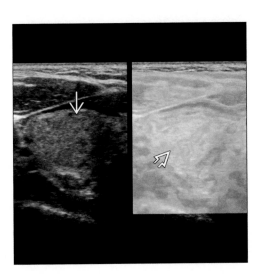 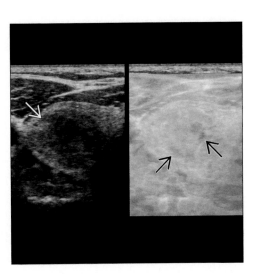

(Left) Transverse strain elastography of FA ➡ shows it to be predominantly green/purple ➡, indicating soft on this color map. *(Right)* Transverse elastography of the lower section of the same lesion ➡ shows intermediate stiffness ➡ with scattered areas of red within. Stiffness in FA is variable and may range from soft to intermediate in stiffness.

COLLOID CYST OF THYROID

Key Facts

Imaging

- Common (15-25% of thyroid nodules)
- Benign lesion without malignant potential
- Typically, unilocular thin-walled cyst
- Anechoic content with posterior acoustic enhancement
- Echogenic foci with "comet tail" artifacts are characteristic
  - Represent suspended colloid aggregates
- If previous hemorrhage into cyst
  - Thick-walled cysts with debris ± fluid level
  - Thick septa ± "comet tail" artifacts
- If colloid cyst arises from hyperplastic nodule
  - Background solid nodule
  - Cystic spaces of variable sizes
  - Solid, well-defined, oval, isoechoic nodule; no punctate calcification
  - Colloid aggregates seen scattered in cystic spaces

- USG-guided FNAC is not necessary for diagnosis

Top Differential Diagnoses

- Thyroid adenoma
- Simple thyroid cyst
- Differentiated thyroid carcinoma

Diagnostic Checklist

- Colloid crystals mimic echogenic foci from punctate calcification seen in papillary thyroid carcinoma
- Newer generation US machine may show "comet tail" artifacts behind punctate calcification due to axial compounding
  - Scanning in fundamental mode helps to distinguish "comet tail" vs. posterior shadowing
- Consider cystic malignant nodule (not colloid cyst) if cystic lesion contain suspicious solid area ± vascularity ± abnormal lymph node

(Left) Longitudinal grayscale US shows a typical colloid nodule with multiple echogenic foci and "comet tail" artifacts suspended in the cyst ➡. These represent colloid particles in viscous fluid concentrated with thyroglobulin. (Right) Axial T1WI MR demonstrates a large, well-defined mass ➡ within the left thyroid lobe that is hyperintense to cerebrospinal fluid ➡. The high signal probably represents proteinaceous content (colloid, thyroglobulin) within the lesion.

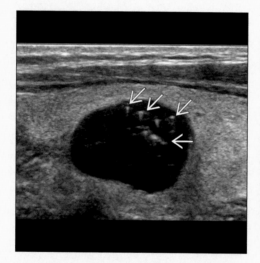
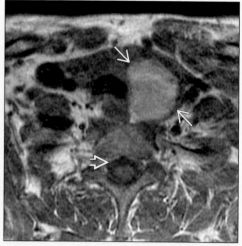

(Left) Longitudinal grayscale US shows debris ➡ and septa in a colloid cyst. This is often due to previous hemorrhage within the colloid cyst. Note the echogenic rim ➡ of "comet tail" artifacts in the colloid cyst. (Right) Longitudinal grayscale US (same patient) better shows the colloid cyst with internal septa ➡ and colloid aggregates represented by echogenic foci with "comet tail" artifacts ➡. Aspiration of such lesions usually has poor yield as the fluid is viscous and orange in color.

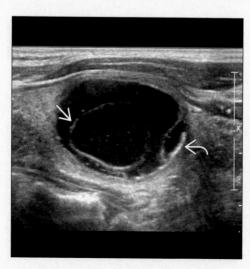
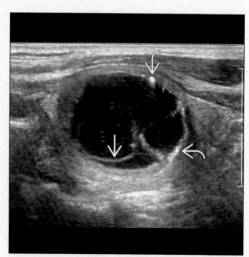

COLLOID CYST OF THYROID

TERMINOLOGY

Synonyms
- Colloid nodule

Definitions
- Fluid lesion of thyroid containing stored form of thyroid hormone (colloid)

IMAGING

General Features
- Best diagnostic clue
  - Thin-walled cysts with "comet tail" artifacts
- Location
  - Intrathyroid, often multiple and bilateral
- Size
  - Variable (a few mm to 4 cm)

Imaging Recommendations
- Best imaging tool
  - Ultrasound

Ultrasonographic Findings
- Grayscale ultrasound
  - Unilocular thin-walled cyst is typical
    - Thin, echogenic wall
    - Anechoic content with posterior acoustic enhancement
    - Echogenic foci with "comet tail" artifacts are characteristic, represents suspended colloid aggregates
    - ± colloid clumps (irregular, echogenic, avascular debris)
  - If previous hemorrhage into cyst
    - Thick-walled cysts with debris ± fluid level
    - Thick septi ± "comet tail" artifacts
  - If cyst arises from hyperplastic nodule
    - Background solid nodule
    - Cystic spaces of variable sizes
    - Solid, well-defined, oval, isoechoic nodule
    - No punctate calcification
    - Colloid aggregates scattered in cystic spaces
- Power Doppler
  - Thin-walled colloid cyst is avascular
  - Colloid cyst arising from adenomatous nodule shows vascularity in solid component
- USG-guided FNAC is not necessary for diagnosis
  - Decompression is often unsuccessful even with large bore (16-18 gauge) because of viscous fluid
  - Colloid clumps cause needle clogging

CT Findings
- CECT
  - Low-density, sharply defined, round to oval nodule

MR Findings
- T1WI
  - Hyper-, iso-, or hypointense depending on concentration of fluid
- T2WI
  - Well-defined hyperintense nodule
- No significant enhancement

DIFFERENTIAL DIAGNOSIS

Thyroid Adenoma
- Hemorrhagic degeneration mimics colloid cyst

Simple Thyroid Cyst
- True thyroid cyst with epithelial lining is rare
- No echogenic foci with "comet tail" artifacts

Differentiated Thyroid Carcinoma
- Rarely predominantly cystic mass
- Solid components are hypoechoic with punctate calcifications ± vascularity
- Regional metastatic lymphadenopathy

Thyroglossal Duct Cyst
- Solitary nodule, usually infrahyoid in location
- Can occur anywhere from tongue base to thyroid

PATHOLOGY

Gross Pathologic & Surgical Features
- Colloid accumulation as nodule or as areas of colloid aggregates in hyperplastic goitre

CLINICAL ISSUES

Presentation
- Most are incidentally detected on ultrasound
- May present as palpable nodule when large or as rapidly enlarging nodule if bleeding in cyst
- Airway deviation and compression if large

Demographics
- Common (15-25% of thyroid nodules)
- Occurs primarily in adults; also reported in children

Natural History & Prognosis
- Benign lesions without malignant potential

DIAGNOSTIC CHECKLIST

Image Interpretation Pearls
- Newer-generation ultrasound machine may show "comet tail" artifacts behind punctate calcification due to axial compounding
  - Scanning in fundamental mode helps to distinguish
  - Use color Doppler as grayscale (scans in fundamental mode)
- Think cystic malignant nodule (not colloid cyst) if cystic lesion contains suspicious solid area ± vascularity ± abnormal lymph node

SELECTED REFERENCES

1. Cibas ES et al: The Bethesda System For Reporting Thyroid Cytopathology. Am J Clin Pathol. 132(5):658-65, 2009
2. Frates MC et al: Management of thyroid nodules detected at US: Society of Radiologists in Ultrasound consensus conference statement. Radiology. 237(3):794-800, 2005
3. Ahuja A et al: Clinical significance of the comet-tail artifact in thyroid ultrasound. J Clin Ultrasound. 24(3):129-33, 1996

COLLOID CYST OF THYROID

(Left) Longitudinal grayscale US shows a small colloid cyst ➡ (measuring only 3 mm). Many of these small colloid cysts are incidentally detected on thyroid US due to its high resolution. *(Right)* Longitudinal grayscale US demonstrates a thyroid colloid cyst with a thin septum ➡, probably related to previous intracystic hemorrhage. Note colloid aggregates with "comet tail" artifacts ➡.

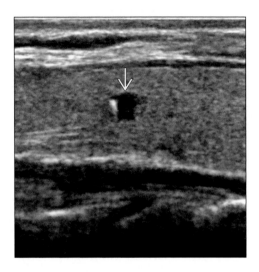 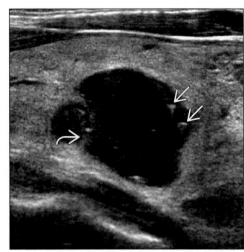

(Left) Longitudinal grayscale US shows a thin-walled, anechoic, unilocular colloid cyst ➡ with a "comet tail" artifact ➡. *(Right)* Corresponding longitudinal US of the same lesion using fundamental mode shows persisting "comet tail" artifact ➡. In case of punctate calcification, a fundamental scan using higher scanning frequency and magnification often demonstrates fine posterior acoustic shadow.

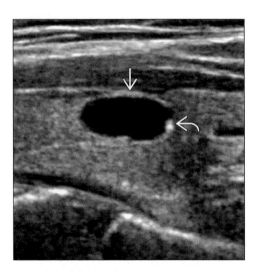 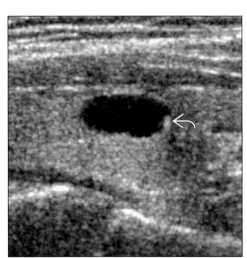

(Left) Longitudinal grayscale US shows a thyroid gland with a colloid cyst. Eccentric debris ➡ are often seen adherent to the nondependent part. Unlike cystic papillary thyroid carcinoma, they contain no punctate calcification. Note the echogenic focus with a "comet tail" artifact ➡ suggesting the colloid nature of the nodule. *(Right)* Power Doppler US (same patient) shows no vascularity in the debris ➡ as opposed to solid tumoral growth. Note the normal vascularity in thyroid parenchyma ➡.

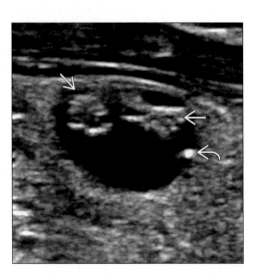 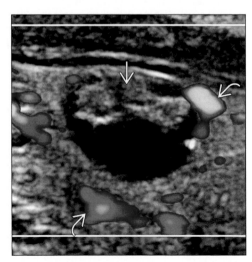

COLLOID CYST OF THYROID

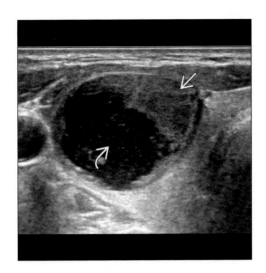

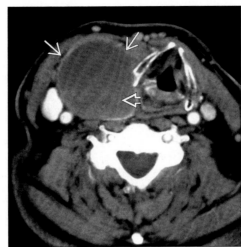

(Left) Transverse grayscale US shows a right lobe thyroid nodule with adherent ➡ and mobile debris ➡. These are often seen in patients with rapid enlargement of a preexisting colloid cyst, representing intracystic bleeding. Unlike viscous colloid content, such hemorrhagic content is readily aspirated. *(Right)* Axial CECT in another patient shows a large, well-defined, thin-walled cystic thyroid mass ➡. Note the subtle higher density in its dependent portion ➡, which suggests recent hemorrhage.

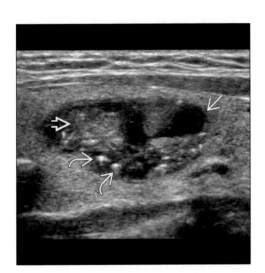

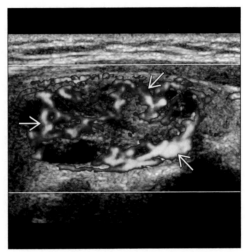

(Left) US shows colloid elements in an adenomatous nodule. Note multiple cystic areas ➡ and echogenic foci with "comet tail" artifacts ➡ scattered throughout the cyst. The solid component is isoechoic ➡ and the border is well defined, as opposed to a malignant thyroid nodule. *(Right)* Power Doppler US (same patient) shows a vascular solid component ➡ in the hyperplastic/adenomatous portion. Such nodules may bleed, and patients often present with a recently enlarging nodule ± pain.

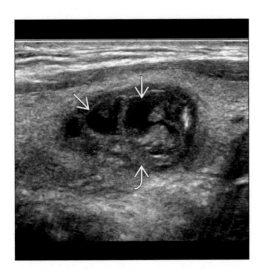

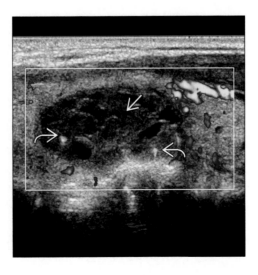

(Left) Longitudinal grayscale US of the thyroid gland shows a colloid cyst arising from a hyperplastic nodule. Note multiple cystic areas ➡ against a background isoechoic to mildly hypoechoic nodule ➡. *(Right)* Power Doppler US (same patient) shows an avascular solid component ➡, likely representing a blood clot. Note echogenic foci with "comet tail" artifacts, characteristics of a colloid aggregate ➡. No posterior shadowing is seen on this Doppler scan in fundamental mode.

HEMORRHAGIC THYROID CYST

Key Facts

Terminology
- Hemorrhage into preexisting thyroid nodules

Imaging
- Well-defined, predominantly cystic thyroid nodule containing blood products of various age ± fluid level
- NECT: Hyperdense thyroid cyst
- CECT: Rim enhancement
- MR: Variable signal intensity consistent with blood product of various age; no internal enhancement
- Ultrasound: Predominantly cystic thyroid nodule with echogenic debris
  - ± fluid level, avascular septi, or avascular solid component
- FNAC invariably yields altered blood

Top Differential Diagnoses
- Colloid cyst
- Adenomatous thyroid nodule
- Cystic differentiated thyroid carcinoma

Clinical Issues
- Rapidly enlarging painful thyroid nodule
- Odynophagia, dysphagia
- Acute airway compression uncommon
- Initial rapid enlargement → firm nodule static in size
- Occasional spontaneous resolution
- Simple FNA: Recurrence rate ≤ 58%
- Sclerotherapy with ethanol, tetracycline, or OK-432: Recurrence rate ≤ 90%; ethanol ablation lowest cost

Diagnostic Checklist
- FNAC is unnecessary for diagnosis if benign-looking on US but is useful for decompression
- Presence of vascular/suspicious solid component and lymph node should raise suspicion of malignant thyroid nodule

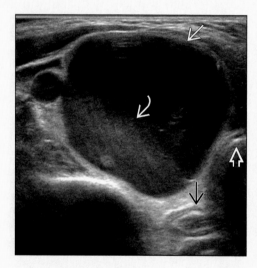
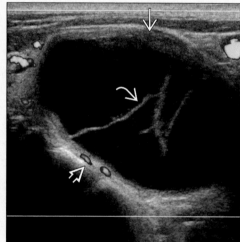

(Left) Transverse grayscale US shows a large, cystic thyroid nodule ➡ with internal debris ➡ (mobile on Doppler) and posterior enhancement. Note mass effect on the trachea ➡ and esophagus ➡. *(Right)* Power Doppler US shows a large, predominantly cystic nodule ➡ with internal debris and septi ➡. Note perinodular vascularity ➡ with no vascularity within septi.

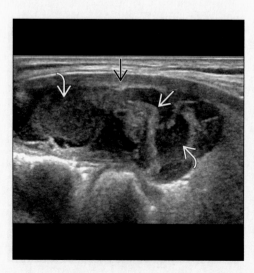
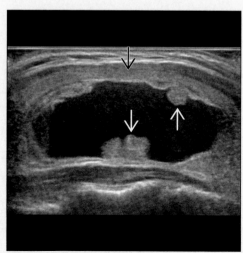

(Left) Longitudinal grayscale US shows typical, heterogeneous-looking hemorrhagic thyroid nodule ➡. Note the multiple thick, irregular internal septi ➡ and loculated cystic areas with internal debris ➡ giving it an isoechoic appearance. *(Right)* Longitudinal grayscale US shows a hemorrhagic thyroid nodule ➡ with multiple mural nodules ➡ within. On Doppler, these mural nodules are invariably avascular and represent intranodular blood clots.

HEMORRHAGIC THYROID CYST

TERMINOLOGY

Definitions
- Hemorrhage into preexisting thyroid nodules

IMAGING

General Features
- Best diagnostic clue
  - Well-defined, predominantly cystic thyroid nodule containing blood products of various age
  - Layering and fluid level; no solid component
  - Confined by thyroid capsule; no local invasion
  - Background multinodular goitre (MNG) common
  - Mass effect on trachea, common carotid artery, and internal jugular vein if large
- Location
  - Thyroid lobes or isthmus; lower pole > upper pole
- Size
  - Commonly 2-5 cm
  - May be large and cause acute airway obstruction

Ultrasonographic Findings
- Grayscale ultrasound
  - Predominantly cystic thyroid nodule with
    - Mobile echogenic debris
    - ± fluid level
    - ± thin or thick septum/septi
    - ± echogenic, solid component in dependent or nondependent area represents blood clot; soft in consistency on FNAC (avascular on Doppler)
- Power Doppler
  - Internal contents including debris, septi, and mural nodules are avascular
- US-guided FNAC invariably yields altered blood

CT Findings
- NECT: Hyperdense thyroid cyst ± fluid-fluid level
- CECT: Rim enhancement; normal enhancement of background thyroid parenchyma or background MNG

MR Findings
- Variable signal intensity on T1WI and T2WI consistent with blood product of various ages ± fluid level
- No internal enhancement

Imaging Recommendations
- Best imaging tool
  - US ± US-guided aspiration

Nuclear Medicine Findings
- Tc-99m pertechnetate thyroid scan: Cold nodule

DIFFERENTIAL DIAGNOSIS

Colloid Cyst
- Echogenic foci with "comet tail" artifacts representing colloid crystals; gel-like, amber-colored aspirate

Thyroid Adenoma (Adenomatous Nodule)
- Vascular halo, smooth margin, ± coarse calcification, perinodular vascularity, no abnormal neck nodes

Cystic Differentiated Thyroid Carcinoma
- Vascular solid component ± punctate calcification ± abnormal neck nodes

Acute Suppurative Thyroiditis
- Septic, pediatric patient
- Thyroid/perithyroid abscess, left lobe > right lobe
- ± ↑ vascularity in inflammatory areas

PATHOLOGY

General Features
- Etiology
  - Intranodular hemorrhage or hemorrhagic infarct
  - Thin-walled aberrant vessels or arteriovenous shunting in thyroid nodule

Gross Pathologic & Surgical Features
- Firm, cystic thyroid mass containing altered blood and blood clots ± multiple chambers
- Content: Venous blood → chocolate-colored fluid (most common) → olive-colored fluid → translucent, amber-colored fluid dependent on age of hemorrhage

Microscopic Features
- Red blood cells

CLINICAL ISSUES

Presentation
- Rapidly enlarging painful thyroid nodule
  - Spontaneous hemorrhage or in association with exertional events such as coughing, choking on food or straining, trauma, or FNAC (1.9-6.4%)
- Odynophagia, dysphagia
- Rarely acute airway compression

Natural History & Prognosis
- Initial rapid enlargement → firm nodule static in size
- Occasional spontaneous resolution
- Recurrence after simple aspiration ≤ 58%

Treatment
- Simple FNA: Recurrence rate ≤ 58%
- Sclerotherapy with ethanol, tetracycline, or OK-432: Recurrence rate ≤ 90%; ethanol ablation lowest cost

DIAGNOSTIC CHECKLIST

Consider
- FNAC unnecessary for diagnosis if benign-looking on ultrasound but may be performed for decompression
- Presence of vascular/suspicious solid component + lymph node should raise suspicion of malignant thyroid nodule

SELECTED REFERENCES

1. Polyzos SA et al: Systematic review of cases reporting blood extravasation-related complications after thyroid fine-needle biopsy. J Otolaryngol Head Neck Surg. 39(5):532-41, 2010
2. Roh JL: Intrathyroid hemorrhage and acute upper airway obstruction after fine needle aspiration of the thyroid gland. Laryngoscope. 116(1):154-6, 2006

HEMORRHAGIC THYROID CYST

(Left) Longitudinal grayscale US shows a hemorrhagic thyroid nodule ➔ with fluid level ➔ in its dependent portion. Note adjacent heterogeneous nodule ➔, suggesting evidence of a background multinodular goitre (MNG), a common feature. *(Right)* Longitudinal power Doppler US shows a hemorrhagic thyroid nodule with sharply defined fluid level ➔ (indicating layering of debris in its dependent portion) and marked posterior enhancement ➔. Note the absence of any intranodular vascularity.

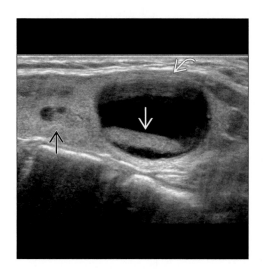
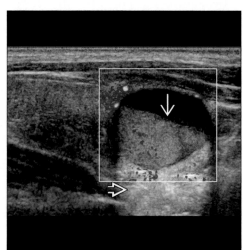

(Left) Transverse grayscale US shows typical hemorrhagic thyroid nodule in the thyroid isthmus. Note multiple intranodular mural nodules ➔. *(Right)* Corresponding power Doppler US shows absence of vascularity within mural nodules. These mural nodules represent blood clots adherent to walls and are soft on FNAC. They are often mobile and adhere to needle tips, making aspiration difficult. Note the location of the trachea ➔ and CCAs ➔.

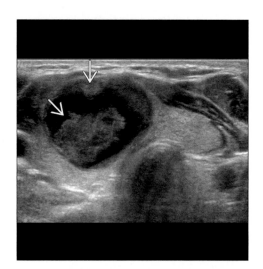
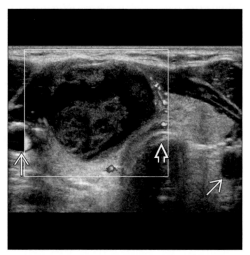

(Left) Longitudinal grayscale US shows a large hemorrhagic thyroid nodule ➔ with fine isoechoic appearance and internal septi ➔. Isoechoic nature is due to fine internal debris ➔ within cystic portion. On power Doppler, such fine internal debris is often mobile, shows swirling motion, and is readily aspirated on FNAC. *(Right)* Corresponding power Doppler US shows no vascularity within the hemorrhagic thyroid nodule. Initially, grayscale appearance may raise suspicion of differentiated thyroid cancer.

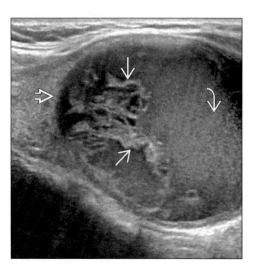
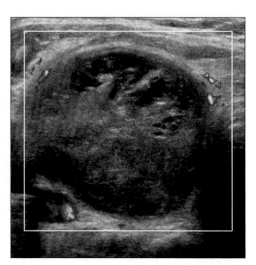

HEMORRHAGIC THYROID CYST

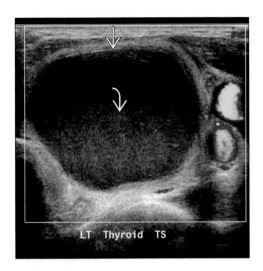

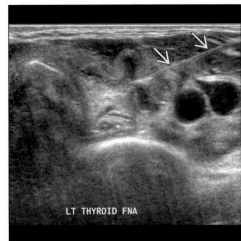

(Left) Transverse power Doppler US shows a large, hemorrhagic, left thyroid nodule ➡ with fine internal debris ➡ in its dependent portion. Intranodular hemorrhage is a common cause of a rapidly enlarging painful thyroid nodule ± obstructive symptoms. The presence of such fine mobile debris suggests the nodule can be readily aspirated. *(Right)* Corresponding US-guided aspiration with fine needle ➡ shows a complete collapse of the nodule. The recurrence rate after simple aspiration is ≤ 58%.

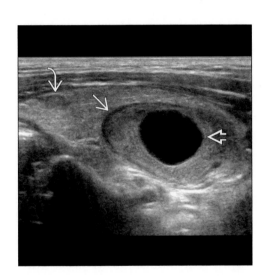

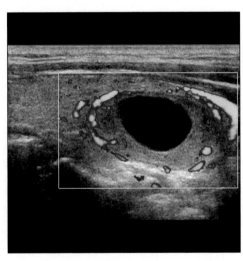

(Left) Longitudinal grayscale US shows a well-defined, haloed ➡ thyroid nodule with a homogeneous, noncalcified, solid component and central cystic change ➡. Note the presence of an adjacent small nodule ➡ indicating multinodularity. *(Right)* Corresponding power Doppler US shows prominent vascular halo with no significant vascularity within the solid component. To evaluate the nodule's nature, FNAC of solid component was performed under power Doppler US guidance.

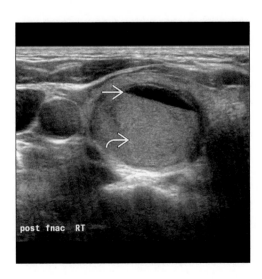

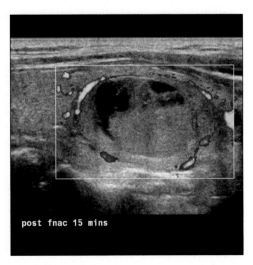

(Left) Transverse grayscale US (same patient) shows fine echogenic debris ➡ with fluid level ➡ within the nodule, immediately after guided FNAC indicated an acute hemorrhage confined to the nodule. *(Right)* Corresponding longitudinal power Doppler US (15 minutes after FNAC) shows the presence of a vascular halo and intranodular debris, but no intranodular vascularity. Note that the nodule appears larger compared to pre-FNAC image but no adjacent hematoma is present.

POST-ASPIRATION THYROID NODULE

Key Facts

Imaging

- Small, heterogeneous, markedly hypoechoic > isoechoic nodule, ± taller than wide shape
- Poorly defined/crenated margin (58%) > well-defined margin (36%) > spiculated border (6%)
- Markedly hypoechoic perilesional halo
  - May represent encapsulation or peripheral fibrosis
- Inner isoechoic rim may be seen
- Small echogenic nonshadowing foci within (may represent strong refractive interface or calcification)
- May show mild to prominent posterior shadowing (refractive shadow due to uneven interface of collapsed cyst wall)
- Majority reduce in size on follow-up
- Avascular ± perilesional vascularity as part of inflammatory response

Top Differential Diagnoses

- Papillary thyroid carcinoma
- Medullary thyroid carcinoma
- Follicular thyroid nodule

Clinical Issues

- History of FNAC for decompression of cystic thyroid nodule with benign aspirate
- Patient presents for routine follow-up or recurrent goiter due to ↑ size of other thyroid nodules in multinodular goiter
- Benign, asymptomatic; majority ↓ in size

Diagnostic Checklist

- Post-aspiration thyroid nodule closely mimics malignant thyroid nodule
- Familiarity with US findings ↓ incidence of unnecessary repeated FNAC
- Although spontaneous collapse of thyroid cyst may occur, differentiated thyroid carcinoma must be excluded in patients without history of prior FNAC

(Left) Transverse grayscale US shows a post-FNAC collapsed nodule ➡ appearing ill defined, hypoechoic, and heterogeneous with faint nonshadowing echogenic foci within, mimicking a small papillary thyroid carcinoma. Note common carotid artery ➡. (Right) Longitudinal US shows a post-FNAC nodule ➡. Note isoechoic rim with dense posterior shadowing ➡ (thought to be due to refractive shadowing from uneven interface of collapsed cyst wall) and adjacent heterogeneous, cystic nodule ➡ in multinodular goiter.

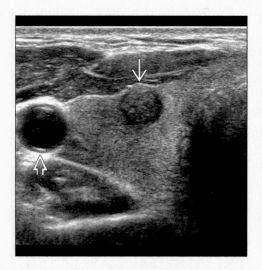
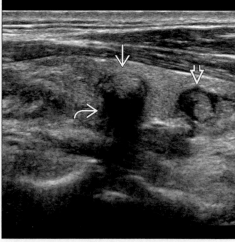

(Left) Longitudinal power Doppler US shows a post-aspiration cystic thyroid nodule. It is diffusely hypoechoic with a small nonshadowing echogenic focus ➡ within (representing strong refractive interface or calcification). Perilesional vascularity may be postinflammatory response. (Right) Longitudinal grayscale US shows a post-aspiration cystic thyroid nodule ➡ with ill-defined borders and an echogenic rim within the nodule. Prior history of FNAC is key to the diagnosis.

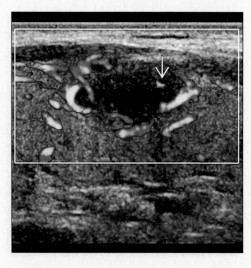
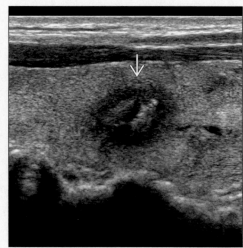

POST-ASPIRATION THYROID NODULE

TERMINOLOGY

Definitions
- Residual thyroid nodule after percutaneous FNAC for benign, predominantly cystic thyroid nodule

IMAGING

General Features
- Best diagnostic clue
  - Small, markedly hypoechoic thyroid nodule
  - Seen weeks to years after FNA
- Location
  - Site of previously aspirated thyroid cyst
- Size
  - Small; range: 0.3-1.8 cm (average: 0.8 cm)

Ultrasonographic Findings
- Grayscale ultrasound
  - Small, heterogeneous, markedly hypoechoic > isoechoic nodule that may be taller than wide
  - Poorly defined/crenated margin (58%) > well-defined margin (36%) > spiculated border (6%)
  - Markedly hypoechoic perilesional halo: Encapsulation or peripheral fibrosis
    - Inner isoechoic rim may be seen
  - Small, echogenic foci (> 60%), most without shadow
    - May represent strong refractive interface or calcification
  - May show mild to prominent posterior shadowing
    - Refractive shadow due to uneven interface of collapsed cyst wall
  - Majority (88%) reduce in size on follow-up
- Power Doppler
  - Avascular ± perilesional vascularity as part of inflammatory response

DIFFERENTIAL DIAGNOSIS

Papillary Thyroid Carcinoma
- Small papillary thyroid carcinoma appears very similar to post-aspiration thyroid cyst
  - Except for posterior shadowing from punctate calcification, internal vascularity, interval enlargement (could be slow), ± hyperechoic lymph nodes

Medullary Thyroid Carcinoma
- Ill-defined hypoechoic nodule, ± calcification, ± hypoechoic lymph nodes
- May appear identical to papillary thyroid carcinoma

Follicular Thyroid Nodule
- Oval, well circumscribed, noncalcified, homogeneous, iso-/hyper-/hypoechoic
- Typically perinodular vascularity with "spoke wheel" appearance

Solitary Thyroid Metastasis
- Rare; seen in patients with disseminated metastasis

PATHOLOGY

Etiology
- Residual nodule of benign thyroid hemorrhagic cyst after percutaneous FNA
  - Possibly collapsed cystic lumen → inflammatory reaction and fibrosis

Microscopic Features
- Fibrosis ± background nodular hyperplasia

CLINICAL ISSUES

Presentation
- Most common signs/symptoms
  - History of FNAC for decompression of cystic thyroid nodule
    - Patient aware of benign pathology of aspirate
    - Often background multinodular goiter (MNG)
  - Asymptomatic
- Other signs/symptoms
  - Patient presents for routine follow-up of MNG or recurrent goiter due to ↑ size of other thyroid nodules in MNG

Natural History & Prognosis
- Benign, asymptomatic; majority reduce in size

Treatment
- No treatment is required

DIAGNOSTIC CHECKLIST

Consider
- History of percutaneous FNAC for decompression of thyroid nodule/goiter
- Hypoechoic halo ± inner isoechoic rim and interval reduction in size

Image Interpretation Pearls
- Post-aspiration thyroid nodule closely mimics malignant thyroid nodule
- Familiarity with US findings decreases incidence of unnecessary repeated FNAC
- Although spontaneous collapse of thyroid cyst may occur, differentiated thyroid carcinoma must be excluded in patients without history of prior FNAC

SELECTED REFERENCES

1. Ko MS et al: Collapsing benign cystic nodules of the thyroid gland: sonographic differentiation from papillary thyroid carcinoma. AJNR Am J Neuroradiol. 33(1):124-7, 2012
2. Wong KT et al: Ultrasound of thyroid and parathyroid glands. In Sofferman RA et al: Benign Thyroid Conditions. New York: Springer. 61-106, 2012
3. Koo JH et al: Cystic thyroid nodules after aspiration mimicking malignancy: sonographic characteristics. J Ultrasound Med. 29(10):1415-21, 2010
4. Alexander EK et al: Natural history of benign solid and cystic thyroid nodules. Ann Intern Med. 138(4):315-8, 2003
5. Kuma K et al: Fate of untreated benign thyroid nodules: results of long-term follow-up. World J Surg. 18(4):495-8; discussion 499, 1994

HASHIMOTO THYROIDITIS

Key Facts

Imaging

- Features vary with different stages of disease and extent of involvement (i.e., diffuse vs. focal)
- Grayscale US
  - Acute, focal: Discrete nodules occur in equal frequency against normal or altered background thyroid parenchyma
  - Acute, diffuse: Diffuse, hypoechoic, heterogeneous, micronodular echo pattern involving entire gland
  - Chronic: Enlarged, hypoechoic, micronodular gland with lobulated outlines; diffuse, hypoechoic, parenchymal echoes (ghost-like thyroid) ± echogenic fibrous septa
  - Atrophic/end-stage: small, hypoechoic gland with heterogeneous echo pattern
- Color Doppler US
  - Acute focal/diffuse: Variable vascularity, focal nodule may mimic benign/malignant thyroid nodule

- Chronic: Hypervascular when patient is hypothyroid, reflecting hypertrophic action of TSH; following treatment when TSH returns to normal, hypervascularity decreases
  - Atrophic/end-stage: Avascular/hypovascular gland
- Hypervascularity is never as marked as Graves disease and flow velocities are within normal limits
- Increased risk of non-Hodgkin lymphoma (NHL) & papillary carcinoma in Hashimoto thyroiditis
- US ± FNAC for monitoring & early detection of
  - Thyroid NHL & papillary carcinoma
  - Lymphomatous/malignant nodes in adjacent neck

Top Differential Diagnoses

- Thyroid NHL
- Graves disease
- de Quervain thyroiditis
- Riedel thyroiditis (invasive fibrosing thyroiditis)

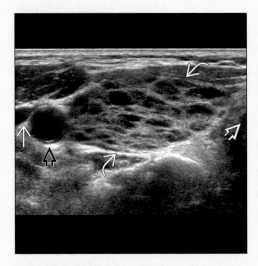
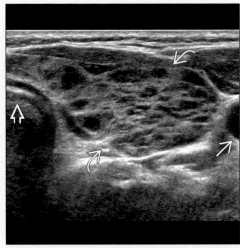

(Left) Transverse grayscale US of the right thyroid lobe in a patient with Hashimoto thyroiditis (HT) shows diffuse heterogeneous pattern with focal hypoechoic areas producing "swiss cheese/ leopard skin" appearance of thyroid ➡. Note the common carotid artery (CCA) ⮕, internal jugular vein (IJV) ➡, and location of trachea ➡.
(Right) Transverse grayscale US of contralateral lobe (same patient) shows similar "swiss cheese/leopard skin" appearance of thyroid gland ➡. Note the CCA ➡ and trachea ➡.

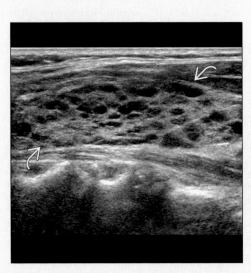
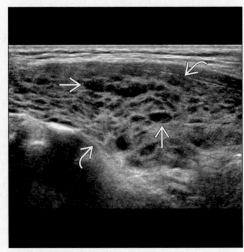

(Left) Corresponding longitudinal grayscale US of the right lobe shows the diffuse nature of "swiss cheese/ leopard skin" involvement of the thyroid gland ➡.
(Right) Longitudinal grayscale US of the left lobe (same patient) shows similar, symmetric "swiss cheese/ leopard skin" appearance of the thyroid gland ➡. Focal hypoechoic areas ➡ in thyroid parenchyma represent lymphocytic infiltration and are clearly demonstrated due to the high resolution of modern US transducers.

HASHIMOTO THYROIDITIS

TERMINOLOGY

Abbreviations
- Hashimoto thyroiditis (HT)

Definitions
- Chronic, autoimmune-mediated lymphocytic inflammation of thyroid gland

IMAGING

General Features
- Best diagnostic clue
  - Diffuse, moderately enlarged, hypoechoic gland with lobulated outlines and heterogeneous echo pattern with fine, bright, fibrotic streaks within
    - Vascularity depends on stage and type of involvement

Ultrasonographic Findings
- Grayscale ultrasound
  - Features vary with different stages of disease and extent of involvement (i.e., diffuse vs. focal)
  - Acute focal HT: Discrete nodules occur in equal frequency against normal or altered background thyroid parenchyma
    - ~ 5% of all biopsied nodules, may sonographically simulate both benign and malignant thyroid nodules
  - Acute diffuse HT: Diffuse, hypoechoic, heterogeneous, micronodular echo pattern involving entire gland
    - Micronodular pattern represents lymphoid infiltration and bright edges due to fibrous septa
  - Chronic HT
    - Enlarged, hypoechoic, micronodular gland with lobulated outlines
    - Diffuse, hypoechoic, parenchymal echoes (ghost-like thyroid) ± echogenic fibrous septa
  - Atrophic/end stage HT: Small, hypoechoic gland with heterogeneous echo pattern
- Color Doppler
  - Acute focal/diffuse: Variable vascularity, focal nodule may mimic benign/malignant thyroid nodule
  - Chronic
    - Hypervascular when patient is hypothyroid, reflecting hypertrophic action of TSH
    - Following treatment when TSH returns to normal, hypervascularity decreases
  - Atrophic: Avascular/hypovascular gland
  - Hypervascularity is never as marked as Graves disease and flow velocities are within normal limits

Imaging Recommendations
- Best imaging tool
  - Diagnosis of HT is made on clinical & biochemical tests of thyroid function; imaging not necessary for diagnosis
  - Increased risk of non-Hodgkin lymphoma (NHL) and papillary carcinoma in HT
    - US is ideal imaging modality to monitor gland and for early detection of NHL and papillary carcinoma
    - US evaluates thyroid gland and adjacent neck nodes and is readily combined with fine-needle aspiration cytology (FNAC) for confirmation
- Protocol advice
  - When scanning patients with HT, always evaluate thyroid (± FNAC) for developing NHL and papillary carcinoma, seen as
    - Focal bulge in contour of gland, calcification in nodule associated with HT
      - Calcification in any nodule with HT has 50% risk of malignancy (compared to 4.7% in noncalcified nodule)
    - Developing areas of ill-defined hypoechogenicity, focal or diffuse, ± mass effect
    - Lymphomatous/malignant nodes in adjacent neck

DIFFERENTIAL DIAGNOSIS

Thyroid Non-Hodgkin Lymphoma
- Focal/diffuse hypoechoic parenchymal echo pattern, ± extrathyroid spread, ± lymphomatous adenopathy
- Most patients with primary thyroid lymphoma have history of antecedent Hashimoto thyroiditis

Graves Disease
- Diffuse, hypoechoic, spotty, heterogeneous parenchymal echo pattern with increased vascularity

de Quervain Thyroiditis
- Focal, ill-defined hypoechoic area within thyroid, ± increased vascularity; progressive on serial examination
- Patient has fever, raised white cell count, and presents with painful thyroid lump, ± thyrotoxicosis

Riedel Thyroiditis (Invasive Fibrosing Thyroiditis)
- Benign fibrosis of part or all of thyroid gland; diffuse enlargement and extension to surrounding tissues

Anaplastic Thyroid Carcinoma
- Heterogeneous, ill-defined, hypoechoic infiltrative mass against a background of multinodular goiter with associated necrotic nodes

CLINICAL ISSUES

Presentation
- Most common signs/symptoms
  - Gradual, painless enlargement of thyroid
    - Patients most often euthyroid with normal T3 and T4 hormones (subclinical HT)
  - Other signs/symptoms
    - 20% present with hypothyroidism, 5% have early hashitoxicosis

Natural History & Prognosis
- Most important complication is increased incidence of thyroid malignancy
  - NHL most frequent, mucosa-associated lymphoid tissue (MALT)-type
  - Also papillary and Hürthle cell tumors, leukemia, and plasmacytoma

SELECTED REFERENCES

1. Sofferman RA et al: Ultrasound of the Thyroid and Parathyroid Glands. New York: Springer. 61-106, 2012

HASHIMOTO THYROIDITIS

(Left) Transverse grayscale US in HT shows diffuse hypoechogenicity of thyroid gland and bright streaks ➡ corresponding to ↓ intraglandular fibrosis. ↓ in echogenicity strongly predicts autoimmune thyroid disease, occurs early, and the degree of hypoechogenicity correlates with circulating thyroid antibody levels. Note prominent pretracheal node ➡ and trachea ➡.
(Right) Transverse grayscale US shows prominent paratracheal nodes ➡, commonly seen with HT. Note trachea ➡ & CCA ➡.

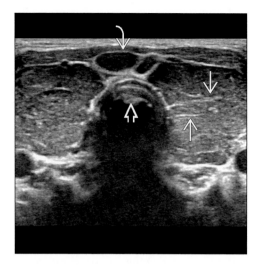
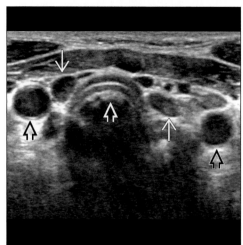

(Left) Transverse grayscale US in HT shows diffuse nodular change ➡ in the background of altered thyroid echo pattern. Nodular HT occurs equally against background of diffuse HT vs. otherwise normal thyroid parenchyma. In nodular HT with diffuse HT, the nodule is solid, haloed, hyperechoic, and noncalcified. Without diffuse HT, the nodule may have cystic change and eggshell calcification.
(Right) Corresponding power Doppler US shows ↑ thyroid parenchymal vascularity.

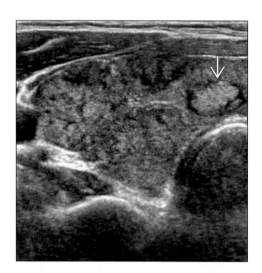
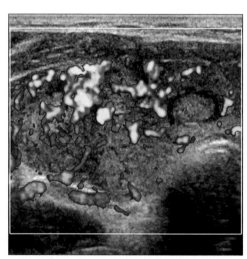

(Left) Transverse power Doppler US shows thyroid hypervascularity in HT. Note trachea ➡ and CCA ➡. *(Right)* Corresponding longitudinal Doppler US shows marked thyroid parenchymal vascularity. Hypervascularity in HT is due to hypertrophic action of TSH and ↓ when TSH normalizes. Thyroid vascularity in HT is variable, from hypovascular to glandular hypervascularity. Flow velocities are normal vs. Graves disease where PSV in inferior thyroid artery may be increased up to 120 cm/sec.

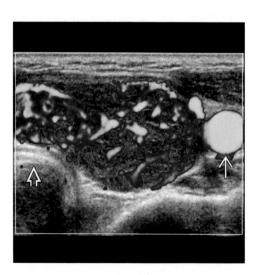
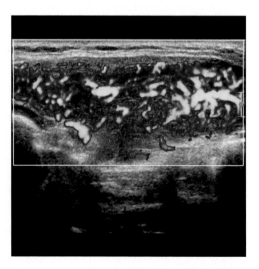

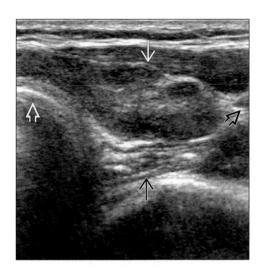

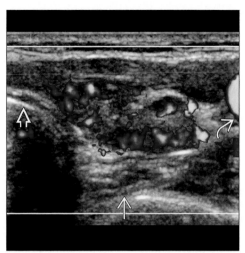

(Left) Transverse grayscale US in atrophic HT shows reduction in thyroid size/volume & hypoechogenicity of the left lobe of the thyroid ➡. Note the trachea ➡, left CCA ➡, and esophagus ➡. *(Right)* Corresponding power Doppler US shows slight prominence of thyroid vascularity in the left lobe. The thyroid gland in atrophic HT is usually hypovascular on power Doppler US. Note the trachea ➡, left CCA ➡, and esophagus ➡.

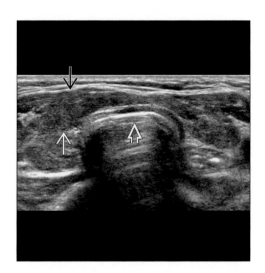

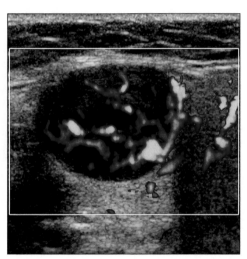

(Left) Transverse grayscale US in atrophic HT shows a focal, hypoechoic right thyroid nodule ➡ with subtle bulge in contour ➡. Note background change of HT and trachea ➡. Development of a thyroid nodule, or recent ↑ in thyroid size in HT is suspicious, as NHL and papillary carcinoma are associated with HT. US neck node examination ± FNAC are indicated. *(Right)* Power Doppler US shows presence of a lymphomatous node in the neck on serial follow-up in a patient with HT.

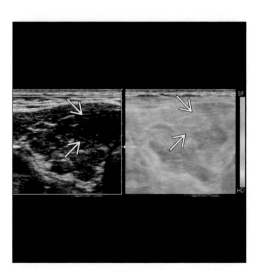

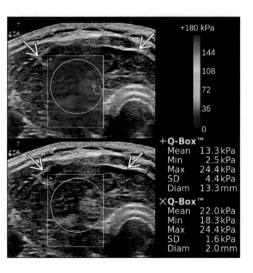

(Left) Transverse grayscale US and qualitative strain elastogram show HT. Strain color scale ranges from purple (elastic, soft) to red (inelastic, hard). It is mixed red & yellow (mixed elasticity). The very hypoechoic area anteriorly ➡ appears more green (elastic) than other parenchyma posteriorly. *(Right)* Transverse grayscale US & SWE show HT ➡. SWE color scale ranges from blue (0 kPa, soft) to red (180 kPa, stiff). It appears diffusely blue with maximum SWE value of 24.4 kPa, which is low.

GRAVES DISEASE

Key Facts

Imaging

- Mild/moderate diffuse, symmetric enlargement of thyroid gland, including isthmus
- Increase in volume of thyroid ≤ 90 mL
- Hypoechoic, heterogeneous, "spotty" parenchymal echo pattern
- Parenchymal hypoechogenicity is due to ↓ colloid content & ↑ cellularity with reduction of colloid-cell interface ± hypervascularity
- Persistence of parenchymal hypoechogenicity on cessation of medical treatment associated with relapse of hyperthyroidism
- Marked increase in parenchymal vascularity (turbulent flow with A-V shunts): "Thyroid inferno"
- Increased vascularity does not correlate with thyroid function but reflects inflammatory activity
- Spectral Doppler: Increase in peak flow velocity (≤ 120 cm/s) as measured in inferior thyroid artery

- ↑ vascularity tends to ↓ in response to treatment
- Increase in vascularity seen in patients with relapse

Top Differential Diagnoses

- Hashimoto thyroiditis
- de Quervain thyroiditis
- Nodular goiter

Diagnostic Checklist

- Imaging in Graves disease is usually not required
- Thyroid US may be necessary to rule out other types of thyroiditis or in patients who fail medical treatment or undergo radioactive iodine treatment (to establish thyroid volume)
- Some institutions may choose technetium thyroid scans over US, depending on expertise available
- In patients with thyroid-associated ophthalmopathy (TAO), CT or MR may be indicated to confirm diagnosis if it cannot be established clinically

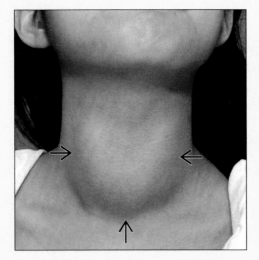
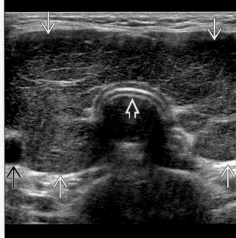

(Left) Clinical photograph shows diffuse thyroid enlargement ➡ in a patient with Graves disease (GD). Diagnosis of GD is based on clinical features and laboratory tests. US is usually not indicated for patient management. (Right) Transverse grayscale US shows enlarged thyroid ➡ with rounded contour & markedly hypoechoic, heterogeneous thyroid parenchymal echo pattern. Normal thyroid demonstrates fine, bright parenchymal echo pattern. Note the right CCA ➡ and trachea ➡.

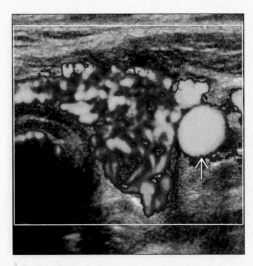
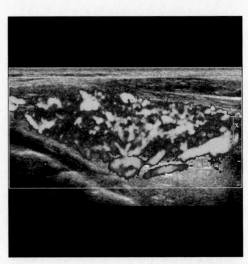

(Left) Transverse power Doppler US shows marked hypervascularity in the left thyroid lobe. Note the left CCA ➡. (Right) Corresponding longitudinal power Doppler US shows diffuse hypervascularity in thyroid gland ("thyroid inferno"). The hypervascularity reflects the inflammatory process in the thyroid and does not correlate with thyroid function. Thyroid vascularity reduces in patients who respond to treatment and increases again if patient relapses.

GRAVES DISEASE

TERMINOLOGY

Definitions
- Autoimmune disorder with long-acting thyroid stimulating antibodies (LATS) producing hyperplasia and hypertrophy of thyroid gland

IMAGING

General Features
- Best diagnostic clue
  - Enlarged gland, hypoechoic, heterogeneous echo pattern, and ↑ in parenchymal vascularity
- Size
  - Mild/moderate increase in thyroid gland size

Ultrasonographic Findings
- Grayscale ultrasound
  - Mild/moderate diffuse, symmetric enlargement of thyroid gland, including isthmus
  - Increase in volume of thyroid ≤ 90 mL
    - Normal volume: Neonate 0.4-1.4 mL, ↑ by 1.0-1.3 mL for each 10 kg weight up to normal volume of 10-11 (± 3-4) mL in adults
  - Hypoechoic, heterogeneous, "spotty" parenchymal echo pattern
    - Parenchymal hypoechogenicity is due to ↓ colloid content & ↑ cellularity with reduction of colloid-cell interface ± hypervascularity
    - Parenchymal hypoechogenicity associated with ↑ frequency of TRAb positivity
  - Persistence of parenchymal hypoechogenicity on cessation of medical treatment associated with relapse of hyperthyroidism
- Color Doppler
  - Marked increase in parenchymal vascularity (turbulent flow with A-V shunts): "Thyroid inferno"
  - Increased vascularity does not correlate with thyroid function but reflects inflammatory activity
  - Spectral Doppler: Increase in peak flow velocity (≤ 120 cm/s) as measured in inferior thyroid artery
  - Increased vascularity tends to ↓ in response to treatment; also seen in patients with relapse

Imaging Recommendations
- Best imaging tool
  - Imaging is usually not required
    - Diagnosis based on clinical signs & symptoms and laboratory findings
  - Imaging of thyroid may be necessary in patients who fail medical treatment and in whom other types of thyroiditis are considered
    - In such instances, US of thyroid is only imaging necessary
  - Thyroid US indicated in patients who undergo radioactive iodine treatment to establish thyroid volume

DIFFERENTIAL DIAGNOSIS

Hashimoto Thyroiditis
- Rounded contours, and hypoechoic, heterogeneous echo pattern with bright fibrotic streaks in parenchyma; atrophic gland in end-stage disease

- Risk of developing NHL, which is seen as hypoechoic nodules in thyroid ± associated lymphomatous nodes

de Quervain Thyroiditis
- Ill-defined, focal hypoechoic areas within thyroid ± increased vascularity; raised white cell count (WCC), fever, and tender thyroid
- Appearances evolve over time to subsequently involve the entire gland; thyroid may revert to normal echo pattern on successful treatment

Nodular Goiter
- Multiple, heterogeneous nodules, cystic change, septa, "comet tail" artifact, dense shadowing calcification
- Biochemical tests are usually normal & patients present with thyroid enlargement ± palpable nodules

CLINICAL ISSUES

Presentation
- Most common signs/symptoms
  - Patients often present with palpitations, loss of weight despite increased appetite, sweating, and wet palms
  - Cardiovascular: Hypermetabolic state → hyperdynamic circulatory state
    - Cardiomegaly, pulmonary edema, peripheral edema, tachycardia, mitral valve prolapse, and increased cardiac output
  - Thyroid-associated ophthalmopathy (TAO), periorbital edema, lid retraction, ophthalmoplegia, proptosis, malignant exophthalmos
    - Extraocular muscle and orbital connective tissue inflammation and swelling due to autoimmune response
  - Common complaints: Muscular weakness and fatigue; rarely muscle wasting

Demographics
- Age
  - 3rd-4th decade
- Gender
  - M:F = 1:7

DIAGNOSTIC CHECKLIST

Image Interpretation Pearls
- Imaging is usually not required in patients with clinical & laboratory evidence of GD
- US of thyroid may be indicated if goiter is nodular or if other thyroiditis is suspected
- US of thyroid also indicated in patients who undergo radioactive iodine treatment (to establish thyroid volume)
- Some institutions may choose technetium thyroid scans over US, depending on expertise available

SELECTED REFERENCES

1. Sofferman RA et al. Ultrasound of the thyroid and parathyroid glands. New York: Springer, 61-106, 2012
2. Abraham P et al: A systematic review of drug therapy for Graves' hyperthyroidism. Eur J Endocrinol. 153(4):489-98, 2005
3. Harnsberger HR et al: Diagnostic Imaging: Head & Neck. Salt Lake City: Amirsys, Inc. II-1-70-73, 2004

GRAVES DISEASE

(Left) Transverse grayscale US shows patchy, hypoechoic, heterogeneous thyroid parenchymal echo pattern in Graves disease. The gland is enlarged ➡ with slight rounding of its contours. Note the right CCA ➡ and location of the trachea ➡. *(Right)* Longitudinal grayscale US (same patient) shows diffuse, patchy, hypoechoic thyroid parenchymal echo pattern. Thyroid hypoechogenicity is due to ↓ colloid content with ↑ cellularity and ↓ cell-colloid interface &/or ↑ blood flow.

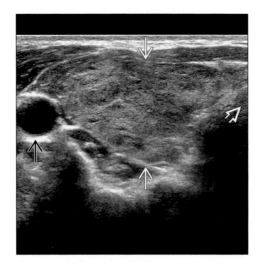
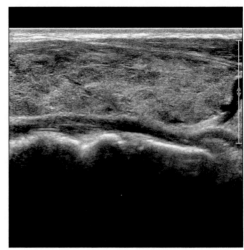

(Left) Transverse power Doppler shows thyroid parenchymal hypervascularity ("thyroid inferno"). Note the right CCA ➡ and location of the trachea ➡. *(Right)* Corresponding longitudinal power Doppler US shows "thyroid inferno," which represents turbulent flow within A-V shunts. Spectral Doppler will show increase in peak systolic velocity (≤ 120 cm/sec) as measured in the inferior thyroid artery. Such increased flow velocity is not seen in Hashimoto thyroiditis.

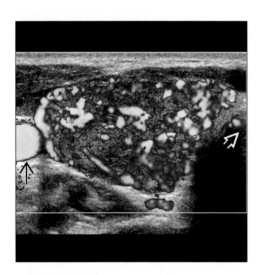
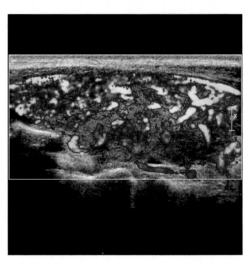

(Left) Transverse grayscale US shows a patient with Graves disease relapse. The thyroid gland ➡ is not enlarged but has a diffuse, hypoechoic, heterogeneous parenchymal echo pattern. Echogenicity is similar to the adjacent strap muscles ➡. The presence of hypoechogenicity correlates with ↑ frequency of TRAb positivity and its persistence upon cessation of treatment associates with relapse. Note the CCA ➡ and trachea ➡. *(Right)* Corresponding power Doppler US shows "thyroid inferno" consistent with relapse.

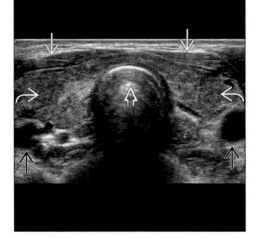
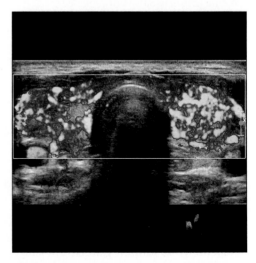

GRAVES DISEASE

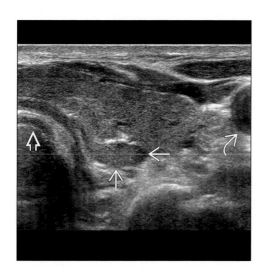

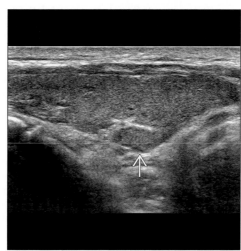

(Left) Transverse grayscale US in a patient with Graves disease shows a diffuse, fine, hypoechoic parenchymal echo pattern. The gland is not significantly enlarged and maintains its normal contour. Note the pseudoparathyroid appearance ⬈ posteriorly, a common pitfall in patients with Graves disease. Note the left CCA ⮕ and trachea ⮕. *(Right)* Longitudinal grayscale US shows the pseudoparathyroid ⬈ tongue of hypertrophied thyroid tissue continuous with the rest of the gland.

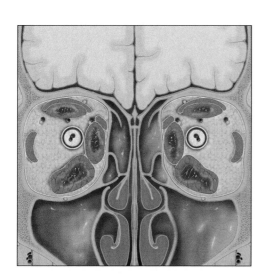

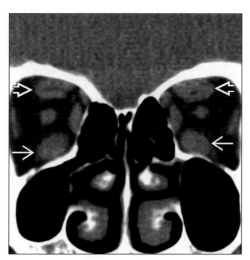

(Left) Coronal graphic shows bilateral enlargement of EOM. Graves disease may present with TAO & have exophthalmos with bilateral enlargement of EOM. Predilection for muscle bellies sparing tendons. *(Right)* Coronal NECT in Graves disease shows inferior ⮕ & superior recti ⮕ enlarged bilaterally. Probable CT findings (not shown) include ↑ ocular fat, enlargement of EOMs (inferior ≥ medial ≥ superior ≥ lateral ≥ oblique), enlarged lacrimal glands & superior ophthalmic veins, and stretched optic nerve.

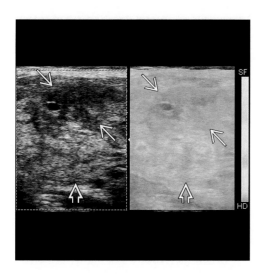

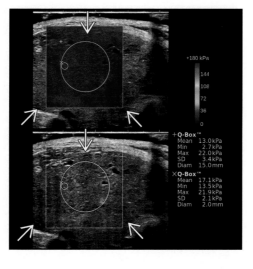

(Left) Transverse grayscale US & qualitative strain elastogram show GD. Relative strain color ranges from purple (elastic, soft) to red (inelastic, hard). Hypoechoic area of more severe involvement ⮕ is more elastic (softer) than less-involved parenchyma posteriorly ⮕. *(Right)* Transverse grayscale US & SWE show GD ⮕. SWE color scale ranges from blue (0 kPa, soft) to red (180 kPa, stiff). This diffusely involved gland has low SWE stiffness (maximum 22.0 kPa), similar to normal thyroid parenchyma.

DE QUERVAIN THYROIDITIS

Key Facts

Terminology
- Self-limited inflammatory disease of thyroid gland

Imaging
- Acute phase: Focal, ill-defined, nodular, hypoechoic, avascular/hypovascular area in subcapsular region
- Subacute phase: Diffuse enlargement of 1 lobe or entire thyroid gland with multifocal, patchy/confluent, ill-defined, hypoechoic, avascular/hypovascular areas
- Radioactive iodine uptake test or Tc-99m pertechnetate thyroid scan: Focal defect or large area of ↓/absent uptake due to failure of iodine trapping

Top Differential Diagnoses
- Hemorrhagic thyroid cyst
- Graves disease
- Hashimoto thyroiditis
- Malignant thyroid nodule

Clinical Issues
- Uncommon in adults, rare in children
- Viral prodrome followed by high-grade fever and exquisite tender goiter, 50% with thyrotoxicosis
- ↑ ESR, ↑ CRP, ↑ serum Tg, thyroid antibodies (-)
- Most recover without complication in 6-12 months
- Permanent hypothyroidism in up to 4-22%
- Recurrent disease in up to 2%, most within 1 year

Diagnostic Checklist
- Diagnosis is usually made by clinical and laboratory findings
- Ill-defined, patchy/heterogeneous, hypoechoic and hypovascular/avascular thyroid lesion in patients with viral prodrome and exquisitely tender goiter
- Typical sonographic features aid in diagnosis of atypical cases and helps to avoid unnecessary biopsy

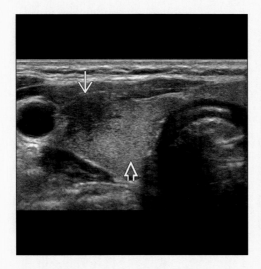

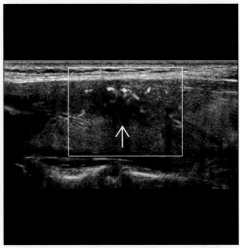

(Left) Transverse grayscale US shows a focal, hypoechoic, heterogeneous, noncalcified, ill-defined area in the thyroid gland, anteriorly & subcapsular in location ➡. A normal, fine, bright, adjacent parenchymal echo pattern ➡ is seen.
(Right) Corresponding power Doppler US shows vascularity within the focal hypoechoic area ➡. Appearances mimic a malignant thyroid nodule. This patient presented with fever & pain. Laboratory tests showed ↑ ESR, C-reactive protein (CRP). Clinical & sonographic appearances are typical for de Quervain thyroiditis (DQT).

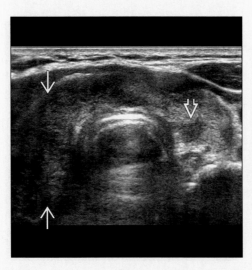

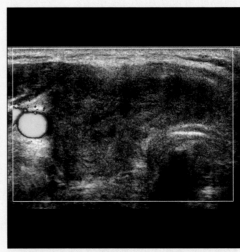

(Left) Transverse grayscale US of a patient presenting with tenderness over thyroid shows that the right thyroid lobe ➡ and isthmus are enlarged with a rounded contour and diffuse hypoechoic heterogeneous echo pattern. Note the small focal area of hypoechogenicity ➡ in the left lobe. *(Right)* Corresponding transverse power Doppler US performed 10 days later shows progressive enlargement of the right lobe and isthmus with a hypoechoic heterogeneous echo pattern and no significant vascularity. FNAC confirmed DQT.

DE QUERVAIN THYROIDITIS

TERMINOLOGY

Abbreviations
- de Quervain thyroiditis (DQT)

Synonyms
- Subacute thyroiditis, subacute granulomatous thyroiditis, painful subacute thyroiditis, subacute nonsuppurative thyroiditis, giant cell thyroiditis, pseudogranulomatous thyroiditis, pseudotuberculous thyroiditis

Definitions
- Self-limited, nonsuppurative inflammatory disease of thyroid gland

IMAGING

General Features
- Best diagnostic clue
  - Ill-defined, hypoechoic, avascular, subcapsular thyroid nodule in patient with tender goiter and viral prodrome
  - Diffuse goiter with patchy, hypoechoic, heterogeneous, hypovascular/avascular appearance in subacute phase
- Location
  - Focal, subcapsular in acute phase
  - Multifocal or diffuse, involves the entire gland > 1 lobe in subacute phase

Ultrasonographic Findings
- Characteristic sonographic features vary
- Acute phase
  - Focal, ill-defined, hypoechoic, nodular area in thyroid; subcapsular in location
  - Normal/hypoechoic, heterogeneous surrounding thyroid parenchyma
  - Tender on transducer pressure
  - Involved areas are avascular or hypovascular on Doppler US
  - ± inflammatory nodes in central compartment and lower internal jugular chain
- Subacute phase
  - Progression of focal involvement to diffuse enlargement of 1 lobe or entire thyroid gland
  - Patchy or confluent, ill-defined hypoechoic areas
  - Residual tenderness on transducer pressure
  - Involved areas are avascular or hypovascular on Doppler US
  - ± inflammatory nodes in vicinity of thyroid gland
- Recovery phase: Return to normal appearance
  - ± glandular atrophy or residual thyroid nodule

CT Findings
- Not indicated for diagnosis of thyroiditis: Administration of iodinated contrast may result in falsely decreased iodine uptake on scintigraphy
- If performed, NECT shows diffusely enlarged thyroid with low attenuation (~ 45 HU); CECT shows moderate enhancement indicating inflammatory process

MR Findings
- Not indicated for diagnosis

- If performed during acute phase, MR shows enlarged thyroid with irregular margins and higher than normal signal intensity on both T1W and T2W sequences

Imaging Recommendations
- Protocol advice
  - Follow-up scan in 1-2 weeks would show progression of DQT and avoid unnecessary FNAC

Nuclear Medicine Findings
- Radioactive iodine uptake test (RAIU) or technetium (Tc-99m) pertechnetate thyroid scan and uptake
  - Acute/subacute phase: Focal defect or large area of decreased/absent uptake due to failure of iodine trapping
  - Recovery phase: Increased uptake before returning to normal thyroid function

DIFFERENTIAL DIAGNOSIS

Hemorrhagic Thyroid Cyst
- Differential of rapid-onset painful goiter ± preceding history of URI with repeated coughing
- Well-defined, predominantly cystic nodule with internal debris and fluid level ± thick, avascular septa

Graves Disease
- Differential of diffuse goiter and thyrotoxicosis ± associated orbitopathy
- Diffusely enlarged, hypoechoic, heterogeneous thyroid gland with "thyroid inferno"
- Positive antithyroid antibody
- Intense homogeneous uptake on thyroid scintigraphy (superscan)

Hashimoto Thyroiditis
- Asymptomatic, painless goiter ± hypothyroidism
- May show nodular, patchy, or diffuse hypoechoic heterogeneous echo pattern, "leopard skin/Swiss cheese" appearance, linear fibrotic streaks, variable vascularity with normal flow velocities on Doppler
- Atrophic, diffuse hypoechoic, heterogeneous, and hypovascular appearance during late/end stage

Malignant Thyroid Nodule
- Noncalcified differentiated thyroid carcinoma (DTCa) or thyroid lymphoma may mimic acute phase of DQT with ill-defined, hypoechoic, nodular appearance
- Usually hypervascular, cystic change ± calcification and regional lymphadenopathy of DTCa
- Asymptomatic when nodule is small, euthyroid

Acute Suppurative Thyroiditis
- Much more common cause of acute thyroiditis in children
- Due to bacterial infection; associated with pyriform sinus fistula
- Intra-/perithyroid abscess; unilateral, left > > > right
- Clinically more toxic, ↑ leukocytes, usually euthyroid

Silent Thyroiditis
- Painless thyroiditis characterized by transient hyperthyroidism followed by transient hypothyroidism
- Mildly enlarged thyroid with heterogeneous hypoechoic pattern

DE QUERVAIN THYROIDITIS

- Decreased uptake on thyroid scintigraphy, similar to DQT

Riedel Thyroiditis
- Rare, chronic, fibroinflammatory thyroiditis
- Nontender, firm to hard goiter
- Diffuse hypoechogenicity described in limited reports

PATHOLOGY

General Features
- Etiology
  - Exact etiology unknown
  - Viral infection in genetically predisposed individual is postulated due to viral prodrome, microscopic findings, and reports on genetic correlation
- Genetics
  - HLA-B35 positive in 2/3 of patients
  - Correlation with HLA-B15/62 and B67 has also been reported
- Associated abnormalities
  - Mumps, adenovirus, EBV, coxsackie virus, CMV, influenza, echovirus, and enterovirus infection reported

Microscopic Features
- Varying stages of follicular cell destruction in patchy distribution
- Initial mononuclear cells, lymphocytes and neutrophils infiltrate → later granuloma formation → interfollicular fibrosis → return to normal with minimal residual fibrosis after resolution

CLINICAL ISSUES

Presentation
- Most common signs/symptoms
  - Low-grade fever and flu-like symptoms followed by high-grade fever and exquisitely tender goiter
    - Goiter may be symmetric or asymmetric, diffuse in 2/3 of adults and 1/2 of affected children or nodular in 1/4 of affected adults
    - Pain initially unilateral then spreads to contralateral thyroid lobe; may radiate to ipsilateral jaw, ear, occiput, or chest
  - 50% present with thyrotoxic symptoms
  - Cervical lymphadenopathy rarely palpable
- Other signs/symptoms
  - Odynophagia, dysphagia, airway obstruction
  - Thyroid storm
- Laboratory findings
  - ↑ erythrocyte sedimentation rate (ESR): usually > 50 mm/h, frequently > 100 mm/h
  - ↑ C-reactive protein (CRP)
  - Leucocytes count normal to mildly elevated
  - Thyrotoxicosis in about 50%: ↑ T3, ↑ T4, ↓ thyroid-stimulating hormone (TSH) initially
  - ↑ serum thyroglobulin (Tg): Consistent with follicular destruction
  - Thyroid antibodies: Usually absent

Demographics
- Age
  - Peak at 4th-5th decades, rare in children
- Gender

  - F:M = 4.7:1
- Epidemiology
  - Most common cause of painful thyroid disease in adults
  - May account for up to 5% of acute thyroid disease
  - Incidence: 12.1 cases per 100,000/year

Natural History & Prognosis
- Classically 4 phases
  - Initial thyrotoxic phase (lasts weeks to 2 months)
    - Due to release of thyroid hormone from inflamed gland
    - Thyroid tender and enlarged
  - Brief euthyroid phase (lasts 1-3 weeks)
  - Hypothyroid phase (lasts weeks to months)
    - Failure to trap iodine by destroyed thyroid gland → failed biosynthesis of thyroxin
    - Reported in 20-56% of adult patients
  - Recovery phase (euthyroid)
    - Thyroid gland returning to normal function
  - Takes 6-12 months if all 4 phases occur
- Most patients recover without complication
- Permanent hypothyroidism in up to 4-22%, could be late onset
- Recurrent disease reported in up to 2%, most within 1 year

Treatment
- Symptomatic treatment with nonsteroidal anti-inflammatory drugs
- ± corticosteroid therapy in severely ill patients
- May require annual monitoring of thyroid function after recovery to exclude development of subclinical hypothyroidism

DIAGNOSTIC CHECKLIST

Consider
- Ill-defined, patchy/heterogeneous, hypoechoic, and hypovascular/avascular thyroid lesion in patients with viral prodrome and exquisitely tender goiter

Image Interpretation Pearls
- Diagnosis is usually made by clinical and laboratory findings
- Typical sonographic features aid in diagnosis of atypical cases; however, condition is rare and may be unexpected; recognition of typical sonographic appearance may avoid unnecessary biopsy

SELECTED REFERENCES

1. Frates MC et al: Subacute granulomatous (de Quervain) thyroiditis: grayscale and color Doppler sonographic characteristics. J Ultrasound Med. 32(3):505-11, 2013
2. Wong KT et al: Benign thyroid conditions. In Sofferman et al: Ultrasound of the Thyroid and Parathyroid Glands. Springer. 61-106, 2012
3. Engkakul P et al: Eponym : de Quervain thyroiditis. Eur J Pediatr. 170(4):427-31, 2011
4. Sarkar SD: Benign thyroid disease: what is the role of nuclear medicine? Semin Nucl Med. 36(3):185-93, 2006
5. Fatourechi V et al: Clinical features and outcome of subacute thyroiditis in an incidence cohort: Olmsted County, Minnesota, study. J Clin Endocrinol Metab. 88(5):2100-5, 2003

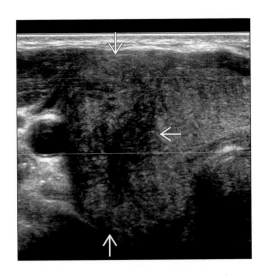
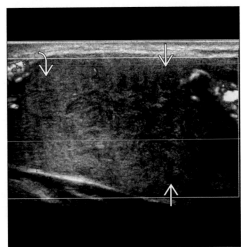

(Left) Transverse grayscale US in a patient with DQT shows an ill-defined, hypoechoic, heterogeneous parenchymal echo pattern ➡ in the right thyroid lobe, subcapsular in location. Adjacent parenchyma appears bright with minimal heterogeneity. (Right) Corresponding longitudinal power Doppler US shows no significant vascularity in the hypoechoic heterogeneous area ➡ in the thyroid gland. Note the apical thyroid parenchyma ➡ shows faint heterogeneity but remains bright.

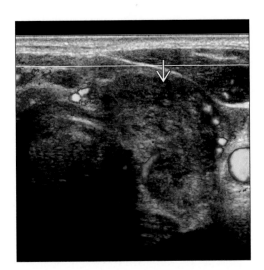
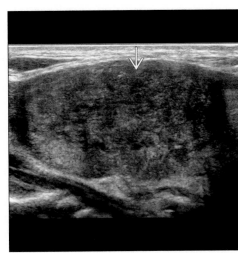

(Left) Transverse power Doppler US of the left lobe ➡ (same patient) also shows a diffuse, hypoechoic, heterogeneous parenchymal echo pattern with no significant increase in vascularity. (Right) Corresponding grayscale US of the left lobe (same patient) shows a similar but more extensive hypoechoic, heterogeneous parenchymal echo pattern ➡ compared with the right lobe. Differential diagnoses include lymphoma, Hashimoto thyroiditis, and Graves disease.

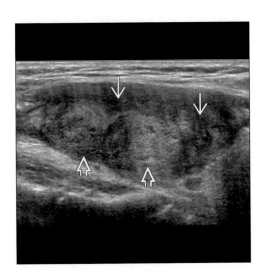
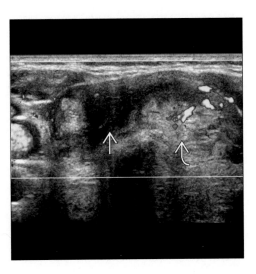

(Left) Longitudinal grayscale US in a patient presenting with tenderness over the thyroid shows background evidence of multinodularity ➡. Against this background, there is diffuse thyroid parenchymal hypoechogenicity ➡. (Right) Corresponding transverse power Doppler US shows no significant vascularity within hypoechoic region ➡. The thyroid nodule ➡ shows perinodular and intranodular vascularity. US-guided FNAC of the hypoechoic area confirmed DQT against this multinodular background.

ACUTE SUPPURATIVE THYROIDITIS

Key Facts

Terminology

- Acute bacterial infection of thyroid gland

Imaging

- Typically left-sided (95%) perithyroid &/or intrathyroid inflammation ± abscess, gas locule, &/or air-fluid level (due to underlying PSF)
- If due to other predisposing condition, begins as intrathyroid phlegmon, no lobar predilection
- Abscess may extend deep to parapharyngeal space, retropharyngeal space, or mediastinum, or discharge into subcutaneous tissue ± discharging sinus
- US is ideal for initial assessment if patient is stable, particularly as most patients are children
- US identifies AST as cause of neck swelling, guides FNAC for diagnosis & microbial analysis
- If AST confirmed on USG, cross-sectional imaging to evaluate full extent of inflammation/abscess

Top Differential Diagnoses

- Subacute thyroiditis
- Aggressive thyroid cancer
- Hemorrhagic thyroid cyst

Clinical Issues

- Acute anterior neck swelling (left > right side), pain and fever in children or young adults

Diagnostic Checklist

- Thyroid gland is extremely resistant to infection; underlying predisposing condition should be excluded in any case of bacterial infection of thyroid
- Exclusion of infection to deep cervical space or mediastinum is essential
- Imaging identification of PSF is best performed after acute episode by barium swallow (100% detection rate) or CECT with trumpet maneuver (68-83% detection rate)

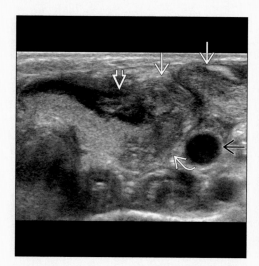
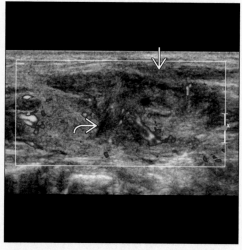

(Left) Transverse US shows typical appearances of acute suppurative thyroiditis (AST). Note perithyroid inflammation ➡, tongue of infection extending into left lobe ➡, and intrathyroid abscess formation ➡. US quickly establishes Dx, guides needle for aspiration, and is ideally suited for follow-up to evaluate temporal change. Note CCA ➡. *(Right)* Corresponding longitudinal power Doppler US shows intrathyroid extension of infection ➡, perithyroid inflammation ➡, and vascularity within inflammatory process.

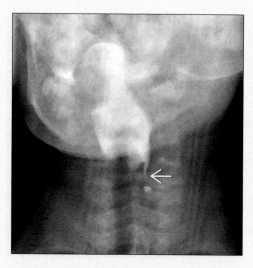
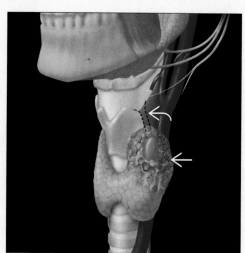

(Left) Barium swallow after remission shows pyriform sinus fistula (PSF) ➡, which is best identified by barium after initial acute episode has subsided (100% detection rate). CECT with trumpet maneuver has a 68-83% detection rate. However, CT better delineates extent of inflammation/abscess and presence of any airway compromise. *(Right)* Graphic shows the relationship of pyriform sinus fistula ➡ to acute suppurative thyroiditis ➡.

ACUTE SUPPURATIVE THYROIDITIS

TERMINOLOGY

Abbreviations
- Acute suppurative thyroiditis (AST)

Synonyms
- Acute pyogenic thyroiditis

Definitions
- Acute bacterial infection of thyroid gland

IMAGING

General Features
- Best diagnostic clue
  - Typically left sided peri- &/or intrathyroid inflammation ± abscess, gas locule, &/or air-fluid level (due to underlying pyriform sinus fistula [PSF])
  - If due to other predisposing condition, begins as intrathyroid inflammatory phlegmon without lobar predilection
- Location
  - 95% left sided, due to underlying PSF
    - Upper pole > lower pole
    - Upper pole first affected
    - Upper end may communicate with or be adherent to pyriform sinus
    - Abscess may extend deep to parapharyngeal space, retropharyngeal space, or mediastinum, or discharge superficially into subcutaneous tissue ± discharging sinus
- Size
  - Variable

Ultrasonographic Findings
- Begins as hypoechoic, thickened soft tissue in perithyroidal region = edema and inflammation
  - → obliteration of fascial planes between thyroid and adjacent tissue
  - → thick-walled perithyroidal abscess with internal debris ± echogenic foci representing gas
  - Tongue of ill-defined hypoechoic area extends from perithyroid to intrathyroid tissue = thyroiditis
  - Abscess may discharge superficially into subcutaneous layer or through a cutaneous sinus
  - Rarely, PSF is seen as fluid-filled, tubular structure
  - Peripheral vascularity
- AST related to other predisposing factors tends to start as a hypoechoic, hypovascular area in thyroid lobe before spreading to perithyroid tissue unless thyroid gland is secondarily involved by neck abscess
- Deep tissue extension may be obscured on US, CT, or MR should be performed after diagnosis made on ultrasound
- Infective/reactive lymphadenopathy in central or lateral cervical compartments

Fluoroscopic Findings
- Barium swallow
  - False-negative during acute phase
    - Detection rate of PSF reported to be 50-70%
  - 100% detection rate for PSF after remission
  - PSF appears as a barium-filled sinus tract extending from apex of left pyriform sinus to anterior lower neck

CT Findings
- NECT
  - Loss of iodine in affected lobe
  - Swelling of thyroid &/or perithyroid tissue with poorly defined margin
  - ± gas locule within perithyroid tissue, thyroid gland, and rarely within sinus tract
  - After barium swallow, may see PSF (barium-filled tract extending from apex of pyriform sinus to lower anterior neck)
- CECT
  - Trumpet maneuver improves detection of sinus tract
  - Ill-defined hypoenhancing area in perithyroid &/or intrathyroid tissue + inflammatory focus
  - Rim-enhancing collection = abscess
  - CT superior in demonstrating anatomical relationship of sinus with surrounding structures

MR Findings
- Hypoenhancing peri-/intrathyroid area = perithyroid infection/thyroiditis
- Rim enhancing abscess ± deep tissue extension
- Signal void area = gas

Nuclear Medicine Findings
- I-123 or Tc-99m thyroid scan: Very low isotope uptake in affected lobe; does not differentiate from de Quervain thyroiditis or thyroid malignancy and no longer appears justified in this disease

Imaging Recommendations
- Best imaging tool
  - CECT is preferred initial imaging modality in most medical centers, particularly if airway is compromised
  - Ultrasound is ideal for initial assessment if patient is stable, particularly as most patients are children
    - Differentiates AST from other common causes of acute swelling, does not involve ionizing radiation, guides FNAC for cytology and culture, and assesses feasibility for US-guided drainage
  - If AST confirmed on US, perform cross-sectional imaging to evaluate full extent of inflammation/abscess
  - Barium or CECT with trumpet maneuver after acute episode to identify PSF

DIFFERENTIAL DIAGNOSIS

Subacute Thyroiditis
- More common than AST in adults, rare in children
- USG: Ill-defined, hypoechoic, avascular area in subcapsular region of thyroid gland → rapid progression to multifocal ± bilobed involvement
- Perithyroid involvement is not a feature

Aggressive Thyroid Cancer
- Rarely, medullary carcinoma of thyroid, anaplastic carcinoma of thyroid, or thyroid lymphoma may grow rapidly and cause local infarction, necrosis, and thyroid tenderness mimicking AST or serve as a predisposing nidus for secondary infection
- Ill-defined, hypoechoic, hypervascular mass in thyroid lobe before invasion to perithyroidal tissue
- Family history of medullary thyroid carcinoma, elevated serum calcitonin level

ACUTE SUPPURATIVE THYROIDITIS

Neck Trauma

- Blunt or penetrating injury (e.g., FNAC)
- Ill-defined, hypoechoic, avascular area at site of injury
- ± edema, bruising, or laceration in overlying skin

Hemorrhagic Thyroid Cyst

- Well-defined cystic nodule with internal debris
- Confined within thyroid capsule
- Rupture of thyroid cyst is exceedingly rare
- Painful if recent hemorrhage or rapid ↑ in size

Parathyroid Hemorrhage

- Underlying parathyroid adenoma
- Cystic nodule posterior or inferior to thyroid capsule

PATHOLOGY

General Features

- Etiology
  - Thyroid gland is extremely resistant to infection
    - Due to intrinsic trophic factors (iodine) and anatomical characteristics (encapsulated, rich vascular, and lymphatic supply)
  - Any bacterial infection of thyroid warrants exclusion of underlying predisposing condition
    - PSF is most common predisposing condition
    - Other predisposing factors for infection
      - Through lymphatics from local infections, contamination of contagious infection, blunt or penetrating injuries, persistent thyroglossal duct
      - ± immunocompromised state
      - Abnormal thyroid structures (e.g., nodules, malignancies) have also been postulated as predisposing factors

Gross Pathologic & Surgical Features

- Perithyroid &/or intrathyroid inflammation ± abscess
- PSF
  - Congenital internal sinus extends from apex of pyriform sinus to upper aspect of left thyroid lobe/perithyroid tissue
  - Controversies on the embryological origin
    - Recent literature suggests course of sinus tract does not follow theoretical tract for 3rd or 4th branchial cleft remnant; 4th branchial apparatus cyst may be remnant of 3rd branchial pouch

Microscopic Features

- Gram-positive aerobes (staphylococci & streptococci) (39%) > polymicrobial infection (30%) > gram-negative aerobes (25%) > anaerobic organisms (12%)

CLINICAL ISSUES

Presentation

- Most common signs/symptoms
  - Acute anterior neck swelling, pain, and fever
    - Occur in previously healthy individual or after upper respiratory tract infection, blunt trauma, or high pressure to hypopharynx (e.g., trumpet blowing)
  - Previous similar episodes, multiple neck scars due to recurrent incision and drainage for neck abscesses
- Other signs/symptoms
  - Stridor, respiratory distress in infant

- Cystic neck mass of variable size as it discharges into pharynx
- Overlying skin may be erythematous and spontaneously ulcerate to discharge pus
- Transient thyrotoxicosis due to destruction of thyroid follicles and release of T3 and T4

Demographics

- Age
  - 80% of patients with AST due to PSF present < 10 years of age; remainder are spread across wide age range
- Epidemiology
  - Rare; 0.1-0.7% of all thyroid disease

Natural History & Prognosis

- Complete resolution to > 12% mortality (e.g., due to suppurative mediastinitis) in absence of immediate intervention
- If PSF unrecognized and untreated, recurrent suppurative thyroiditis results

Treatment

- Intubation if airway compromised
- Antibiotics ± urgent transcutaneous or open surgical drainage of abscess
- Elective surgical resection or obliteration of sinus tract, if present

DIAGNOSTIC CHECKLIST

Consider

- Thyroid gland is extremely resistant to infection; any bacterial infection of thyroid gland warrants exclusion of underlying predisposing factor

Image Interpretation Pearls

- Exclusion of infection to deep cervical space or mediastinum is essential
- Imaging identification of PSF is best after acute episode by barium swallow (100% detection rate) or CECT with trumpet maneuver (68-83% detection rate)
- Recent studies show excellent (100%) identification rate of PSF ± endoscopic sinus occlusion

SELECTED REFERENCES

1. Cha W et al: Chemocauterization of the internal opening with trichloroacetic acid as first-line treatment for pyriform sinus fistula. Head Neck. 35(3):431-5, 2013
2. Wong KT et al: Benign thyroid conditions. In Sofferman et al: Ultrasound of the Thyroid and Parathyroid Glands. New York: Springer. 61-106, 2012
3. Masuoka H et al: Imaging studies in sixty patients with acute suppurative thyroiditis. Thyroid. 21(10):1075-80, 2011
4. Koch B: 4th branchial cleft cyst. In Harnsberger R et al: Diagnostic Imaging: Head and Neck. 2nd ed. Salt Lake City: Amirsys, Inc. III-1-36-39, 2010
5. Paes JE et al: Acute bacterial suppurative thyroiditis: a clinical review and expert opinion. Thyroid. 20(3):247-55, 2010
6. Miyauchi A et al: Computed tomography scan under a trumpet maneuver to demonstrate piriform sinus fistulae in patients with acute suppurative thyroiditis. Thyroid. 15(12):1409-13, 2005

ACUTE SUPPURATIVE THYROIDITIS

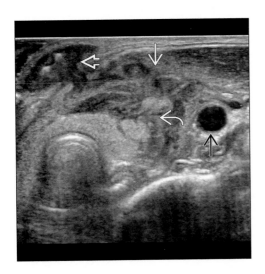

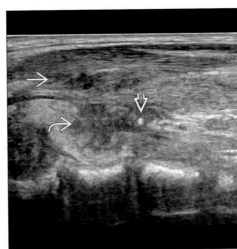

(Left) Transverse grayscale US shows the variety of imaging findings in AST. Note perithyroid inflammation ➡ (and its relation to CCA ➡), intrathyroid extension into left lobe producing AST ➡, and extension of the abscess into subcutaneous tissues ➡. This patient presented with discharging sinus. (Right) Corresponding longitudinal grayscale US clearly demonstrates an intrathyroid abscess ➡ with an echogenic focus ➡ representing gas and perithyroid inflammation ➡.

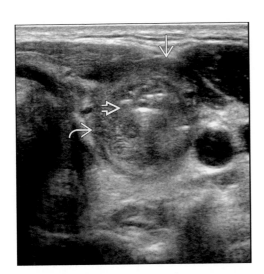

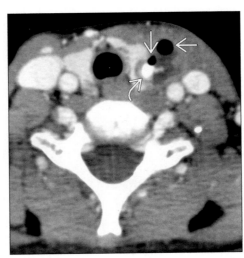

(Left) Transverse US shows perithyroid inflammation ➡ with a typical left-sided intrathyroid abscess ➡ containing multiple echogenic streaks ➡ representing gas within the abscess cavity. (Right) CECT after oral contrast & trumpet maneuver shows left intrathyroid abscess with locules of air ➡ & dense contrast ➡ (oral contrast to demonstrate PSF) within. Although US readily identifies AST, CECT better shows the extent of inflammation/abscess & excludes mediastinum involvement.

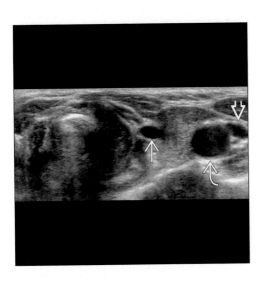

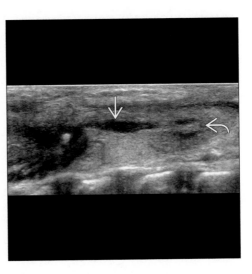

(Left) Transverse grayscale US in a child with AST shows a round, cystic, fluid-filled structure representing a tract of PSF ➡. Note the CCA ➡ and the IJV ➡. (Right) Corresponding longitudinal grayscale US shows tubular tract of PSF ➡ originating from apex of pyriform sinus and extending to lower anterior neck. Note the associated intrathyroid abscess ➡. This tract is not often seen on US and is best demonstrated by barium and CECT with trumpet maneuver.

ECTOPIC THYROID

Key Facts

Terminology
- Ectopic thyroid tissue in base of tongue (BOT) or floor of mouth (FOM)

Imaging
- Well-circumscribed, round or oval midline BOT mass with imaging characteristics similar to thyroid tissue
- Ultrasound
  - Homogeneously hyper-/isoechoic mass
  - Echopattern similar to that of normal thyroid tissue
  - ± other sites of ectopic thyroid in anterior neck
  - Scattered peripheral vascularity; may be profuse
  - Thyroid bed is empty or with small volume residual
  - May show multinodular (uncommon) or malignant (exceedingly rare) change
- Tc-99m pertechnetate scan
  - Avid tracer accumulation in midline BOT ± other sites of ectopic thyroid tissue and thyroid bed
- Best imaging tool: Thyroid scintigraphy

- US is reasonable alternative; no ionizing radiation
- Scan through entire thyroglossal duct to exclude other sites of thyroid ectopics

Top Differential Diagnoses
- Thyroglossal duct cyst
- Epidermoid/dermoid cyst
- Venous vascular malformation

Pathology
- Arrest of thyroid anlage migration in 1st trimester
  - 90% present in BOT
  - In cases of complete arrest (75%), lingual thyroid is the only functioning thyroid tissue

Diagnostic Checklist
- Must comment on status of cervical thyroid tissue
- Ectopic thyroid as only functioning thyroid tissue in 70-80% of cases; important for preoperative planning

(Left) Axial graphic depicts a lingual thyroid ⮕ in the posterior midline of the tongue, just deep to the foramen cecum. The sharply defined contour and midline location in the floor of mouth or tongue base are typical of lingual thyroid. (Right) Axial grayscale US shows a lingual thyroid ⮕ located at the tongue base, appearing as a solid, well-defined, noncalcified, homogeneous mass with fine bright parenchymal echopattern reminiscent of thyroid parenchymal echogenicity.

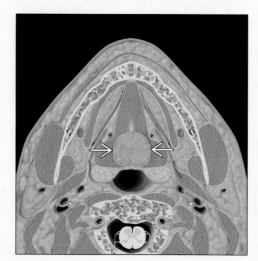

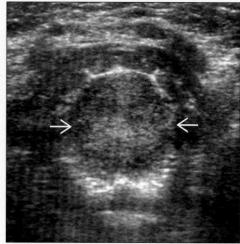

(Left) Corresponding power Doppler US (same patient) shows no significant vascularity within the lingual thyroid ⮕. Vascularity within a lingual thyroid is variable, ranging from scattered peripheral vascularity to profuse intranodular vascularity. (Right) Transverse grayscale US of the thyroid bed in the same patient shows no thyroid tissue in its normal location in the paratracheal thyroid bed ⮕. Note the trachea ⮕, common carotid artery (CCA) ⮕, and strap muscles ⮕.

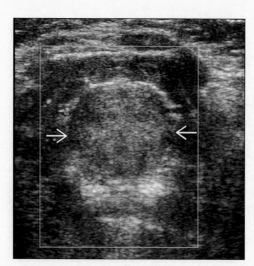

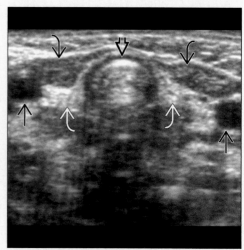

ECTOPIC THYROID

TERMINOLOGY

Definitions
• Ectopic thyroid tissue at base of tongue (BOT) or floor of mouth (FOM)

IMAGING

General Features
• Best diagnostic clue
  ○ Well-circumscribed, round or oval midline BOT mass with imaging characteristics similar to thyroid tissue
    ▪ 75% complete arrest = empty thyroid bed
    ▪ 25% partial arrest = high cervical thyroid
• Size
  ○ 1-3 cm

Ultrasonographic Findings
• Grayscale ultrasound
  ○ Well-defined, round/oval, homogeneously hyper- to isoechoic mass in midline BOT/FOM
  ○ Fine echopattern, similar to normal thyroid gland
  ○ Thyroid bed is empty or contains subnormal to normal thyroid tissue
  ○ ± other sites of ectopic thyroid in anterior neck
  ○ Rarely contains well-defined nodules and cysts
    ▪ Similar to multinodular thyroid (uncommon, 3%)
  ○ May contain punctate calcification or ill-defined hypoechoic, hypervascular nodule if malignant change (exceedingly rare)
• Power Doppler
  ○ Scattered peripheral vascularity; may be profuse

CT Findings
• NECT: Hyperdense due to iodine content
• CECT: Avid homogeneous enhancement

MR Findings
• T1WI: Iso- to mildly hyperintense
• T2WI: Mildly to strikingly hyperintense
• T1WI C+: Most often shows homogeneous enhancement

Nuclear Medicine Findings
• Tc-99m pertechnetate or radioiodine scan
  ○ Avid tracer accumulation in midline BOT ± other sites of ectopic thyroid tissue and thyroid bed

Imaging Recommendations
• Best imaging tool: Thyroid scintigraphy
  ○ US is reasonable alternative; no ionizing radiation
• Scan entire thyroglossal duct to exclude other sites of thyroid ectopics

DIFFERENTIAL DIAGNOSIS

Thyroglossal Duct Cyst
• Anechoic/pseudosolid, avascular, commonly in vicinity of hyoid bone
• Orthoptic thyroid and euthyroid function

Epidermoid/Dermoid Cyst
• Well-defined, round/oval mass in midline FOM
• Appearance depends on content: Homogeneously hyperechoic, pseudosolid, fluid-level, or "sack of marbles" appearance

Venous Vascular Malformation
• Septated, serpiginous, cystic spaces with slow-flow debris on grayscale imaging ± phleboliths

Infantile Hemangioma, Upper Airway
• Cavernous > capillary (infantile)
• Highly vascular, hypoechoic mass
• Rapid enlargement in early months
• Orthoptic thyroid

PATHOLOGY

General Features
• Etiology
  ○ Arrest of thyroid anlage migration in 3rd-7th week of gestation
    ▪ Can be anywhere along thyroglossal duct but is most common (90%) in BOT
• Associated abnormalities
  ○ Other thyroid migration anomalies, such as thyroglossal duct cyst

CLINICAL ISSUES

Presentation
• Majority are hypothyroid (60%) or euthyroid
• Many are asymptomatic and found incidentally
• May present with mass effect or primary hypothyroidism during puberty
  ○ High physiologic demand for thyroxin leading to thyroid hyperplastic response
  ○ Pinkish nodule in posterior tongue
• Accounts for up to 25% of congenital hypothyroidism cases in infants

Demographics
• Epidemiology
  ○ Estimated incidence: 1:10,000-100,000
  ○ F:M = 4:1

Natural History & Prognosis
• Nodular change (uncommon) and malignancy (rare) have been reported
  ○ Estimated risk similar to that of orthoptic thyroid

Treatment
• Hormone replacement
• Excision if obstructive symptoms or bleeding

DIAGNOSTIC CHECKLIST

Reporting Tips
• Must comment on status of cervical thyroid tissue
  ○ Ectopic thyroid as only functioning thyroid tissue in 70-80% of cases; important for preoperative planning

SELECTED REFERENCES

1. Shatzkes DR: Lingual thyroid. In Harnsberger R et al: Diagnostic Imaging: Head and Neck. 2nd ed. Salt Lake City: Amirsys, Inc. 1206, 2011
2. Gupta M et al: Lingual thyroid. Ear Nose Throat J. 88(6):E1, 2009
3. Lai YT et al: Lingual thyroid. Otolaryngol Head Neck Surg. 140(6):944-5, 2009

ECTOPIC THYROID

(Left) Axial image from a Tc-99m pertechnetate nuclear scan demonstrates activity within a mass at the base of the tongue ➡. Expected radionuclide uptake is also evident in the parotid glands ➡. *(Right)* Axial CECT shows a round, well-delineated, enhancing mass in the midline of the tongue base ➡ with minimal distortion of genioglossus muscles ➡. Lingual thyroid is markedly hyperdense relative to a minimally enhancing lingual tonsil ➡.

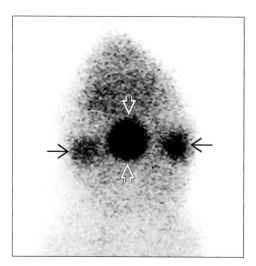
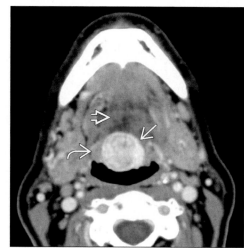

(Left) Coronal image from a Tc-99m pertechnetate nuclear scan demonstrates activity within a mass at the base of the tongue ➡. *(Right)* Sagittal T1WI C+ MR shows avid, homogeneous enhancement within the lingual thyroid ➡.

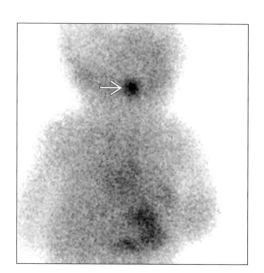
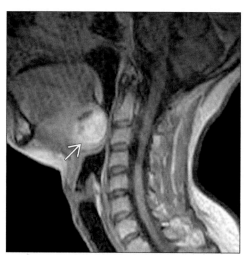

(Left) Grayscale US shows a well-defined, heterogeneous mass ➡ with multiple faint foci of "comet tail" artifacts within ➡, reminiscent of thyroid parenchymal tissue and consistent with lingual thyroid. *(Right)* Corresponding transverse grayscale US of the thyroid bed in the same patient shows no thyroid tissue in its normal location in the paratracheal thyroid bed ➡. Note the trachea ➡, CCA ➡, and strap muscles ➡. Empty thyroid bed suggests complete arrest of thyroid tissue.

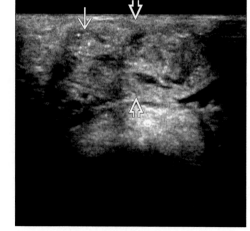
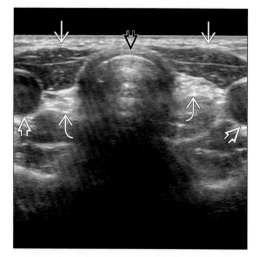

ECTOPIC THYROID

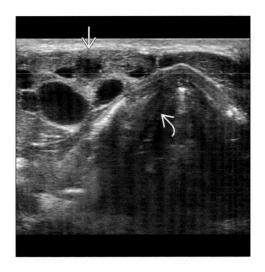

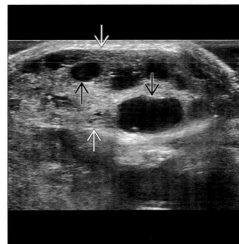

(Left) Transverse grayscale US shows ectopic thyroid ➘, high paramidline in location, at the level of the glottis/vocal cord ➚. *(Right)* Corresponding longitudinal grayscale US (same patient) shows multiple well-defined, anechoic, cystic nodules ➡ scattered throughout the parenchyma of ectopic thyroid tissue ➘, reminiscent of multinodular change seen in orthoptic thyroid glands.

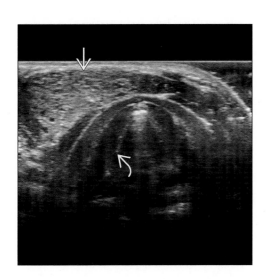

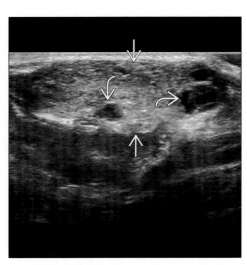

(Left) Transverse grayscale US (different patient) shows ectopic thyroid ➘, high paramidline in location, at the level of the glottis/vocal cord ➚. *(Right)* Corresponding longitudinal grayscale US (same patient) shows a diffuse, heterogeneous parenchymal echopattern ➡ with small, focal cystic nodules ➘ with septa in ectopic thyroid tissue. Sonographic features are reminiscent of a multinodular change seen in orthoptic thyroid glands and uncommonly seen in ectopic thyroid tissue.

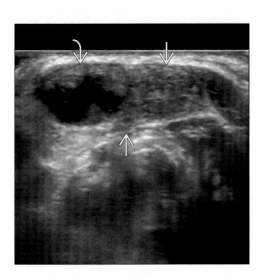

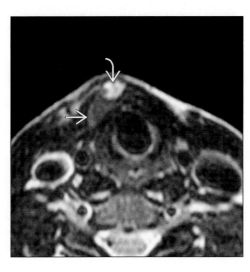

(Left) Transverse grayscale US (different patient) shows ectopic thyroid ➘, high paramidline in location, at supraglottic level. Note the focal, cystic, noncalcified, heterogeneous nodule ➘, similar to a hyperplastic nodule in a nodular goiter in orthoptic thyroid. *(Right)* Corresponding axial T2WI FS MR confirms the location of ectopic thyroid tissue ➘ and focal cystic nodule ➘ within. Always comment on the status of orthoptic thyroid tissue as ectopic thyroid may be the only functioning tissue in 70-80% of cases.

PARATHYROID ADENOMA IN VISCERAL SPACE

Key Facts

Imaging

- Most are hypoechoic to thyroid (due to uniform hypercellularity) and have echogenic capsule
- Some show cystic degeneration
- Calcification is rare; more common in carcinoma or hyperplasia due to hyperparathyroidism (HPT)
- Intrathyroid parathyroid adenomas (PTAs) are rare (2-5%), completely intrathyroid + echogenic edge with thyroid gland
- Parathyroid carcinoma appears similar to PTA + local invasion, calcification, and immobility on swallowing
- Color Doppler: PTAs (including intrathyroid) are hypervascular, commonly with central blunt-ending vessel; if branching, it mimics lymph node
- Combination of Tc-99m sestamibi and US ideal to evaluate most PTAs
- Some suggest scintigraphy as 1st-choice examination and US complementary
- Other start with US; if PTA is identified (incidence of multiple PTAs is low [2-3%]), localize, mark skin surface for limited access surgery ± intraoperative use of gamma probe, parathormone estimation
- US safely guides needle for alcohol ablation and parathyroid hormone (PTH) estimation in suspected intrathyroid PTA
- US identifies concurrent thyroid pathology (2% thyroid malignancy) that may be treated at same surgical procedure
- Scintigraphy better evaluates ectopic gland
- Combined Tc-99m sestamibi scintigraphy and MR likely best approach in postoperative neck (recurrent/persistent HPT, failed previous surgery)

Top Differential Diagnoses

- Thyroid nodule
- Paratracheal lymph node
- Parathyroid carcinoma

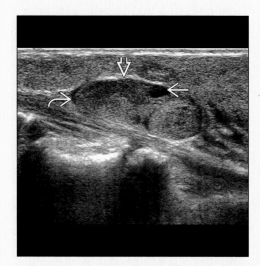
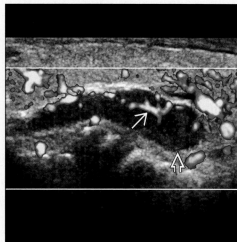

(Left) Longitudinal grayscale US shows well-circumscribed hypoechoic (due to uniform hypercellularity) parathyroid adenoma (PTA) ➡ behind a thyroid gland. Note small focal cystic area ➡ and echogenic line ⇨ separating PTA from thyroid. *(Right)* Longitudinal power Doppler US shows large PTA ⇨ with central vessel ➡, which are often short segment and blunt ending. Note arrowhead appearance of PTA pointing superiorly. Retrothyroid PTAs may be oval or flat as glands here develop within longitudinally aligned fascial planes.

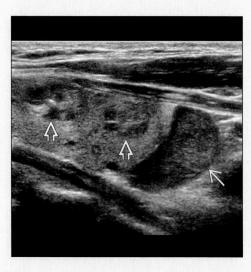
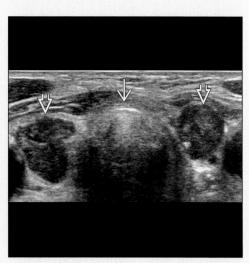

(Left) Longitudinal grayscale US shows PTA ➡ below the lower pole of the thyroid gland. Note multiple nodules ⇨ are seen within the thyroid (frequently seen with modern high-resolution US transducers). Concurrent thyroid malignancy is reported in 2%. If identified preoperatively, both thyroid and parathyroid lesions can be addressed in a single surgical procedure. *(Right)* Transverse grayscale US shows multiple PTAs ⇨ on either side of the trachea ➡. Of patients with primary hyperparathyroidism, 2-3% may have multiple PTAs.

PARATHYROID ADENOMA IN VISCERAL SPACE

TERMINOLOGY

Abbreviations
- Parathyroid adenoma (PTA)

IMAGING

General Features
- Best diagnostic clue
  - US shows well-defined, hypoechoic extrathyroid nodule with bright capsule and vascularity in vicinity of thyroid gland
- Location
  - Upper parathyroid glands: Posterior to upper midpole of thyroid
    - Rarely located posterior to pharynx or esophagus
  - Lower parathyroid glands: 65% inferior, lateral to lower pole of thyroid
    - 35% of lower parathyroid glands are variably located along thymopharyngeal duct tract, extending from angle of mandible to lower anterior mediastinum
  - ≤ 20% in ectopic location: Hyoid, carotid sheath, mediastinum, intrathyroid
- Size
  - Typically 1-3 cm in size
- Morphology
  - Round or oval, well-circumscribed, solid mass
  - Usually homogeneous, but cystic degeneration and hemorrhage may occur

Ultrasonographic Findings
- PTA: Well-defined mass adjacent to thyroid gland
  - Most are hypoechoic to thyroid (due to uniform hypercellularity) and have echogenic capsule
  - Some show cystic degeneration
  - Calcification is rare; more common in carcinoma or hyperplasia due to hyperparathyroidism (HPT)
- Intrathyroid PTAs
  - Usually round
    - Retrothyroid PTAs may be oval, arrowhead-shaped (pointing superiorly on longitudinal scan), or flat (as parathyroid glands in this position develop in longitudinally aligned planes) medial to common carotid artery (CCA)
  - Rare (2-5%), completely intrathyroid + echogenic edge with thyroid gland
  - In mid to lower 1/3 of thyroid and aligned in long axis of thyroid
- Retrotracheal PTAs may not be detected by US as they are obscured by shadowing from tracheal cartilage
- Parathyroid carcinoma appears similar to PTA + local invasion, calcification, and immobility on swallowing
- Color Doppler: PTAs (including intrathyroid) are hypervascular, commonly with a central blunt-ending vessel; if branching, it mimics lymph node
  - Inferior thyroid artery is principal vascular supply of superior & inferior parathyroids

Imaging Recommendations
- Best imaging tool
  - Combination of Tc-99m sestamibi and US is ideal for evaluating most PTAs
    - Some suggest scintigraphy as 1st-choice examination with US complementary
- Others start with US; if PTA is identified (incidence of multiple PTAs is low [2-3%]), localize, mark skin surface for limited access surgery ± intraoperative use of gamma probe, parathormone estimation
  - US safely guides needle for alcohol ablation and PTH estimation in suspected intrathyroid PTA
  - US identifies concurrent thyroid pathology (2% thyroid malignancy) that may be treated at same surgical procedure
- Scintigraphy better evaluates ectopic gland
- Combined Tc-99m sestamibi scintigraphy + MR likely best approach in postoperative neck (recurrent, persistent HPT, failed previous surgery)
- Protocol advice
  - US best performed in transverse plane starting above level of thyroid to clavicle caudally
    - Patient lies supine with neck hyperextended as this elevates low-lying PTAs into neck
    - Limited in obese patients with short necks, ectopic PTAs, and postoperative necks
    - PTA may be confused with longus colli muscle, blood vessels, lymph nodes, and esophagus

DIFFERENTIAL DIAGNOSIS

Thyroid Nodule
- Solitary/multiple, hypoechoic, heterogeneous, cystic change, debris, septa, peripheral/intranodular vascularity, ± calcification

Paratracheal Lymph Node
- Ovoid, hypoechoic nodule in tracheoesophageal groove with hilar echopattern and vascularity

Thymic Cyst
- Inferior to left thyroid, anechoic, thin walls

Parathyroid Cyst
- Anechoic cystic lesion in parathyroid location; cyst fluid has high PTH and low T3, T4 levels

Parathyroid Carcinoma
- Invasive mass in parathyroid location; hypoechoic with calcification and fixed on swallowing

CLINICAL ISSUES

Demographics
- Epidemiology
  - PTA responsible for 75-85% of primary HPT cases
    - HPT occurs in 1/700 adults
    - Other causes of HPT include
      - Parathyroid hyperplasia: 10-15%
      - Multiple PTAs: 2-3%
      - Parathyroid carcinoma: < 1%

Treatment
- Surgical excision
- US-guided percutaneous ethanol ablation

SELECTED REFERENCES

1. Sofferman RA et al: Parathyroid Ultrasound. In Sofferman RA et al: Ultrasound of the Thyroid and Parathyroid Glands. New York: Springer. 157-186, 2012

PARATHYROID ADENOMA IN VISCERAL SPACE

(Left) Longitudinal grayscale US in a patient with HPT shows a large, teardrop-shaped PTA ➡ posterior to the lower pole of the left thyroid gland ⬌. Note that focal areas of cystic degeneration ➡ are occasionally seen within PTA. (Right) Corresponding coronal T2WI FS MR shows a large left PTA ➡ with cystic degeneration. CECT and MR are useful if there are discordant US and scintigraphic findings or for persistent/recurrent postoperative parathyroid hormone (PTH) elevation.

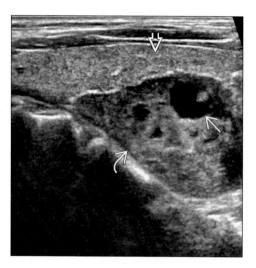
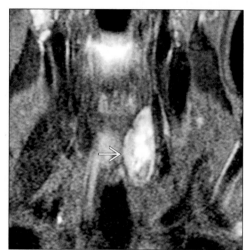

(Left) Multiple projections of Tc-99m sestamibi scan show persistent, intense focus of uptake ⬌ in region of left thyroid gland in this patient with HPT, suggesting PTA. (Right) Corresponding transverse grayscale US (same patient) shows a well-defined, solid, hypoechoic, noncalcified nodule ➡ in the left lobe of the thyroid ⬌, posteriorly located. In view of HPT, scintigraphic, & US findings, intrathyroid parathyroid adenoma was suspected. The trachea ➡, esophagus ➡, and CCA ⬌ are also shown.

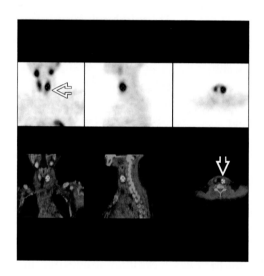
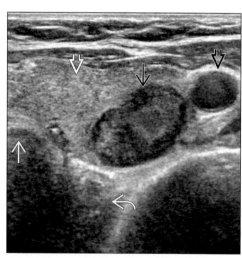

(Left) Longitudinal grayscale US (same patient) shows a nodule ➡ aligned along long axis of the thyroid in the lower pole and completely intrathyroid in location. (Right) Corresponding power Doppler shows multiple intranodular vessels. Normally, but not always, PTA has a solitary blunt ending vessel. Surgery confirmed intrathyroid PTA (occurs in 2-5% of cases). For PTA to qualify as intrathyroid, it must be completely intrathyroid, as in this case.

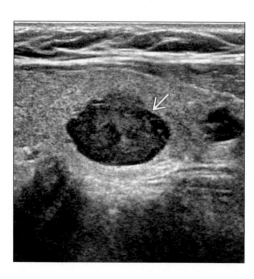
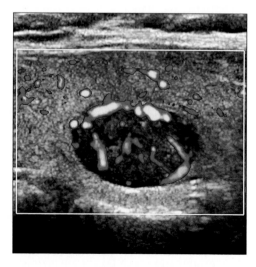

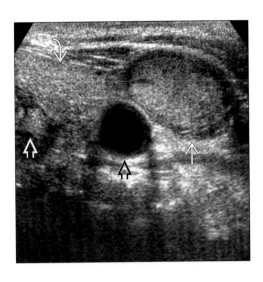

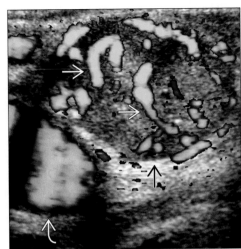

(Left) Transverse grayscale US shows an ectopic PTA ➜ in the carotid sheath location. The CCA ➜, trachea ➜, and thyroid ➜ are also shown. (Courtesy A. Momin, MD.) (Right) Corresponding power Doppler US confirms location of the PTA ➜ next to the CCA ➜ and shows the presence of multiple vessels ➜ within (not a single vessel as commonly reported). Ectopic locations include carotid sheath, intrathyroid, pyriform sinus, in thyrothymic ligament, and mediastinum. (Courtesy A. Momin, MD.)

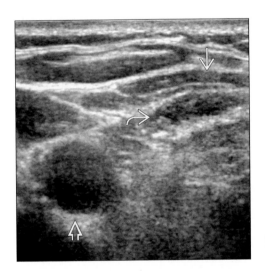

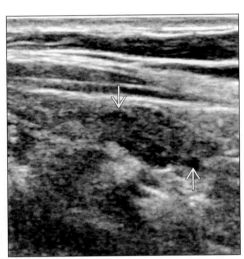

(Left) Transverse grayscale US shows a small, flat PTA ➜ in the sternal notch, just under the strap muscles ➜. The right CCA ➜ is also shown. (Right) Corresponding longitudinal US confirms PTA ➜ alignment in the long axis and well away from the thyroid gland (not seen on these scans). This PTA initially was seen as faint uptake on Tc-99m sestamibi scan. US helped in localizing PTA, facilitating limited access surgery under local anesthesia. US is also useful to guide needle position for ethanol injection of PTA.

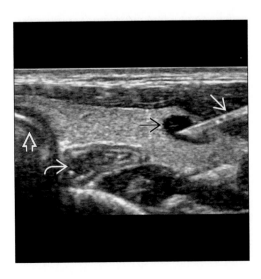

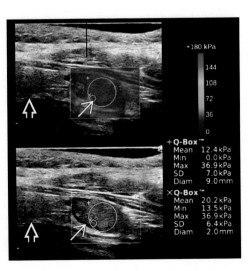

(Left) Transverse grayscale US shows needle aspiration ➜ of a suspected small intrathyroid PTA ➜. Although cytology may not be definitive, even moderate elevation of PTH supports the diagnosis of intrathyroid PTA. Note the trachea ➜ and esophagus ➜. (Right) Longitudinal grayscale US & SWE of PTA ➜ are shown. SWE color scale ranges from blue (0 kPa, soft) to red (180 kPa, stiff). The PTA appears blue, mean and maximum SWE of 12.4 kPa & 36.9 kPa, respectively, which suggests a soft lesion. Note the thyroid ➜.

PARATHYROID CARCINOMA

Key Facts

Terminology

- Low-grade malignancy arising from one of the parathyroid glands

Imaging

- Often indistinguishable from parathyroid adenoma (PTA)
- Typically larger than PTA at presentation
- Behavior of tumor (metastases) may be only indicator of malignancy
- Typically posterior to thyroid gland but can be within
- Hypoechoic nodule posterior to thyroid lobe
- Infiltrative border and calcification are highly specific, seen in ~ 50% of cases
- Thick capsule is much more commonly seen in carcinoma than in adenoma
- Heterogeneity is common but seen with both benign and malignant parathyroid tumors
- US: Cystic change and irregular shape are nonspecific
  - Irregular vessels extending from periphery are more suggestive of malignant than benign lesion
  - PTA is typically hypervascular, blunt-ending intratumoral vessel
- CECT: Useful for carcinoma arising in ectopic glands; evaluate extent of local invasion and lung metastasis
- Tc-99m sestamibi confirms presence and localizes disease; confirm with sonography or CECT

Top Differential Diagnoses

- Parathyroid adenoma
- Thyroid adenoma
- Thyroid differentiated carcinoma

Diagnostic Checklist

- Rare malignancy
- Mimics PTA clinically and radiographically
- Brown tumors of hyperparathyroidism should not be mistaken for bone metastases

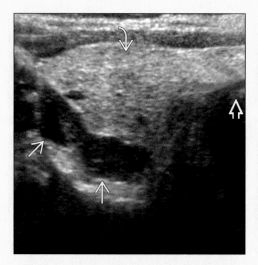
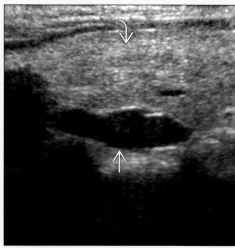

(Left) Axial grayscale US in a patient with proven PTCa shows solid, hypoechoic, well-defined, noncalcified nodule ➡ posterior to right lobe of thyroid ➡. With known hyperparathyroidism and hypercalcemia, this would be invariably reported as parathyroid adenoma (PTA). Note trachea ➡. *(Courtesy A. Momin, MD.)* *(Right)* Longitudinal grayscale US *(same patient)* shows proven PTCa ➡ is well-defined with no extension into adjacent soft tissues or thyroid gland anteriorly ➡. *(Courtesy A. Momin, MD.)*

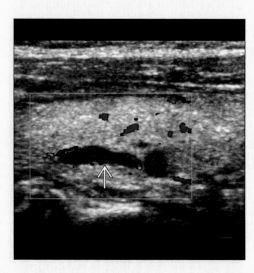
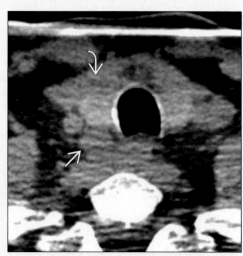

(Left) Longitudinal color Doppler US *(same patient)* shows no significant vascularity within PTCa ➡. PTA is most common cause of hyperparathyroidism, with PTCa being very rare (0.1% of hyperparathyroidism). Diagnosis of PTCa is made following surgery, and metastases (brown tumors should not be mistaken for metastases) may be the only indicators of malignancy preoperatively. *(Courtesy A. Momin, MD.)* *(Right)* Axial NECT in another patient with PTCa ➡ shows PTCa posterior to the thyroid gland ➡.

PARATHYROID CARCINOMA

TERMINOLOGY

Abbreviations
- Parathyroid carcinoma (PTCa)

Definitions
- Low-grade malignancy arising from parathyroid gland

IMAGING

General Features
- Location
  - Usually posterior to thyroid gland but may be within
  - Rarely arises from ectopic parathyroid gland
- Size
  - Typically larger than parathyroid adenoma (PTA) at presentation
  - Usually > 3 cm, rarely < 15 mm

Ultrasonographic Findings
- Grayscale ultrasound
  - Hypoechoic nodule posterior to thyroid lobe
  - Infiltrative border and calcification are highly specific, seen in ~ 50% of cases
  - Thick capsule is much more commonly seen in carcinoma than in adenoma
  - Heterogeneity is common but seen with both benign and malignant parathyroid tumor
  - Cystic change and irregular shape are nonspecific
- Power Doppler
  - Irregular vessels extending from periphery are more suggestive of malignant rather than benign lesion
  - PTA is typically hypervascular, blunt-ending intratumoral vessel

CT Findings
- CECT
  - Useful for carcinoma arising in ectopic glands
  - Evaluate extent of local invasion and lung metastasis

Nuclear Medicine Findings
- Tc-99m sestamibi
  - Localizes source of hyperparathyroidism
  - Insensitive for lung metastasis and localized mediastinal recurrence

Imaging Recommendations
- Best imaging tool
  - Tc-99m sestamibi
    - Confirms presence and localizes disease
  - Confirm with sonography or CECT

DIFFERENTIAL DIAGNOSIS

Parathyroid Adenoma
- Usually indistinguishable from PTCa

Thyroid Adenoma
- Intrathyroidal, well-defined mass with variable echogenicity, perinodular vascularity, ± cystic change

Thyroid Differentiated Carcinoma
- Ill-defined mass with abnormal vascularity ± nodes, ± calcification, ± cystic change, ± extrathyroid extension
- Usually appears more aggressive than PTCa

PATHOLOGY

General Features
- Difficult to distinguish from adenoma
  - Behavior of tumor (metastases) may be only indicator of malignancy

Staging, Grading, & Classification
- 80% well differentiated, 10% moderately differentiated, 8% poorly differentiated, 2% undifferentiated

CLINICAL ISSUES

Presentation
- Most common signs/symptoms
  - Related to severe hyperparathyroidism and hypercalcemia
    - Serum PTH level > 4-5x upper limit of normal
    - Serum calcium level higher than that of PTA
    - Weakness, vomiting, anorexia, constipation, polydipsia, polyuria, weight loss, renal stone
    - Recurrent severe pancreatitis, peptic ulcer, and anemia in severe cases
- Other signs/symptoms
  - Described as seen with 15% of hyperparathyroidism-jaw tumor syndrome (HPT-JT)
    - Associated with fibroosseous tumors in jaw ± renal hamartoma, polycystic kidneys, Wilms tumor, etc.

Demographics
- Age
  - No age predilection; range: 8-85 years
- Gender
  - F = M, whereas F > > M for adenomas
- Epidemiology
  - Very rare, < 1,000 cases in English literature
  - ~ 0.1% of hyperparathyroidism
- 90% of carcinoma are functional

Natural History & Prognosis
- Slow, indolent growth; 5-year survival rate: 70-85%
- Tumor size and nodes are not predictive of outcome
- Death is more likely from hypercalcemia than tumor

Treatment
- En bloc resection is mainstay of treatment
  - Adjuvant radiation is controversial

DIAGNOSTIC CHECKLIST

Image Interpretation Pearls
- Rare malignancy
- Mimics PTA clinically and radiographically
- Rate of false-positive suspicion should be kept low

Reporting Tips
- Brown tumors of hyperparathyroidism should not be mistaken for bone metastases

SELECTED REFERENCES
1. Halenka M et al: Four ultrasound and clinical pictures of parathyroid carcinoma. Case Rep Endocrinol. 2012:363690, 2012
2. Digonnet A et al: Parathyroid carcinoma: a review with three illustrative cases. J Cancer. 2:532-7, 2011

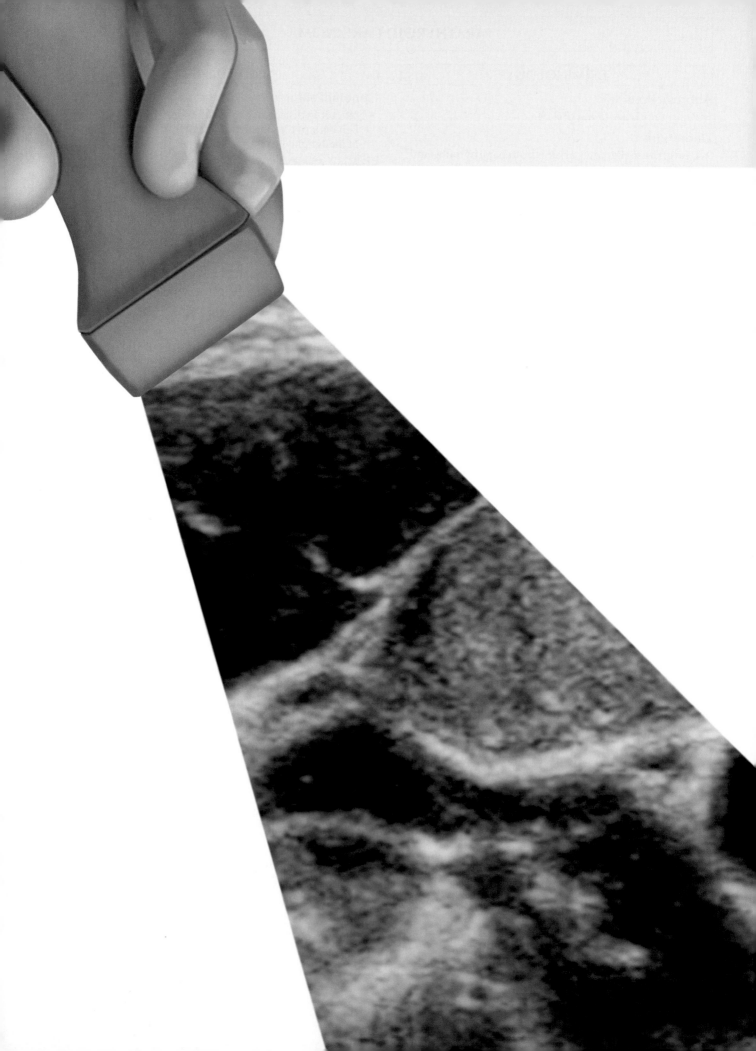

SECTION 3
Lymph Nodes

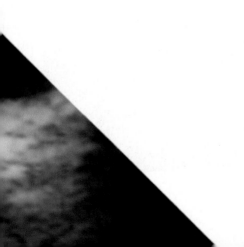

REACTIVE ADENOPATHY

Key Facts

Imaging

- Normal or mildly enlarged node in its known anatomical location
- Other reactive nodes in neck, unilateral or bilateral
- Hypoechoic cortex compared with adjacent muscle, ± cortical hypertrophy
- Oval in shape except for submandibular nodes which are usually round
- Preserved hilar architecture
- Reactive nodes may be ill-defined due to periadenitis, which blurs nodal margins
- Absence of intranodal necrosis or nodal matting
- Adjacent soft tissue is not obviously inflamed
- Color Doppler: Hilar vascularity
- Often may not clearly display an echogenic hilum on grayscale US but displays prominent hilar vessels on Doppler

- Spectral Doppler: Low vascular resistance (resistive index [RI] < 0.8, pulsatility index [PI] < 1.6)
- US is ideal imaging modality for initial assessment of enlarged lymph node & readily identifies reactive nodes based on grayscale & Doppler features
- US is quick, nonionizing, and does not require contrast or sedation; ideal in children as reactive/enlarged nodes are common clinical dilemma

Top Differential Diagnoses

- Metastatic node: Hypoechoic, round, ± necrosis, absent hilum, peripheral vascularity
- Tuberculous node: Intranodal necrosis, matting, soft tissue edema, displaced vascularity/avascular
- Metastatic node from papillary thyroid carcinoma: Hyperechoic, nodal necrosis, punctate calcification
- Non-Hodgkin lymphoma nodes: Solid, hypoechoic, round, pseudocystic/reticulated echo pattern, marked hilar and peripheral vascularity

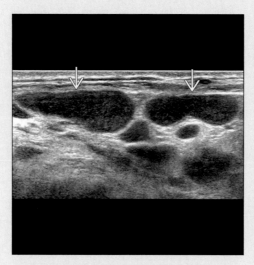
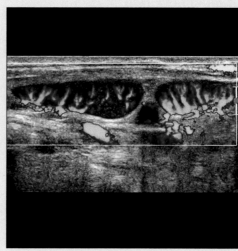

(Left) Longitudinal grayscale US shows a chain of accessory nodes ➡ in the posterior triangle. They are elongated in shape, solid, and noncalcified with a hypoechoic cortex and no obvious hilar architecture. No nodal matting or associated soft tissue edema is seen.
(Right) Corresponding power Doppler US shows prominent, radiating hilar vascularity (despite nonvisualization of hilum on grayscale US) with no peripheral vascularity. These are typical vascular features of reactive nodes.

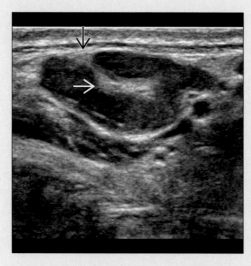
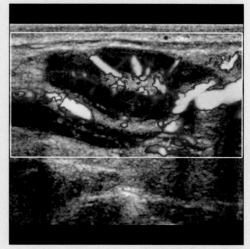

(Left) Transverse grayscale US shows an enlarged node in the submandibular region with normal hilar architecture ➡ (continuation with adjacent soft tissues ➡) and a hypertrophied cortex. Note ill-defined edges, a feature of reactive/inflammatory nodes, as these excite periadenitis, which blurs lymph node margins. *(Right)* Corresponding power Doppler US shows radiating hilar vascularity, which is typically low resistance, RI < 0.8 & PI < 1.6 (not used/limited use in routine clinical practice).

REACTIVE ADENOPATHY

TERMINOLOGY

Synonyms
- Reactive adenopathy, reactive lymphoid hyperplasia, nodal hyperplasia

Definitions
- Reactive implies benign etiology
- Benign, reversible enlargement of nodes in response to antigen stimulus
  - Nodal involvement may be acute or chronic, localized or generalized

IMAGING

General Features
- Best diagnostic clue
  - Normal or mildly enlarged node in its known anatomical location
  - Other reactive nodes in neck, unilateral or bilateral
  - Multiple well-/ill-defined, oval-shaped nodes
- Location
  - Known anatomical location of nodes in neck
    - Submental nodes, submandibular nodes, internal jugular nodes (from skull base to clavicle)
    - Retropharyngeal nodes, spinal accessory nodes (above clavicle, posterior to sternomastoid and anterior to trapezius muscle)
    - Anterior compartment nodes (between hyoid and sternal notch, and between carotid sheaths), upper mediastinal nodes (below sternal notch)
  - Any nodal groups of head and neck depending on site of antigen stimulus
- Size
  - Wide range
    - Adult: Often ≤ 1.5 cm
    - Child: Reactive node may be ≥ 2 cm
- Morphology
  - Node is typically oval rather than round

Ultrasonographic Findings
- Hypoechoic cortex compared with adjacent muscle, ± cortical hypertrophy
- Oval in shape except for submandibular nodes, which are usually round
- Enlarged node, preserved hilar architecture
  - Hilum; intranodal, linear, echogenic, and continuous with soft tissues around lymph node
  - Hilar echogenicity is due to multiple sound-reflecting surfaces from hilar afferent and efferent lymphatics, artery and vein
- May be ill-defined due to periadenitis, which blurs lymph node margins
- Absence of intranodal necrosis or nodal matting
- Adjacent soft tissue is not obviously inflamed
  - No evidence of associated cellulitis, abscess
- Color Doppler: Hilar vascularity
  - Often may not clearly display echogenic hilum on grayscale US but display prominent hilar vessels on Doppler
  - Hilar vascularity may be prominent with vessels reaching periphery of node (i.e., originates in hilum and reaches periphery)
  - Must be distinguished from peripheral vascularity in malignant and lymphomatous nodes; tumor neovascularity originates peripherally
- Spectral Doppler: Low vascular resistance (resistive index [RI] < 0.8, pulsatility index [PI] < 1.6)
  - Evaluation of nodes using spectral Doppler is not routinely necessary to evaluate reactive nodes

CT Findings
- NECT
  - Homogeneous, well-defined nodes, isodense or hypodense to muscle
  - Stranding of adjacent fat frequently associated with acute infectious cause
- CECT
  - Variable enhancement, minimal to mild, homogeneous
  - Linear enhancement within node characteristic
  - Hyperplasia of pharyngeal lymphoid tissue (Waldeyer ring) often associated

MR Findings
- T1WI
  - Homogeneous low to intermediate signal
- T2WI
  - Homogeneous intermediate to high signal intensity
  - Cystic change suggests suppuration or tumoral necrosis
- DWI
  - Benign nodes tend to have higher ADC values than neoplastic nodes
- T1WI C+
  - Variable enhancement, usually mild & homogeneous
  - Linear central enhancement favors benign node
  - Tonsillar enlargement (Waldeyer ring) may be found

Nuclear Medicine Findings
- PET
  - Mild FDG uptake may be seen
    - Marked uptake more likely with active granulomatous disease or tumor

Imaging Recommendations
- Best imaging tool
  - US is ideal imaging modality for initial assessment of enlarged lymph node and readily identifies reactive nodes based on grayscale and Doppler features
    - Quick, nonionizing, and does not require contrast or sedation; ideal in children as reactive/enlarged nodes are common clinical dilemma
    - Differentiates reactive from suppurative nodes and cellulitis from abscess
  - Limitations of US in assessing neck lymph node
    - Unable to evaluate retropharyngeal nodes and upper mediastinal nodes
    - Nodes in anterior compartment may be obscured by shadowing/artifact from tracheal rings and air in trachea
    - MR and CT overcome these limitations

DIFFERENTIAL DIAGNOSIS

Metastatic Node
- Enlarged, round, hypoechoic lymph node

REACTIVE ADENOPATHY

- Commonly solid but may show intranodal cystic necrosis (squamous cell carcinoma, papillary thyroid carcinoma)
- Absent echogenic hilum
- Peripheral vascularity and RI > 0.8, PI > 1.6

Tuberculous Node

- Round, hypoechoic, intranodal necrosis
- Clumped/nodal matting with absence of normal soft tissues between nodes
- Soft tissue edema, ± cellulitis, ± abscess
- Color Doppler: Displaced hilar vascularity or avascular

Metastatic Node From Papillary Thyroid Carcinoma

- Hyperechoic (characteristic), ± intranodal necrosis
- Punctate calcification, representing psammoma bodies
- Color Doppler: Increased chaotic peripheral vascularity, variable intravascular resistance

Non-Hodgkin Lymphoma (NHL) Node

- Multiple chains involved ± enlarged lymph nodes in rest of body
- Solid, hypoechoic, round, pseudocystic/reticulated echo pattern
- Marked hilar and peripheral vascularity
  - Hilar > peripheral

PATHOLOGY

General Features

- Enlarged node may be due to nonspecific or specific histologic reaction to both noninfectious or infectious agents
- Most children 2-12 years have lymphadenopathy at some time

CLINICAL ISSUES

Presentation

- Most common signs/symptoms
  - Firm, sometimes fluctuant, freely mobile subcutaneous nodal masses
  - Other signs/symptoms
    - Bacterial adenitis and cat scratch disease usually painful
    - Nontuberculous mycobacteria (NTM) usually nontender
- Clinical profile
  - Most frequently, enlarged nodes in young patient with pharyngeal or systemic viral infection
  - Pediatric or teenage presentation with nodal enlargement
  - Patient with known primary neoplasm may have borderline-sized nodes that are only reactive

Demographics

- Age
  - Any, but most common in pediatric age group
    - Neonatal neck nodes not palpable
  - Children: Organisms have predilection for specific ages
    - < 1 year: *Staphylococcus aureus*, group B *Streptococcus*
    - 1-5 years: *Staphylococcus aureus*, group A β-hemolytic *Streptococcus*, atypical mycobacteria

- 5-15 years: Anaerobic bacteria, toxoplasmosis, *Bartonella* (cat scratch disease), tuberculosis
- Ethnicity
  - High incidence of *Mycobacterium tuberculosis* in developing countries
- Epidemiology
  - Common clinical problem in pediatric age group
    - Pediatric nodes not often imaged
    - Most children 2-12 years have lymphadenopathy at some time
    - Most adenopathy is result of infection, though organism may not be identified
  - Less common in adults
    - Most important differential considerations are malignancy or HIV infection

Treatment

- Nodal aspiration or biopsy may be necessary if
  - Failed response to antibiotics
  - Rapid increase in nodal size
  - Associated systemic adenopathy or unexplained fever and weight loss
  - Features concerning for malignancy
    - Nodes feel hard &/or matted to examination
    - Supraclavicular or posterior cervical node location
- If needle aspiration shows nonspecific reactive changes, follow clinically for 3-6 months
- Persistent adenopathy requires repeat needle aspiration to rule out lymphoma, metastasis, or TB

DIAGNOSTIC CHECKLIST

Consider

- Oval-shaped nodes likely to be benign and reactive
- Preserved internal nodal architecture and hilar vascularity is suggestive of reactive node
- Adjacent cellulitis suggests bacterial infection
- Always consider metastatic disease, NHL, and HIV in nonpediatric age group
- Certain locations should raise concern
  - Postauricular nodes in child > 2 years are likely clinically significant
  - Supraclavicular nodes are neoplastic in ~ 60% and the primary infraclavicular in location
  - Posterior cervical nodes suggest NHL, skin nodal metastases, or nasopharyngeal carcinoma

SELECTED REFERENCES

1. Sofferman RA et al: Ultrasound of the Thyroid and Parathyroid Glands. USA: Springer, 211-228, 2012
2. Abdel-Galiil K et al: Incidence of sarcoidosis in head and neck cancer. Br J Oral Maxillofac Surg. 46(1):59-60, 2008
3. Chan JM et al: Ultrasonography of abnormal neck lymph nodes. Ultrasound Q. 23(1):47-54, 2007
4. Ahuja AT et al: Sonographic evaluation of cervical lymph nodes. AJR Am J Roentgenol. 184(5):1691-9, 2005
5. Leung AK et al: Childhood cervical lymphadenopathy. J Pediatr Health Care. 18(1):3-7, 2004
6. Ahuja A et al: Sonography of neck lymph nodes. Part II: abnormal lymph nodes. Clin Radiol. 58(5):359-66, 2003
7. Ahuja AT et al: Distribution of intranodal vessels in differentiating benign from metastatic neck nodes. Clin Radiol. 56(3):197-201, 2001

REACTIVE ADENOPATHY

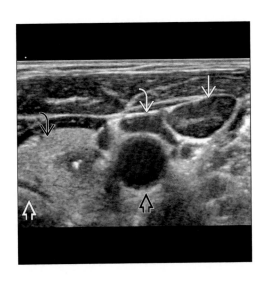
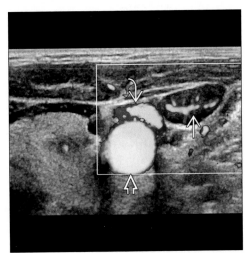

(Left) Transverse grayscale US shows a solitary solid, noncalcified, hypoechoic node ➡ with cortical hypertrophy and echogenic hilum along deep cervical/jugular chain. Note its relation to IJV ➡ & CCA ➡. This is a common site of reactive nodes, often bilateral & symmetrical. Note thyroid ➡ (with small nodule with "comet tail" artifact) & trachea ➡. *(Right)* Corresponding power Doppler US of reactive node clearly defines radiating hilar vascularity ➡ and relation to IJV ➡ and CCA ➡.

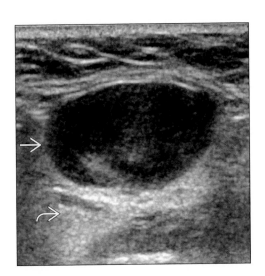
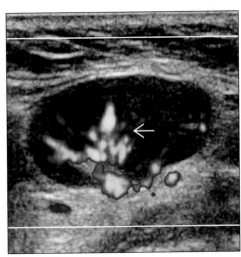

(Left) Transverse grayscale US shows a prominent, oval-shaped, solid, hypoechoic, noncalcified node ➡ with a markedly hypertrophied cortex, posterior enhancement ➡ and faint hilar echo pattern. US features are equivocal and lymphoma should be ruled out (fine-needle/core/excision biopsy). *(Right)* Corresponding power Doppler US shows isolated hilar vascularity ➡, unusual for lymphoma, which has mixed vascularity (hilar > peripheral). Biopsy confirmed reactive lymphadenopathy.

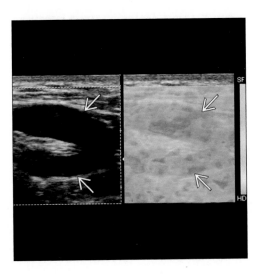
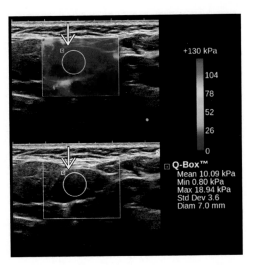

(Left) Longitudinal grayscale US & qualitative strain elastogram show a reactive node ➡. Strain color scale ranges from purple (elastic, soft) to red (inelastic, hard). It displays a mosaic color pattern of mostly purple & green, similar to the adjacent tissue, suggestive of an elastic node. *(Right)* Longitudinal grayscale US & SWE shows a reactive node ➡. SWE color scale ranges from blue (0 kPa, soft) to red (130 kPa, stiff). It appears blue with mean & maximum SWE values of 10.1 kPa & 18.9 kPa, which are low.

SUPPURATIVE ADENOPATHY

Key Facts

Terminology

- Adenitis, acute lymphadenitis, intranodal abscess
- Pus formation within nodes from bacterial infection

Imaging

- Enlarged node with surrounding inflammation (cellulitis), often multiple
- ↑ cortical echogenicity, hypertrophy, absent echogenic hilum, central hypoechogenicity ± anechoic areas
- Peripheral hypervascularity and soft tissue edema
- Ultrasound characterizes nature of adenopathy and provides image guidance for aspiration of abscesses
- Contrast CT best evaluates extent of suppurative changes and complications

Top Differential Diagnoses

- Tuberculosis lymph nodes
- Non-TB *Mycobacterium* lymph nodes
- Metastatic nodes
- Non-Hodgkin lymphoma nodes

Pathology

- *Staphylococcus aureus* and group A *Streptococcus* most frequent causative organisms
- Pediatric infections show clustering of organisms by age range
- Dental infections are typically polymicrobial and predominantly anaerobic

Diagnostic Checklist

- Look for primary infectious source on images
  - Pharyngitis, dental infection, salivary gland calculi
- With any neck infection, must evaluate for
  - Airway compromise
  - Thrombophlebitis or pseudoaneurysm
- In children, consider non-TB mycobacterial adenitis if no significant inflammatory changes

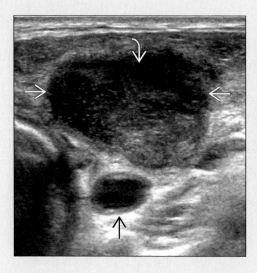
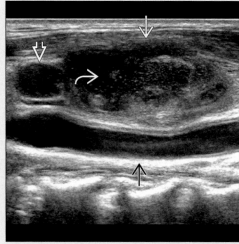

(Left) Transverse grayscale US of the left upper neck reveals a 4 cm, ill-defined, hypoechoic lymph node at the upper internal jugular chain ➡, anterior to common carotid artery (CCA) ➡. Note the loss of hilar architecture and intranodal necrosis ➡. (Right) Corresponding longitudinal grayscale US clearly shows a hypoechoic, heterogeneous node ➡ with intranodal necrosis ➡. Note its proximity to the CCA ➡ and the presence of an adjacent smaller cystic node ➡. Guided aspiration of the cystic area yielded pus.

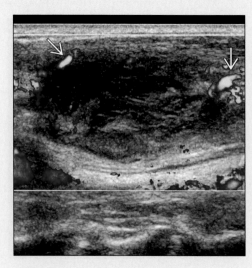
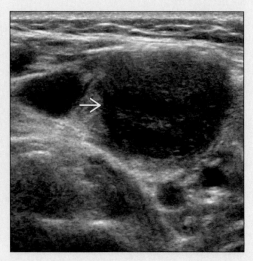

(Left) Longitudinal power Doppler US (same patient) shows hypervascularity of the surrounding inflamed tissues ➡, consistent with suppurative lymph node. TB node may have a similar appearance. (Right) Transverse grayscale US of another patient shows similar findings in an enlarged, ill-defined hypoechoic node ➡ with the cystic component located in the left upper neck. This patient presented with a painless mass and biopsy revealed lymphoma. Intranodal necrosis is uncommon in lymphoma.

SUPPURATIVE ADENOPATHY

TERMINOLOGY

Synonyms
- Adenitis, acute lymphadenitis, intranodal abscess

Definitions
- Pus formation within nodes from bacterial infection

IMAGING

General Features
- Best diagnostic clue
  - Enlarged node with intranodal fluid and surrounding inflammation (cellulitis), may be multiple
- Location
  - Any of nodal groups of head and neck
    - Most often: Jugulodigastric, submandibular, retropharyngeal
  - Unilateral or bilateral
- Size
  - Typically enlarged node or confluence of nodes
  - 1-4 cm range
- Morphology
  - Ovoid to round, large node
  - Often poorly defined margins

Ultrasonographic Findings
- Grayscale ultrasound
  - Enlarged, hypoechoic nodes with ill-defined margins
  - Cortical hypertrophy, ± increased echogenicity
  - Loss of echogenic hilum
  - Central hypoechogenicity ± anechoic cystic areas with posterior acoustic enhancement
  - Cellulitis in surrounding soft tissue
    - Hypervascular thickening of skin and subcutaneous layers
    - Presence of fluid/edema: Hypoechoic strands, "cobblestone" appearance
- Color Doppler
  - Increased vascularity, predominantly at nodal periphery and in inflamed soft tissues
  - Central avascularity due to intranodal necrosis
  - Low resistance and pulsatility indices

CT Findings
- CECT
  - Enhancing nodal wall with central hypodensity/lack of enhancement
  - Stranding of adjacent fat and subcutaneous tissues
  - If progresses to abscess: Irregular, ill-defined, peripherally enhancing, low-density collection

MR Findings
- T1WI
  - Node with central low signal intensity
- T2WI
  - Node with diffuse or central high signal intensity
  - Fat saturation best demonstrates surrounding hyperintense tissues
- T1WI C+
  - Marked peripheral enhancement with poorly defined margin
  - Absent central enhancement

Imaging Recommendations
- Best imaging tool
  - Ultrasound
    - Commonly first-line imaging modality for investigation of neck swelling
    - Good for characterizing nature of adenopathy
    - Provides image guidance for aspiration of any abscesses
  - CECT is required if any deep extension is suspected and to look for any primary cause for infection
    - To evaluate anatomical extent of large abscesses, extensive infection, deep extension
    - Identify source of infection and possible complications (airway compromise, thrombophlebitis)
- Protocol advice
  - Contrast should be administered to best appreciate extent of suppurative changes

DIFFERENTIAL DIAGNOSIS

Tuberculosis Lymph Nodes
- Painless, unilateral, low jugular and posterior cervical low-density nodes
- Matted nodes with cystic necrosis ± surrounding inflammation
- Calcification present in recurrent or treated disease
- Strongly reactive tuberculosis (PPD) skin test

Non-TB Mycobacterium Lymph Nodes
- Asymmetric enlarged nodes with adjacent subcutaneous necrotic ring-enhancing masses
- Minimal or absent subcutaneous fat stranding
- PPD skin test weakly reactive in ~ 55%
- Pediatric age group; usually ≤ 5 years of age

Metastatic Nodes
- Usually painless, hard nodes; no hot overlying skin
- Round nodes with absent echogenic hilum ± internal necrosis, ± abnormal vascularity
- Typically no adjacent inflammation unless extracapsular spread
- Primary tumor mass often evident

Non-Hodgkin Lymphoma Nodes
- Solid, round, well defined, hypoechoic with pseudocystic/reticulated pattern
- Marked hilar > peripheral hypervascularity
- No inflammation of surrounding tissues
- Multiple chains involved ± enlarged nodes in rest of body

Fatty Nodal Metaplasia
- Chronic inflammation results in fatty change of nodal hilus
- Fat density on CT; fat intensity on MR
- Well-defined node, no inflammatory change

PATHOLOGY

General Features
- Etiology
  - Primary head and neck infection
    - Adjacent lymph nodes enlarge in reaction to pathogen: Reactive nodes

SUPPURATIVE ADENOPATHY

- ▪ Intranodal exudate forms containing protein-rich fluid with dead neutrophils (pus): Suppurative nodes
- ▪ If untreated or incorrectly treated, suppurative nodes rupture, then interstitial pus is walled-off by immune system: Abscess in soft tissues
- ○ Reactive nodes from viral pathogen may have 2° bacterial superinfection creating suppurative nodes
- • Associated abnormalities
- ○ Primary causes of head and neck infection include pharyngitis, salivary gland ductal calculus, dental decay ± mandibular osteomyelitis

Gross Pathologic & Surgical Features
- • Fluctuant neck mass with erythematous, warm skin
- • Aspiration of pus is diagnostic

Microscopic Features
- • Acute inflammatory cell infiltrate in necrotic background
- ○ Presence of neutrophils and macrophages
- ○ Negative staining for acid-fast bacilli
- • Staphylococcus aureus and group A *Streptococcus* most frequent organisms
- • Pediatric infections show clustering of organisms by age
- ○ Infants < 1 year: *Staphylococcus aureus*, group B *Streptococcus*
- ○ Children 1-4 years: *Staphylococcus aureus*, group A β-hemolytic *Streptococcus*, atypical mycobacteria
- ○ 5-15 years: Anaerobic bacteria, toxoplasmosis, *Bartonella* (cat scratch disease), tuberculosis
- • Dental infections: Typically polymicrobial; predominantly anaerobic organisms

CLINICAL ISSUES

Presentation
- • Most common signs/symptoms
- ○ Painful neck mass(es)
- ▪ Often reddened, hot overlying skin
- ○ Fever, poor oral intake
- ○ Elevated WBC and ESR
- • Other signs/symptoms
- ○ Other symptoms referable to primary source of infection
- ▪ Pharyngeal/laryngeal infection: May have drooling, respiratory distress
- ▪ Peritonsillar infection: May have trismus
- ▪ Retropharyngeal or paravertebral infection: May have neck stiffness
- • Clinical profile
- ○ Young patient presents with acute/subacute onset of tender neck mass and fever

Demographics
- • Age
- ○ Most commonly seen in pediatric and young adult population
- ○ Odontogenic neck infections: Adults > > children

Natural History & Prognosis
- • Conglomeration of suppurative nodes or rupture of node results in abscess formation
- ○ Superficial neck abscesses: Anterior or posterior cervical space, submandibular space

- ○ Deep neck abscesses: Retropharyngeal or parapharyngeal space
- • Deep space abscesses can rapidly progress with airway compromise

Treatment
- • Antibiotics only for small suppurative nodes and primary infection
- • Incision and drainage for large suppurative nodes or abscesses
- • Nodes from atypical mycobacteria should be excised to prevent recurrence or fistula/sinus tract

DIAGNOSTIC CHECKLIST

Consider
- • Pediatric patient
- ○ Consider nontuberculous mycobacterial adenitis if no significant inflammatory changes
- • Adult patient
- ○ If infective cause not evident, look for tooth infection ± mandibular osteomyelitis
- ○ Consider metastatic disease with necrotic or cystic nodes
- ▪ Especially if inflammatory history or signs are absent

Image Interpretation Pearls
- • Look for primary infectious source on CT images
- ○ Pharyngitis, dental infection, salivary gland calculi
- • Evaluate airway for compromise with any neck infection
- ○ Bigger problem in deep infections
- • Evaluate vascular structures for thrombophlebitis, pseudoaneurysm

SELECTED REFERENCES

1. Ludwig BJ et al: Imaging of cervical lymphadenopathy in children and young adults. AJR Am J Roentgenol. 199(5):1105-13, 2012
2. Guss J et al: Antibiotic-resistant Staphylococcus aureus in community-acquired pediatric neck abscesses. Int J Pediatr Otorhinolaryngol. 71(6):943-8, 2007
3. Koç O et al: Role of diffusion weighted MR in the discrimination diagnosis of the cystic and/or necrotic head and neck lesions. Eur J Radiol. 62(2):205-13, 2007
4. Niedzielska G et al: Cervical lymphadenopathy in children--incidence and diagnostic management. Int J Pediatr Otorhinolaryngol. 71(1):51-6, 2007
5. Luu TM et al: Acute adenitis in children: clinical course and factors predictive of surgical drainage. J Paediatr Child Health. 41(5-6):273-7, 2005
6. Coticchia JM et al: Age-, site-, and time-specific differences in pediatric deep neck abscesses. Arch Otolaryngol Head Neck Surg. 130(2):201-7, 2004
7. Leung AK et al: Childhood cervical lymphadenopathy. J Pediatr Health Care. 18(1):3-7, 2004
8. Franzese CB et al: Peritonsillar and parapharyngeal space abscess in the older adult. Am J Otolaryngol. 24(3):169-73, 2003
9. Handa U et al: Role of fine needle aspiration cytology in evaluation of paediatric lymphadenopathy. Cytopathology. 14(2):66-9, 2003
10. Kendi T et al: MR spectroscopy in a cervical abscess. Neuroradiology. 45(9):631-3, 2003

SUPPURATIVE ADENOPATHY

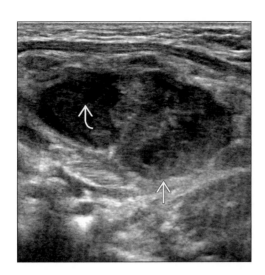

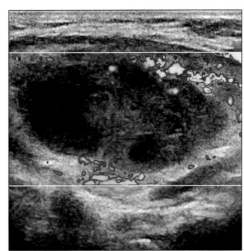

(Left) Longitudinal grayscale US in a patient presenting with fever and painful left neck swelling shows an enlarged, heterogeneous, hypoechoic lymph node ➡ with intranodal necrosis ➡ in apex of left posterior triangle. Note marked perinodal soft tissue edema. (Right) Corresponding power Doppler US reveals marked peripheral vascularity in soft tissues around inflamed node, often seen with suppurative lymph nodes. Note absence of intranodal vascularity. Aspiration yielded Staphylococcus aureus.

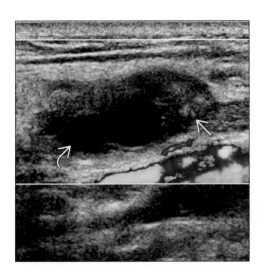

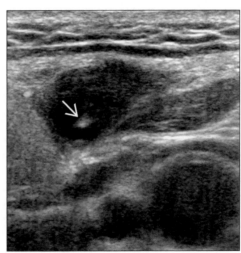

(Left) Longitudinal power Doppler US of a suppurative node shows minimal peripheral vascularity ➡ but no intranodal vascularity due to necrosis ➡ within the node. In an adult patient, metastatic lymph node should be considered, especially in the absence of inflammatory symptoms and signs. (Right) Corresponding transverse grayscale US shows the presence of a needle tip within the necrotic portion of the node ➡ during guided aspiration to differentiate metastatic from inflammatory node.

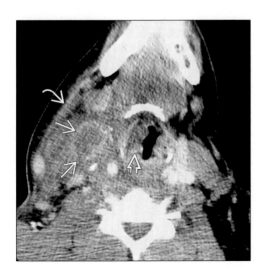

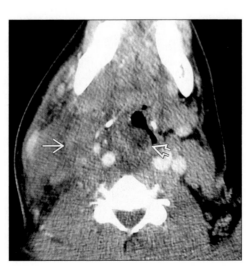

(Left) Axial CECT shows a rim-enhancing upper cervical suppurative node ➡ with extensive surrounding inflammatory change and thickened platysma muscle ➡. Deep extension of inflammation to the supraglottis ➡ is narrowing the airway in this very sick patient. (Right) Axial CECT at a slightly higher plane (same patient) shows a suppurative node ➡ and hypopharyngeal edema ➡. Both sites yielded group A Streptococcus. CECT evaluates deep extent and primary source of infection.

TUBERCULOUS ADENOPATHY

Key Facts

Terminology
- Cervical lymphadenitis due to *Mycobacterium tuberculosis* infection

Imaging
- Cervical nodes most common site of extrapulmonary tuberculous adenopathy
- Multiple hypoechoic, round nodes in posterior triangle and supraclavicular fossa (SCF), unilateral/bilateral
- Intranodal cystic/caseous necrosis, producing posterior enhancement
- Multiple matted nodes with no normal intervening soft tissues between involved nodes
- TB adenitis incites periadenitis resulting in affected nodes being clumped/matted together
- Associated adjacent soft tissue edema, response to adjacent inflamed node
- Nodal calcification is not seen in acute disease
- Calcification may be seen in nodes following treatment or in recurrent disease in previously affected/treated node
- Hilar vascularity in 50%, vessels are displaced by focal areas of necrosis: Displaced hilar vascularity
- No vascularity detected on power Doppler (19%)
- Capsular vascularity (12%) due to supply from perinodal inflammatory tissues
- ↑ vascularity in adjacent inflamed soft tissue
- Spectral Doppler: Low intranodal vascular resistance
  - Intranodal vascular resistance: Malignant nodes > tuberculous nodes > reactive nodes
- US identifies abnormal nodes, suggests diagnosis, and guides cytology/biopsy for confirmation

Top Differential Diagnoses
- Suppurative lymph nodes
- Non-Hodgkin lymphoma nodes
- Squamous cell carcinoma (SCCa) nodal metastases

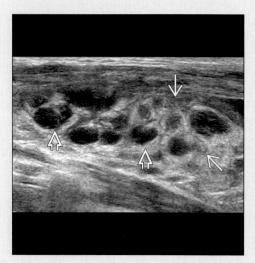
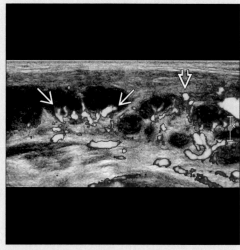

(Left) Longitudinal grayscale US shows multiple small, necrotic nodes in the posterior triangle ⇒. Note that they are clumped/matted together, with no normal soft tissue between them, and there is extensive edema in the adjacent soft tissue ➡. Their location and grayscale appearances are characteristic of tuberculous lymphadenitis. *(Right)* Corresponding power Doppler US shows typical displaced hilar vessels ➡ in some necrotic nodes and in the adjacent inflamed soft tissues ➡.

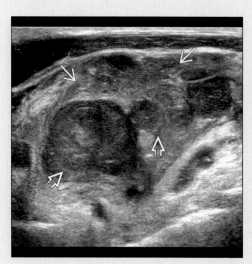
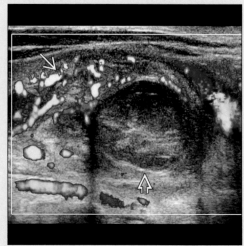

(Left) Transverse grayscale US shows multiple, matted nodes ➡ with marked adjacent soft tissue edema ➡ in the posterior triangle of the neck. TB produces periadenitis, causing nodes to be clumped/matted together. The presence of an adjacent inflamed node excites soft tissue inflammation around affected nodes, another hallmark of TB. *(Right)* Corresponding power Doppler US shows marked vascularity in inflamed soft tissues ➡ around a TB node ➡. Radiation to the neck may also cause soft tissue edema.

TUBERCULOUS ADENOPATHY

TERMINOLOGY

Synonyms
- Cervical lymphadenitis, scrofula

Definitions
- Enlargement of ≥ 1 cervical lymph nodes (LNs) due to *Mycobacterium tuberculosis* infection

IMAGING

General Features
- Location
  - Usually unilateral, involving level V nodes
  - Cervical nodes are the most common site of extrapulmonary TB adenopathy

Ultrasonographic Findings
- Grayscale ultrasound
  - Multiple hypoechoic, round nodes in posterior triangle, supraclavicular fossa (SCF)
  - Intranodal cystic/caseous necrosis, producing posterior enhancement
  - Multiple matted nodes with no normal intervening soft tissues between involved nodes
    - TB adenitis incites periadenitis, resulting in affected nodes being clumped/matted together
  - Associated adjacent soft tissue edema, response to adjacent inflamed node
  - Nodal calcification is not seen in acute disease
    - Calcification may be seen in nodes following treatment or in recurrent disease in previously affected/treated node
- Power Doppler
  - Hilar vascularity in 50%, but such vessels are displaced by focal areas of necrosis: Displaced hilar vascularity
  - No vascularity detected on power Doppler (19%)
    - Necrotizing granulomatous lesions may obliterate intranodal vessels
    - During healing phase, fibrosis and hyalinization obliterate intranodal vessels
  - Capsular (12%) vascularity due to supply from perinodal inflammatory tissues
  - Prominent vascularity in adjacent inflamed soft tissue
- Spectral Doppler: Low intranodal vascular resistance
  - Intranodal vascular resistance: Malignant nodes > tuberculous nodes > reactive nodes

CT Findings
- CECT
  - Node or nodal cluster with cystic changes
  - Rim enhancement typically thick and irregular
  - ± nodal calcification, adjacent soft tissue inflammatory changes

MR Findings
- T1WI C+ FS
  - Centrally necrotic nodal mass or multiple nodes
  - Thick, irregular enhancing periphery of nodes

Imaging Recommendations
- Best imaging tool
  - US identifies abnormal nodes, suggests diagnosis, and guides cytology/biopsy for confirmation

DIFFERENTIAL DIAGNOSIS

Suppurative Lymph Nodes
- Cystic component with adjacent inflammation
- Systemically unwell with fever and painful mass

Non-Hodgkin Lymphoma Nodes
- Hypoechoic, solid, nonnecrotic, reticulated/pseudocystic echo pattern
- Hilar > peripheral vascularity

SCCa Nodal Metastases
- Round, well-defined, hypoechoic nodes
- Intranodal necrosis and peripheral vascularity

Reactive Lymph Nodes
- Elliptical, solid, hypoechoic nodes with normal echogenic hilus and hilar vascularity

PATHOLOGY

General Features
- Etiology
  - Infection due to *M. tuberculosis* and other members of its complex: *M. bovis*, *M. africanum*, and *M. microti*

Microscopic Features
- Caseating granulomas, smear for acid-fast bacilli (AFB)
- Excisional biopsy more sensitive than FNA

CLINICAL ISSUES

Presentation
- Most common signs/symptoms
  - Solitary or multiple enlarged cervical masses in posterior triangle and SCF, unilateral or bilateral
- Other signs/symptoms
  - Constitutional symptoms and concomitant pulmonary tuberculosis (frequently absent)
    - Fever, night sweats, weight loss, cough

Demographics
- Age
  - Any age group; young children are more prone
- Epidemiology
  - More common in developing and southeast Asian countries due to overcrowding, poverty, poor living conditions, malnutrition
    - Often encountered in developed countries with increased incidence of HIV and AIDS

Treatment
- Antituberculous therapy
- LN excision by functional lymph node dissection
  - Lack of response from nodes despite adequate anti-TB therapy probably due to drug resistance

SELECTED REFERENCES

1. Ahuja AT et al: Sonographic evaluation of cervical lymph nodes. AJR Am J Roentgenol. 184(5):1691-9, 2005
2. Ahuja A et al: Power Doppler sonography to differentiate tuberculous cervical lymphadenopathy from nasopharyngeal carcinoma. AJNR Am J Neuroradiol. 22(4):735-40, 2001

TUBERCULOUS ADENOPATHY

(Left) Longitudinal grayscale US shows a solitary node in the posterior triangle ➡. Note that it appears almost completely cystic with loss of internal hilar architecture. *(Right)* Corresponding power Doppler US shows a large focal area of avascularity ➡ with displaced hilar vessels ➡. Avascularity is due to necrotizing granulomatous change obliterating intranodal vessels. In the healing phase, fibrosis and hyalinization may also cause occlusion of intranodal vessels.

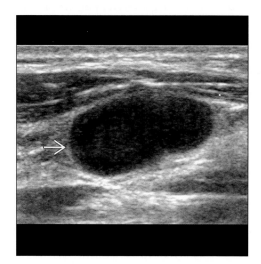
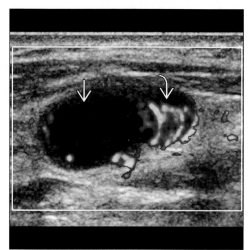

(Left) Clinical photo shows a patient with skin erythema and persistent discharge from the sinus ➡. *(Right)* Corresponding grayscale US shows multiple necrotic nodes matted together ➡. Note large areas of cystic necrosis within nodes (FNAC yields pus) and avascularity in some nodes and displaced vessels ➡ in others. One of the nodes ➡ has ruptured through subcutaneous tissue, discharging on to the skin surface, corresponding to the sinus opening seen in the clinical photo.

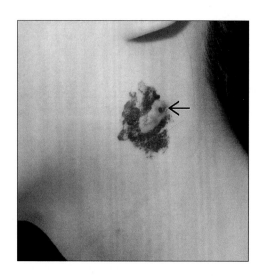
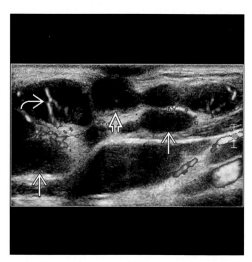

(Left) Transverse grayscale US shows typical "collar stud" tuberculous abscess ➡. It is necrotic with internal debris and locule formation. No vascularity is detected within the abscess cavity on Doppler. Note its proximity to adjacent major vessels (CCA ➡, IJV ➡). *(Right)* Transverse grayscale US shows a small node with dense intranodal calcification and posterior shadowing, better seen on Doppler scan (using its grayscale feature). Calcification is often seen in post-treatment tuberculous nodes.

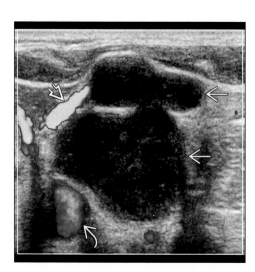
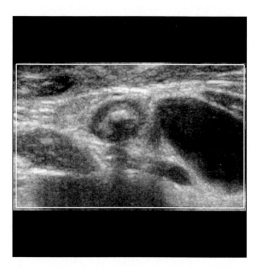

TUBERCULOUS ADENOPATHY

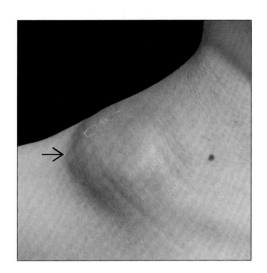

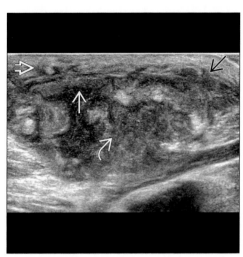

(Left) Clinical photo shows a patient presenting with fever and a warm, tender right supraclavicular mass ➡, clinically suggestive of TB lymphadenitis. *(Right)* Corresponding oblique grayscale US shows a large, ill-defined, hypoechoic, noncalcified heterogeneous mass ➡ with thick walls ➡, internal debris ➡, and adjacent soft tissue edema ➡. US features suggest tuberculous abscess. Guided aspiration yielded pus, and diagnosis of TB was subsequently confirmed.

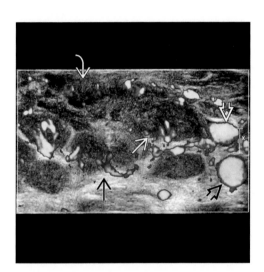

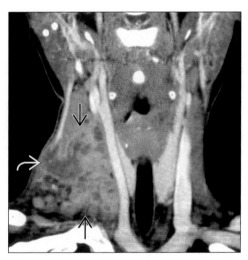

(Left) Transverse power Doppler US of the same patient shows a large abscess ➡ with areas of vascularity ➡ within and in adjacent soft tissues ➡. Large parts of the abscess are expectedly avascular due to tissue necrosis. Note the CCA ➡, IJV ➡. *(Right)* Corresponding coronal reformat CECT shows location and extent of right SCF abscess ➡ seen as a large, ill-defined, noncalcified, heterogeneous mass with areas of necrosis ➡ and enhancement.

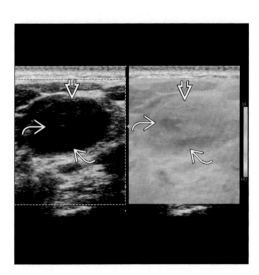

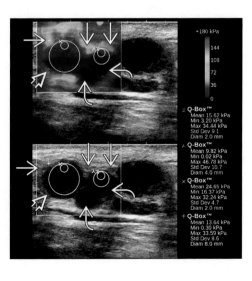

(Left) Transverse grayscale US and qualitative strain EI show a TB node ➡. Strain color scale ranges from purple (elastic, soft) to red (inelastic, hard). It has heterogeneous medium-high elasticity ➡, possibly due to necrosis and softening. *(Right)* Transverse grayscale US and SWE show necrotic TB nodes ➡. SWE color scale ranges from blue (0 kPa, soft) to red (180 kPa, stiff), displaying low SWE values (< 46 kPa) and a few dark areas lacking signal ➡. Perinodal fat is stiffer ➡, possibly due to dense matting.

HISTIOCYTIC NECROTIZING LYMPHADENITIS (KIKUCHI-FUJIMOTO DISEASE)

Key Facts

Terminology

- Synonym: Kikuchi-Fujimoto disease

Imaging

- Majority (> 80%) oval or elliptical; minority rounded
- Multiple but discrete, rarely matted with conglomerate appearance
- Most with unsharp border (67%) due to inflammatory periadenitis
- Echogenic surrounding rim is common (76%); may represent perinodal inflammatory change
- Intranodal necrosis is usually microscopic and gross intranodal necrosis is uncommon (mimics TB)
- Majority (67-87%) show preserved echogenic hilum, sometimes with ill-defined "shaggy" appearance
- Hypoechoic (100%) with hilar vascularity (83-92%)
- Overall sonographic appearances may be very similar to reactive lymphadenopathy

Top Differential Diagnoses

- Reactive lymph nodes
- Tuberculosis lymph nodes
- Non-Hodgkin lymphoma nodes
- Systemic nodal metastases

Clinical Issues

- F:M = 1-2:1
- High prevalence among Asians, particularly Japanese
- Benign, self-limiting disease with spontaneous resolution of adenopathy

Diagnostic Checklist

- Unilateral, oval/elliptical, mildly enlarged, hypoechoic, discrete (nonmatted) lymph nodes (levels II-V) in young Asian female patients
- Cytology or biopsy to confirm diagnosis if imaging features overlap with other differential diagnosis & prolonged disease course

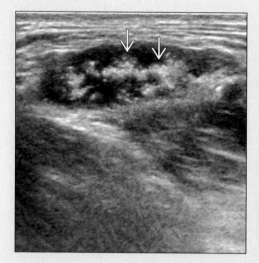
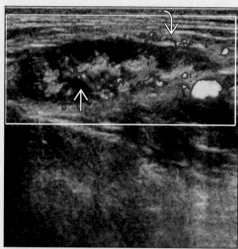

(Left) Longitudinal grayscale US shows prominent, hyperechoic shaggy-looking hilar architecture ➡ in an otherwise elliptical, solid, hypoechoic node. Such hilar architecture may be seen in histiocytic necrotizing lymphadenitis (HNL).
(Right) Corresponding power Doppler US shows sparse but predominantly hilar vascularity ➡ with no obvious peripheral vascularity. Faint vascularity adjacent to the node ➡ may be due to inflammatory periadenitis.

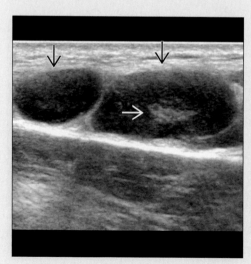
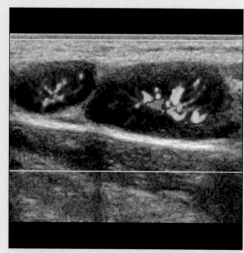

(Left) Longitudinal grayscale US in a patient with HNL shows enlarged, hypoechoic nodes ➡ with marked cortical hypertrophy. Note the presence of normal echogenic hilus ➡ in the larger node. Nodal edges appear blurred, reflecting periadenitis. *(Right)* Corresponding power Doppler image shows prominent hilar vascularity in enlarged HNL nodes. Note the absence of any peripheral vascularity in an otherwise hypertrophied, hypoechoic nodal cortex.

HISTIOCYTIC NECROTIZING LYMPHADENITIS (KIKUCHI-FUJIMOTO DISEASE)

TERMINOLOGY

Abbreviations
- Histiocytic necrotizing lymphadenitis (HNL)

Synonyms
- Kikuchi disease
- Kikuchi-Fujimoto disease

Definitions
- Necrotizing lymphadenitis with predominant histiocytic infiltration

IMAGING

General Features
- Best diagnostic clue
  - Unilateral, oval/elliptical, mildly enlarged, hypoechoic, discrete (nonmatted) lymph nodes (levels II-V) in young Asian female patient
- Location
  - Posterior triangle or internal jugular chain
    - Majority in level II and V
  - Unilateral > bilateral
- Size
  - Usually 0.5-4 cm (mean: 1.6 cm)
  - Smaller than lymphoma nodes

Ultrasonographic Findings
- Grayscale ultrasound
  - Majority (> 80%) oval or elliptical, minority rounded
    - Multiple but discrete, rarely matted with conglomerate appearance
  - Shape
    - Elliptical (short axis:long axis [S:L] ratio < 0.5) in 50-83%
    - Oval (S/L ratio 0.5-0.7) in up to 44%
    - Rounded shape is uncommon
    - Occasionally matted with conglomerate appearance
  - Border
    - Most with unsharp border (67%), due to inflammatory periadenitis
    - Echogenic surrounding rim is common (76%); may represent perinodal inflammatory change
  - Echogenicity
    - All are hypoechoic (100%)
    - Intranodal necrosis is usually microscopic and gross intranodal necrosis uncommon (may mimic tuberculosis if present)
    - Reticular pattern is rare (may mimic lymphoma)
  - Hilum
    - Majority (67-87%) show preserved echogenic hilum, sometimes with ill-defined "shaggy" appearance
  - No calcification
- Power Doppler
  - Hilar vascular pattern (83-92%)
  - Apparently avascular (7-17%) less common
  - Occasionally displaced hilar vascularity, if gross intranodal necrosis present
  - Peripheral vascular pattern not a typical feature
- Overall sonographic appearances may be very similar to reactive lymphadenopathy
- Generally distinct from metastatic lymphadenopathy

CT Findings
- CECT
  - Variable imaging appearances reported depending on degree of necrosis
    - Homogeneously enhancing solid nodes
    - Rim-enhancing centrally hypodense nodes
  - Perinodal inflammatory changes

MR Findings
- T2WI
  - Central nonenhancing necrotic-looking areas are not hyperintense
- T1WI C+ FS
  - Solidly enhancing or peripherally enhancing nodes

Nuclear Medicine Findings
- PET/CT
  - Increased FDG uptake in enlarged nodes

DIFFERENTIAL DIAGNOSIS

Reactive Lymph Nodes
- Looks similar to HNL nodes, often bilateral and symmetrical
- HNL longer clinical course

Tuberculosis Lymph Nodes
- Necrosis is early and common; displaced hilar vascularity
- Matting and collar stud abscess
- ± intranodal calcification in post-treatment nodes

Non-Hodgkin Lymphoma Nodes
- Older patient group, larger, rounder nodes
- Majority with reticular/pseudosolid pattern
- Mixed vascularity, hilar > peripheral

Systemic Nodal Metastases
- Round, solid, nodes with absent hilum, ± intranodal necrosis, ± calcification
- Peripheral vascular pattern and known primary

Cat Scratch Disease
- Regional adenopathy following scratch incident; arm > neck commonly in children and teens

PATHOLOGY

General Features
- Etiology
  - Viral or autoimmune causes speculated: Possibly exuberant T-cell-mediated immune response to several organisms or stimuli in genetically prone people
    - *Toxoplasma*, *Yersinia*, HHV-6, HHV-8, EBV, parvovirus B19 reported; all have supportive and contrary data
- Genetics
  - Higher incidence of HLA class II genes, particularly DPA*01 and DPB1*0202 alleles
  - Extremely rare in Caucasians but relatively common in Asians, which is consistent with Asian-predominant epidemiology
- Associated abnormalities

HISTIOCYTIC NECROTIZING LYMPHADENITIS (KIKUCHI-FUJIMOTO DISEASE)

- Well-reported increased incidence of systemic lupus erythematosis (SLE)
- Associated with other autoimmune disorders
  - Hashimoto, polymyositis, mixed connective tissue disease
  - Still disease, autoimmune hepatitis, antiphospholipid syndrome

Microscopic Features

- Cortical and paracortical coagulative necrosis
  - Necrosis is microscopic, not often macroscopic
- Cellular infiltrate of histiocytes and immunoblasts

CLINICAL ISSUES

Presentation

- Most common signs/symptoms
  - Acute to subacute onset tender cervical lymphadenopathy
    - ~ 90% involve posterior triangle, ~ 90% unilateral
    - Lymph node size ranges 0.5-4 cm in majority
  - 30-50% have low-grade fever
  - Upper respiratory prodrome
  - Laboratory test usually normal
    - May have leukopenia, raised ESR, serum LDH & AST
    - May have atypical peripheral blood lymphocytes
- Other signs/symptoms
  - Generalized lymphadenopathy (1-22%)
  - Weight loss, nausea, vomiting, night sweats
  - Pyrexia of unknown origin reported
  - Extranodal involvement (30-50%)
    - Skin or bone marrow involvement, hepatosplenomegaly, liver dysfunction
    - Cutaneous manifestation
      - More common in male patients
      - Wide variety of dermatological pattern ranging from rash to maculopapular eruptions
      - Mainly affecting face and upper body

Demographics

- Age
  - Young adults
  - Mean age: 25 years
- Gender
  - Female predominance in adults
    - F:M = 1-2:1
  - In children, M > F
- Epidemiology
  - High prevalence among Asians, particularly Japanese

Natural History & Prognosis

- Benign, self-limiting disease
  - Lasts 1-4 months
  - Spontaneous resolution of adenopathy
- Low recurrence rate of 3-4%
- Rarely complicated course with poor outcome
  - More frequent when extranodal involvement is present
  - Pulmonary hemorrhage, heart failure, fatal hemophagocytic syndrome

Treatment

- Symptomatic: Analgesics, antipyretics, rest

DIAGNOSTIC CHECKLIST

Consider

- Symptoms, imaging, and histology may mimic lymphoma

Image Interpretation Pearls

- Consider HNL in young female Asian patient with tender, unilateral, small to medium-sized cervical lymphadenopathy localized to level II or V
- Cytology or biopsy to confirm diagnosis if
  - Imaging features overlap with other differential diagnosis
  - Prolonged disease course

SELECTED REFERENCES

1. Ohta K et al: Axillary and intramammary lymphadenopathy caused by Kikuchi-Fujimoto disease mimicking malignant lymphoma. Breast Cancer. 20(1):97-101, 2013
2. Lo WC et al: Ultrasonographic differentiation between Kikuchi's disease and lymphoma in patients with cervical lymphadenopathy. Eur J Radiol. 81(8):1817-20, 2012
3. Yoo JL et al: Gray scale and power Doppler study of biopsy-proven Kikuchi disease. J Ultrasound Med. 30(7):957-63, 2011
4. Ito K et al: F-18 FDG PET/CT findings showing lymph node uptake in patients with Kikuchi disease. Clin Nucl Med. 34(11):821-2, 2009
5. Lee DH et al: Disseminated Kikuchi-Fujimoto disease mimicking malignant lymphoma on positron emission tomography in a child. J Pediatr Hematol Oncol. 31(9):687-9, 2009
6. Nomura Y et al: Phenotype for activated tissue macrophages in histiocytic necrotizing lymphadenitis. Pathol Int. 59(9):631-5, 2009
7. Pilichowska ME et al: Histiocytic necrotizing lymphadenitis (Kikuchi-Fujimoto disease): lesional cells exhibit an immature dendritic cell phenotype. Am J Clin Pathol. 131(2):174-82, 2009
8. Chase SP et al: Cervical lymphadenopathy secondary to Kikuchi-Fujimoto disease in a child: case report. Ear Nose Throat J. 87(6):350-3, 2008
9. Kaicker S et al: PET-CT scan in a patient with Kikuchi disease. Pediatr Radiol. 38(5):596-7, 2008
10. Kampitak T: Fatal Kikuchi-Fujimoto disease associated with SLE and hemophagocytic syndrome: a case report. Clin Rheumatol. 27(8):1073-5, 2008
11. Pace-Asciak P et al: Case Series: raising awareness about Kikuchi-Fujimoto disease among otolaryngologists: is it linked to systemic lupus erythematosus? J Otolaryngol Head Neck Surg. 37(6):782-7, 2008
12. Papla B et al: Histiocytic necrotizing lymphadenitis without granulocytic infiltration (the so called Kikuchi-Fujimoto disease). Pol J Pathol. 59(1):55-61, 2008
13. Youk JH et al: Sonographic features of axillary lymphadenopathy caused by Kikuchi disease. J Ultrasound Med. 27(6):847-53, 2008
14. Bosch X et al: Enigmatic Kikuchi-Fujimoto disease: a comprehensive review. Am J Clin Pathol. 122(1):141-52, 2004
15. Kwon SY et al: CT findings in Kikuchi disease: analysis of 96 cases. AJNR Am J Neuroradiol. 25(6):1099-102, 2004
16. Ying M et al: Grey-scale and power Doppler sonography of unusual cervical lymphadenopathy. Ultrasound Med Biol. 30(4):449-54, 2004
17. Na DG et al: Kikuchi disease: CT and MR findings. AJNR Am J Neuroradiol. 18(9):1729-32, 1997

HISTIOCYTIC NECROTIZING LYMPHADENITIS (KIKUCHI-FUJIMOTO DISEASE)

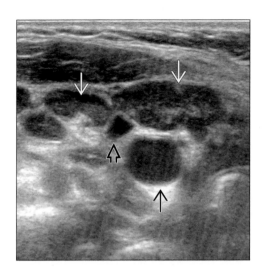
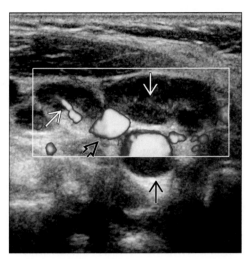

(Left) Axial grayscale US in a patient with HNL shows multiple, solid, hypoechoic nodes ➡ in the upper cervical area. Enlarged nodes maintain their normal hilar architecture. Despite their multiplicity, there is no associated matting or adjacent soft tissue edema. Note the CCA ⇨ and IJV ⬦. *(Right)* Corresponding power Doppler US shows hilar vascularity ➡ with no evidence of intranodal peripheral vascularity. Overall US features mimic reactive nodes. Note the CCA ⇨ and IJV ⬦.

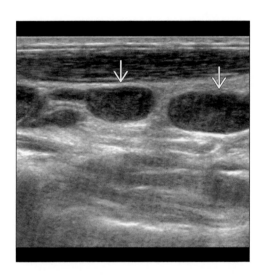
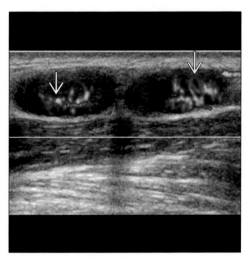

(Left) Longitudinal grayscale US in a patient with HNL shows a chain of nodes ➡ in the posterior triangle. Their location is similar to the distribution of TB nodes, but there is no obvious intranodal necrosis, matting, or soft tissue edema. Overall US features mimic reactive nodes, and diagnosis of HNL is suggested in combination with clinical features and patient's sex and ethnicity. Cytology may be required to confirm the diagnosis. *(Right)* Corresponding power Doppler US shows prominent hilar vascularity ➡.

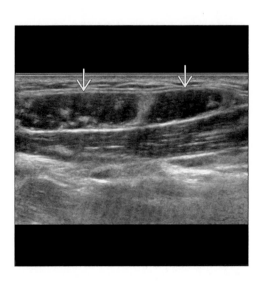
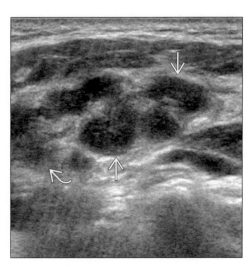

(Left) Longitudinal grayscale US in a patient with HNL shows multiple, elliptical hypoechoic nodes ➡ with "shaggy" hilar architecture. Note normal adjacent soft tissues. *(Right)* Grayscale US in a patient with tuberculous adenitis shows multiple, hypoechoic, heterogeneous nodes ➡ in the posterior triangle. Note associated nodal matting/clumping and soft tissue edema ➡, features of tuberculous lymphadenitis. Compare this with normal soft tissues and discrete nodes in HNL.

SQUAMOUS CELL CARCINOMA NODES

Key Facts

Imaging

- New neck mass in adult patient with head and neck (H&N) squamous cell carcinoma (SCCa) should raise suspicion of malignant node
- In patients with known H&N SCCa, ↑ in nodal size on serial examination is highly suggestive of metastatic involvement
- Metastatic nodes are commonly round
- Malignant nodes tend to have sharp borders
- In a proven metastatic node, presence of an unsharp nodal border suggests extracapsular spread
- Loss of normal echogenic hilar architecture (69-95%)
- Metastatic nodes from H&N SCCa are hypoechoic, compared to adjacent muscle
- Calcification is rare
- Intranodal cystic necrosis is commonly found
- Color Doppler: May have both peripheral and mixed (hilar & peripheral) vascularity

- Presence of peripheral vascularity regardless of hilar vascularity is highly suggestive of metastases
- US cannot evaluate primary tumor site, retropharyngeal and mediastinal nodes

Top Differential Diagnoses

- Non-Hodgkin lymphoma nodes
- Neoplastic nodes from papillary thyroid cancer
- Tuberculous nodes

Clinical Issues

- Nodal metastasis is single most important prognostic factor for H&N SCCa
- Single unilateral node reduces prognosis by 50%; bilateral nodes reduce prognosis by 75%
- Presence of extranodal spread reduces prognosis by further 50%; risk of recurrence ↑ 10x
- Carotid artery encasement: ~ 100% mortality

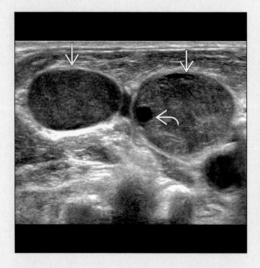
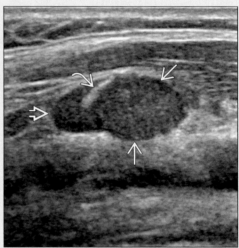

(Left) Transverse grayscale US shows typical metastatic squamous cell carcinoma (SCCa) nodes ➡. They are round, predominantly solid, well defined, and hypoechoic with loss of normal hilar architecture. A tiny area of cystic necrosis is seen in 1 node ➡. *(Right)* Longitudinal grayscale US shows a metastatic SCCa node ➡. Note that it maintains a reniform shape and its hilar ➡ architecture. However, there is focal tumor deposition ➡ causing eccentric cortical hypertrophy, a feature of an abnormal node.

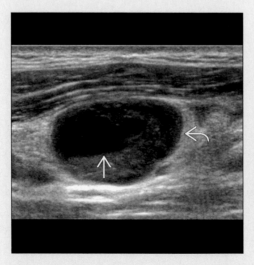
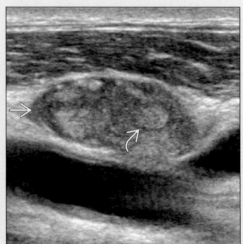

(Left) Longitudinal grayscale US shows a metastatic SCCa node ➡ with intranodal cystic necrosis ➡, which is pathological irrespective of nodal size. It is seen in metastatic SCCa nodes, metastatic nodes from thyroid papillary cancer, and in tuberculous nodes. *(Right)* Longitudinal grayscale US shows a metastatic SCCa node ➡ with coagulation necrosis ➡, appearing as an ill-defined hyperechoic area within the node. Unlike nodal hilus, these hyperechoic areas are not continuous with surrounding soft tissue.

SQUAMOUS CELL CARCINOMA NODES

TERMINOLOGY

Abbreviations
- Squamous cell carcinoma (SCCa) nodes

Synonyms
- SCCa nodal metastases

IMAGING

General Features
- Best diagnostic clue
  - Round, hypoechoic, heterogeneous node in expected nodal drainage level(s) of primary H&N SCCa
  - New neck mass in adult patient with H&N SCCa should raise suspicion of malignant node
- Location
  - Levels I-VI of neck, retropharyngeal, and parotid space
  - Level IIA (jugulodigastric group) is most frequently involved nodal group
- Size
  - Size alone cannot be used as absolute criteria as inflammatory nodes may be large and malignancy may be found in small nodes
    - In patients with known H&N SCCa, an increase in nodal size on serial examination is highly suggestive of metastatic involvement
- Morphology
  - Rounded contour
    - Loss of hilar architecture, eccentric cortical hypertrophy and peripheral vessels suggest malignant node
  - Intranodal cystic/coagulation necrosis is often seen in metastases from H&N SCCa
  - Extranodal spread suggested by indistinct nodal margins, infiltration of adjacent fat ± invasion of adjacent structures

Ultrasonographic Findings
- Metastatic nodes are commonly round
  - However, if there is focal intranodal tumor deposition, node may show eccentric cortical hypertrophy
- Malignant nodes tend to have sharp borders
  - Tumor deposition in nodes results in greater difference in acoustic impedance between node and surrounding soft tissues leading to sharp nodal border
  - In a proven metastatic node, presence of an unsharp nodal border suggests extracapsular spread
- Loss of normal echogenic hilar architecture (69-95%)
- Metastatic nodes from H&N SCCa are hypoechoic, compared with adjacent muscle
  - Metastatic nodes from thyroid papillary carcinoma tend to be hyperechoic to adjacent muscle
- Calcification in metastatic H&N SCCa nodes is rare
  - Calcification is common in metastatic nodes from thyroid papillary and medullary carcinoma
- Intranodal cystic necrosis is commonly found in metastatic nodes from H&N SCCa
  - Intranodal coagulation necrosis (seen as echogenic area) may be found in both malignant and inflammatory nodes
- Color Doppler: Metastatic nodes may have both peripheral or mixed (hilar & peripheral) vascularity
  - Presence of peripheral vascularity regardless of hilar vascularity is highly suggestive of metastases
- Spectral Doppler: High intranodal vascular resistance (resistive index [RI] > 0.8, pulsatility index [PI] > 1.6)
  - Evaluation of intranodal vascular resistance is time consuming and not routinely indicated

Imaging Recommendations
- Best imaging tool
  - US is ideal imaging modality to screen neck nodes below angle of mandible and is readily combined with guided FNAC
  - US is unable to evaluate primary tumor site
    - Does not evaluate retropharyngeal and mediastinal nodes
  - Either CECT or MR stage primary tumor and nodes simultaneously

DIFFERENTIAL DIAGNOSIS

Non-Hodgkin Lymphoma Nodes
- Multiple, round, hypoechoic, well defined, pseudocystic, or reticulated echo pattern
- Marked hilar and peripheral vascularity

Neoplastic Nodes From Papillary Thyroid Cancer
- Hyperechoic, solid/cystic, punctate calcification, & peripheral vascularity

Tuberculous Nodes
- Multiple, hypoechoic, heterogeneous nodes with intranodal necrosis, nodal matting, soft tissue edema, avascular or displaced hilar vessels

2nd Branchial Cleft Cyst
- Anechoic, ± pseudosolid pattern, thin/thick walls with faint internal debris, ± septa & characteristic location in neck

CLINICAL ISSUES

Presentation
- Most common signs/symptoms
  - Painless, firm neck mass, may be fixed to adjacent tissues, especially if large
  - Neck mass (enlarged node) may be presenting feature of H&N SCCa

Demographics
- Epidemiology
  - Presence of nodal metastasis at time of diagnosis varies by primary tumor site
    - Nasopharyngeal most often (~ 85%), laryngeal (glottic) primary least often (< 10%)

Natural History & Prognosis
- Nodal metastasis is single most important prognostic factor for H&N SCCa
  - Single unilateral node reduces prognosis by 50%; bilateral nodes reduce prognosis by 75%
  - Presence of extranodal spread reduces prognosis by further 50%; risk of recurrence ↑ 10x
- Carotid artery encasement: ~ 100% mortality

SELECTED REFERENCES

1. Ahuja AT et al: Ultrasound of malignant cervical lymph nodes. Cancer Imaging. 8:48-56, 2008

SQUAMOUS CELL CARCINOMA NODES

(Left) Transverse grayscale US shows metastatic SCCa node ⇨ with irregular borders ⇨, suggesting extracapsular spread. Metastatic nodes have sharp borders due to the sharp, attenuating interface between malignant tissue & surrounding soft tissue. Inflammatory nodes excite periadenitis and have irregular borders. (Right) Transverse grayscale US shows a metastatic SCCa node ⇨ with ill-defined edge ⇨, suggestive of extracapsular spread, a sign of poor prognosis. Note CCA ⇨ and IJV ⇨.

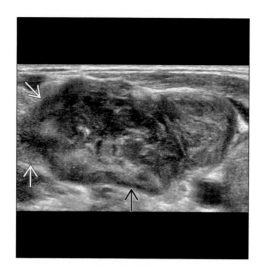
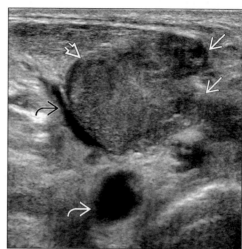

(Left) Transverse grayscale US in a patient with a metastatic SCCa node ⇨ shows a metastatic node with ill-defined borders suggesting extracapsular spread. Note its relation to the carotid sheath containing the CCA ⇨ and vagus nerve ⇨. Normal IJV is not seen. (Right) Corresponding longitudinal grayscale US shows long-segment thrombus ⇨ in the IJV ⇨, obliterating its lumen. Thrombosis may be due to tumor invasion or venous stasis. Presence of thrombus vascularity on Doppler suggests tumor thrombus.

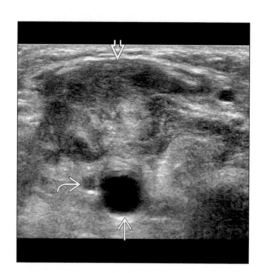
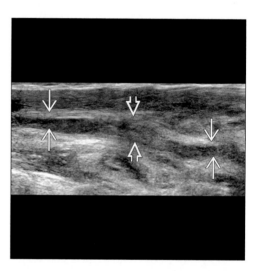

(Left) Transverse power Doppler US shows a metastatic SCCa node ⇨ with markedly chaotic intranodal vascularity (hilar and peripheral), a hallmark of an abnormal node. (Right) Longitudinal grayscale US shows metastatic SCCa nodes with a rim of typical peripheral vascularity ⇨, commonly found in metastatic nodes and thought to be due to angiogenesis recruiting peripheral vessels into lymph nodes. Benign nodes tend to have central, hilar vascularity.

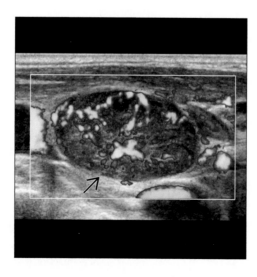
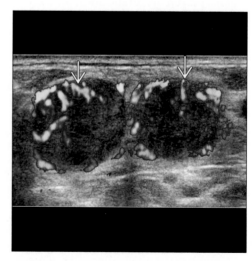

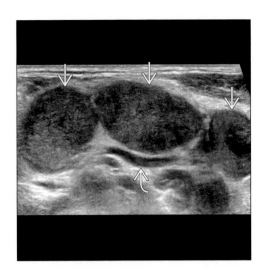

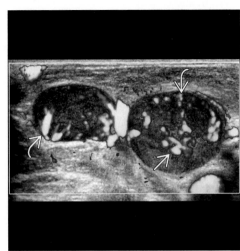

(Left) Transverse grayscale US shows metastatic nodes ➜ in a patient with H&N SCCa. Note IJV ➜. (Right) Corresponding power Doppler US shows typical abnormal intranodal vascularity, hilar ➜ & peripheral ➜. Combination of grayscale features (round shape, absent hilum, intranodal necrosis) and peripheral vascularity is highly accurate in distinguishing benign from malignant nodes in neck. Features are easily assessed by US, and guided FNAC readily confirms diagnosis.

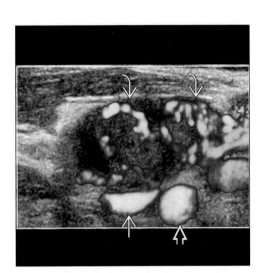

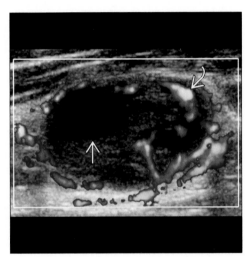

(Left) Transverse power Doppler US shows marked abnormal vascularity in metastatic SCCa nodes ➜. Note CCA ➜, IJV ➜. (Right) Longitudinal power Doppler US shows metastatic SCCa node with focal area of cystic necrosis ➜ and abnormal peripheral vascularity ➜. Although malignant nodes have high intranodal vascular resistance (RI > 0.8 & PI > 1.6), these indices are not usually measured in routine clinical practice. Distribution of intranodal vessels is most commonly investigated and will usually suffice.

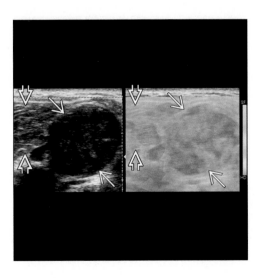

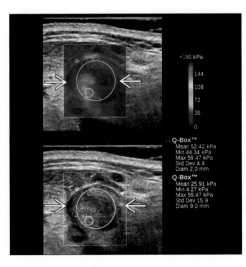

(Left) Transverse grayscale US and qualitative strain EI show an SSCa node ➜. Strain color scale ranges from purple (elastic, soft) to red (inelastic, hard). It appears heterogeneous and mostly inelastic relative to adjacent tissues. Note the sternocleidomastoid muscle ➜. (Right) Transverse grayscale US & SWE show SCCa node ➜. SWE color scale ranges from blue (0 kPa, soft) to red (180 kPa, stiff). It appears heterogeneous dark and light blue with maximum SWE value of 59.5 kPa; higher than normal reactive nodes.

NODAL DIFFERENTIATED THYROID CARCINOMA

Key Facts

Imaging

- Location: Most often levels VI, III, and IV
- PTCa: 80% hyperechoic to muscle (vs. hypoechoic in MTCa); FTCa: Hypoechoic
- Cystic necrosis is common (in 25%) in PTCa, nodal metastases; occasionally, these nodes may be entirely cystic/septate
- PTCa: Punctate calcification with fine acoustic shadow (50%); represents psammoma bodies
  - MTCa: Microcalcification mimics PTCa, more often dense and coarse with acoustic shadow; represents amyloid and associated calcification
- Chaotic/disorganized intranodal vascularity, peripheral vascularity
- NECT: Preferred over CECT, as iodinated contrast delays I-131 radioablation
- MR: Nodes heterogeneous in size and signal; variable T1 intensity on MR

- FDG PET: Best for recurrence when ↑ thyroglobulin with negative iodide scan
- I-123 & I-131 scans show low sensitivity, high specificity

Top Differential Diagnoses

- Nodal SCCa, tuberculosis, and non-Hodgkin lymphoma

Clinical Issues

- Papillary = 80-90% of all thyroid malignancies
- Follicular = 5% of thyroid malignancies
- PTCa: > 50% nodal metastasis at presentation
- 21-65% of primary or recurrent PTCa (& MTCa) metastasize to ipsilateral central and lateral compartments before contralateral neck and mediastinum
- Nodes more likely with larger primary
- Up to 64% of patients have primary tumor < 1 cm

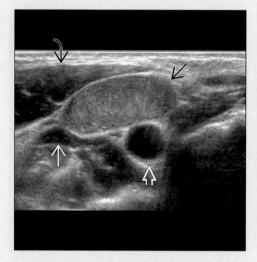
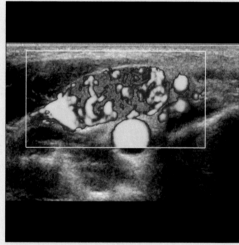

(Left) Transverse grayscale US shows a typical metastatic node ⇥ from PTCa. It is solid, hyperechoic (vs. sternomastoid muscle ⇥), well defined, homogeneous, and located along the CCA ⇥ and compressed IJV ⇥. *(Right)* Corresponding power Doppler US shows markedly chaotic/disorganized intranodal vascularity. In the absence of a known primary, presence of such a bright, vascular, abnormal node should prompt a search for ipsilateral thyroid papillary cancer. In some cases, primary PTCa may be small or occult.

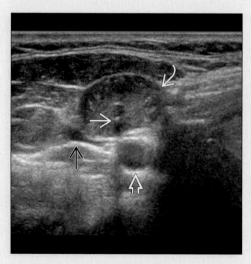
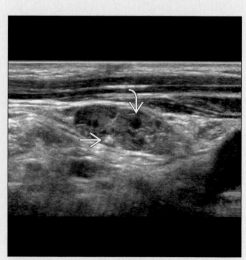

(Left) Transverse grayscale US in a patient with known PTCa shows a round, heterogeneous, hyperechoic node ⇥ with loss of echogenic hilum and characteristic punctate calcification ⇥ with fine posterior acoustic shadowing. Note CCA ⇥ and compressed IJV ⇥. *(Right)* Longitudinal grayscale US of metastatic node shows hyperechogenicity, fine echogenic calcification ⇥, and multiple small areas of intranodal necrosis ⇥. These features are characteristic of nodal metastases from PTCa.

NODAL DIFFERENTIATED THYROID CARCINOMA

TERMINOLOGY

Abbreviations
- Differentiated thyroid carcinoma (DTCa)

Definitions
- Metastatic node(s) from papillary or follicular thyroid carcinoma

IMAGING

General Features
- Best diagnostic clue
  - Papillary thyroid carcinoma (PTCa): Hyperechoic > hypoechoic nodes with punctate calcification ± cystic necrosis and peripheral/chaotic vascularity
  - Medullary thyroid carcinoma (MTCa): Hypoechoic nodes with coarse or microcalcification and peripheral/chaotic vascularity
  - Follicular thyroid carcinoma (FTCa): Solid, hypoechoic, noncalcified, homogeneous nodes with peripheral vascularity
- Location
  - Anywhere in neck; most often levels VI, III, and IV
- Size
  - Variable between patients and in single patient
    - Nodes may be 2-3 cm, but commonly < 1 cm

Ultrasonographic Findings
- Grayscale ultrasound
  - Size
    - Generally, cervical lymph nodes with short axis diameter (SAD) > 1 cm are regarded as abnormal
      - However, many metastatic DTCa nodes are < 1 cm in SAD, and normal submandibular and jugulodigastric nodes may be > 1 cm
    - Size of lymph node alone cannot be used as independent predictor of malignancy
    - At site of expected drainage, cut-off for abnormal nodes is lowered (> 4 mm SAD)
  - Shape
    - Round (short:long axis ratio [S:L ratio] > 0.5) more than oval (S:L ratio < 0.5)
  - Border
    - Most are well defined (due to sharp attenuating interface between malignant tissue and surrounding soft tissue)
    - Ill-defined border indicates extracapsular spread
    - Invasion of surrounding structures invariably represents extracapsular spread
  - Echogenic hilus
    - Typically loss of echogenic hilus
    - In case of early metastatic disease, before invasion of medullary sinus, echogenic hilus may be preserved
  - Echogenicity
    - PTCa: 80% hyperechoic to muscle (vs. hypoechoic in MTCa)
    - FTCa: Hypoechoic
  - Necrosis
    - Cystic necrosis is common (in 25%) in PTCa nodal metastases, and occasionally these nodes may be entirely cystic/septated
  - Calcification
    - PTCa: Punctate calcification with fine acoustic shadow (50%); represents psammoma bodies

- MTCa: Microcalcification may mimic PTCa, but more often calcification is dense and coarse with strong acoustic shadow; represents amyloid and associated calcification
- Power Doppler
  - In case of early metastasis before invasion of medullary sinus, hilar vessels may be preserved
  - Chaotic/disorganized intranodal vascularity, peripheral vascularity
- Although intranodal necrosis, calcification, and peripheral vascularity are independent predictors, sonographic features should be used in combination

CT Findings
- Overall sensitivity poor as metastases often small
- NECT: Nodes heterogeneous: Solid, cystic, calcified
- CECT: Variable enhancement: Minimal to marked

MR Findings
- T1WI
  - Variable signal intensity
  - Frequently bright from thyroglobulin or colloid
- T2WI
  - Variable, most often hyperintense
  - Cystic nodes may have fluid-fluid levels

Nuclear Medicine Findings
- PET/CT
  - Not useful for differentiated thyroid carcinoma
  - Best for nodal recurrence when ↑ thyroglobulin with negative iodide scan
- I-123 and I-131 scans
  - Focal uptake in metastatic nodes
  - Poor sensitivity, near 100% specificity

Imaging Recommendations
- Best imaging tool
  - US-guided biopsy
    - Improves diagnostic sensitivity to 89-98%, specificity to 95-98%, and accuracy to 95-97%
    - Needle tip should be targeted toward abnormal areas, including calcification, solid component in a cystic lymph node, and eccentric cortical hypertrophy
  - US with guided FNA is ideal for detecting malignant cervical nodal metastasis in H&N cancer patients
    - Superior to CT & MR in detecting and characterizing small thyroid primary
  - MR/CT is superior in demonstrating deep tissue (retrotracheal) extension, retropharyngeal and mediastinal lymphadenopathy
- Protocol advice
  - CECT should be avoided because iodinated contrast delays I-131 radioablation

DIFFERENTIAL DIAGNOSIS

Nodal Squamous Cell Carcinoma
- Hypoechoic, solid; cystic necrosis common
- Calcification is rare
- T1 MR iso- to low intensity unless aspiration hematoma

Nodal Tuberculosis
- Necrosis is common; cystic or coagulative
- Matting early → "collar stud" abscess
- Inflammatory changes around node(s)

NODAL DIFFERENTIATED THYROID CARCINOMA

- ± calcification in post-treatment node

Nodal Non-Hodgkin Lymphoma

- Usually multiple, large, hypoechoic nodes with reticulated/pseudosolid pattern
- Intranodal necrosis is uncommon
- ± calcification in post-treatment node

Systemic Nodal Metastases

- Small, round, solid hypoechoic nodes in SCF, low posterior triangle
- Adenocarcinoma metastases may have calcifications

PATHOLOGY

General Features

- Etiology
  - Metastatic disease from DTCa

Microscopic Features

- Papillary
  - Formation of papillae with "orphan Annie eye" nuclei
  - Psammomatous calcifications common (vs. MTCa; stroma has amyloid deposits from calcitonin, coarse calcifications)
- Follicular
  - Look like follicular adenomas but capsule invasion

Staging, Grading, & Classification

- < 45 years: Nodal disease does not alter staging
- > 45 years: Higher locoregional recurrence
  - N1a = level VI
  - N1b = I-V, retropharynx or superior mediastinum

CLINICAL ISSUES

Presentation

- Most common signs/symptoms
  - May present as slow-growing nodal mass

Demographics

- Age
  - Most patients 25-65 years
- Gender
  - F > M
- Epidemiology
  - Papillary: 80-90% of all thyroid malignancies
  - Follicular: 5% of all thyroid malignancies
  - PTCa: > 50% nodal metastasis at presentation
    - 21-65% of primary or recurrent PTCa (and MTCa) metastasize to ipsilateral central and lateral compartments before contralateral neck and mediastinum
    - Nodes more likely with larger primary
    - Up to 64% of patients have primary tumor < 1 cm

Natural History & Prognosis

- Nodes prognostically significant only in patients > 45 years old

Treatment

- Surgical and oncological literature debates management of cervical metastases
- If nodes are palpable, many advocate selective dissection (levels II-VI) with thyroidectomy

DIAGNOSTIC CHECKLIST

Image Interpretation Pearls

- Metastatic lymphadenopathy from DTCa involves level VI, III, and IV, a distribution that differs from suprahyoid and infraclavicular primary
  - Presence of suspicious nodes at these sites should prompt exclusion of malignant thyroid primary
- Characteristic features of PTCa lymphadenopathy (hyperechoic, microcalcification ± cystic necrosis) should alert sonologist to carefully search thyroid for PTCA, sonographically positive or occult
  - US-guided FNA should be performed for cytological confirmation

SELECTED REFERENCES

1. Lee YYP et al: Ultrasound in head and neck cancer. In Glastonbury CM et al: Head and Neck Cancer: State of the Art Diagnosis, Staging, and Surveillance. Specialty Imaging. Philadelphia: Lippincott Williams & Wilkins, 1-18-25, 2012
2. Lim YC et al: Occult lymph node metastases in neck level V in papillary thyroid carcinoma. Surgery. 147(2):241-5, 2010
3. Kaplan SL et al: The role of MR imaging in detecting nodal disease in thyroidectomy patients with rising thyroglobulin levels. AJNR Am J Neuroradiol. 30(3):608-12, 2009
4. Roh JL et al: Use of preoperative ultrasonography as guidance for neck dissection in patients with papillary thyroid carcinoma. J Surg Oncol. 99(1):28-31, 2009
5. Ahuja AT et al: Ultrasound of malignant cervical lymph nodes. Cancer Imaging. 8:48-56, 2008
6. Roh JL et al: Central cervical nodal metastasis from papillary thyroid microcarcinoma: pattern and factors predictive of nodal metastasis. Ann Surg Oncol. 15(9):2482-6, 2008
7. Soler ZM et al: Utility of computed tomography in the detection of subclinical nodal disease in papillary thyroid carcinoma. Arch Otolaryngol Head Neck Surg. 134(9):973-8, 2008
8. Sugitani I et al: Prospective outcomes of selective lymph node dissection for papillary thyroid carcinoma based on preoperative ultrasonography. World J Surg. 32(11):2494-502, 2008
9. Yanir Y et al: Regional metastases in well-differentiated thyroid carcinoma: pattern of spread. Laryngoscope. 118(3):433-6, 2008
10. de Bondt RB et al: Detection of lymph node metastases in head and neck cancer: a meta-analysis comparing US, USgFNAC, CT and MR imaging. Eur J Radiol. 64(2):266-72, 2007
11. Leboulleux S et al: Ultrasound criteria of malignancy for cervical lymph nodes in patients followed up for differentiated thyroid cancer. J Clin Endocrinol Metab. 92(9):3590-4, 2007
12. Wong KT et al: Ultrasound of thyroid cancer. Cancer Imaging. 5:157-66, 2005
13. Ahuja AT et al: Metastatic cervical nodes in papillary carcinoma of the thyroid: ultrasound and histological correlation. Clin Radiol. 50(4):229-31, 1995
14. Evans RM et al: The linear echogenic hilus in cervical lymphadenopathy--a sign of benignity or malignancy? Clin Radiol. 47(4):262-4, 1993
15. van den Brekel MW et al: Lymph node staging in patients with clinically negative neck examinations by ultrasound and ultrasound-guided aspiration cytology. Am J Surg. 162(4):362-6, 1991
16. Tohnosu N et al: Ultrasonographic evaluation of cervical lymph node metastases in esophageal cancer with special reference to the relationship between the short to long axis ratio (S/L) and the cancer content. J Clin Ultrasound. 17(2):101-6, 1989

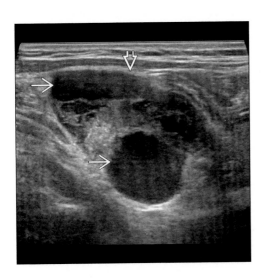

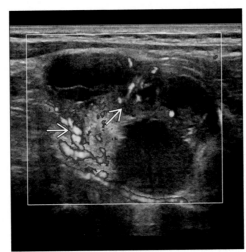

(Left) Transverse grayscale US shows a metastatic node ➡ from PTCa. Note the large areas of intranodal necrosis ➡. (Right) Corresponding power Doppler US shows marked vascularity within the solid component of the node ➡. US-guided FNA should be targeted toward solid portion (with vascularity) to ↑ diagnostic yield. In metastatic PTCa, nodes that are completely cystic, fluid aspirated from completely cystic PTCa nodes can be sent for thyroglobulin estimation, which also helps in predicting diagnosis.

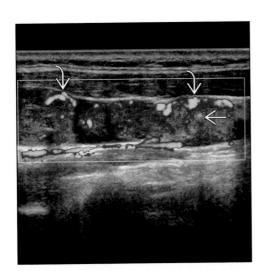

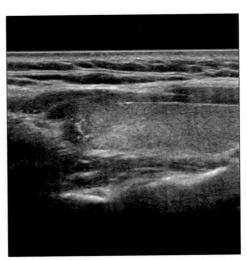

(Left) Longitudinal power Doppler US shows multiple malignant-looking nodes in the lower jugular chain. Disorganized vascularity ➡ and characteristic punctate calcification ➡ are typical of metastatic nodes from PTCa. (Right) Corresponding longitudinal grayscale US reveals a 5 mm nodule with characteristic sonographic features of primary PTCa in the ipsilateral thyroid (ill-defined, punctate echogenic foci). Thyroid primary may be small or occult and FNAC may be nondiagnostic in small lesions.

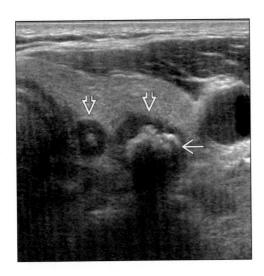

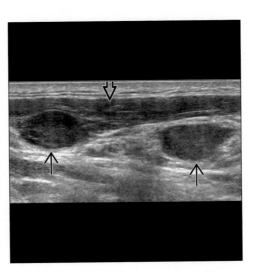

(Left) Axial grayscale US shows well-defined, solid, hypoechoic nodules ➡ in the left lobe of a thyroid with central dense shadowing calcification in a larger nodule ➡. These were confirmed to be MTCa. (Right) Corresponding longitudinal grayscale US (same patient) shows multiple, solid nodes ➡ with loss of echogenic hilum, consistent with metastasis from MTCa. Note hypoechoic appearance (compared to sternomastoid muscle ➡), as opposed to lymphadenopathy from PTCa.

SYSTEMIC METASTASES IN NECK NODES

Key Facts

Terminology
- Cervical metastatic adenopathy from systemic, particularly infraclavicular, primary tumor

Imaging
- Deep cervical, transverse cervical (supraclavicular), and spinal accessory nodes most commonly involved
- Nodes are generally clustered toward lower neck, especially on left as thoracic duct empties on left
- Solid, hypoechoic, well-defined node with loss of normal echogenic hilum
- Eccentric cortical hypertrophy may be seen
- Intranodal coagulation/cystic necrosis
- Internal cystic or hyperechoic areas within enlarged node
- Color Doppler: Peripheral, or hilar & peripheral, vascularity
- Spectral Doppler: High intranodal vascular resistance (resistive index [RI] > 0.8, pulsatility index [PI] > 1.6)

- If a node is confirmed as malignant on FNAC & has ill-defined borders, it suggests extracapsular spread
- Do not mistake neck nodes for brachial plexus elements, which may be prominent in post-radiation neck
- Irrespective of size/number, any solid, round, hypoechoic node with abnormal architecture & vascularity, located in lower neck, in a patient with known systemic malignancy, is considered metastatic unless proven otherwise

Top Differential Diagnoses
- Reactive adenopathy
- Metastatic adenopathy, head & neck primary squamous cell carcinoma
- Non-Hodgkin lymphoma, nodal

Clinical Issues
- Disseminated disease associated with poor prognosis

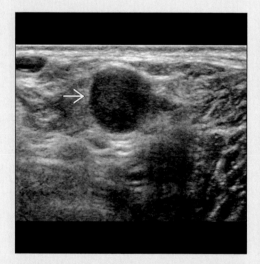
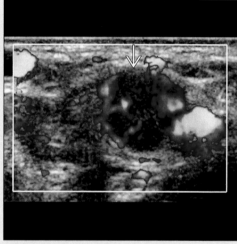

(Left) Transverse grayscale US shows a solid, solitary, round, hypoechoic node with absent hilar architecture in left supraclavicular fossa (SCF). US features are suggestive of a metastatic node ➡. Location of a solitary node in the SCF suggests an infraclavicular primary tumor. *(Right)* Corresponding power Doppler US shows abnormal vascularity within the node ➡, consistent with metastasis. It may not always be possible to evaluate intranodal vascularity at this site due to pulsations from adjacent major vessels.

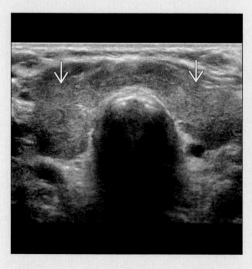
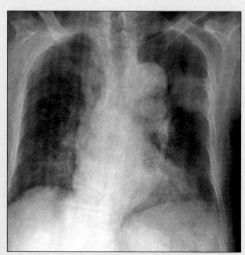

(Left) Transverse grayscale US of thyroid gland (same patient) shows a hypoechoic parenchymal echo pattern ➡ but no significant enlargement or focal nodule. In view of associated malignant-looking nodes this was considered suspicious for thyroid metastases and FNAC confirmed diagnosis. *(Right)* Corresponding chest x-ray shows a large mass in the left upper lobe and guided biopsy confirmed primary carcinoma of the lung, a common malignancy to metastasize to the SCF.

SYSTEMIC METASTASES IN NECK NODES

TERMINOLOGY

Definitions
- Cervical metastatic adenopathy from systemic, particularly infraclavicular, primary tumor
- Virchow node is left supraclavicular nodal metastases
  - Usually abdominal or pelvic primary malignancy

IMAGING

General Features
- Best diagnostic clue
  - Enlarged ± necrotic cervical lymph node or nodal cluster in patient with systemic malignancy
- Location
  - Deep cervical, transverse cervical (supraclavicular), and spinal accessory nodes most commonly involved
  - Most often lower neck (infrahyoid)
  - Frequently unilateral
- Size
  - Variable sizes, often > 1.5 cm
  - May form conglomerate mass > 5-6 cm

Ultrasonographic Findings
- Solid, hypoechoic, well-defined node with loss of normal echogenic hilum
- Eccentric cortical hypertrophy may be seen
- Intranodal coagulation/cystic necrosis
  - Internal cystic or hyperechoic areas within enlarged node
- Color Doppler: Peripheral, or hilar & peripheral, vascularity
- Spectral Doppler: High intranodal vascular resistance (resistive index [RI] > 0.8, pulsatility index [PI] > 1.6)

CT Findings
- CECT
  - Size: > 1.5 cm, especially if node is round, suggests metastatic node
  - Enhancement pattern variable; homogeneous, peripheral enhancement seen
  - Nodes generally clustered toward lower neck, especially on left as thoracic duct empties on left

MR Findings
- T1WI
  - Cervical nodal mass usually isointense to muscle
- T2WI
  - Nodes slightly hyperintense compared to muscle
- T1WI C+
  - Minimal/mild enhancement common; peripherally when nodes necrotic

Imaging Recommendations
- Best imaging tool
  - US is ideal imaging modality as it evaluates most commonly involved part of neck and readily combines with guided FNAC
  - If node is confirmed as malignant on FNAC and has ill-defined borders, it suggests extracapsular spread
- Protocol advice
  - Do not mistake neck nodes for brachial plexus elements, which may be prominent in post-radiation neck

- Irrespective of size/number, any solid, round, hypoechoic node with abnormal architecture and vascularity, located in lower neck, in patient with known systemic malignancy, is considered metastatic unless proven otherwise

DIFFERENTIAL DIAGNOSIS

Reactive Adenopathy
- Elliptical, solid, hypoechoic node with echogenic hilus and hilar vascularity

Metastatic Adenopathy, Head & Neck Primary Squamous Cell Carcinoma
- Round, hypoechoic, cystic necrosis, absent hilum and presence of peripheral vascularity

Nodal Non-Hodgkin Lymphoma
- Large, round, solid hypoechoic node with reticulated or pseudosolid pattern, hilar > peripheral vascularity

PATHOLOGY

General Features
- Etiology
  - Represents disseminated malignancy
  - Systemic malignancy sites that more commonly create cervical neck metastatic nodes
    - Melanoma, esophagus, breast or lung carcinoma; occasionally unknown primary

CLINICAL ISSUES

Presentation
- Most common signs/symptoms
  - Low cervical neck mass in patient with known systemic malignancy

Demographics
- Epidemiology
  - Metastatic nodes from head and neck (H&N) primary more common than nodes from systemic malignancy

Natural History & Prognosis
- Disseminated disease associated with poor prognosis

Treatment
- If cervical node is only metastatic disease, selective neck dissection may be performed
- Otherwise chemotherapy ± XRT

DIAGNOSTIC CHECKLIST

Consider
- Cervical nodal metastases if patient with known primary presents with new infrahyoid neck mass
- If infrahyoid/supraclavicular nodal metastasis, suspect systemic or intraabdominal primary
- When nodes are calcified, suspect thyroid carcinoma or systemic adenocarcinoma

SELECTED REFERENCES

1. Ahuja AT et al: Sonographic evaluation of cervical lymph nodes. AJR Am J Roentgenol. 184(5):1691-9, 2005

SYSTEMIC METASTASES IN NECK NODES

(Left) Transverse grayscale US shows 2 predominantly solid, round, heterogeneous, hypoechoic nodes ➡ with absent hilar architecture in the right lower neck, adjacent to the CCA ⬧➤ and IJV ➤. No other abnormal looking neck nodes were detected. *(Right)* Corresponding power Doppler US on the larger node shows abnormal intranodular vascularity, consistent with metastatic node. Patient had known history of primary breast carcinoma and FNAC confirmed metastatic nodes in lower neck.

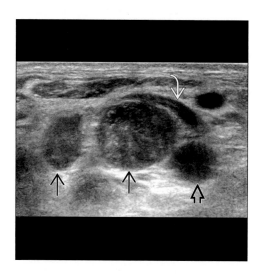
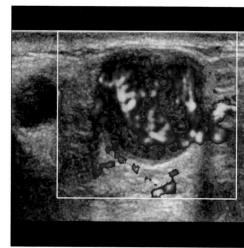

(Left) Transverse grayscale US of a patient with known primary carcinoma of colon shows a solitary large node ➡ in the left lower neck/ SCF in proximity to the CCA ⬧➤ and IJV ➤. It is solid, hypoechoic, well-defined, and noncalcified with absent hilar architecture, suggestive of a metastatic node. *(Right)* Corresponding power Doppler US shows abnormal intranodal vascularity ➡. At this site, pulsations from major vessels produce artifacts and limit the quality/ reliability of Doppler US.

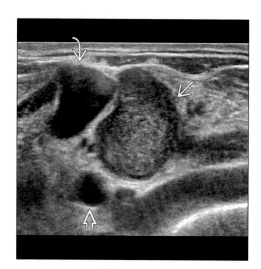
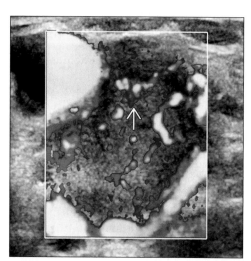

(Left) Axial CECT of the same patient shows the location of a metastatic node ➡ in the left lower neck. *(Right)* Corresponding CECT of the mediastinum also shows an abnormal mediastinal node ➡. Guided biopsy of the left lower neck node confirmed nodal metastasis from primary carcinoma colon. Malignancies from the esophagus, lung, and breast are the most common to metastasize the to the lower neck/SCF. Malignant cervical nodes from the infraclavicular primary represent distant metastatic disease.

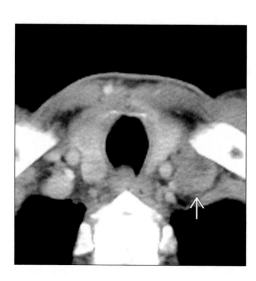
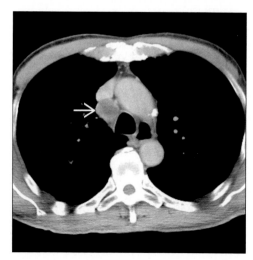

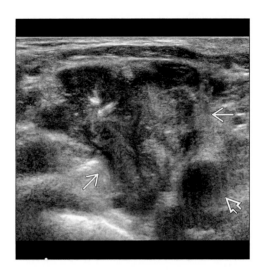

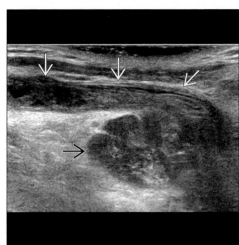

(Left) Transverse grayscale US of a patient with lung carcinoma shows a solid, hypoechoic, ill-defined mass ➡ in the right lower neck, adjacent to the CCA ➡. US features suggest a conglomerate of metastatic nodes. *(Right)* Corresponding longitudinal grayscale US shows metastatic nodes ➡ and their relation to the IJV ➡, which has a long segment of the thrombus within. Intrathrombus vascularity differentiates tumor thrombus vs. bland thrombus (avascular) due to venous stasis.

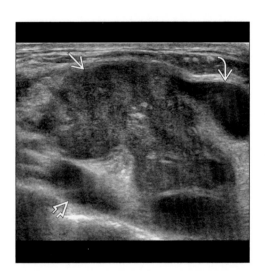

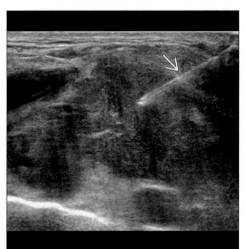

(Left) Transverse grayscale US shows a large, solid mass in the right lower neck, which is suggestive of a matted group of abnormal lymph nodes ➡. Differential diagnosis includes metastatic nodes from an infraclavicular primary and TB lymphadenitis. Note the subclavian vein ➡ and IJV ➡. *(Right)* Corresponding US-guided biopsy confirmed metastatic nodes from an unknown primary. US readily guides the needle ➡ for biopsy to confirm the nature of nodes at this site, particularly in patients with no known primary.

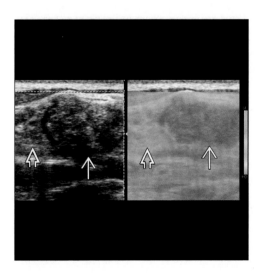

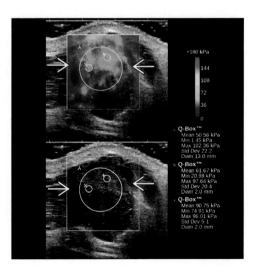

(Left) Transverse grayscale US and qualitative strain EI show a metastatic node from uterine cancer. Strain color scale is from purple (elastic, soft) to red (inelastic, hard). It appears inelastic ➡ compared to adjacent tissues ➡. *(Right)* Transverse grayscale US and SWE show a metastatic node ➡. SWE color scale ranges from blue (0 kPa, soft) to red (180 kPa, stiff). It is heterogeneous with high stiffness foci (maximum ~ 102 kPa). Nodal stiffness varies according to precise histology.

NON-HODGKIN LYMPHOMA NODES

Key Facts

Imaging

- Multiple, bilateral, nonnecrotic enlarged nodes in usual & unusual (RPS, SMS, occipital) nodal chains
- NHL nodes are commonly round with sharp borders
- Unsharp border indicates extracapsular spread implying aggressive disease
- Solid node, absent normal echogenic hilum (72-73%)
- Using modern high-resolution transducers, despite their solid nature, NHL nodes tend to show posterior enhancement
- NHL nodes show intranodal reticular/micronodular pattern using newer high-resolution transducers
- Calcification rare; if present, usually after radiation Rx
- Despite large nodal size, cystic necrosis is uncommon; if present, suggests aggressive NHL
- Color Doppler: Mixed vascularity, with prominent hilar vessels & presence of peripheral vascularity
- Peripheral vascularity alone is rare in NHL nodes

Top Differential Diagnoses

- Nodal metastases, systemic primary
- Reactive adenopathy
- Tuberculous adenitis

Clinical Issues

- Incidence increases with age and in immunocompromised patients
- Increased association with EBV or HTLV-1, especially African Burkitt & AIDS-associated lymphomas

Diagnostic Checklist

- If NHL suspected on US, a core biopsy may be performed instead of FNAC
- Choice of core biopsy, excision biopsy, or FNAC in NHL depends on local practice and expertise
- US does not evaluate retropharyngeal & mediastinal involvement
- CECT or PET/CT to determine disease extent

(Left) Longitudinal grayscale US shows well-defined, solid, hypoechoic nodes with a reticular/micronodular echo pattern ➡ within. Note the marked posterior enhancement ➡ often seen in NHL nodes. (Right) Corresponding power Doppler US shows a combination of hilar ➡ & peripheral vascularity ➡, a feature of NHL nodes, and clearly demonstrates posterior enhancement ➡.

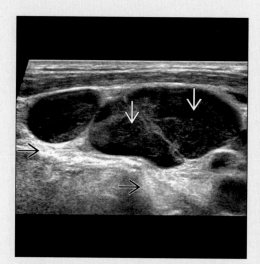
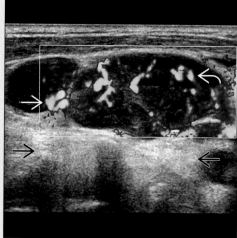

(Left) Longitudinal grayscale US shows solid, hypoechoic nodes with a reticular/micronodular pattern ➡. Note the ill-defined edges ➡ anteriorly, suggesting extracapsular spread and implying aggressive disease. (Right) Corresponding power Doppler US shows typical NHL intranodal vascularity, both hilar ➡ & peripheral ➡ in distribution. Note the posterior enhancement ➡ despite the solid nature of the nodes.

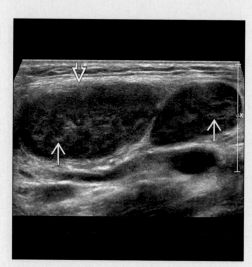
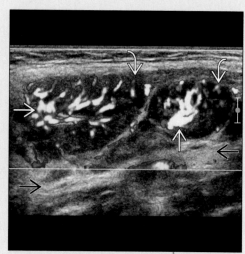

NON-HODGKIN LYMPHOMA NODES

TERMINOLOGY

Abbreviations
- Non-Hodgkin lymphoma (NHL)

Definitions
- Cancer developing in lymphoreticular system, thought to arise from lymphocytes and their derivatives

IMAGING

General Features
- Best diagnostic clue
  - Multiple, bilateral, nonnecrotic enlarged nodes in usual (jugular chain, posterior triangle) and unusual (retropharyngeal space [RPS], submandibular space [SMS], occipital) nodal chains
  - May also present as single dominant nonnecrotic node with multiple smaller surrounding nodes
- Location
  - Nodal disease occurs in cervical chains
    - Levels II, III, and IV often involved
    - Superficial adenopathy, level V, and spinal accessory nodes are also common

Ultrasonographic Findings
- NHL nodes are commonly round with sharp borders
  - Tumor deposition in nodes produces greater acoustic impedance between node and adjacent soft tissues leading to sharp border
  - Unsharp border indicates extracapsular spread implying aggressive disease
- Solid node, absent normal echogenic hilum (72-73%)
- Commonly hypoechoic compared to adjacent muscle
  - Previously described as "pseudocystic" nodes with posterior enhancement
    - Using older transducers, internal echoes in nodes were very low, almost anechoic, resembling cyst
  - Using modern high-resolution transducers, despite their solid nature, NHL nodes tend to show posterior enhancement
    - Uniform cellular infiltration within nodes produces fewer interfaces and facilitates passage of sound
      - This, combined with low internal echoes, produces so-called pseudocystic pattern
  - NHL nodes show intranodal reticular/micronodular pattern using newer high-resolution transducers
- Calcification rare; if present, usually after radiation Rx
- Despite large nodal size, cystic necrosis is uncommon; if present, suggests aggressive NHL
- Color Doppler: Mixed vascularity with prominent hilar vessels and presence of peripheral vascularity
  - Peripheral vascularity alone is rare in NHL nodes
- Spectral Doppler: Variable intranodal intravascular resistance, nonspecific

Imaging Recommendations
- Best imaging tool
  - US is ideal initial imaging modality to evaluate nodes below angle of mandible
    - Core biopsy may be performed instead of FNAC if NHL is suspected on US
    - Choice of core biopsy or excision biopsy or FNAC in NHL depends on local practice and expertise
  - US does not evaluate retropharyngeal and mediastinal involvement
- CECT or PET/CT to determine disease extent

DIFFERENTIAL DIAGNOSIS

Nodal Metastases, Systemic Primary
- Multiple, hypoechoic nodes in areas of known drainage site of the primary tumor; hypoechoic, round, ± intranodal necrosis, peripheral vascularity
- If history of primary tumor is not known, US appearances may be indistinguishable from NHL

Reactive Adenopathy
- Solid, hypoechoic, elliptical nodes with echogenic hilar echo pattern and low-resistance hilar vascularity

Tuberculous Adenitis
- Multiple, round, necrotic, matted nodes ± echogenic hilum, avascular or displaced hilar vascularity

Sarcoidosis
- Diffuse cervical nodes that may exactly mimic NHL, associated with mediastinal nodes ± calcification

Hodgkin Lymphoma
- Nodal-type NHL cannot be differentiated from nodal Hodgkin lymphoma; NHL: More common, presents in older patients ± extranodal disease

CLINICAL ISSUES

Presentation
- Most common signs/symptoms
  - Large, painless, small rubbery neck mass(es)
  - Systemic symptoms: Night sweats, recurrent fever, unexplained weight loss, fatigue, and pruritic skin rash
- Clinical profile
  - Painless neck mass in patient with AIDS most commonly NHL

Demographics
- Epidemiology
  - NHL is 2nd most common neoplasm of head and neck
  - NHL = 5% of all head and neck cancers
  - NHL risk factors
    - ↑ incidence with age and in immunocompromised
    - ↑ association with EBV or HTLV-1, especially African Burkitt and AIDS-associated lymphomas

Natural History & Prognosis
- Prognosis depends on stage and response to therapy
  - Outcome very poor in AIDS-related NHL

DIAGNOSTIC CHECKLIST

Consider
- Imaging reveals multiple cervical nodes in multiple nodal chains, especially if nonnecrotic
- NHL in AIDS patient with neck mass

SELECTED REFERENCES

1. Ahuja AT et al: Sonographic evaluation of cervical lymph nodes. AJR Am J Roentgenol. 184(5):1691-9, 2005

(Left) Longitudinal grayscale US shows typical features of NHL node: Well-defined, solid, and hypoechoic, with micronodular internal architecture and posterior enhancement. Despite its large size, there is no intranodal necrosis, which is uncommon in NHL nodes. *(Right)* Longitudinal grayscale US shows a reticular/micronodular ➡ appearance & posterior enhancement ⬇ in NHL nodes. Modern high-resolution transducers make it possible to see internal architecture even in small nodes.

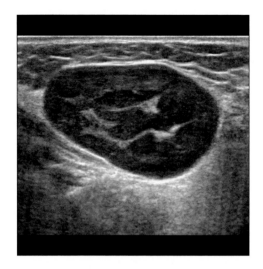
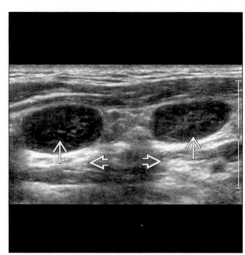

(Left) Longitudinal grayscale US shows typical NHL nodes ➡, which are solid, well-defined, and hypoechoic with micronodular architecture within. Note the absence of normal echogenic hilum. *(Right)* Corresponding power Doppler US shows profuse intranodal vascularity, hilar ➡ & peripheral ➡.

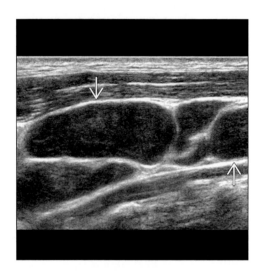
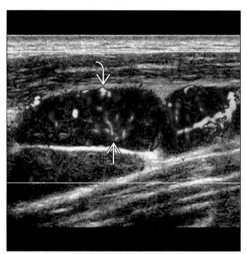

(Left) Longitudinal grayscale US of NHL nodes shows them to be solid, hypoechoic, & well-defined with a granular micronodular echo pattern within. Note absence of echogenic hilum in 1 node and its presence ➡ in another. Note posterior enhancement ⬇ despite their solid nature (pseudocystic appearance). *(Right)* Corresponding power Doppler US shows marked abnormal peripheral vascularity ➡. Peripheral vascularity alone is rare in NHL, usually hilar & peripheral, hilar > peripheral.

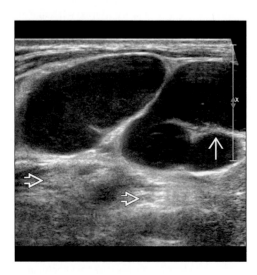
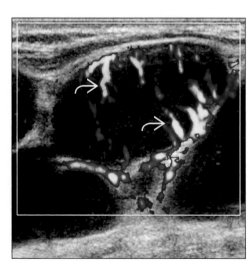

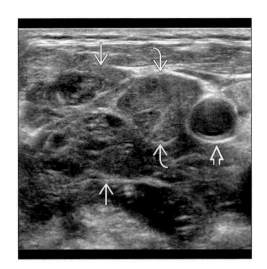

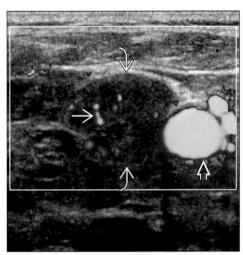

(Left) Transverse grayscale US in a patient with nodal NHL shows a large conglomerate of nodes ➡ in the vicinity of the CCA ➡. There is suggestion of thrombus within the bulging IJV ➡. Note that the normal bright carotid walls are maintained. *(Right)* Corresponding power Doppler US shows an IJV ➡ thrombus with vascularity ➡ within, suggesting tumor thrombus rather than bland venous thrombosis. Despite their large size, NHL nodes commonly displace rather than infiltrate adjacent structures. CCA ➡ is shown.

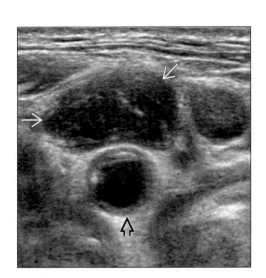

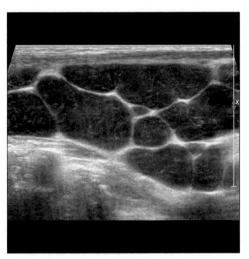

(Left) Transverse grayscale US shows heterogeneous, hypoechoic, and cystic node ➡ anterior to CCA ➡ in a patient with NHL. Cystic necrosis is seldom seen in NHL nodes even when they are large. *(Right)* Longitudinal grayscale US shows NHL nodes in posterior triangle. Each node is discrete, well defined, solid, & hypoechoic with micronodular echo pattern. Despite their multiplicity, location, and proximity, there is no periadenitis (i.e., nodal matting & soft tissue edema), commonly seen in TB nodes.

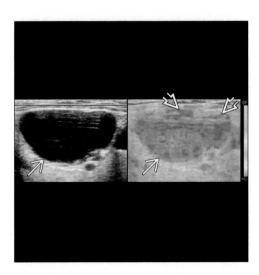

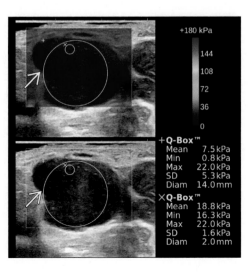

(Left) Longitudinal grayscale US & qualitative strain elastogram show a pseudocystic NHL node ➡. Strain color scale ranges from purple (elastic, soft) to red (inelastic, hard). It appears mostly purple & green, similar to adjacent fascia, suggesting soft node. Superficial compression artifacts are present ➡. *(Right)* Transverse US grayscale & SWE show a NHL node ➡. SWE color scale ranges from blue (0 kPa, soft) to red (180 kPa, stiff). It appears blue with a maximum SWE value of 22.0 kPa, which is low.

CASTLEMAN DISEASE

Key Facts

Terminology

- Rare, benign lymph node disease of unknown cause characterized by distinctive histology

Imaging

- In neck, UCD > MCD, solitary > multicentric
- Cervical lymph node (80%) > parotid gland (9%) > oral base, submandibular/parapharyngeal space
- Most common in level I lymph nodes
- Markedly enlarged, well-demarcated, rounded, noncalcified, hypoechoic lymph node with cortical hypertrophy and compressed echogenic hilum
- Mixed hilar > peripheral vascularity
- Involvement of parotid gland typically as solitary enlarged intraparotid node
- Differentiation from benign chronic lymphadenitis or lymphoma usually difficult based on imaging, FNA, or core needle biopsy; diagnosis is often established on excision biopsy

Top Differential Diagnoses

- Lymphadenitis
- Lymphoma
- Metastatic lymphadenopathy
- Tuberculous lymphadenitis

Clinical Issues

- Typically affects mediastinal compartment > neck > retroperitoneum > axilla
- Most common in adults; affects both sexes equally
- UCD: Painless, enlarging mediastinal/ neck mass
- MCD: Constitutional symptoms + multicentric lesion

Diagnostic Checklist

- CD is rare and often difficult to diagnose on imaging due to its lack of unique signs; awareness of disease in patients with painless, expanding neck mass may prevent delayed diagnosis and treatment

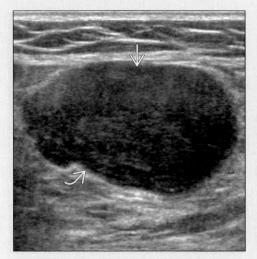
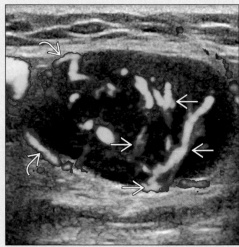

(Left) Transverse grayscale US shows abnormal node ⇨ in anterior submandibular space in patient with unicentric Castleman disease. Lymph node is enlarged, round, solid, noncalcified, and hypoechoic. Note well-defined border ⇨ and normal surrounding tissue. (Right) Corresponding power Doppler US shows prominent hilar ⇨ > peripheral ⇨ vascularity. This appearance of CD mimics lymphoma (hilar > peripheral vascularity) or metastatic lymphadenopathy (predominant peripheral vascularity), which are more common.

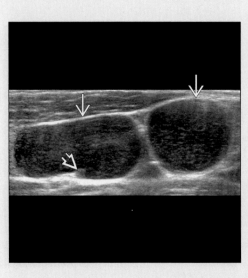
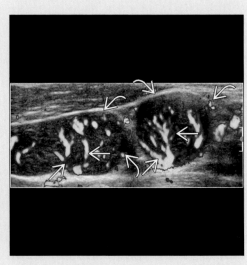

(Left) Longitudinal grayscale US shows multiple enlarged nodes ⇨ in the upper internal jugular chain in a patient with MCD. Note cortical hypertrophy, compressed echogenic hilum ⇨, and normal adjacent soft tissues. (Right) Corresponding longitudinal power Doppler US shows profuse hilar ⇨ & peripheral ⇨ vascularity. Note the hilar vascularity is greater than peripheral vascularity, a finding consistent with most reported cases of CD, mimicking lymphoma. Diagnosis of CD is usually made at histology.

CASTLEMAN DISEASE

TERMINOLOGY

Abbreviations
- Castleman disease (CD), unicentric Castleman disease (UCD), multicentric Castleman disease (MCD)

Definitions
- Rare, benign lymphoproliferative disorder of uncertain cause characterized by distinctive pattern of hypervascular lymphoid hyperplasia

IMAGING

General Features
- Best diagnostic clue
  ○ In neck, UCD > MCD, typically solitary, enlarging lymphadenopathy in otherwise asymptomatic patient
- Location
  ○ Cervical lymph node (80%) > parotid gland (9%) > oral base, submandibular gland, parapharyngeal space
- Size
  ○ Average: 5-10 cm

Ultrasonographic Findings
- Grayscale ultrasound
  ○ Cervical lymphadenopathy
    ▪ Level I > level V; solitary > multiple, bilateral
    ▪ Markedly enlarged, well circumscribed, rounded, solid, hypoechoic lymph node with cortical hypertrophy ± slit-like echogenic hilum
    ▪ No internal necrosis, matting, or calcification
    ▪ No involvement of surrounding tissue
    ▪ Differentiation from chronic lymphadenitis or lymphoma usually not possible
  ○ Parotid involvement
    ▪ Usually seen as solitary, well-defined nodule (intraparotid lymphadenopathy); ill-defined margin reported, mimics salivary gland neoplasm
  ○ Guided FNA helps to narrow differential diagnosis
- Power Doppler
  ○ Most reported cases show prominent mixed hilar and peripheral vascularity, with hilar vascularity dominant

CT Findings
- Homogeneous nodal mass; moderate to marked enhancement

MR Findings
- T1 hypointense, T2 hyperintense; rarely, hypointense linear signals within lesion due to calcification, fibrous septation, or vessels

DIFFERENTIAL DIAGNOSIS

Chronic Lymphadenitis
- Related to dental infection (level I) or connective tissue disease (close mimic and more common)

Lymphoma
- Similar imaging & FNA, need histology for differentiation

Metastatic Lymphadenopathy
- Multiple ± necrosis ± extracapsular spread; known 1°

Tuberculosis
- Posterior triangle; early necrosis, matting, and abscess

Nerve Sheath Tumor
- Reported mimic of UCD; continuation with involved nerve = nerve sheath tumor

PATHOLOGY

General Features
- Affects mediastinum (60%) > neck (14%) > retroperitoneum (11%) > axilla (4%); can affect any part of body that contains lymphoid tissue
- Associated abnormalities
  ○ UCD: Lymphoma, paraneoplastic pemphigus
  ○ MCD: HIV infection (→ rapid symptom development), Kaposi sarcoma (13%), NHL (15-20%), POEMS

Microscopic Features
- 2 histological subgroups
  ○ Hyaline vascular variant (90%): Abnormal follicle with "regressed" germinal centers and broad mantle zone organized in "onion-skin" arrangement; majority of UCD is hyaline vascular type
  ○ Plasma cell variant (10%): Regressed follicles + hyperplastic germinal centers, interfollicular hypervascularity, and plasma cell sheets; most of MCD is plasma/mixed plasma-hyaline vascular type

CLINICAL ISSUES

Presentation
- 2 clinical forms: Vastly different clinical features
  ○ UCD: Solitary painless, enlarging mass in mediastinum or neck; systemic symptom is rare
  ○ MCD: Systemic symptoms include fever, night sweats, fatigue + multifocal peripheral > central lymphadenopathy; ↑ IL6

Demographics
- Rare; affects both sexes equally; UCD peaks at 2nd–4th decade while MCD peaks at 6th–7th

Natural History & Prognosis
- UCD: Benign, nonprogressive disease course
- MCD: Comorbidity is common and prognosis is guarded

DIAGNOSTIC CHECKLIST

Image Interpretation Pearls
- CD is rare and often difficult to diagnose on imaging because it lacks unique signs
- FNA or core needle biopsy are easily misread as reactive change or lymphoma
  ○ Usually, pathologic diagnosis is achieved by excisional biopsy
- Awareness of CD in patients with painless, expanding neck mass may prevent delayed diagnosis & treatment

SELECTED REFERENCES

1. Puram SV et al: Castleman disease presenting in the neck: report of a case and review of the literature. Am J Otolaryngol. 34(3):239-44, 2013

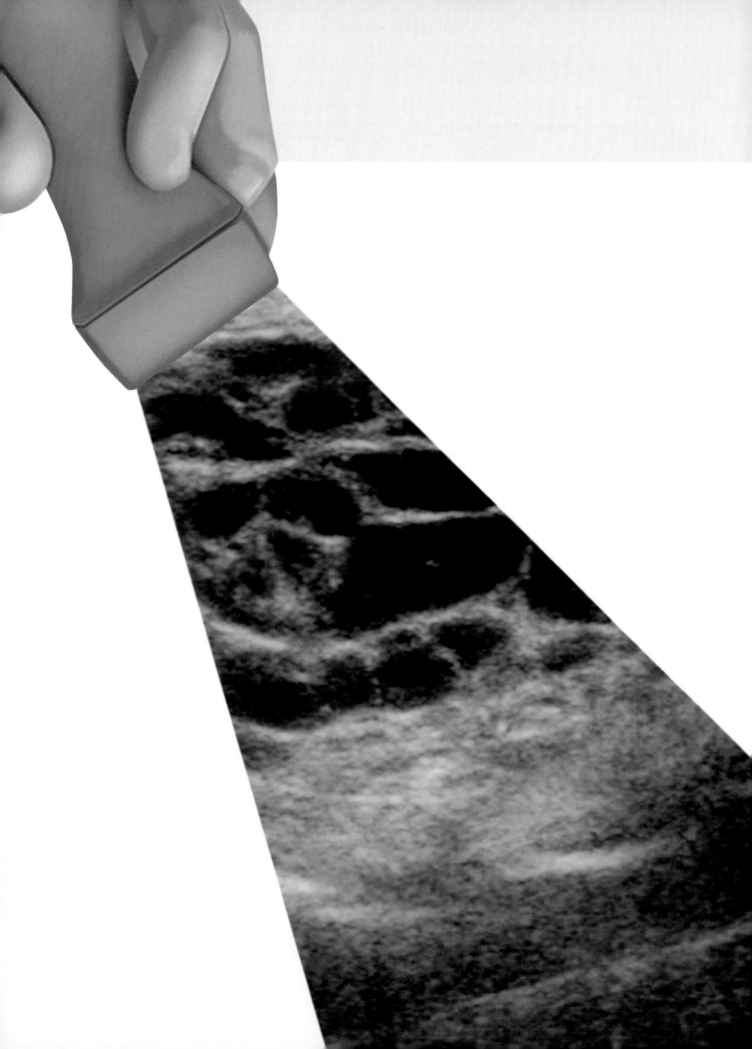

SECTION 4
Salivary Glands

Parotid Space

Submandibular Space

General Lesions

PAROTID BENIGN MIXED TUMOR

Key Facts

Imaging

- Well-defined, solid, & hypoechoic compared to adjacent salivary tissue
- Homogeneous internal echoes with posterior enhancement
- Large tumors may show heterogeneous internal echo pattern due to hemorrhage and necrosis
- Heterogeneous BMT may have ill-defined edges mimicking malignant mass
- No abnormal adjacent intra-/periparotid node
- No infiltration of overlying skin/subcutaneous tissue
- ↑ peripheral vessels, mainly venous; often sparse
- Spectral Doppler: Low intra-BMT vascular resistance (resistive index [RI] < 0.8, pulsatility index [RI] < 2.0)
- If left untreated, BMTs will undergo malignant transformation
- Intratumoral calcification implies longstanding tumor & should raise suspicion

- Risk of malignant transformation: 1.5% at 5 years, 9.5% at 15 years
- Rapid ↑ in size of known BMT raises concern for malignant transformation
- Most parotid BMTs are located in superficial parotid; US is ideal initial imaging modality for such lesions
- BMT from apex of superficial lobe of parotid at angle of mandible is in proximity to submandibular gland (SMG) & should not be mistaken for SMG BMT
- Multicentric BMT rare (< 1%); multiple lesions often seen at surgical site in recurrent BMT ("cluster of grapes")

Top Differential Diagnoses

- Warthin tumor
- Primary parotid carcinoma
- Non-Hodgkin lymphoma, parotid
- Parotid nodal metastasis

(Left) Transverse grayscale US shows a well-defined, solid, hypoechoic (vs. parotid parenchyma ➡), homogeneous mass ➡ with intense posterior enhancement ➡ in the superficial parotid lobe. Note the mandible ➡. (Right) Corresponding longitudinal grayscale US shows its lobulated nature with no extraparotid extension. Note the intense posterior enhancement ➡ despite its solid homogeneous nature, typical of parotid benign mixed tumor (BMT), which offers few interfaces and allows sound to penetrate easily.

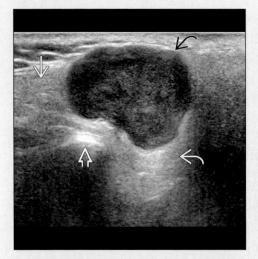
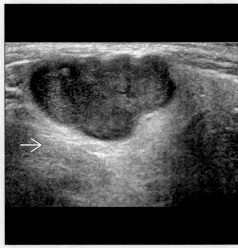

(Left) Transverse grayscale US shows a small parotid BMT ➡ in the superficial lobe. Note its lobulated outline and small focus of calcification ➡ within (shadowing is better seen on fundamental scans). Note the mandible ➡. Calcification is seen in longstanding BMTs and is unusual in other salivary neoplasms. (Right) Longitudinal grayscale US shows a large parotid BMT ➡ in the superficial lobe ➡. Large BMTs have a heterogeneous echo pattern, and if edges appear blurred/ill-defined, they mimic malignant salivary tumor.

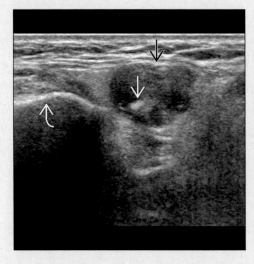
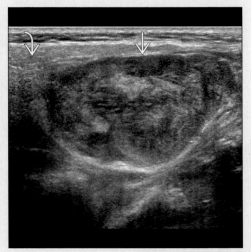

PAROTID BENIGN MIXED TUMOR

TERMINOLOGY

Abbreviations
- Benign mixed tumor (BMT)

Synonyms
- Pleomorphic adenoma

IMAGING

General Features
- Best diagnostic clue
  - Small BMT: Sharply marginated, lobulated/bosselated, intraparotid mass with homogeneous, hypoechoic echo pattern and posterior enhancement
  - Large BMT (> 2 cm): Lobulated mass with heterogeneous, hypoechoic echo pattern, ± ill-defined edges

Ultrasonographic Findings
- Grayscale ultrasound
  - Specificity 87%, accuracy 89%
  - Well-defined, solid, and hypoechoic compared with adjacent salivary tissue
  - Homogeneous internal echoes with posterior enhancement
    - Tumor offers few interfaces and allows sound to penetrate easily, producing posterior enhancement
  - Large tumors may show heterogeneous internal echo pattern due to hemorrhage and necrosis
  - Heterogeneous BMT may have ill-defined edges mimicking malignant mass
  - Calcification is unusual, seen in longstanding BMT
    - Calcification is dense and dysmorphic with posterior shadowing
  - No abnormal adjacent intra-/periparotid node
  - No infiltration of overlying skin/subcutaneous tissue
- Color Doppler
  - ↑ peripheral vessels, mainly venous; often sparse
  - Spectral Doppler: Low intra-BMT vascular resistance (resistive index [RI] < 0.8, pulsatility index [RI] < 2.0)

Imaging Recommendations
- Best imaging tool
  - Most parotid BMTs are located in superficial parotid; US is ideal initial imaging modality for such lesions
  - US is readily combined with guided fine-needle aspiration cytology (FNAC), which has sensitivity of 83%, specificity of 86%, and accuracy of 85% for salivary gland tumors; FNAC ↑ specificity of US
  - Although facial nerve cannot be seen on ultrasound, its location is inferred by identifying retromandibular vein (RMV) or external carotid artery (ECA) as they run together in parotid gland
  - US is unable to evaluate deep lobe masses or deep lobe extension of superficial lobe masses
  - CECT, or preferably MR (DWI, ↑ ADC value compared to other tumors and cancers), indicated to fully evaluate parotid masses, their deep extension, and relationship to facial nerve
    - DWI not yet accurate enough to avoid biopsy
- Protocol advice
  - In evaluating parotid masses, carefully assess
    - Edge: Benign lesions have well-defined edges and malignant tumors are ill defined
    - Internal architecture: Benign tumors have homogeneous internal echo pattern, malignant tumors have heterogeneous architecture
  - Malignant tumors are more likely associated with skin, subcutaneous, and nodal involvement
  - Malignant tumors show prominent vessels with high resistance, resistance index (RI) > 0.8, pulsatility index (PI) > 2.0
  - BMT from apex of superficial lobe of parotid at angle of mandible is in close proximity to submandibular gland (SMG) and should not be mistaken for SMG BMT
    - Always identify origin of tumor as surgical incisions for parotid BMT and SMG BMT are different
    - Pattern of displacement of adjacent structures/vessels help in differentiating them
  - Always evaluate both parotid and SMGs

DIFFERENTIAL DIAGNOSIS

Warthin Tumor
- Smoker, 20% multifocal, unilateral/bilateral
- Hypoechoic, heterogeneous with solid and cystic component in superficial lobe of parotid gland

Primary Parotid Carcinoma
- ± pain, facial nerve palsy, and skin/subcutaneous induration
- Ill-defined, heterogeneous internal echoes, ± associated nodes, ± extraglandular infiltration
- Low-grade malignancy may be well defined, homogeneous, and mimic BMT

Parotid Non-Hodgkin Lymphoma
- Chronic systemic NHL may already be present
- Solitary, multiple, or bilateral; round, solid, hypoechoic/reticulated nodes with abnormal vascularity

Parotid Nodal Metastasis (Systemic or Skin SCCa or Melanoma, Nasopharyngeal Carcinoma)
- Known primary; multiple, round, solid, ± cystic nodes with abnormal peripheral vascularity

CLINICAL ISSUES

Demographics
- Age
  - Most common > 40 years
- Epidemiology
  - Most common parotid space tumor (80%)
  - 80% of BMTs arise in parotid glands
    - 8% in SMGs; 6.5% arise from minor salivary glands in nasopharyngeal mucosa
  - 80-90% of parotid BMTs involve superficial lobe
  - Multicentric BMT is rare (< 1%); multiple lesions are often seen at surgical site in recurrent BMT ("cluster of grapes")
    - Recurrent tumor typically due to incomplete resection or cellular spillage at surgery

SELECTED REFERENCES

1. Lee YY et al: Imaging of salivary gland tumours. Eur J Radiol. 66(3):419-36, 2008

PAROTID BENIGN MIXED TUMOR

(Left) Transverse grayscale US shows a parotid BMT in the superficial lobe, well defined with intratumoral cystic ➡ area, thick walls, and no extraparotid extension. Note the mandible ➡. Cystic change is more frequently seen in malignant tumors but may also be seen in BMT, usually larger tumors, and may be a result of ischemic infarction ± associated abrupt onset of pain. *(Right)* Corresponding power Doppler US shows a large intratumoral vessel within, which is usually of low resistance.

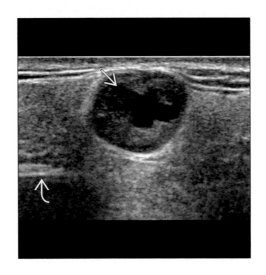
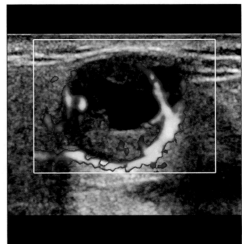

(Left) Longitudinal grayscale US shows a parotid BMT ➡. It is hypoechoic with heterogeneous internal architecture, and margins are not well delineated. Note the presence of posterior enhancement ➡. *(Right)* Corresponding power Doppler US shows marked intratumoral vascularity and posterior enhancement ➡. US features are very similar to a malignant salivary mass. Therefore, FNA/biopsy is often indicated to confirm diagnosis and is ideally performed under US guidance.

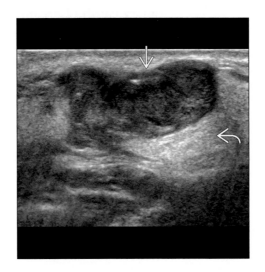
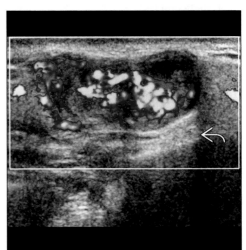

(Left) Transverse power Doppler US of parotid BMT shows central ➡ and peripheral ➡ tumor vascularity. *(Right)* Transverse power Doppler US of a parotid BMT in another patient shows central ➡ & peripheral ➡ vascularity. Although peripheral vascularity is described in the literature (venous and low resistance in nature), the distribution of vascularity in BMT is variable. It does not significantly contribute toward its diagnosis nor is it accurate enough to avoid biopsy.

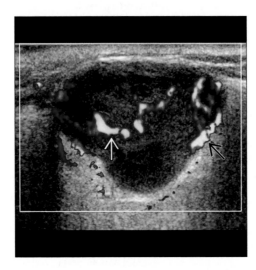
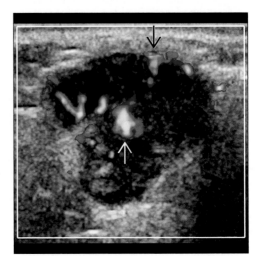

PAROTID BENIGN MIXED TUMOR

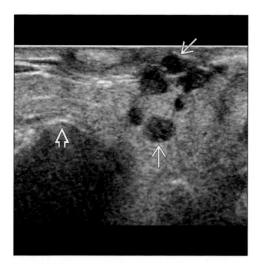

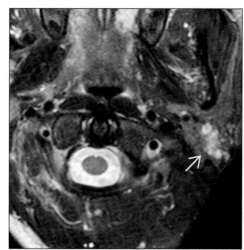

(Left) Transverse grayscale US of a patient with previous history of surgery for parotid BMT shows multiple small, solid, hypoechoic nodules (intra- & periparotid) ➡ at the surgical site. Note the mandible ⮕. US features are characteristic of recurrent BMTs, which are often multiple/multifocal ("cluster of grapes") and are due to incomplete resection or spillage at surgery. *(Right)* Corresponding axial T2WI MR clearly shows multiple high-signal BMTs ➡ at surgical site.

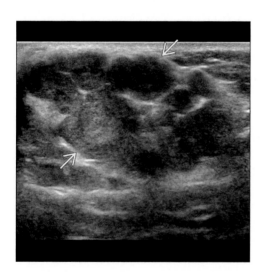

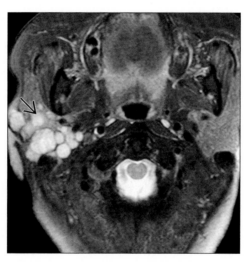

(Left) Longitudinal grayscale US shows a cluster of solid, hypoechoic nodules, some of which are bosselated at the postoperative site, in a patient with previous surgery for BMT. Multifocal BMTs by themselves are rare (< 1%) but are often seen in recurrent BMT ➡, as in this case. *(Right)* Corresponding T2WI MR shows high-signal BMTs ➡, their extent, & anatomical relations better than US, which readily identifies the lesion and suggests diagnosis but may not define the entire extent of the abnormality.

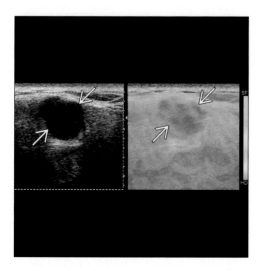

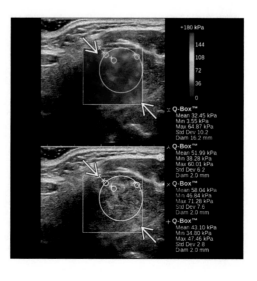

(Left) Grayscale US and qualitative strain elastogram show a parotid BMT ➡. Strain color scale ranges from purple (elastic, soft) to red (inelastic, hard). It is mixed with green & mostly red areas, signifying moderate inelasticity compared to normal parenchyma. *(Right)* Transverse grayscale US & SWE show a parotid BMT ➡. SWE color scale ranges from blue (0 kPa, soft) to red (180 kPa, stiff). It is mixed dark & light blue, with a maximum SWE value of 71.3 kPa (intermediate stiffness).

PAROTID WARTHIN TUMOR

Key Facts

Imaging

- Large Warthin tumor: Clinically obvious
  - Well-defined, hypoechoic, noncalcified mass in apex of superficial lobe of parotid
  - Heterogeneous internal architecture with cystic and solid components
  - Multiseptated with thick walls and debris ± posterior enhancement
- Small Warthin tumor: Incidental finding
  - Elliptical, solid reniform mass in known location of intraparotid lymph node
  - Heterogeneous architecture and echogenic hilus mimic appearance of lymph node
- Color Doppler: Prominent hilar (in small solid tumors) and septal (may be striking) vessels

Top Differential Diagnoses

- Parotid benign mixed tumor
- Parotid malignant tumor

- Nodal metastasis
- Benign lymphoepithelial lesions (BLEL)-HIV

Pathology

- Smoking-induced, benign tumor arising from salivary lymphoid tissue in intraparotid and periparotid nodes
- Theorized heterotopic salivary gland parenchyma present in preexisting intra-/periparotid nodes
- Parotid gland undergoes late encapsulation, incorporating lymphoid tissue nodes within superficial layer of deep cervical fascia
  - Warthin tumor arises within this lymphoid tissue
- Submandibular gland undergoes early encapsulation with no lymphoid tissue nodes in glandular parenchyma and no Warthin tumor in submandibular gland
- 5-10% may arise in extraparotid locations (periparotid and upper neck lymph nodes)

(Left) Clinical photograph of a smoker demonstrates a soft, painless mass ➡ at the angle of the mandible, a common nondiscriminatory presentation for most benign salivary masses. *(Right)* Transverse grayscale US shows a well-defined, predominantly cystic mass ➡ with internal septa ➡ and debris ➡ located at the angle of the mandible ➡, in the left superficial parotid gland. The location, US features, and history are fairly typical of Warthin tumor. Note its anatomical location in relation to the retromandibular vein (RMV) ➡.

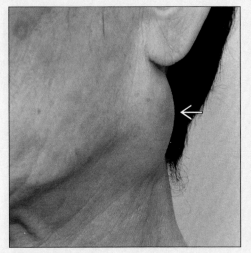
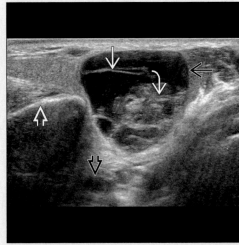

(Left) Longitudinal grayscale US (same patient) clearly shows smooth outlines, no extraparotid extension, posterior enhancement ➡, and internal debris ➡ and septa ➡. Aspirates from the cystic component may only yield fluid containing debris, resulting in nondiagnostic smears. US-guided aspiration of the solid component helps. *(Right)* Corresponding power Doppler shows no vascularity in the septa and solid debris. Internal fine debris is usually mobile, and aspiration of fluid reduces the nodule size.

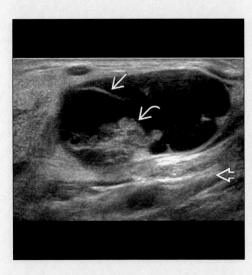
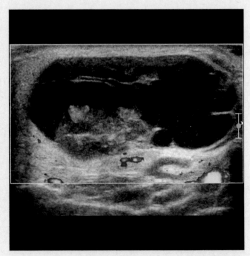

PAROTID WARTHIN TUMOR

TERMINOLOGY

Abbreviations
- Papillary cystadenoma lymphomatosum, adenolymphoma, lymphomatous adenoma

IMAGING

General Features
- Best diagnostic clue
  - Sharply marginated parotid tail mass with heterogeneous echo pattern and solid and cystic components within
- Location
  - Intraparotid > > periparotid > upper cervical nodes
  - When intraparotid, most commonly within parotid tail superficial to angle of mandible

Ultrasonographic Findings
- Grayscale US: Specificity 91%, accuracy 89%
  - Large Warthin tumor: Clinically obvious
    - Well-defined, hypoechoic, noncalcified mass in apex of superficial lobe of parotid
    - Heterogeneous internal architecture with cystic and solid components
    - Multiseptated with thick walls and debris ± posterior enhancement
  - Small Warthin tumor: Incidental finding
    - Small, elliptical, solid reniform mass in known location of intraparotid lymph node
    - Heterogeneous architecture and echogenic hilus
      – Mimics appearance of lymph node
  - Multiplicity of lesions, unilateral or bilateral (20%)
  - No skin or subcutaneous tissue infiltration
- Color Doppler: Prominent hilar (in small solid tumors) and septal (may be striking) vessels
- Spectral Doppler: Low-resistance vessels (resistive index [RI] < 0.8, pulsatility index [PI] < 2.0)

Imaging Recommendations
- Best imaging tool
  - Most Warthin tumors are in superficial lobe, and US is ideal initial imaging modality
  - US may be unable to evaluate the entire extent and anatomical relationships of large tumors
  - As these lesions rarely turn malignant (< 1%), US is ideal for surveillance in patients who refuse surgery
  - US is readily combined with FNAC, which has sensitivity of 83%, specificity of 86%, and accuracy of 85% for salivary gland tumors
  - Facial nerve cannot be seen on US, but its location is inferred by identifying retromandibular vein or external carotid artery as they run together in parotid
- Protocol advice
  - Use of high-resolution transducer (scanning frequency ≥ 7.5 MHz) is essential
    - Use low-resolution transducer (5 MHz) with standoff gel to evaluate size & extent of large masses

DIFFERENTIAL DIAGNOSIS

Benign Mixed Tumor, Parotid
- Well-circumscribed, bosselated, homogeneous, solid intraparotid mass with posterior enhancement

- Larger lesions may show cystic change (hemorrhage or necrosis) and mimic Warthin tumor

Malignant Tumor, Parotid
- Ill-defined, solid, hypoechoic, heterogeneous echo pattern ± nodes and extraglandular infiltration
- Low-grade parotid malignancy may be well defined and homogeneous

Nodal Metastasis
- Primary malignancy on or around skin of ear, nasopharyngeal carcinoma (NPC)
- Single or multiple hypoechoic, heterogeneous intraparotid nodes with abnormal vascularity

Benign Lymphoepithelial Lesions (BLEL)-HIV
- When unilateral and solitary, may strongly mimic Warthin tumor
- Tonsillar enlargement and cervical lymphadenopathy help differentiate

PATHOLOGY

General Features
- Etiology
  - Smoking-induced, benign tumor arising from salivary lymphoid tissue in intraparotid and periparotid nodes
  - Theorized heterotopic salivary gland parenchyma present in preexisting intra-/periparotid nodes
- Embryology
  - Parotid gland undergoes late encapsulation, incorporating lymphoid tissue nodes within superficial layer of deep cervical fascia
    - Warthin tumor arises within this lymphoid tissue
  - Submandibular gland (SMG) undergoes early encapsulation with no lymphoid tissue nodes in glandular parenchyma, no Warthin tumor in SMG

CLINICAL ISSUES

Demographics
- Epidemiology
  - 2nd most common benign parotid tumor
  - 10% of all salivary gland epithelial tumors
  - 12% of benign parotid gland tumors
  - 20% are multicentric, unilateral or bilateral, and synchronous or metachronous
  - 5-10% may arise in extraparotid locations (periparotid and upper neck lymph nodes)

DIAGNOSTIC CHECKLIST

Image Interpretation Pearls
- Always examine for multiplicity and bilaterality
- 5-10% may arise in extraparotid locations (periparotid and upper neck lymph nodes) but not in SMG
- US appearance of Warthin tumor depends on tumor size

SELECTED REFERENCES

1. Lee YY et al: Imaging of salivary gland tumours. Eur J Radiol. 66(3):419-36, 2008

PAROTID WARTHIN TUMOR

(Left) Transverse grayscale US shows a predominantly cystic tumor ➡ with thick walls, posterior enhancement ⇢, and internal debris ➡ (with layering) in the superficial lobe of the parotid gland. Note the mandible ⬧. *(Right)* Longitudinal grayscale US (same patient) shows that the tumor is confined to the superficial parotid gland ⬧. US appearances are consistent with Warthin tumor. Transverse scans show the location and anatomical relation to RMV, whereas longitudinal scans allow better Doppler interrogation.

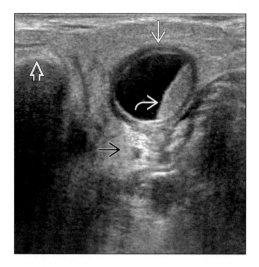
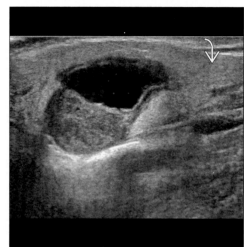

(Left) Transverse grayscale US of a Warthin tumor ➡ shows well-defined outlines, uniform internal debris, and intense posterior enhancement ➡, confirming the cystic nature of the tumor. Such uniformly distributed debris is usually mobile and readily aspirated. Note the mandible ⬧. *(Right)* Longitudinal grayscale US shows a large Warthin tumor ➡ in its typical location in the superficial parotid ➡ extending inferiorly. Note its predominantly cystic nature with internal septa, debris, & posterior enhancement ⬧.

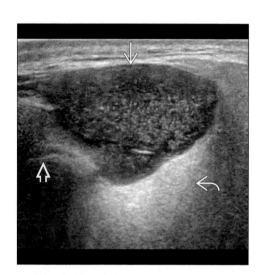
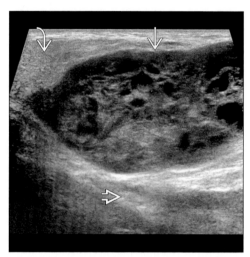

(Left) Longitudinal grayscale US shows a Warthin tumor ➡ at its typical location in the superficial lobe at the parotid tail ⬧, a common location of known intraparotid node. Note its elliptical shape, well-defined outlines, and hilar architecture ⬧ reminiscent of lymph node. Embryologically, the parotid incorporates lymphoid tissue nodes, and Warthin tumor arises within this lymphoid tissue. *(Right)* Power Doppler US (same patient) shows hilar vascularity ➡ within the Warthin tumor.

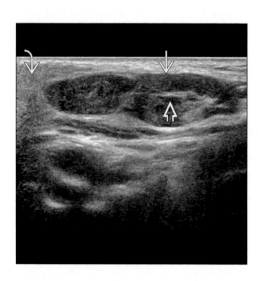
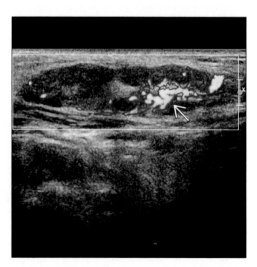

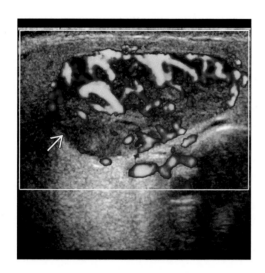
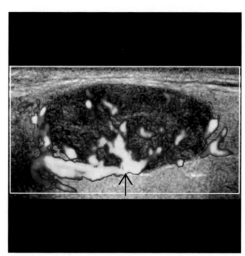

(Left) Transverse power Doppler US shows marked intratumoral vascularity in this Warthin tumor ➡. These are generally low-resistance vessels, RI < 0.8 and PI < 2.0. Intravascular resistance in salivary neoplasms is usually routinely measured in clinical practice. *(Right)* Longitudinal power Doppler US shows a Warthin tumor with typical nodal type of hilar vascularity ➡. Such vascularity is often seen in solid Warthin tumors before they have undergone cystic change.

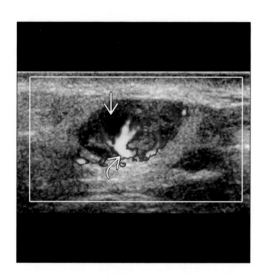
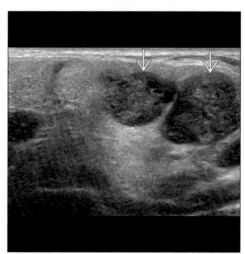

(Left) Longitudinal power Doppler US shows a small Warthin tumor with a focal cystic area ➡ and hilar vascularity ➡. Note its striking resemblance to a small lymph node & its typical location in superficial lobe of parotid tail. High-resolution US often picks up small lesions. US-guided FNA confirms diagnosis. *(Right)* Longitudinal US shows multiple small tumors ➡ in the superficial lobe of parotid tail; 20% of Warthin tumors are multiple, unilateral/bilateral, & synchronous or metachronous.

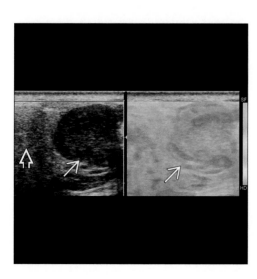
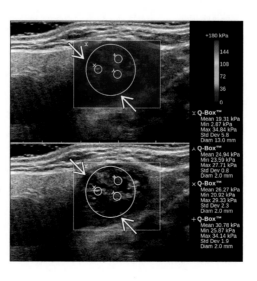

(Left) Longitudinal grayscale US and qualitative strain elastogram show a Warthin tumor ➡. Strain color scale ranges from purple (elastic, soft) to red (inelastic, hard). It displays mostly purple & green colors, appearing more elastic (softer) than adjacent parotid tissue ➡. *(Right)* Longitudinal grayscale US and SWE show a Warthin tumor ➡. SWE color scale ranges from blue (0 kPa, soft) to red (180 kPa, stiff). It displays blue with a maximum SWE of 34.8 kPa, which is low relative to many other salivary tumors.

PAROTID MUCOEPIDERMOID CARCINOMA

Key Facts

Imaging

- MECa; superficial lobe > > deep lobe parotid
- Imaging appearance based on MECa histologic grade
- Low-grade MECa
  - Solid mass with well-defined margin
  - Predominantly homogeneous echo pattern
  - No extraglandular invasion or lymphadenopathy
- High-grade MECa
  - Solid mass with ill-defined margin
  - Hypoechoic with heterogeneous architecture (due to necrosis & hemorrhage)
  - Extraglandular invasion of adjacent soft tissue ± skin involvement
- High-grade MECa: ± associated intraparotid & jugulodigastric lymph node metastases
- Color Doppler: Pronounced intratumoral vascularity
- Spectral Doppler: Increased intravascular resistance
  - Resistive index > 0.8; pulsatility index > 2.0

- As MECa commonly involves superficial lobe of parotid, US is ideal initial imaging modality
- US identifies malignancy ± metastatic nodes, guides biopsy but cannot differentiate between various types of malignant parotid lesions
- US cannot visualize CN7; position inferred by RMV/ECA as they run together in parotid gland
- US cannot evaluate deep extent of superficial lobe MECa and may miss a deep lobe tumor
- MR best delineates MECa local/regional extension & perineural spread
- Remember to look for nodal metastases

Top Differential Diagnoses

- Benign mixed tumor
- Warthin tumor
- Adenoid cystic carcinoma
- Malignant intraparotid nodes: Metastases, non-Hodgkin lymphoma

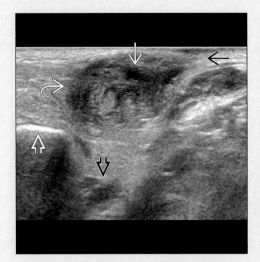
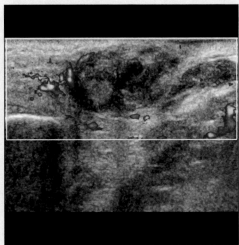

(Left) Transverse US shows a hypoechoic, heterogeneous mass ➡ in the superficial parotid. Note ill-defined edges, internal cystic change ➡, and subtle extraparotid extension into subcutaneous tissue ➡. The mandible ➡ & RMV/ECA ➡ are shown. (Right) Corresponding power Doppler US shows no significant vascularity in the tumor (hypervascularity and ↑ RI & PI described in malignant tumors). Ill-defined edges, tumor heterogeneity & extrasalivary extension suggested malignancy, and biopsy confirmed MECa.

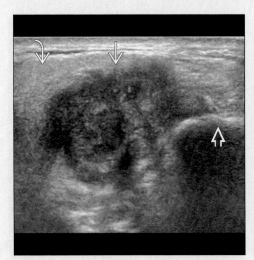
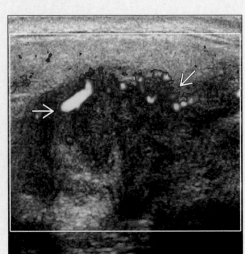

(Left) Transverse grayscale US in a patient presenting with constant facial pain shows an ill-defined, solid, hypoechoic, heterogeneous mass ➡ in the superficial parotid lobe ➡. US features are strongly suspicious of malignant salivary tumor, and biopsy confirmed MECa. Note the mandible ➡. (Right) Corresponding longitudinal power Doppler US shows moderate intratumoral vascularity ➡. In patients with parotid malignancy, prognosis is worse in those presenting with constant pain.

PAROTID MUCOEPIDERMOID CARCINOMA

TERMINOLOGY

Abbreviations
- Mucoepidermoid carcinoma (MECa)

Definitions
- Malignant epithelial salivary gland neoplasm composed of variable admixture of epidermoid and mucus-secreting cells arising from ductal epithelium

IMAGING

General Features
- Best diagnostic clue
  - Imaging appearance based on MECa histologic grade
    - Low-grade MECa: Well-defined, solid, hypoechoic, homogeneous/heterogeneous parotid mass
    - High-grade MECa: Ill-defined, hypoechoic, heterogeneous mass, ± infiltration into adjacent soft tissues and associated malignant nodes
    - Malignant adenopathy often present with high-grade tumors (readily assessed by US)
      - 1st order nodes = jugulodigastric nodes (level 2)
      - Intrinsic parotid nodes and parotid tail nodes also involved (simulate nodal parotid metastases)
- Superficial lobe > > deep lobe parotid (amenable to US)

Ultrasonographic Findings
- Grayscale ultrasound
  - US features depend on tumor grade; low grade similar to benign mixed tumor (BMT)
  - Low-grade MECa
    - Solid mass with well-defined margin
    - Predominantly homogeneous echo pattern
    - No extraglandular invasion or lymphadenopathy
  - High-grade MECa
    - Solid mass with ill-defined margin
    - Hypoechoic with heterogeneous architecture (due to necrosis and hemorrhage)
    - Extraglandular invasion into adjacent soft tissue ± skin involvement
  - High-grade MECa: ± associated intraparotid and jugulodigastric lymph node metastases
- Color Doppler
  - Pronounced intratumoral vascularity
- Spectral Doppler
  - Increased intravascular resistance
    - Resistive index (RI) > 0.8; pulsatility index (PI) > 2.0

Imaging Recommendations
- Best imaging tool
  - As MECa commonly involves superficial lobe of parotid, US is ideal initial imaging modality
  - US identifies malignancy ± metastatic nodes and guides biopsy but cannot differentiate between various malignant parotid lesions
  - US is readily combined with guided fine-needle aspiration cytology (FNAC) to ↑ specificity
  - US cannot visualize facial nerve: Position is inferred by identifying retromandibular vein (RMV) or external carotid artery as they run together in parotid gland
  - US cannot evaluate deep extent of superficial lobe MECa and may miss a deep lobe tumor
  - MR best delineates MECa local/regional extension and perineural spread
- Protocol advice
  - In evaluating parotid masses, assess
    - Edge: Benign tumors have well-defined edges; malignant tumors have ill-defined edges; low-grade MECa may have well-defined edges mimicking benign lesions
      - If associated sialadenitis, benign tumors may show ill-defined edges
    - Internal architecture: Benign tumors have homogeneous internal echoes, whereas malignant tumors have heterogeneous echo pattern due to necrosis and hemorrhage; low-grade MECa may have homogeneous echo pattern
    - Malignant tumors are more likely associated with adjacent soft tissue and nodal involvement
    - Malignant tumors have prominent vessels and high resistance (RI > 0.8, PI > 2.0)

DIFFERENTIAL DIAGNOSIS

Benign Mixed Tumor (BMT)
- Well-defined, lobulated, solid, hypoechoic, homogeneous echo pattern, posterior enhancement, and sparse vascularity

Warthin Tumor
- 20% multicentric, well-defined, hypoechoic with solid & cystic elements, thick septa, occur in parotid tail

Adenoid Cystic Carcinoma (ACCa)
- Well/ill defined, hypoechoic, homogeneous/heterogeneous echo pattern, prominent vascularity
- Prone to perineural spread

Non-Hodgkin Lymphoma (NHL)
- Primary parotid NHL: Invasive parenchymal tumor simulating high-grade MECa or ACCa
- Primary nodal NHL: Multiple bilateral, solid hypoechoic nodes with abnormal vascularity

Metastases to Parotid Nodes
- Primary lesion on or around skin of ear (SCCa, melanoma), nasopharyngeal carcinoma
- Solitary/multiple parotid masses with ill-defined, hypoechoic, heterogeneous architecture

DIAGNOSTIC CHECKLIST

Image Interpretation Pearls
- Low-grade MECa closely mimics BMT, always has high degree of suspicion
- High-grade MECa has nonspecific invasive appearance
- General evaluation of parotid space masses
  - Decide whether lesion is intraparotid or extraparotid
    - If intraparotid, distinguish superficial vs. deep lobe
      - Divided by facial nerve plane, just lateral to RMV
  - Sharpness of margin, internal architecture, and vascularity help distinguish benign from malignant lesions
  - Remember to look for nodal metastases

SELECTED REFERENCES

1. Lee YY et al: Imaging of salivary gland tumours. Eur J Radiol. 66(3):419-36, 2008

PAROTID MUCOEPIDERMOID CARCINOMA

(Left) Longitudinal grayscale US shows a high-grade parotid MECa ➡. It is ill defined, solid, hypoechoic, and heterogeneous with presence of an associated malignant level II lymph node ➡. *(Right)* Corresponding power Doppler US shows abnormal vascularity within the primary tumor ➡ and metastatic node ➡. Recurrence & survival rates depend on tumor grade. High grade: 78% local recurrence, 27% 10-year survival rate. Distant metastases in high grade > > low/intermediate grade.

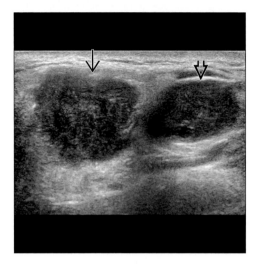
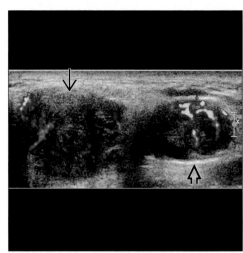

(Left) Axial T1WI MR (same patient) shows a solid, intermediate signal infiltrative parotid mass ➡. T1 unenhanced scans best delineate the tumor, as high signal fat of the normal parotid provides natural contrast. *(Right)* Axial T1WI MR (same patient) shows a malignant node associated with high-grade parotid MECa ➡. Jugulodigastric/level II nodes are 1st-order nodes of involvement. Intraparotid nodes are other commonly involved nodes.

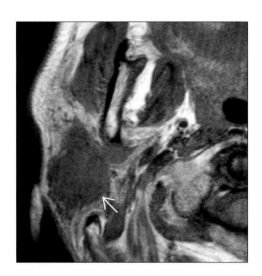
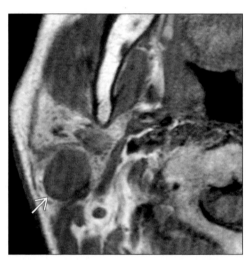

(Left) Transverse grayscale US shows a well-defined, hypoechoic, heterogeneous mass ➡ in the superficial lobe of the parotid ➡. Note intratumoral cystic areas ➡ and mandible ➡. *(Right)* Corresponding power Doppler US shows large intratumoral vessels in the solid portion of the tumor ➡. US features resemble Warthin tumor. Biopsy confirmed MECa. Presence of vascularity in the solid component distinguishes it from Warthin where the "solid" portion is avascular on Doppler.

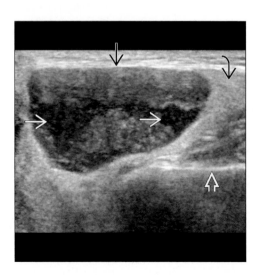
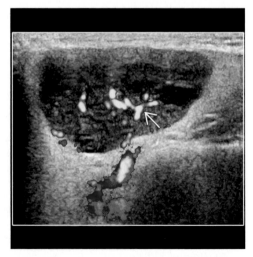

PAROTID MUCOEPIDERMOID CARCINOMA

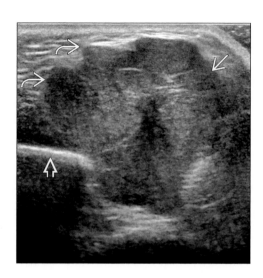

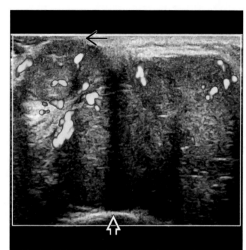

(Left) Transverse US shows recurrent MECa ➡️. Note that it is solid, hypoechoic, "bosselated" ➡️, and fairly homogeneous in architecture. US features mimic parotid BMT. Mandible ⟱ is shown. *(Right)* Corresponding longitudinal power Doppler US shows large intratumoral vascularity and subtle extension to skin and subcutaneous tissue ➡️. Note mandible ⟱. Although US safely guides needle for biopsy, it does not delineate anatomical extent and involvement of adjacent structures.

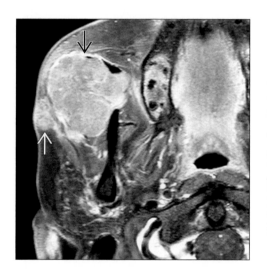

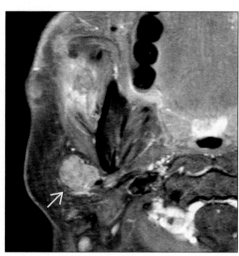

(Left) Corresponding axial T1WI C+ FS MR (same patient) shows solid, homogeneous (vs. heterogeneous) enhancement, and clearly delineates the extent of MECa ➡️ and cutaneous/subcutaneous involvement ➡️. *(Right)* Axial T1WI C+ FS MR (same patient) shows another intensely enhancing tumor ➡️ in the right parotid gland. This lesion was seen on US, and guided biopsy confirmed high-grade MECa, which has high recurrence rates (78% local recurrence).

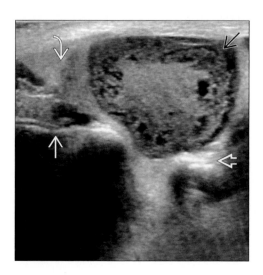

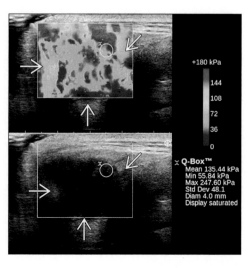

(Left) Transverse grayscale US shows an unusual looking lesion ➡️ in superficial parotid ➡️: Well-defined, hypoechoic, heterogeneous with small cystic areas & posterior enhancement ➡️. Note mandible ➡️. Tumor heterogeneity raised suspicion; guided biopsy confirmed MECa. *(Right)* Transverse grayscale US & SWE show parotid MECa ➡️. SWE color scale ranges from blue (0 kPa, soft) to red (180 kPa, stiff). It has a heterogeneous SWE pattern with several red areas & max SWE of 247.6 kPa (very stiff).

PAROTID ADENOID CYSTIC CARCINOMA

Key Facts

Imaging

- US is unable to differentiate adenoid cystic carcinoma (ACCa) from other salivary gland malignancies
- Low-grade tumors may be well defined with homogeneous internal architecture
- High-grade tumors are ill defined with invasive edges and heterogeneous areas of necrosis/hemorrhage
- ± extraglandular invasion of soft tissues, perineural spread
- ± adjacent nodal, disseminated metastases
- Spectral Doppler: Increased intravascular resistance
- US is useful in identifying tumor, predicting malignancy, and guiding biopsy
  - However, US cannot accurately delineate extent of large tumors or detect perineural spread
- MR best delineates extent of tumor and perineural spread

Top Differential Diagnoses

- Benign mixed tumor
- Parotid mucoepidermoid carcinoma
- Warthin tumor
- Parotid nodal metastasis

Clinical Issues

- 2nd most frequent parotid malignancy (after mucoepidermoid carcinoma)
- Painful, hard parotid mass; present months to years
- Peak: 5th to 7th decades; rare < 20 years
- 33% present with pain and CN7 paralysis
- Greatest propensity of all head & neck tumors to spread via perineural pathway
- Favorable short-term but poor long-term prognosis
- Late local recurrence common, ≤ 20 years after Dx
- Metastatic spread to lungs and bones > > lymph nodes
- Predictors of distant metastases: Tumor > 3 cm, solid pattern, local recurrence, nodal disease

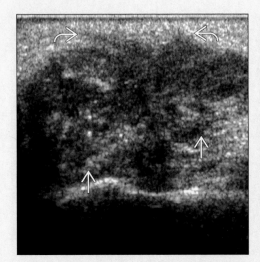
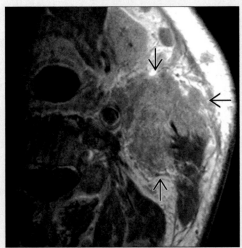

(Left) Transverse grayscale US shows a high-grade adenoid cystic carcinoma (ACCa) ➡ seen as a solid, ill-defined, hypoechoic mass with extraglandular extension ➡. US predicts malignancy but cannot differentiate between types. *(Right)* Corresponding T1WI C+ MR shows the extent of the ill-defined, parotid ACCa ➡. Although US can detect tumors in the superficial lobe, identify malignancy, and guides biopsy, MR best detects perineural spread and delineates anatomical relations and extent of tumor.

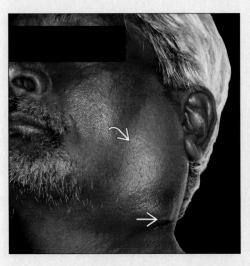
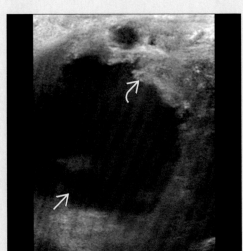

(Left) Clinical photograph shows a patient with a large, parotid region mass ➡, present for many years and now causing pain. Note skin infiltration over mass ➡. (Courtesy Suresh, MD and Anbarasu, MD.) *(Right)* Corresponding grayscale US shows a large, predominantly cystic tumor ➡ with a solid component at its periphery ➡. Guided biopsy confirmed ACCa. US visualized a large parotid mass and a guided biopsy for confirmatory diagnosis was performed, but did not evaluate the extent and anatomical location.

PAROTID ADENOID CYSTIC CARCINOMA

TERMINOLOGY

Abbreviations
- Parotid adenoid cystic carcinoma (ACCa)

Definitions
- Malignant salivary gland neoplasm arising in peripheral parotid ducts

IMAGING

General Features
- Best diagnostic clue
  - Low-grade ACCa: Well-defined, homogeneous, hypoechoic mass
  - High-grade ACCa: Ill-defined, heterogeneous, hypoechoic mass with extraglandular invasion
- Location
  - May involve superficial or deep parotid lobes

Ultrasonographic Findings
- Grayscale ultrasound
  - US is unable to differentiate ACCa from other salivary gland malignancies
  - Low-grade tumors may be well defined with homogeneous internal architecture
  - High-grade tumors are ill defined with invasive edges and heterogeneous areas of necrosis/hemorrhage
  - ± extraglandular invasion of soft tissues, perineural spread
  - ± adjacent nodal, disseminated metastases
- Color Doppler
  - Color Doppler: Pronounced intratumoral vascularity
  - Spectral Doppler: Increased intravascular resistance
    - Resistive index > 0.8, pulsatility index > 2.0

CT Findings
- CECT
  - Low grade: Homogeneously enhancing, well-circumscribed mass
  - High grade: Enhancing mass with poorly defined margins

MR Findings
- T1WI
  - Low to intermediate signal intensity
- T2WI
  - Moderate signal intensity
  - High grade tend to be lower in signal intensity
- T1WI C+
  - Solid homogeneous enhancement of mass
  - Perineural tumor on CN7 &/or CN5

Imaging Recommendations
- Best imaging tool
  - US evaluates superficial parotid but is unable to evaluate deep lobe masses or deep extension of superficial lobe lesions
  - US combined with guided fine-needle aspiration cytology (FNAC) has sensitivity of 83%, specificity of 86%, and accuracy of 85% for salivary gland masses
- Protocol advice
  - Carefully evaluate tumor edge, extraglandular/nodal involvement, internal heterogeneity
  - US is useful in identifying tumor, predicting malignancy, and guiding biopsy
    - However, US cannot accurately delineate extent of large tumors or detect perineural spread
  - MR best delineates tumor extent and perineural spread

DIFFERENTIAL DIAGNOSIS

Benign Mixed Tumor
- Well-defined, homogeneous, hypoechoic mass with posterior enhancement
- Lobulated/bosselated when large
- May be indistinguishable from low-grade ACCa

Parotid Mucoepidermoid Carcinoma
- Well defined or infiltrative, depending on tumor grade
- Malignant nodes present with high-grade tumors

Warthin Tumor
- Parotid tail in location, well defined, hypoechoic, solid with cystic component and septa
- May be multicentric and bilateral

Parotid Nodal Metastasis
- Known primary draining into parotid nodes; ill-defined, solid, hypoechoic mass, ± intranodal necrosis
- ± multiple nodal involvement

PATHOLOGY

General Features
- Superficially located, slow-growing neoplasm with propensity for perineural extension and late recurrence

Staging, Grading, & Classification
- Tumor grading based on dominant histologic pattern
  - Grade 1 = tubular; grade 2 = cribriform; grade 3 = solid

CLINICAL ISSUES

Presentation
- Most common signs/symptoms
  - Painful, hard parotid mass; present months to years
  - 33% present with pain and CN7 paralysis

Demographics
- Age
  - Peak: 5th to 7th decades; rare < 20 years
- Epidemiology
  - 7-18% of parotid tumors are ACCa (higher percentage in smaller salivary glands)
  - Greatest propensity of all head & neck tumors to spread via perineural pathway

Natural History & Prognosis
- Favorable short-term but poor long-term prognosis
- Late local recurrence common, ≤ 20 years after diagnosis
- Metastatic spread to lungs and bones more frequent than lymph nodes
- Predictors of distant metastases: Tumor > 3 cm, solid pattern, local recurrence, nodal disease

SELECTED REFERENCES

1. Lee YY et al: Imaging of salivary gland tumours. Eur J Radiol. 66(3):419-36, 2008

PAROTID ADENOID CYSTIC CARCINOMA

(Left) Transverse grayscale US of parotid ACCa shows a heterogeneous, infiltrative mass ➤ in proximity to the intraparotid portion of CN7 (as inferred by the location of retromandibular vein [RMV] ➤). Note that its extent behind the mandible ➤ cannot be evaluated. *(Right)* Corresponding longitudinal grayscale US clearly defines the intraparotid origin of the mass ➤ with no extension into overlying subcutaneous tissue. Note its infiltrative edges ➤, characteristic of malignant salivary tumor.

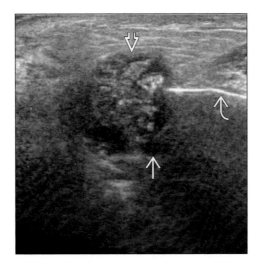
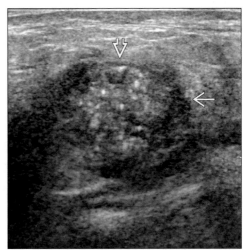

(Left) Transverse power Doppler US (same patient) shows no significant intratumoral vascularity. Note the location of the RMV ➤, which is closely related to intraparotid CN7. *(Right)* Axial T2WI MR clearly defines the location and extent of the parotid ACCa, seen as a hyperintense mass ➤ in the right parotid gland. Although the US identified the mass, suggested the malignant nature of the mass, and guided biopsy for confirmation, MR best delineates the tumor's extent.

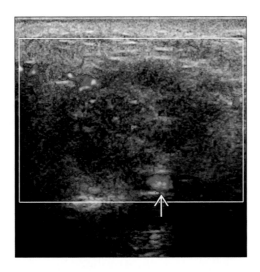
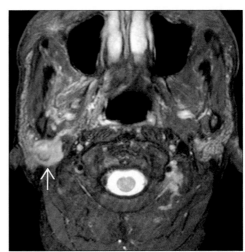

(Left) Corresponding axial T1WI C+ FS MR shows a solid, homogeneous enhancement of the mass ➤ and ill-defined borders. *(Right)* Oblique T1WI C+ MR (same patient) clearly shows perineural spread along CN7 ➤. Although imaging may be unable to differentiate between various parotid malignancies, ACCa has the greatest propensity of all head & neck tumors to spread via the perineural pathway. It also explains facial pain and paralysis in such patients.

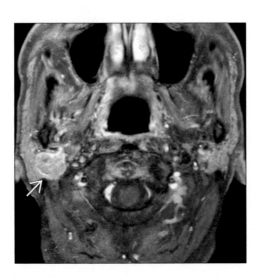
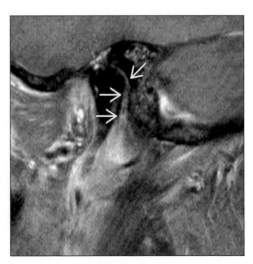

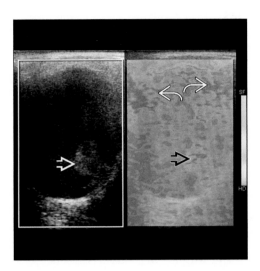

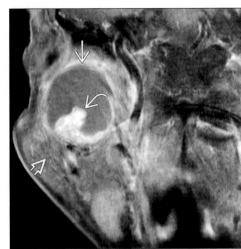

(Left) Transverse grayscale US and qualitative strain elastogram show cystic parotid ACCa with a small mural nodule ➔. Strain color scale ranges from purple (elastic, soft) to red (inelastic, hard). The nodule appears inelastic ➔ although strain EI is unreliable in markedly cystic nodules. Note compression artifacts in the near field ➔. *(Right)* Corresponding coronal T1WI C+ MR defines the location of mass ➔ in relation to the parotid ➔ and delineates the cystic component from solid-enhancing mural nodule ➔.

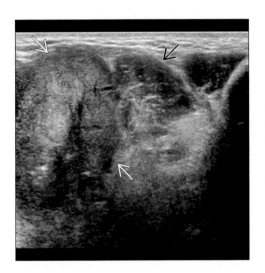

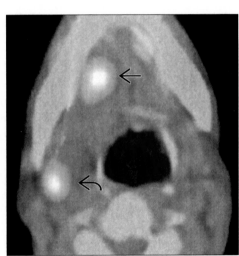

(Left) Transverse grayscale US shows a large mass ➔, submental in location, displacing the anterior belly of the digastric muscle ➔. It is solid, hypoechoic, and ill defined. Biopsy confirmed ACCa. *(Right)* Corresponding PET/CT shows FDG-avid masses in the sublingual region ➔ and right upper neck ➔, consistent with sublingual ACCa with nodal metastases. ACCa accounts for 12% of submandibular gland tumors, 15% of sublingual gland tumors, and 30% of minor salivary gland tumors.

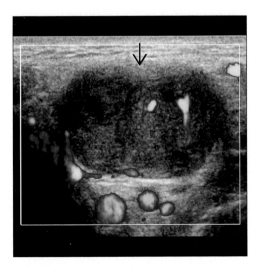

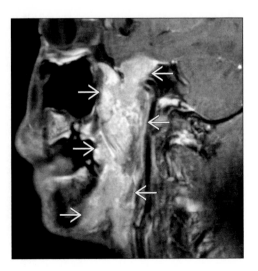

(Left) Transverse power Doppler US (same patient) shows a metastatic jugulodigastric node ➔ corresponding to the FDG-avid node seen on PET/CT. In high-grade ACCa, metastases to lungs and bone > > lymph nodes. *(Right)* Corresponding longitudinal T1WI C+ FS MR shows marked perineural spread ➔ of sublingual ACCa extending to the skull base. In large tumors, MR better delineates tumor origin, extent, and perineural spread, which is hallmark of ACCa in head & neck.

PAROTID ACINIC CELL CARCINOMA

Key Facts

Imaging

- Almost 80% occur in parotid gland
- Can be multifocal and bilateral; 3% involve both parotid glands
- 2nd most common multiple/bilateral primary salivary gland tumor after Warthin
- Usually well marginated
- Ill-defined borders are occasionally seen
- Heterogeneously hypoechoic solid mass
- May contain cystic or necrotic components
- Infrequently appears as a predominantly cystic lesion with mural nodule
- ± metastatic cervical lymph nodes
- Moderate to marked intralesional flow signal

Top Differential Diagnoses

- Warthin tumor
- Metastatic disease to parotid gland
- Other primary parotid carcinomas

- Non-Hodgkin lymphoma

Clinical Issues

- Most commonly presents in 5th to 6th decades of life
- 4% of patients < 20 years of age
- 2nd most common pediatric parotid malignancy after mucoepidermoid carcinoma
- Acinic cell carcinoma (AciCC) is an indolent malignancy with better prognosis compared to other salivary gland cancers
- Tumors in minor salivary glands tend to be less aggressive than those in major salivary glands
- Recurrence rates of 30-50% have been reported
- Initially metastasizes to cervical lymph nodes

Diagnostic Checklist

- May be indistinguishable from benign or other malignant salivary gland neoplasms on imaging
- Diagnosis often made by biopsy/surgery

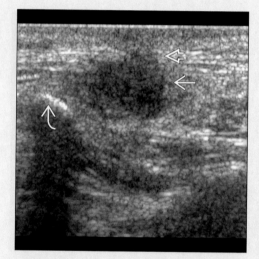
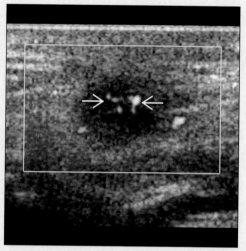

(Left) Transverse grayscale US of a patient with acinic cell carcinoma (AciCC) shows a hypoechoic mass with ill-defined borders ➡, located within the superficial lobe of the right parotid gland. Note subtle extraglandular extension ➡ into subcutaneous tissue. Mandible ➡ is also shown. *(Right)* Corresponding power Doppler US of the same lesion shows moderate disorganized hypervascularity within ➡. In clinical practice, vascular distribution and intravascular resistance are not consistent predictors of malignancy in salivary masses.

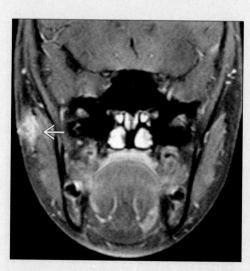
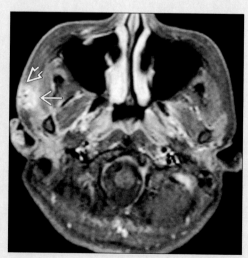

(Left) Coronal T1WI C+ FS MR of the same patient reveals moderate post-contrast enhancement of the tumor ➡. *(Right)* Corresponding axial T1WI FS MR again shows an ill-defined enhancing mass in superficial lobe of right parotid gland ➡. Here, there is local infiltration of muscular and subcutaneous layers ➡. AciCC can have nonspecific imaging features shared by other parotid malignancies. MR delineates deep lobe & evaluates multiplicity/bilaterality.

PAROTID ACINIC CELL CARCINOMA

TERMINOLOGY

Abbreviations
- Acinic cell carcinoma (AciCC)

Synonyms
- Acinic cell adenocarcinoma
- Acinous cell carcinoma

Definitions
- Malignant epithelial neoplasm of salivary glands in which neoplastic cells demonstrate acinar differentiation

IMAGING

General Features
- Location
  - Almost 80% occur in parotid gland
  - ~ 17% are found in intraoral minor salivary glands
  - Uncommonly found in other major salivary glands
    - 4% submandibular
    - < 1% sublingual
  - Can be multifocal and bilateral; 3% involve both parotid glands
    - AciCC is 2nd most common multiple or bilateral primary salivary gland tumor following Warthin tumor
- Size
  - Usually 1-3 cm
- Morphology
  - Most commonly well defined
  - Can occasionally be ill defined with irregular borders

Ultrasonographic Findings
- Grayscale ultrasound
  - Usually well marginated
  - Ill-defined borders are occasionally seen
  - Heterogeneously hypoechoic solid mass
    - May contain cystic or necrotic components
    - Infrequently appears as predominantly cystic lesion with mural nodule
  - Not uncommonly multifocal and bilateral lesions
  - ± metastatic cervical lymph nodes
- Color Doppler
  - Moderate to marked intralesional flow signal

CT Findings
- NECT
  - Mildly hyperattenuating to background parotid parenchyma
  - Low-attenuation components represent cystic or necrotic areas
- CECT
  - Mild to moderate intralesional enhancement

MR Findings
- T1WI
  - Hypointense signal relative to background parotid parenchyma
- T2WI
  - Both hypointense and hyperintense signals have been reported
    - Cystic and necrotic components appear markedly hyperintense
  - Heterogeneous signal intensity may correspond with hemorrhage and necrosis
- STIR
  - Cystic and necrotic areas appear more conspicuous
- T1WI C+
  - Mild to moderate intralesional enhancement

Imaging Recommendations
- Best imaging tool
  - US
    - Optimal characterization of lesions in superficial lobe
    - Capability of guiding fine-needle aspiration or biopsy for pathological diagnosis
  - MR
    - Required to fully assess deep lobe of parotid (particularly multiplicity) and evaluate any extraglandular spread

DIFFERENTIAL DIAGNOSIS

Warthin Tumor
- Well defined with cystic components
- Frequently bilateral
- When circumscribed, AciCC can be indistinguishable from Warthin tumor

Metastatic Disease of Parotid Gland
- Multiple ill-defined intraparotid nodes
- Pronounced abnormal vascularity on color Doppler
- Primary malignancy is usually known clinically or apparent

Mucoepidermoid Carcinoma
- Well or ill defined depending on histologic grade; heterogeneous (cystic necrosis/hemorrhage)
- Infrequently multicentric compared with acinic cell carcinoma

Adenoid Cystic Carcinoma
- Well or ill defined depending on histologic grade
- Prone to perineural spread
- Infrequently multicentric

Non-Hodgkin Lymphoma (NHL)
- Bilateral intraparotid nodes with abnormal vascularity (hilar > peripheral)
- Primary NHL of parotid gland appears as infiltrative mass, ± abnormal nodes

PATHOLOGY

Staging, Grading, & Classification
- Several histolomorphologic growth patterns have been described including acinar, intercalated ductal, vacuolated, clear, solid/lobular, papillary-cystic, microcystic, and follicular
  - Although single growth pattern dominates, > 1 type often occurs simultaneously in lesion
  - Grouping plays no significant role in predicting clinical behavior
- Histological grading has been controversial and inconsistent

Gross Pathologic & Surgical Features
- Commonly circumscribed but can be ill-defined

PAROTID ACINIC CELL CARCINOMA

- Cut surface appears lobular and tan to red in color
- Vary in consistency: Cystic, soft to solid

Microscopic Features

- Diagnosis depends on identifying cells with acinar differentiation
  - Acinar cells are large, polygonal cells with mild basophilic cytoplasm and round eccentric nuclei
  - Cytoplasmic zymogen-like granules are periodic acid-Schiff (PAS) positive and resistant to diastase digestion
  - Immunohistochemical staining is nonspecific
- Acinar tumor cells are closely apposed together in sheets, nodules, or aggregates in solid/lobular form (most common subtype)

CLINICAL ISSUES

Presentation

- Most common signs/symptoms
  - Slow, progressive facial swelling
  - ~ 1/3 of patients experience vague intermittent pain
  - 5-10% develop facial nerve paralysis
  - Duration of symptoms can occasionally be prolonged (up to decades) in some cases

Demographics

- Age
  - Most commonly presents in 5th to 6th decades of life
  - 4% of patients < 20 years of age
    - 2nd most common pediatric parotid malignancy after mucoepidermoid carcinoma
- Gender
  - Slight female preponderance
    - F:M ≈ 1.5:1
- Ethnicity
  - No ethnic predilection
- Epidemiology
  - Comprises 1% of all salivary gland neoplasms and ~ 10% of parotid gland malignancies

Natural History & Prognosis

- Majority display indolent growth but recurrence rates of 30-50% have been reported
- Initially metastasizes to cervical lymph nodes
- 7-29% incidence of distant metastasis has been reported
  - Most common site is to lungs
- Relatively good prognosis compared with other salivary gland malignances
  - Reported survival rates vary, with 10-year survival ranging 55-89%
- Tumors in minor salivary glands tend to be less aggressive than those in major salivary glands

Treatment

- Surgical excision
  - Total or superficial parotidectomy with dissection of facial nerve
  - Facial nerve may be sacrificed in patients presenting with nerve palsy, which indicates tumor infiltration
  - Surgery alone is satisfactory for disease control if no extracapsular spread
  - Surgical margin is regarded to have prognostic significance
- Neck dissection

  - Usually only performed with clinically apparent cervical nodal disease
  - Role of routine dissection, even in clinically negative cervical nodes, is controversial
- Radiotherapy
  - Used as adjunct treatment in cases of
    - Tumor recurrence
    - Positive margins or tumor spillage
    - Tumor with deep lobe involvement, or adjacent to facial nerve
    - Large tumors (> 4 cm) or tumors with extraparotid extension
    - Nodal metastasis

DIAGNOSTIC CHECKLIST

Consider

- AciCC is an indolent malignancy with better prognosis compared to other salivary gland cancers
- Patient may experience symptoms for several years, even decades, before clinical presentation

Image Interpretation Pearls

- Nonspecific imaging features
  - Can appear as circumscribed or ill-defined masses
  - May be indistinguishable from benign or other malignant salivary gland neoplasms on imaging
  - Diagnosis often made by biopsy/surgery
- Not infrequently multifocal and bilateral

SELECTED REFERENCES

1. Jia YL et al: Synchronous bilateral multifocal acinic cell carcinoma of parotid gland: case report and review of the literature. J Oral Maxillofac Surg. 70(10):e574-80, 2012
2. Gomez DR et al: Clinical and pathologic prognostic features in acinic cell carcinoma of the parotid gland. Cancer. 115(10):2128-37, 2009
3. Ellis G et al. Tumors of the Salivary Glands AFIP Atlas of Tumor Pathology: Series 4. American Registry of Pathology. 4th ed. 216-8, 2008
4. Lee YY et al: Imaging of salivary gland tumours. Eur J Radiol. 66(3):419-36, 2008
5. Yabuuchi H et al: Parotid gland tumors: can addition of diffusion-weighted MR imaging to dynamic contrast-enhanced MR imaging improve diagnostic accuracy in characterization? Radiology. 249(3):909-16, 2008
6. Thoeny HC: Imaging of salivary gland tumours. Cancer Imaging. 7:52-62, 2007
7. Suh SI et al: Acinic cell carcinoma of the head and neck: radiologic-pathologic correlation. J Comput Assist Tomogr. 29(1):121-6, 2005
8. Federspil PA et al: [Acinic cell carcinomas of the parotid gland. A retrospective analysis.] HNO. 49(10):825-30, 2001
9. Hoffman HT et al: National Cancer Data Base report on cancer of the head and neck: acinic cell carcinoma. Head Neck. 21(4):297-309, 1999
10. Laskawi R et al: Retrospective analysis of 35 patients with acinic cell carcinoma of the parotid gland. J Oral Maxillofac Surg. 56(4):440-3, 1998
11. Sakai O et al: Acinic cell Carcinoma of the parotid gland: CT and MRI. Neuroradiology. 38(7):675-9, 1996

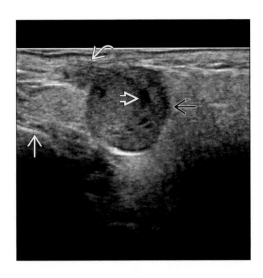

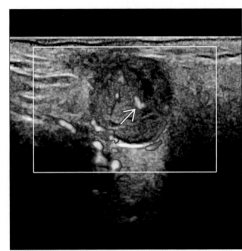

(Left) Transverse grayscale US in a patient with previous excisional biopsy of a left parotid mass reveals AciCC. There is residual tumor in the superficial lobe, which appears as a round, well-defined hypoechoic mass ➡. Note small cystic areas within the lesion ➡ & an ill-defined hypoechoic area in overlying skin, corresponding to postsurgical change ➡. Note the mandible ➡. (Right) Corresponding transverse power Doppler US reveals moderate, nondiscriminatory intralesional vascularity ➡.

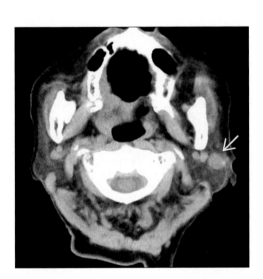

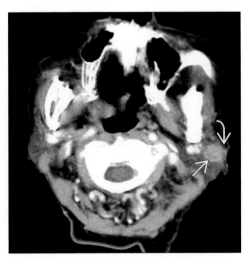

(Left) Axial NECT of the same patient shows residual tumor in the superficial lobe ➡, hyperattenuating relative to the background parotid parenchyma. (Right) Post-contrast CT of the patient shows mild enhancement of the tumor ➡. Subtle mild enhancement of overlying subcutaneous tissue ➡ is also noted, corresponding to changes from previous excisional biopsy. Patient went on to receive total left parotidectomy, which showed clear margins.

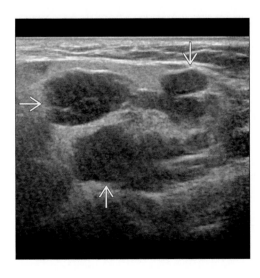

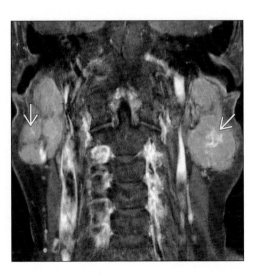

(Left) Longitudinal grayscale US shows numerous hypoechoic masses ➡ in the superficial parotid. (Right) Corresponding coronal T1WI C+ FS MR shows multiple bilateral parotid masses with mild intralesional enhancement ➡. Cytology findings, together with multifocal nature, were suspicious for AciCC. However, it should be stressed that imaging features for AciCC are nonspecific and final histologic diagnosis for this was in fact oncocytoma.

PAROTID NON-HODGKIN LYMPHOMA

Key Facts

Imaging

- Nodal non-Hodgkin lymphoma (NHL): Solitary or multiple enlarged ovoid intraparotid lymph nodes
  - Homogeneously hypoechoic relative to parotid parenchyma, reticulated echo pattern
  - Posterior acoustic enhancement
  - Pronounced hilar hypervascularity
- Mucosa-associated lymphoid tissue lymphoma (MALToma): Diffuse heterogeneous echo pattern, ill-defined hypoechoic mass-like areas
  - Punctate intracystic or parenchymal calcification due to end-stage inflammatory change
  - Small cystic areas due to compression of terminal ducts by lymphoid hypertrophy
  - Multiple small hypoechoic areas (thought to represent lymphoid aggregates) scattered against background salivary tissue
  - Diffuse glandular hypervascularity

- Mimics chronic sialadenitis, with diagnosis often made by biopsy
- ± periparotid and cervical lymphadenopathy
- Bilateral disease with systemic NHL only; MALToma often bilateral, is 30% multiglandular

Top Differential Diagnoses

- Parotid Sjögren syndrome (SS)
- Parotid sialadenitis
- Benign lymphoepithelial lesions-HIV
- Parotid nodal metastatic disease

Diagnostic Checklist

- In patient with new parotid mass, background heterogeneous parotids suggest NHL with SS
- Evaluate contralateral parotid, other salivary and lacrimal glands, and extent of cervical nodes
- Imaging features may be suggestive, but excisional biopsy is frequently required for definitive diagnosis

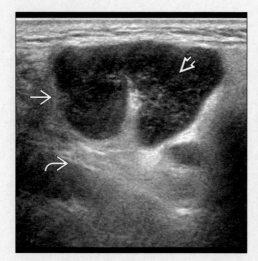
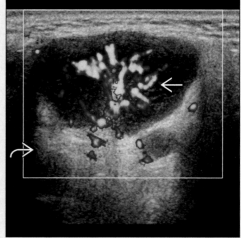

(Left) Oblique grayscale US of the right parotid gland shows a well-defined, solid, enlarged lymph node ➡ with a typical internal reticulated echo pattern ➡. Note posterior acoustic enhancement ➡. *(Right)* Corresponding power Doppler US shows marked hilar ➡ and posterior acoustic enhancement ➡. Hilar vascularity much greater than peripheral vascularity is a feature of lymphomatous nodes. Incisional biopsy of this lesion revealed atypical lymphoid proliferation.

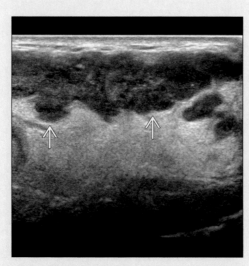
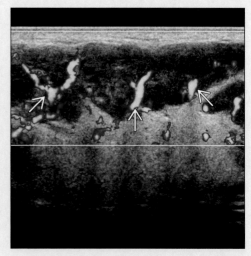

(Left) Longitudinal grayscale US of the right parotid gland in a patient with known cutaneous T-cell lymphoma shows multiple hypoechoic nodular masses that represent a conglomerate of intraparotid nodes ➡. *(Right)* Corresponding power Doppler US displays moderate central vascularity within the parotid nodes ➡. Nodal salivary lymphoma is restricted to parotid glands as embryologically there are no lymph nodes within submandibular gland salivary tissue.

PAROTID NON-HODGKIN LYMPHOMA

TERMINOLOGY

Abbreviations
- Non-Hodgkin lymphoma (NHL)

Definitions
- NHL includes any of various lymphomas, characterized by absence of Reed-Steinberg cells
  - Can be categorized into aggressive/high-grade or indolent/low-grade types
  - Formed by either B cells or T cells
- Different forms of parotid involvement with NHL
  - Nodal NHL
    - Primary nodal NHL
    - Systemic NHL involving parotid nodes
  - Primary parenchymal lymphoma
    - Most often mucosa-associated lymphoid tissue (MALT)-type NHL (MALToma), often associated with Sjögren syndrome (SS) or benign lymphoepithelial lesion (BLEL)

IMAGING

General Features
- Best diagnostic clue
  - Nodal NHL: Multiple homogeneous, well-defined parotid masses and upper cervical adenopathy
  - Parenchymal NHL: Infiltrative parotid mass, background SS, BLEL
- Location
  - Parotid gland ± ipsilateral neck nodes
  - Bilateral disease with systemic NHL only
  - MALToma is often bilateral, 30% are multiglandular
- Size
  - Nodal NHL
    - Usually 1-3 cm
  - Parenchyma NHL
    - May involve most of parotid &/or submandibular gland
- Morphology
  - Nodal NHL
    - Usually well-circumscribed masses
    - Round to ovoid, sometimes lobulated or irregular
    - May occasionally be matted but rarely necrotic
  - Parenchymal NHL
    - Diffusely infiltrating or ill-defined mass
    - May be solid or (less commonly) cystic

Ultrasonographic Findings
- Grayscale ultrasound
  - Nodal NHL
    - Solitary or multiple enlarged ovoid intraparotid lymph nodes
    - Homogeneously hypoechoic relative to parotid parenchyma
    - Reticulated echo pattern
    - Posterior acoustic enhancement
  - Primary parenchyma NHL
    - Diffuse heterogeneous echo pattern, ill-defined hypoechoic mass-like areas
    - Punctate intracystic or parenchymal calcification due to end-stage inflammatory change
    - Small cystic areas due to compression of terminal ducts by lymphoid hypertrophy

- Multiple, small hypoechoic areas (represent lymphoid aggregates) scattered against background salivary tissue
  - Mimic chronic sialadenitis, diagnosis often made by biopsy
  - Look for similar involvement of other salivary and lacrimal glands, background SS, BLEL
- May or may not have periparotid and cervical lymphadenopathy
- Color Doppler
  - Nodal NHL
    - Pronounced central or hilar hypervascularity
  - Parenchyma NHL
    - More diffuse glandular hypervascularity
    - Moderate to marked vascularity within ill-defined masses

CT Findings
- CECT
  - Nodal NHL
    - Multiple well-defined intraparotid masses
    - Mild to moderate homogeneous enhancement
    - Necrosis, calcification, and hemorrhage are rare
  - Primary parenchymal NHL
    - Ill-defined invasive lesion
    - May be difficult to appreciate if diffuse and isodense

MR Findings
- T1WI
  - Homogeneous intermediate-signal nodules or infiltrative mass, relative to hypointense parotid
- T2WI FS
  - Parotid lesions appear more conspicuous with fat saturation
  - Homogeneous intermediate to low signal intensity
- T1WI C+
  - Mild to moderate homogeneous enhancement

Nuclear Medicine Findings
- PET/CT
  - Nodal NHL
    - Typically markedly FDG avid
    - Benign parotid lesions may also be FDG avid
  - Parenchymal/MALT lymphoma
    - Variable, often less hypermetabolic
    - Role of PET is controversial

Imaging Recommendations
- Best imaging tool
  - US optimally characterizes lesions in superficial lobe of parotid and cervical lymphadenopathy and guides biopsy
    - MALToma mimics chronic sialadenitis or Kuttner tumor
      - Maintain high degree of suspicion
  - CECT to evaluate cervical lymphadenopathy and rest of body for staging
    - Isodense intraparotid lesions may not be visible
  - Deep lobe intraparotid lesions are more conspicuous on MR, especially T2 FS/STIR
    - Lesions may appear isointense and less distinct compared with US
  - PET or CT is typically performed for complete staging
- Protocol advice
  - Be sure to image from skull base to clavicles for staging of cervical disease

PAROTID NON-HODGKIN LYMPHOMA

- Not possible with US

DIFFERENTIAL DIAGNOSIS

Parotid Sjögren Syndrome
- Older female with connective tissue disease, dry eyes, dry mouth
- Bilateral enlarged parotid glands, small or large cysts, ± lymphoid aggregates
- Chronic: Atrophied, heterogeneous glands ± calcifications
- Has 40x incidence of NHL

Parotid Sialadenitis
- Diffuse heterogeneous echo pattern and hypervascularity may mimic parenchyma NHL
- May detect ductal dilatation and calculi
- Clinically presents with pain and swelling

Benign Lymphoepithelial Lesions-HIV
- Mixed cystic and solid intraparotid lesions enlarge both parotid glands
- If AIDS patient has NHL, imaging may be complex

Parotid Nodal Metastatic Disease
- Multiple unilateral or bilateral masses with invasive margins and often with central necrosis
- Often other nodal metastases: Levels II and V
- Periparotid skin, scalp, and nasopharynx primaries are frequent

PATHOLOGY

General Features
- Etiology
  - Unknown; possibly multifactorial
    - Environment, genetics, virus, prior radiation
  - Increased incidence with autoimmune disorders
    - SS has 40x incidence of NHL
    - Rheumatoid arthritis, systemic lupus
  - Increased incidence with immunosuppression

Staging, Grading, & Classification
- Modified Ann Arbor staging system is for clinical staging, treatment, and prognosis of NHL
  - Stage I: Single node region or lymphoid structure (e.g., spleen) or single extralymphatic site (IE)
  - Stage II: ≥ 2 node regions on same side of diaphragm (II) or contiguous extranodal organ/site + regional nodes ± other nodes on same side of diaphragm (IIE)
  - Stage III: Node regions on both sides of diaphragm (III), spleen (IIIS), extranodal (IIIE), both (IIISE)
  - Stage IV: Disseminated disease: ≥ 1 extranodal organ or tissue, ± nodes or isolated extralymphatic disease with distant nodes
- World Health Organization histological classification for NHL (2008)
  - Based on immunophenotype and morphology
  - B-cell (≤ 85%), T-cell, and putative NK-cell neoplasms

Gross Pathologic & Surgical Features
- Well-circumscribed, encapsulated, soft fleshy masses

Microscopic Features
- Sheets of homogeneous lymphoid cells arranged in diffuse or follicular pattern

- Subdivided into small-cleaved and large-cell variants
- Primary parotid lymphoma
  - Most often MALT-type NHL
  - Unilateral diffuse invasion of ductal and acinar tissue

CLINICAL ISSUES

Presentation
- Most common signs/symptoms
  - Slowly enlarging painless parotid mass ± cervical lymphadenopathy
  - Occasional systemic B symptoms: Fever, weight loss, night sweats
  - "Rubbery" consistency has been classically described on clinical palpation of lymphomatous nodes

Demographics
- Age
  - Mean age at presentation: 55 years
- Gender
  - M:F = 1.5:1
- Ethnicity
  - Caucasian > > African American, Hispanic, or Asian
  - Rare T-cell lymphomas are more common in young African American males
- Epidemiology
  - Primary parotid NHL; 2-5% of parotid malignancies
  - Systemic NHL involves parotid in 1-8%

Natural History & Prognosis
- Depends on histology, morphology, and stage
- Overall 5-year survival rate: 72%
  - High-grade disease: Rapidly progressive
  - Low-grade lesions: Slow progression over years
    - Best prognosis: Small cleaved cell & follicular forms
- Generally good prognosis with primary parotid NHL, although 35% recur at 5 years
  - Usually diagnosed early: Stage I or II

Treatment
- Tumor debulking may be performed for cosmetic purposes
- Chemotherapy & XRT remain mainstays of treatment

DIAGNOSTIC CHECKLIST

Consider
- In patient with new parotid mass, background heterogeneous parotids suggest NHL + SS

Image Interpretation Pearls
- On US, hypoechoic nodes with reticulated echo pattern are characteristic for parotid nodal NHL
- Parotid parenchymal NHL appears as small, ill-defined, hypoechoic lesions on US; may be indistinct on CT, MR
- Carefully evaluate contralateral parotid glands, other salivary & lacrimal glands, and extent of cervical nodes

Reporting Tips
- Imaging features may be suggestive, but excisional biopsy is frequently required for definitive diagnosis

SELECTED REFERENCES

1. Lee YY et al: Imaging of salivary gland tumours. Eur J Radiol. 66(3):419-36, 2008

PAROTID NON-HODGKIN LYMPHOMA

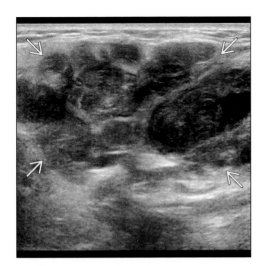

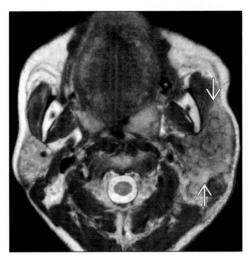

(Left) Longitudinal grayscale US of a patient with diffuse large B-cell lymphoma reveals parenchymal involvement of the left parotid gland. It appears as a large, hypoechoic, infiltrative lesion replacing the superficial lobe ➡. *(Right)* Corresponding axial T2WI MR shows the diffuse, infiltrative appearance of the left parotid lesion ➡ isointense to parotid parenchyma. Nonenhanced T1WI MR better delineates the infiltrative tumor edge as intraparotid fat provides natural background contrast.

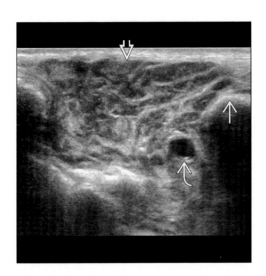

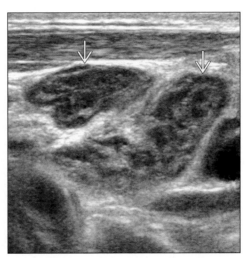

(Left) Transverse grayscale US of a patient with parotid MALToma shows diffuse involvement of the superficial parotid ➡ with multiple small, focal hypoechoic areas thought to represent lymphoid tissue. Note the mandible ➡ and RMV ➡. MALToma is more common in patients with Sjögren syndrome. *(Right)* Transverse grayscale US (same patient) shows multiple solid lymphomatous nodes ➡, typically reticulated. Focal intranodal hypoechoic areas reportedly represent lymphoid tissue.

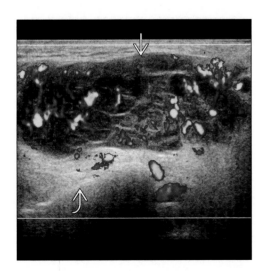

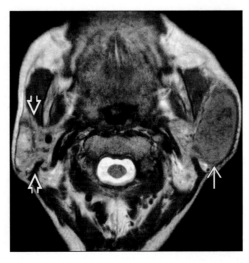

(Left) Transverse power Doppler US of the left parotid gland in a patient with MALToma shows a large, solid, hypoechoic mass in the superficial lobe ➡. The lesion has marked internal vascularity. Mandible ➡ is shown. *(Right)* Corresponding axial T2WI MR reveals a large hypointense mass in the superficial lobe of the left parotid gland ➡. Heterogeneity is also noted in the right parotid ➡. Findings are consistent with parenchymal parotid NHL, which is multiglandular in 30% and often bilateral.

METASTATIC DISEASE OF PAROTID NODES

Key Facts

Terminology

- Lymphatic or hematogenous tumor spread to intraglandular parotid lymph nodes
- Normal parotid has intraglandular lymph nodes (unlike submandibular and sublingual glands)
- Parotid and periparotid nodes: 1st-order nodal station for skin squamous cell carcinoma and melanoma from scalp, auricle, and face

Imaging

- Solitary or multiple hypoechoic masses in known distribution of intraparotid nodes
- Well defined or ill defined (extranodal spread)
- Look for local invasion: Intraparotid external carotid artery, retromandibular vein, extraparotid soft tissue
- Abnormal internal architecture ± echogenic hilus; homogeneous or heterogeneous with internal cystic areas in necrotic nodes
- ± metastatic cervical lymph nodes

- Chaotic/disorganized or predominantly peripheral
- Ultrasound: Optimally characterizes nodes in superficial lobe and guides confirmatory biopsy
- PET/CT: Most sensitive for discerning metastatic nature of small nodes
- MR: Most sensitive for extranodal involvement, especially perineural tumor spread on facial nerve

Top Differential Diagnoses

- For multifocal unilateral parotid masses with cervical adenopathy: Regional metastases, local non-Hodgkin lymphoma (NHL)
- For multifocal unilateral parotid masses without cervical adenopathy: Warthin tumor, recurrent benign mixed tumor, regional metastases
- For multifocal bilateral parotid masses: Systemic metastases, systemic NHL, Warthin tumors, HIV-related benign lymphoepithelial lesions, Sjögren disease

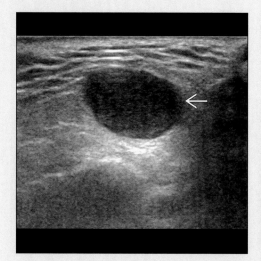
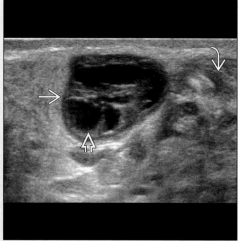

(Left) Transverse grayscale US of the left parotid gland in a patient with eyelid carcinoma reveals a well-defined, hypoechoic mass ➡ in the superficial lobe. *(Right)* Transverse grayscale US of a patient with nasopharyngeal carcinoma (NPC) shows a well-defined mass ➡ with internal cystic/necrotic components ➡ in the left parotid. These lesions were proven to be metastatic intraparotid nodes. Their well-defined nature mimics the benign tumor. However, note heterogeneous infiltrative tumor ➡ in adjacent tissue.

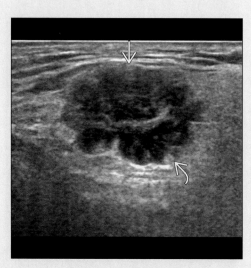
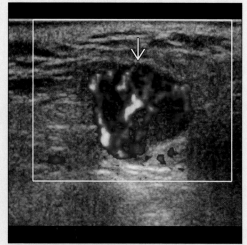

(Left) Grayscale US reveals an ill-defined, hypoechoic mass in the superficial lobe of the right parotid ➡. Note the spiculated margins ➡, typically seen in malignant lesions. *(Right)* Doppler US of another patient shows chaotic hypervascularity in an otherwise well-defined, intraparotid mass ➡. Both patients had a history of NPC, and the intraparotid lesions were confirmed to be nodal metastases. In absence of history of NPC, these lesions may be mistaken for primary salivary gland tumors.

METASTATIC DISEASE OF PAROTID NODES

TERMINOLOGY

Definitions
- Lymphatic or hematogenous tumor spread to intraparotid lymph nodes

IMAGING

General Features
- Best diagnostic clue
  - On its own, imaging features of parotid nodal metastasis are nonspecific
  - Solitary or multiple parotid masses
    - Well defined or ill defined (extranodal spread), homogeneous or heterogeneous with internal necrosis
    - Intranodular vascularity or enhancement
  - Associated with known primary cancer, often in adjacent skin or regional head and neck region
    - Parotid and periparotid nodes: 1st-order nodal station for skin squamous cell carcinoma (SCCa) and melanoma from lateral scalp, auricle/external auditory canal (EAC), and anterior face
- Location
  - Intraparotid ± periparotid
- Size
  - Usually 1-3 cm
- Morphology
  - Ovoid or round
  - Well defined or (if extranodal spread) infiltrative

Ultrasonographic Findings
- Grayscale ultrasound
  - Solitary or multiple hypoechoic masses in known distribution of intraparotid nodes
  - Well defined or poorly marginated (extranodal spread)
  - Extranodal spread
    - Look for local invasion of intraparotid external carotid artery (ECA), retromandibular vein, or extraparotid soft tissue
  - Abnormal internal architecture, ± echogenic hilus
    - Homogeneous or heterogeneous with internal cystic areas in necrotic nodes
  - ± metastatic cervical lymph nodes
- Power Doppler
  - Intralesional vascularity
    - Chaotic/disorganized or predominantly peripheral

CT Findings
- CECT
  - ≥ 1 intraparotid mass with sharp or invasive margins
  - Nodes may be homogeneous or heterogeneous with central necrosis
  - Preauricular ± cervical nodal metastases may also be present

MR Findings
- T1WI
  - Single mass or multiple intermediate signal masses
- T2WI
  - Uniform or heterogeneous (necrosis) high signal
- T1WI C+
  - Solid or rim (central nodal necrosis) enhancement of intraparotid nodal masses
  - If extranodal spread, may appear invasive
    - Best modality for assessing perineural infiltration of facial nerve (CN7), encasement of ECA, and extraparotid soft tissue invasion

Nuclear Medicine Findings
- PET
  - Metastatic intraparotid and cervical lymph nodes show increased metabolic activity
    - Benign parotid lesions can also be hypermetabolic

Imaging Recommendations
- Best imaging tool
  - Ultrasound: Optimally characterizes nodes in superficial lobe and guides confirmatory biopsy
  - PET/CT: Most sensitive for discerning metastatic nature of small nodes
  - MR: Most sensitive for extranodal involvement, especially perineural tumor spread on CN7
- Protocol advice
  - Image primary site, parotid, and remainder of neck nodal chains to clavicles
- MR imaging is best tool to evaluate deep lobe lesions
  - Deep tissue spread and perineural tumor are better defined by MR
  - T1 non-fat-suppressed, unenhanced images often best delineate edges/margins (inherent contrast between mass and fatty gland)
- All patients with invasive skin SCCa or melanoma on skin of face, scalp, and auricle should undergo staging PET/CT for intraparotid nodes ± nodes in cervical neck
- In patients with nasopharyngeal carcinoma (NPC), abnormal ipsilateral intra-/periparotid nodes should be considered malignant unless proven otherwise
  - Compare with contralateral side as metastatic intra-/periparotid nodes are usually unilateral

DIFFERENTIAL DIAGNOSIS

Parotid Non-Hodgkin Lymphoma (NHL)
- Patient usually has systemic NHL
- Multiple solid, bilateral, hypoechoic intraparotid nodes with abnormal reticulated/pseudocystic architecture and hilar > peripheral vascularity
- Difficult to distinguish from metastases if no known primary

Warthin Tumor
- Smokers with painless cheek mass
- Multifocal in 20%
- Heterogeneous with cystic change, internal debris, thick walls

Recurrent Parotid Benign Mixed Tumor (BMT)
- History of BMT surgical removal
- Multifocal masses
- "Cluster of grapes" appearance

Benign Lymphoepithelial Lesions (BLEL)-HIV
- HIV or AIDS patient
- Multiple small, bilateral, parotid cystic and solid lesions

Parotid Sjögren Disease
- Autoimmune disease affecting salivary tissue
- Enlarged salivary ± lacrimal glands
- Micro-/macrocystic dilatation of intraglandular ducts + lymphoid aggregates

METASTATIC DISEASE OF PAROTID NODES

PATHOLOGY

General Features
- Etiology
  - Lymphatic or hematogenous spread of tumor
    - Skin of face, external ear, and scalp (account for 75% of primary tumors)
    - Occasionally from regional head and neck primary (e.g., naso-/oropharynx)
    - Systemic metastases to parotid nodes (rare)
- Parotid has intraglandular lymph nodes (unlike submandibular and sublingual glands)
  - Normal parotid has ~ 20 intraglandular nodes
- Embryology
  - Parotid undergoes late encapsulation, incorporating nodes within its parenchyma

Gross Pathologic & Surgical Features
- Nodes may remain encapsulated or undergo extracapsular spread
- SCCa node: Tan-yellow nodule within parotid
- Melanoma node: Black, brown, or white rubbery mass

Microscopic Features
- Most common skin carcinomas
  - Squamous cell (60%)
  - Melanoma (15%)
- Most common systemic metastases: Lung and breast primaries
- SCCa: Lymph node is partially or entirely replaced by epithelial-lined structure ± central cystic change
  - Epithelium lining of cystic spaces is composed of hypercellular and pleomorphic cell population, with loss of polarity and ↑ mitotic activity
- Melanoma: Diffuse proliferation of epithelioid ± spindle cells with abundant eosinophilic cytoplasm and prominent nucleoli
  - Immunochemistry: S100 protein and HMB-45 positive

CLINICAL ISSUES

Presentation
- Most common signs/symptoms
  - External ear, scalp, upper face skin cancer with enlarging parotid mass
  - CN7 dysfunction
  - Facial pain
  - Nonhealing sore (skin SCCa or melanoma) on skin of face, scalp, or auricle-EAC associated with cheek mass

Demographics
- Age
  - Most frequently occurs in 7th decade
- Gender
  - M:F = 2:1
- Epidemiology
  - Occurs in 1-3% of patients with head and neck SCCa
  - Metastases (4% of all parotid neoplasms)
  - Intraparotid nodes are more common in geographic regions with ↑ sun exposure

Natural History & Prognosis
- Prognosis depends heavily on presence of extracapsular spread (8% vs. 79% local recurrence)
- 5-year parotid control of 78%; overall survival of 54%
- Metastatic SCCa involving parotid gland and neck nodes is aggressive form of SCCa with tendency for infiltrative growth pattern and multiple recurrences
- Some primary subsites (e.g., EAC) have worse prognosis
- Melanoma: Poor prognosis; long-term survival is rare

Treatment
- Varies depending of pathology and location of primary tumor
- SCCa: Parotidectomy and neck dissection dictated by imaging and physical exam
  - Postoperative radiotherapy
- Melanoma: Parotidectomy and neck dissection dictated by lymphatic mapping and sentinel node identification
  - Adjuvant radiotherapy ± chemotherapy

DIAGNOSTIC CHECKLIST

Consider
- If asked to image parotid nodal metastases from skin cancer, also scan cervical nodes to clavicle
- If SCCa or melanoma is found in parotid nodes, check external ear and scalp for primary
- Skin cancer may be hidden above hairline at time of presentation of parotid node

Image Interpretation Pearls
- If solitary, imaging features of parotid nodal metastasis mimic primary salivary gland malignancy
- Multifocal unilateral disease is most suggestive of 1st-order nodal disease from adjacent skin sites or regional head and neck
- Presence of bilateral nodes suggests systemic disease or hematogenous metastatic spread

Reporting Tips
- Differential diagnoses
  - Multifocal, unilateral parotid masses with cervical adenopathy: Regional metastases, local NHL
  - Multifocal, unilateral parotid masses without cervical adenopathy: Warthin tumor, recurrent BMT, regional metastases
  - Multifocal, bilateral parotid masses: Systemic metastases, systemic NHL, Warthin tumors, BLEL-HIV, Sjögren disease

SELECTED REFERENCES

1. Turner SJ et al: Metastatic cutaneous squamous cell carcinoma of the external ear: a high-risk cutaneous subsite. J Laryngol Otol. 124(1):26-31, 2010
2. Dong XR et al: Parotid gland metastasis of nasopharyngeal carcinoma: case report and review of the literature. J Int Med Res. 37(6):1994-9, 2009
3. Hinerman RW et al: Cutaneous squamous cell carcinoma metastatic to parotid-area lymph nodes. Laryngoscope. 118(11):1989-96, 2008
4. Lee YY et al: Imaging of salivary gland tumours. Eur J Radiol. 66(3):419-36, 2008
5. Veness MJ et al: Cutaneous head and neck squamous cell carcinoma metastatic to parotid and cervical lymph nodes. Head Neck. 29(7):621-31, 2007
6. Ch'ng S et al: Parotid metastasis--an independent prognostic factor for head and neck cutaneous squamous cell carcinoma. J Plast Reconstr Aesthet Surg. 59(12):1288-93, 2006

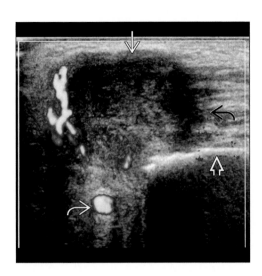

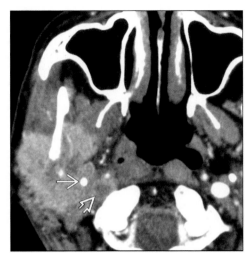

(Left) Doppler US shows parotid metastasis ➡ from laryngeal carcinoma as large, vascular, infiltrative lesion in right parotid gland, invading masseter ➡ and appearing to encase external carotid artery (ECA) ➡. Deep extension is not assessed on US due to posterior shadowing from mandible ➡. *(Right)* Axial CECT (same patient) shows full extent of parotid metastasis. Right ECA is encased but patent ➡; IJV is thrombosed ➡. MR and CECT show the full extent of disease. MR better delineates perineural spread.

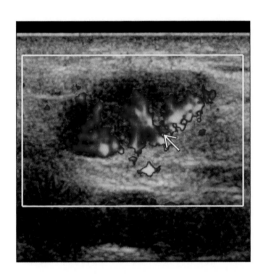

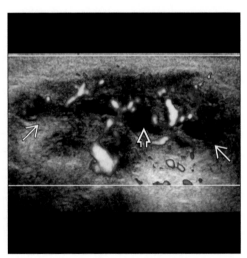

(Left) Longitudinal Doppler US of a right parotid nodal metastasis from scalp carcinoma shows an ill-defined intraparotid node in superficial gland, which contains marked internal vascularity ➡. It maintains a reniform shape, and the presence of adjacent primary was a clue to its diagnosis. *(Right)* Longitudinal Doppler US in a different patient with parotid nodal metastasis from NPC shows an ill-defined conglomerate of nodes ➡ with chaotic internal vascularity and necrotic elements ➡.

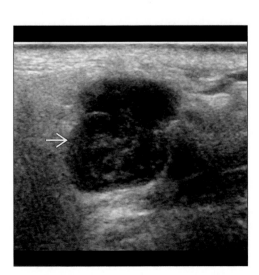

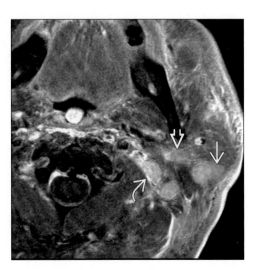

(Left) US of left parotid in another patient depicts an ill-defined, heterogeneous, intraparotid node in the superficial lobe ➡. FNA revealed poorly differentiated carcinoma. *(Right)* Axial T2WI FS MR (same patient) reveals hyperintense nodes in the superficial ➡ and deep lobes ➡ of the left parotid, and upper internal jugular/periparotid lymphadenopathy ➡. MR from skull base to clavicles is recommended for full evaluation of cervical nodes and the possible primary. Note the normal contralateral side.

PAROTID LIPOMA

Key Facts

Imaging

- 15% of all lipomas occur in head and neck
- 5% of all lipomas are multiple
- Most common sites: Posterior cervical and submandibular spaces
- Other sites: Anterior cervical and parotid spaces
- Well-defined, mildly lobulated lesion
- Compressible with ultrasound transducer
- Homogeneously hypoechoic relative to parotid parenchyma; hyperechoic compared with muscle
- Linear hyperechoic striations parallel to transducer
  - Feathered-striped appearance
- Echogenic lines within lesion remain parallel to transducer irrespective of scanning plane
- No posterior acoustic enhancement or shadowing
- No calcification, nodularity, or necrosis
- No significant vascularity in/around mass
- Ultrasound
  - Readily identifies lipoma, and no further imaging necessary if all margins of lipoma are clearly delineated by US
  - May not be able to define extent of large lipomas even in superficial lobe
  - Cannot visualize deep parotid lobe
- CT and MR may occasionally be required to delineate entire extent of large lesions ± deep lobe involvement

Top Differential Diagnoses

- Parotid lymphatic malformation
- Parotid venous vascular malformation
- Liposarcoma

Diagnostic Checklist

- Well-differentiated liposarcoma is indistinguishable from lipoma on imaging
- Liposarcoma if there is nodularity, heterogeneity, stranding, calcification, necrosis, and vascularity

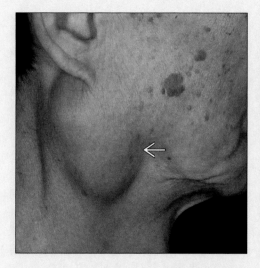
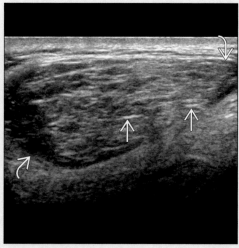

(Left) Clinical photo shows a patient presenting with longstanding right facial swelling. Physical examination reveals a soft mobile mass around the angle of the mandible ➡. (Right) Longitudinal grayscale US depicts a well-defined, hypoechoic lesion ➡ in the superficial lobe of the right parotid gland. Note multiple linear echogenic striations ➡ (feathered-striped appearance) orientated parallel to the transducer. Features are characteristic of parotid lipoma.

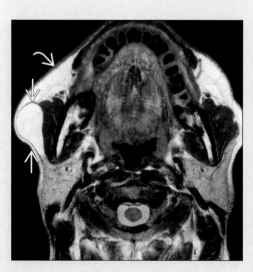
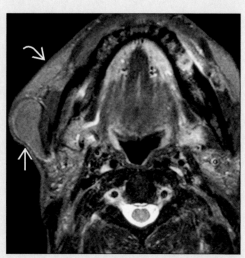

(Left) Axial T2WI MR of the same patient confirms a mass confined to the superficial lobe of the right parotid gland, stretching the parotid capsule ➡. The lipoma is hyperintense, with similar signal to adjacent subcutaneous fat ➡. (Right) Corresponding axial T2WI FS MR reveals that the high signals of the lipoma ➡ and the surrounding subcutaneous fat ➡ are similarly suppressed.

PAROTID LIPOMA

TERMINOLOGY

Synonyms
- Classic parotid lipoma
- Simple parotid lipoma

Definitions
- Encapsulated benign tumor of adipose tissue composed of mature fat cells

Associated Syndromes
- Familial multiple lipomatosis
- Cowden syndrome
- Multiple endocrine neoplasia type 1 (MEN1)
- Dercum disease
- Bannayan syndrome

IMAGING

General Features
- Best diagnostic clue
  - Well defined, hypoechoic, with linear hyperechoic striations parallel to transducer; feathered-striped appearance
  - Fat density on CT or fat signal intensity on MR
- Location
  - 15% of all lipomas occur in head and neck, and 5% are multiple
    - Most common sites: Posterior cervical and submandibular spaces
    - Other common sites: Anterior cervical and parotid spaces
  - Majority (95%) of lipomas are solitary and sporadic
- Size
  - Variable; usually a few centimeters
- Morphology
  - Well defined, reflecting encapsulated nature
  - Mildly lobulated due to thin connective tissue separating lipoma into groups of fat cells

Ultrasonographic Findings
- Grayscale ultrasound
  - Well-defined, mildly lobulated lesion
  - Elliptical in shape, with long axis parallel to skin
  - Compressible with ultrasound transducer
  - Homogeneously hypoechoic relative to parotid parenchyma, hyperechoic compared with muscle
    - Echogenicity of lipomas can vary depending on proportion of fat and water in lesion
  - Linear hyperechoic striations parallel to transducer; feathered-striped appearance
  - No posterior acoustic enhancement or shadowing
  - No calcification, nodularity or necrosis
- Color Doppler
  - No significant vascularity in/around mass

CT Findings
- NECT
  - Homogeneously hypoattenuating
    - Fat density, comparable to adjacent subcutaneous fat
      - Densities range from -140 HU to -50 HU
- CECT
  - No intralesional enhancement
  - May have thin rim enhancement of capsule

MR Findings
- T1WI
  - Homogeneously hyperintense, similar signal to subcutaneous fat
- T2WI
  - Homogeneously hyperintense, similar signal to subcutaneous fat
- T2WI FS
  - High signal of fat is suppressed
- T1WI C+ FS
  - Signal of fat is suppressed
  - No intralesional enhancement
  - May have thin rim enhancement of capsule

Imaging Recommendations
- Best imaging tool
  - Ultrasound
    - Readily identifies lipoma, and no further imaging is necessary if all margins of lipoma are clearly delineated by US
    - May not be able to define extent of large lipomas even in superficial lobe
    - Cannot visualize deep parotid lobe
  - CT and MR may occasionally be required to delineate entire extent of large lesions ± deep lobe involvement
- Protocol advice
  - On US, echogenic lines within lesion remain parallel to transducer irrespective of scanning plane
  - Further imaging is required only if diagnosis is uncertain or to demonstrate extent/deep lobe involvement

DIFFERENTIAL DIAGNOSIS

Parotid Lymphatic Malformation
- Unilocular/multilocular, septate, ± fine internal echoes, trans-spatial, avascular on Doppler

Parotid Venous Vascular Malformation
- Heterogeneous, sinusoidal vascular spaces, ± slow flow on Doppler and grayscale US, ± phleboliths, ± augmentation by Valsalva maneuver

Liposarcoma
- Clinical history of rapid growth; thus, tends to be larger
- Infiltrative margins/stranding on imaging
- Nodularity, septation, cystic necrosis, and vascularity raise suspicion
- Well-differentiated liposarcomas may be indistinguishable from lipomas on imaging and even FNA
- Surgical excision is usually required for definitive histological diagnosis, due to sampling error on routine biopsy

Dermoid
- Dermoid consists of mixture of ectodermal, endodermal, and mesodermal elements
  - Imaging shows heterogeneous, mixed soft tissue
  - Cystic components are commonly present
  - May occasionally detect calcifications

Lipoma Subtypes
- Angiolipomas contain internal vascularity on Doppler

PAROTID LIPOMA

- Echogenic calcifications are frequently detected in chondroid lipomas
- Other variants, such as myelolipomas and fibrolipomas, may be indistinguishable on imaging but are more commonly heterogeneous, containing hypo- and isoechoic constituents
- Lipoma subtypes are much rarer than classic lipoma in salivary glands as well as in rest of body

Sialolipoma

- Rare entity with ductal dilatation

PATHOLOGY

Staging, Grading, & Classification

- Majority of lipomas are classic lipomas, which are purely composed of adipose tissue
- Subclassification into numerous groups, including angiolipoma, myolipoma, fibrolipoma, chondroid lipoma, spindle cell lipoma, etc., depending on type and amount of composite tissue

Gross Pathologic & Surgical Features

- Homogeneous, yellow in color
- Thin fibrous capsule
- Thin connective tissue septa separating aggregates of adipose tissue

Microscopic Features

- Mature adipose cells without atypia
  - Morphologically indistinguishable from normal adipose cells except for increased variation in cell size
  - Lipid in lipomas is not available for metabolism
- Uniform cytoplasmic vacuoles
- Occasionally contains fat necrosis with histiocytes, infarction, or calcification

CLINICAL ISSUES

Presentation

- Most common signs/symptoms
  - Incidental finding
  - Painless facial mass or swelling

Demographics

- Age
  - Most commonly present in 5th-7th decades
- Gender
  - No gender predilection
- Ethnicity
  - No ethnic predilection
- Epidemiology
  - ~ 1% of general population has a lipoma
    - Most common mesenchymal tumor to occur at any site of body
  - Parotid lipoma comprises 10% of all parotid tumors

Natural History & Prognosis

- Lipomas have benign course with little or no growth

Treatment

- Conservative management
- Surgical excision, usually for cosmetic purposes

DIAGNOSTIC CHECKLIST

Consider

- Well-differentiated liposarcoma is indistinguishable from lipoma on imaging, and differentiation requires correlation with clinical history and surgical excision
- Liposarcoma if nodularity, heterogeneity, stranding, calcification, necrosis, and vascularity

Image Interpretation Pearls

- Finding of well-defined hypoechoic lesion with linear echogenic striations internally is characteristic of lipoma
- Typical findings on ultrasound are usually diagnostic
- CT or MR may be occasionally required to evaluate full anatomical extent
- FNA/biopsy should not be relied on to make diagnosis of lipoma

SELECTED REFERENCES

1. Ozturk M et al: Fibrolipoma of the nasal septum; report of the first case. J Otolaryngol Head Neck Surg. 42(1):11, 2013
2. Qayyum S et al: Sialolipoma of the parotid gland: Case report with literature review comparing major and minor salivary gland sialolipomas. J Oral Maxillofac Pathol. 17(1):95-7, 2013
3. Bhatia KS et al: A pilot study evaluating real-time shear wave ultrasound elastography of miscellaneous non-nodal neck masses in a routine head and neck ultrasound clinic. Ultrasound Med Biol. 38(6):933-42, 2012
4. Sah K et al: Non-infiltrating angiolipoma of the upper lip: A rare entity. J Oral Maxillofac Pathol. 16(1):103-6, 2012
5. Bhatia KS et al: Real-time qualitative ultrasound elastography of miscellaneous non-nodal neck masses: applications and limitations. Ultrasound Med Biol. 36(10):1644-52, 2010
6. Hohlweg-Majert B et al: Salivary gland lipomas: ultrasonographic and magnetic resonance imaging. J Craniofac Surg. 18(6):1464-6, 2007
7. Madani G et al: Tumors of the salivary glands. Semin Ultrasound CT MR. 27(6):452-64, 2006
8. Furlong MA et al: Lipoma of the oral and maxillofacial region: Site and subclassification of 125 cases. Oral Surg Oral Med Oral Pathol Oral Radiol Endod. 98(4):441-50, 2004
9. Inampudi P et al: Soft-tissue lipomas: accuracy of sonography in diagnosis with pathologic correlation. Radiology. 233(3):763-7, 2004
10. Zhong LP et al: Ultrasonographic appearance of lipoma in the oral and maxillofacial region. Oral Surg Oral Med Oral Pathol Oral Radiol Endod. 98(6):738-40, 2004
11. Gritzmann N et al: [Lipoma in the parotid gland: typical US and CT morphology.] Ultraschall Med. 24(3):195-6, 2003
12. Ahuja AT et al: Head and neck lipomas: sonographic appearance. AJNR Am J Neuroradiol. 19(3):505-8, 1998
13. Chikui T et al: Imaging findings of lipomas in the orofacial region with CT, US, and MRI. Oral Surg Oral Med Oral Pathol Oral Radiol Endod. 84(1):88-95, 1997
14. Rougraff BT et al: Histologic correlation with magnetic resonance imaging for benign and malignant lipomatous masses. Sarcoma. 1(3-4):175-9, 1997
15. Malave DA et al: Lipoma of the parotid gland: report of a case. J Oral Maxillofac Surg. 52(4):408-11, 1994
16. Fujimura N et al: Lipoma of the tongue with cartilaginous change: a case report and review of the literature. J Oral Maxillofac Surg. 50(9):1015-7, 1992
17. Fornage BD et al: Sonographic appearances of superficial soft tissue lipomas. J Clin Ultrasound. 19(4):215-20, 1991

PAROTID LIPOMA

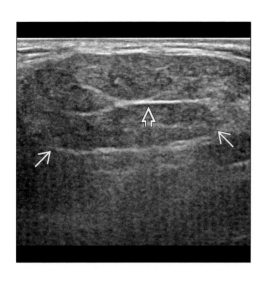

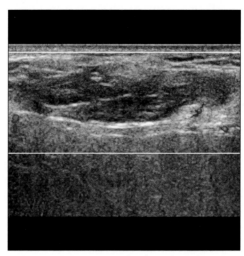

(Left) Longitudinal grayscale US shows a left parotid lipoma as a well-defined hypoechoic mass ➡. Prominent, linear echogenic line is seen within the center ⬆ of the lesion, representing a septum, separating the aggregates of adipose tissue. (Right) Power Doppler US of a lipoma shows no significant intralesional flow. Note that its long axis is parallel to the skin surface. Heterogeneity, vascularity, nodularity, necrosis, stranding, and calcification should raise suspicion for liposarcoma.

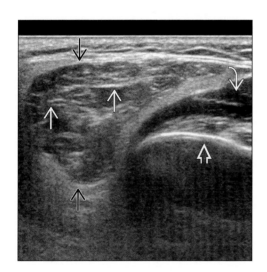

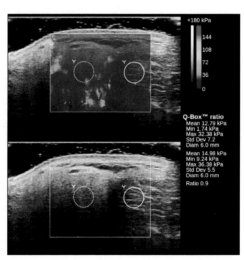

(Left) Transverse grayscale US shows a parotid lipoma ➡ with characteristic echogenic striations ➡. Note that the lesion conforms to the capsule of the parotid gland, reflecting its soft consistency. Note the mandible ⬆ and masseter muscle ➡. (Right) Shearwave elastogram compares the stiffness of a lipoma (solid circle) against the background parotid parenchyma (dotted circle). The stiffness values are shown on the right. Both tissues are comparably soft and appear blue on the chromatic scale.

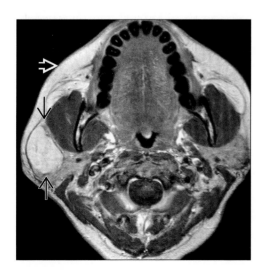

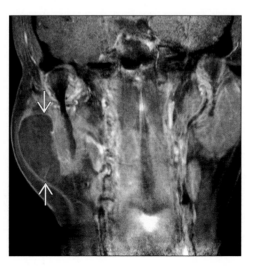

(Left) Axial T1WI MR of a woman with mild facial swelling shows an encapsulated hyperintense mass in the right parotid gland ➡ with signal identical to subcutaneous fat in the cheek ⬆. (Right) Corresponding coronal T1WI C+ FS MR reveals suppression of high fat signal, consistent with lipoma ➡. No significant enhancement is seen within the lesion. Although US readily identifies parotid lipoma, MR/CT may be required to delineate the extent and deep lobe involvement of large lesions.

PAROTID SCHWANNOMA

Key Facts

Imaging

- Well-defined, round to oval mass
- Hypoechoic relative to background parotid parenchyma
- Anechoic cystic components are frequently present
- Posterior acoustic enhancement or through transmission is frequently present even in predominantly solid tumors
- Tapering ends at tumor-nerve interface is characteristic
  - Not commonly seen as facial nerve is usually too small to resolve
- Absence of associated cervical lymphadenopathy
- Mild to moderate degrees of internal hypervascularity (compressed by increasing transducer pressure)

Top Differential Diagnoses

- May be difficult to differentiate from pleomorphic adenoma, even with cytology

- Intraparotid malignancy; ill-defined/infiltrative margins, solid, hypoechoic, ± vascularity, ± abnormal nodes
- Intraparotid neurofibroma is extremely rare but it is indistinguishable from schwannoma on imaging

Diagnostic Checklist

- Parotid schwannomas share common features with other benign parotid tumors on ultrasound
- Tapering ends at tumor-nerve interface is rarely detected, but when present, is highly suggestive of schwannoma
- When direct visualization is not possible, location of tumor in relation with facial nerve can be inferred by its relationship to RMV/ECA, widening of stylomastoid foramen
- When characteristic features are absent on ultrasound, MR or CT should be performed to look for typical avid enhancement

(Left) Clinical photograph shows a woman presenting with right facial swelling & partial facial nerve palsy. She was later confirmed to have right parotid schwannoma. (Right) Coronal T1WI C+ FS MR of the same patient depicts an enhancing mass with central nonenhancing cystic component ➡. The mass tapers toward the facial nerve ➡, which can be seen extending into the stylomastoid foramen. Findings are consistent with parotid schwannoma.

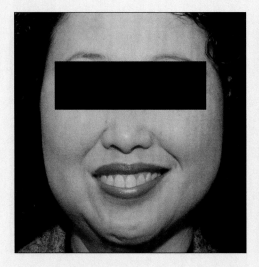
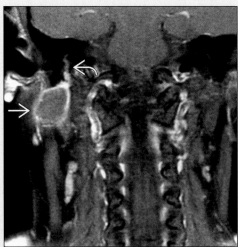

(Left) Grayscale US of the same patient shows a well-defined, heterogeneous, hypoechoic mass with sharply defined internal cystic components ➡ and posterior acoustic enhancement ➡. (Right) Corresponding transverse power Doppler US again displays cystic degeneration ➡, posterior acoustic enhancement ➡, and mild vascularity in the solid component, features commonly encountered in parotid schwannoma. Compared with MR, US is unable to define lesion extent. RMV ➡ is shown.

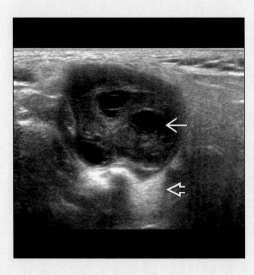
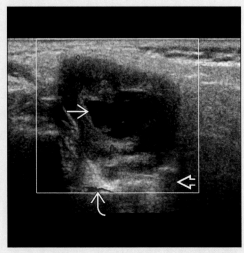

PAROTID SCHWANNOMA

TERMINOLOGY

Synonyms
- Nerve sheath tumor
- Neurilemmoma
- Neurogenic tumor (includes nerve sheath tumor and neurofibroma)

Definitions
- Benign tumor arising from intraparotid facial nerve Schwann cells

Associated Syndromes
- Neurofibromatosis type 2
  - Commonly bilateral and with nerve sheath tumors at other sites of the body

IMAGING

General Features
- Best diagnostic clue
  - Visualization of the tumor-nerve interface
  - Located along known course of intraparotid facial nerve segment (relation to retromandibular vein [RMV] and external carotid artery [ECA])
  - Well-defined, avidly enhancing mass (CT & MR)
  - Internal sharply defined cystic areas ± mild/moderate vascularity on Doppler
- Location
  - Arises from facial nerve sheath along its intraparotid segment
    - Path of facial nerve within parotid gland: Posterolateral to RMV extending from lower facial nerve canal toward stylomastoid foramen
  - Only 9% of facial nerve schwannomas occur in infratemporal, intraparotid segment
  - Most nerve sheath tumors are solitary and sporadic
- Size
  - Variable, can grow to > 5 cm in size
- Morphology
  - Round to oval in shape, occasionally lobulated
  - Well defined, reflecting their encapsulated nature

Ultrasonographic Findings
- Grayscale ultrasound
  - Well defined, round to oval mass
  - Hypoechoic relative to background parotid parenchyma
  - Anechoic cystic components are frequently present
  - Posterior acoustic enhancement or through transmission is frequently present even in predominantly solid tumors
  - Tapering ends at tumor-nerve interface is characteristic
    - Not commonly seen as facial nerve is usually too small to resolve
    - If present, diagnosis of schwannoma is strongly suggested
  - Absence of associated cervical lymphadenopathy
- Color Doppler
  - Mild to moderate degrees of internal hypervascularity (compressed by increasing transducer pressure)

CT Findings
- NECT
  - Hypo- to isoattenuating relative to parotid parenchyma
  - Intralesional cystic areas within larger (> 2 cm) tumors
- CECT
  - Avid contrast enhancement of solid components of lesion
  - Nonenhancing areas representing cystic degeneration or hemorrhage
- Bone CT
  - Widening of stylomastoid foramen in larger lesions

MR Findings
- T1WI
  - Iso- to hypointense relative to parotid parenchyma
- T2WI
  - High signal intensity relative to parotid parenchyma
  - Peripheral hyperintensity with central hypointensity giving a "target" sign
    - Reported to occur in 15% of extracranial schwannomas
    - Outer high-intensity rim corresponds to myxoid content whereas inner region is composed of more cellular components
  - Cystic component displays hyperintense fluid signal
  - Facial nerve is located eccentrically relative to the mass, but is infrequently visible on MR imaging
- T1WI C+
  - Solid components avidly enhance
  - Nonenhancing areas correspond to cystic degeneration or hemorrhage

Imaging Recommendations
- Best imaging tool
  - US is not definitive; diagnosis may be considered if nerve-tumor interface tapering, sharply defined cystic areas within, posterior enhancement, and location along course of facial nerve are seen
  - CT or MR to look for characteristic enhancement and evaluate anatomical location and extent
- Protocol advice
  - T2WI best visualizes cystic components
  - T1WI C+ for identifying avidly enhancing solid tumor

DIFFERENTIAL DIAGNOSIS

Parotid Benign Mixed Tumor
- Similar features to parotid schwannoma on ultrasound (lobulated, predominantly solid, posterior enhancement, ± vascularity)
- Can be difficult to differentiate even with cytology
- Does not arise from facial nerve
  - Relationship with facial nerve is not always evident on imaging
- Less avidly enhancing on contrast CT and MR compared with nerve sheath tumors

Warthin Tumor
- Well defined, solid and cystic components ± posterior enhancement
- Location in parotid tail
- Minimal enhancement on contrast CT and MR

Parotid Malignancy With Perineural Invasion
- On US, ill-defined/infiltrative margins, solid, hypoechoic, ± vascularity, ± abnormal nodes

PAROTID SCHWANNOMA

- Ill-defined soft tissue, increased T2WI signal or hyperenhancement extending along course of facial nerve
- Clinical history of rapid growth and facial nerve palsy

Neurofibroma

- Indistinguishable from schwannoma on imaging but parotid neurofibroma is extremely rare

PATHOLOGY

Staging, Grading, & Classification

- Type A: Exophytic off CN7 branch; no CN7 resection required
- Type B: Intrinsic to CN7 branch; branch resection required
- Type C: Intrinsic to CN7 trunk; resection and reconstruction required
- Type D: Encases main CN7 trunk and branches; resection and reconstruction required

Gross Pathologic & Surgical Features

- Well-defined, encapsulated tumor
  - True capsule composed of epineurium
- Peripherally attached to underlying nerve but can be separable from it
  - Tumor is characteristically eccentric with respect to nerve

Microscopic Features

- Contains mixture of ordered cellular component (Antoni A) and myxoid component (Antoni B)
  - Antoni A areas consist of dense proliferation of nerve sheath cells, and Verocay bodies are commonly present
  - Antoni B areas are composed of vacuolar degeneration and occasional large, irregularly spaced vessels

CLINICAL ISSUES

Presentation

- Most common signs/symptoms
  - Painless facial mass or swelling
  - Facial nerve dysfunction is uncommon
    - When facial nerve palsy is present, it is usually due to stretching effect of a large nerve sheath tumor, rather than infiltration
- Other signs/symptoms
  - Fine-needle aspiration may produce neurapraxia or self-limiting facial nerve palsy

Demographics

- Age
  - Predominantly in 3rd to 6th decade of life
- Gender
  - No significant gender predilection
  - Some series report a slight female preponderance

Natural History & Prognosis

- Benign course
- May be either static or have slow progressive growth

Treatment

- Conservative treatment for asymptomatic patients
- Surgical excision is considered in cases of nerve dysfunction or for cosmetic purposes
- Tumor removal with facial nerve reconstruction can be performed in selected cases

DIAGNOSTIC CHECKLIST

Image Interpretation Pearls

- Parotid schwannomas share common features with other benign parotid tumors on ultrasound
- Cystic areas are frequently present within tumor
- Tapering ends at tumor-nerve interface rarely detected, but when present, highly suggestive of schwannoma
- When direct visualization is not possible, location of tumor in relation with facial nerve can be inferred by its relationship to RMV/ECA, widening of stylomastoid foramen
- When characteristic features are absent on ultrasound, MR or CT should be performed to look for typical avid enhancement

SELECTED REFERENCES

1. Lee DW et al: Diagnosis and surgical outcomes of intraparotid facial nerve schwannoma showing normal facial nerve function. Int J Oral Maxillofac Surg. 42(7):874-9, 2013
2. Gross BC et al: The intraparotid facial nerve schwannoma: a diagnostic and management conundrum. Am J Otolaryngol. 33(5):497-504, 2012
3. Ma Q et al: Diagnosis and management of intraparotid facial nerve schwannoma. J Craniomaxillofac Surg. 38(4):271-3, 2010
4. Tanna N et al: Intraparotid facial nerve schwannoma: clinician beware. Ear Nose Throat J. 88(8):E18-20, 2009
5. Salemis NS et al: Large intraparotid facial nerve schwannoma: case report and review of the literature. Int J Oral Maxillofac Surg. 37(7):679-81, 2008
6. Lee JD et al: Management of facial nerve schwannoma in patients with favorable facial function. Laryngoscope. 117(6):1063-8, 2007
7. Wippold FJ 2nd et al: Neuropathology for the neuroradiologist: Antoni A and Antoni B tissue patterns. AJNR Am J Neuroradiol. 28(9):1633-8, 2007
8. Shimizu K et al: Intraparotid facial nerve schwannoma: a report of five cases and an analysis of MR imaging results. AJNR Am J Neuroradiol. 26(6):1328-30, 2005
9. Assad L et al: Fine-needle aspiration of parotid gland schwannomas mimicking pleomorphic adenoma: a report of two cases. Diagn Cytopathol. 30(1):39-40, 2004
10. Beaman FD et al: Schwannoma: radiologic-pathologic correlation. Radiographics. 24(5):1477-81, 2004
11. Caughey RJ et al: Intraparotid facial nerve schwannoma: diagnosis and management. Otolaryngol Head Neck Surg. 130(5):586-92, 2004
12. Jee WH et al: Extraaxial neurofibromas versus neurilemmomas: discrimination with MRI. AJR Am J Roentgenol. 183(3):629-33, 2004
13. Gritzmann N et al: Sonography of the salivary glands. Eur Radiol. 13(5):964-75, 2003
14. Jaehne M et al: [Clinical aspects and therapy of extratemporal facial neurinoma.] HNO. 49(4):264-9, 2001
15. Chong KW et al: Management of intraparotid facial nerve schwannomas. Aust N Z J Surg. 70(10):732-4, 2000

PAROTID SCHWANNOMA

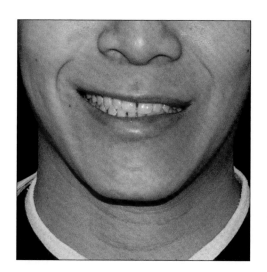

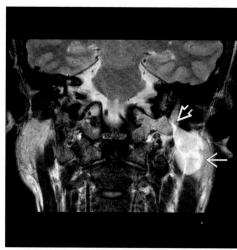

(Left) Clinical photograph shows a patient with parotid schwannoma who presented with partial left facial nerve palsy. Most patients present with a slowly enlarging cheek mass (often asymptomatic for > 10 years), and facial nerve palsy is uncommon. *(Right)* Coronal T2WI FS MR of the same patient reveals a T2 hyperintense mass situated in the left parotid gland ➡. Tapering at the tumor-nerve interface with extension towards the stylomastoid foramen ➡ is noted.

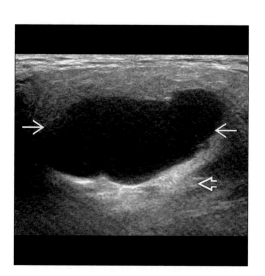

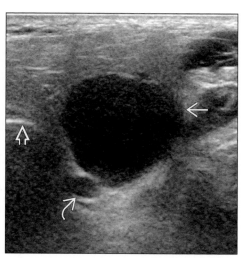

(Left) Longitudinal grayscale US of the same lesion depicts parotid schwannoma as a lobulated mass ➡, which is hypoechoic compared with background parotid parenchyma with posterior enhancement ➡. *(Right)* Corresponding transverse grayscale US shows the schwannoma ➡ is situated at expected course of facial nerve, extending toward the stylomastoid foramen and posterolateral to RMV ➡, which acts as a surrogate marker for the position of the intraparotid facial nerve. Note the mandible ➡.

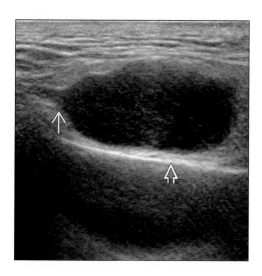

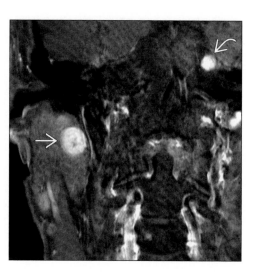

(Left) Longitudinal grayscale US depicts parotid schwannoma as an oval mass in the superficial lobe. Tapering end ➡ at the tumor-nerve interface, an uncommon but characteristic feature on US, is shown. Note the mandible ➡. *(Right)* Coronal T1 C+ FS MR of right parotid schwannoma demonstrates an avidly enhancing nodule ➡, a typical finding of schwannoma. This patient also has a small synchronous trigeminal schwannoma ➡, which could not have been picked up by US.

PAROTID LYMPHATIC MALFORMATION

Key Facts

Imaging

- Parotid LMs may be detected in prenatal US
- More frequently multilocular than unilocular
- Superficial lesions are compressible with transducer
- Nonhemorrhagic/uninfected LM
  - Unilocular/multilocular, anechoic compressible cysts with thin walls and intervening septi
  - Despite large size, there is no significant mass effect
  - Thin imperceptible walls, posterior enhancement
  - Color Doppler: No vascularity within lesion
- Hemorrhagic/infected LM
  - Unilocular/multilocular heterogeneous cysts with irregular walls, internal debris
  - Noncompressible, hypoechoic, thick walls and septi
  - Fluid-fluid levels due to sedimentation and separation of fluids (suggests prior hemorrhage)
  - Color Doppler: If infected, vascularity may be seen in walls, septi, and adjacent soft tissues

- Prior to treating with sclerosant, perform pre-procedure baseline imaging (US and MR)
- US safely guides injection of sclerosant and monitors response after treatment

Top Differential Diagnoses

- Venous malformation, venolymphatic malformation
- 1st branchial cleft cyst
- Parotid abscess

Diagnostic Checklist

- LM is top differential diagnosis in newborn presenting with a cystic facial or neck swelling
- Diagnosis of LM should be considered in infant suspected of parotid abscess, as smaller LMs frequently present during infective episode
- MR should be performed in larger lesions to evaluate full anatomical extent

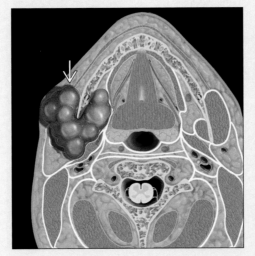
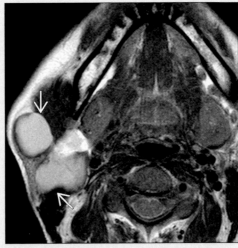

(Left) Schematic axial illustration of a right parotid lymphatic malformation ➡ shows a multilocular lesion with cystic spaces of varying size involving superficial and deep lobes. (Right) Axial T2WI MR shows a hyperintense multiloculated LM ➡ involving both superficial & deep lobes of right parotid gland. Individual locules are > 2 cm³, consistent with macrocystic LM. Note the entire extent of LM is clearly mapped & deep lobe involvement defined by MR. US cannot visualize deep parotid lobe.

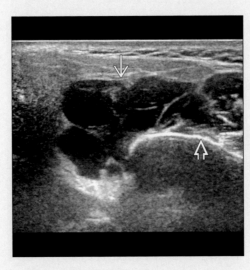
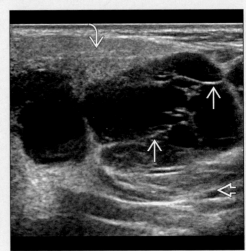

(Left) Transverse grayscale US (same patient) shows LM ➡ in the superficial lobe of the parotid gland. Note deep lobe extension cannot be evaluated as it is obscured by shadowing from the mandibular ramus ➡. This is a major limitation of US assessment of parotid glands. (Right) Corresponding longitudinal grayscale US shows parotid LM as multiseptated, anechoic, cystic lesion in superficial parotid parenchyma ➡. Note internal septations ➡ & posterior acoustic enhancement ➡.

PAROTID LYMPHATIC MALFORMATION

TERMINOLOGY

Abbreviations
- Parotid lymphatic malformation (parotid LM)

Synonyms
- Vascular malformation, lymphatic type
  - Spectrum of diseases
    - Venolymphatic malformation (VLM): Elements of VVM and LM in same mass
- Lymphangioma and cystic hygroma (old terms)

Definitions
- Abnormal collection of dilated lymphatic channels that are lined with endothelial cells
  - Almost all are congenital, resulting from abnormal development of the lymphatic system
  - Very rarely can be secondary to trauma or surgery

Associated Syndromes
- Turner syndrome is most common syndrome association
- Less commonly seen in Down syndrome and fetal alcohol syndrome

IMAGING

General Features
- Location
  - 75% occur in head and neck region (most frequent)
    - In infrahyoid neck, posterior triangle is most common location whereas masticator and submandibular spaces are most common sites of suprahyoid neck
    - Intraparotid location is infrequently encountered
    - Can be trans-spatial, affecting multiple contiguous spaces
  - 20% affect axilla
  - Less commonly affects mediastinum, groin, and retroperitoneum
- Size
  - Variable; may be large and extensive
- Morphology
  - Unilocular or, more commonly, multilocular lesion
  - May contain either rounded or insinuating cystic spaces
  - Tends to invaginate between normal structures without any mass effect

Ultrasonographic Findings
- Grayscale ultrasound
  - Larger parotid LMs may be detected in prenatal ultrasound
  - More frequently multilocular than unilocular
    - Cystic spaces may either be rounded or insinuating
  - Superficial lesions are compressible with ultrasound transducer
  - Appearances depend on whether there was previous hemorrhage/infection
  - Nonhemorrhagic/uninfected LM
    - Unilocular/multilocular (more common) anechoic compressible cysts with thin walls and intervening septi
    - Despite large size, there is no significant mass effect

- Thin imperceptible walls, posterior acoustic enhancement
- Color Doppler: No vascularity within lesion
  - Hemorrhagic/infected LM
    - Unilocular/multilocular heterogeneous cysts with irregular walls, internal debris
    - Noncompressible and hypoechoic, with thick walls and septi
    - Fluid-fluid levels due to sedimentation and separation of fluids, suggests prior hemorrhage
    - Color Doppler: If infected; vascularity may be seen in walls, septi, and adjacent soft tissues

CT Findings
- NECT
  - Well defined, multiseptated
  - Homogeneous low attenuation, near water density
    - Occasionally contains higher density material due to highly proteinaceous content or hemorrhage
  - Not preferred imaging modality as it involves ionizing radiation

MR Findings
- T1WI
  - Low signal intensity relative to parotid parenchyma
- T2WI
  - High signal intensity (near fluid signal) relative to parotid parenchyma
    - Highly proteinaceous or hemorrhagic content will appear lower in signal
    - Fluid-fluid levels due to sedimentation and separation of different fluids (suggests prior hemorrhage)
- FLAIR
  - High signal usually cannot be suppressed due to proteinaceous content of cysts
- T1WI C+
  - No internal enhancement and insignificant enhancement of walls and septa in uncomplicated parotid LMs
  - More pronounced enhancement of walls and septa in cases of superimposed infection

Imaging Recommendations
- Best imaging tool
  - Ultrasound depicts cystic nature of mass and is often diagnostic
  - MR (over CT) is recommended to evaluate lesion's full anatomical extent and relation to adjacent structures and vessels
    - T2WI provides best lesion conspicuity and definition
  - Prior to treating with sclerosant perform pre-procedure baseline imaging (US and MR)
  - US safely guides injection of sclerosant and monitors response after treatment

DIFFERENTIAL DIAGNOSIS

Parotid Venous Vascular Malformation
- VVM and VLM; both contain venous components
- Enhancing soft tissue components intermixed with cystic areas
- May detect phleboliths

PAROTID LYMPHATIC MALFORMATION

Parotid Abscess
- Presentation may be similar as small LMs may be discovered during an infective episode
- Thicker hypervascular walls
- Prominent peripheral hypervascularity

1st Branchial Cleft Cyst
- Rare and usually presents later in life
- Unilocular in nature
- May see beaking of deep portion toward bone-cartilaginous junction of external auditory canal

Cystic Intraparotid Lymph Node
- More rounded in morphology, known anatomical intra- to periparotid locations
- Thick walls ± vascularity

PATHOLOGY

General Features
- Etiology
  - Various hypotheses concerning mechanism of lymphangiogenesis
    - Failure of lymphatic system to connect or separate from venous system
    - Abnormal budding of lymphatic system
    - Benign neoplastic process influenced by lymphangiogenic growth factors

Staging, Grading, & Classification
- Classification according to size of cysts (microcystic, macrocystic, or mixed)
  - Prognostic relevance as macrocystic LMs are successfully treated with sclerotherapy
    - Microcystic LM: Composed of cysts measuring < 2 cm³ in volume
    - Macrocystic LM: Cysts measuring > 2 cm³ in volume
    - Mixed type LM: Contains both microcystic and macrocystic components
- Less commonly, parotid LMs are classified by location (stage)
  - Stage I: Unilateral infrahyoid
  - Stage II: Unilateral suprahyoid
  - Stage III: Unilateral supra and infrahyoid
  - Stage IV: Bilateral suprahyoid
  - Stage V: Bilateral supra and infrahyoid

Gross Pathologic & Surgical Features
- Cystic spaces ± communication with each other
- Contains proteinaceous lymphatic fluid

Microscopic Features
- Cyst-like spaces are lined by a single layer of endothelial cells and connective tissue stroma
- Scattered lymphocytes are commonly detected within cyst content

CLINICAL ISSUES

Presentation
- Most common signs/symptoms
  - Parotid/facial swelling
    - Sudden onset of swelling precipitated by trauma or upper respiratory tract infection may occur

- Functional problems such as dyspnea and dysphagia are uncommon unless lesion extends down into anterior triangle of neck

Demographics
- Age
  - 50-65% present at birth or in utero
  - 80-90% present by age of 2
  - Adult presentation is extremely rare and is usually secondary to trauma or surgery

Natural History & Prognosis
- Spontaneous remission in infants has been described but is relatively uncommon

Treatment
- Surgery
  - Involves risk of facial nerve damage
  - Recurrence rates reported to range from 10-38%
- Sclerosing agents
  - OK-432 and bleomycin are most commonly used
  - Procedure is usually limited to macrocystic lesions
- Aspiration
  - Not recommended
  - Only temporarily effective and can lead to infection

DIAGNOSTIC CHECKLIST

Consider
- Parotid LM is top diagnosis in newborn presenting with a cystic facial or neck swelling
- Diagnosis of parotid LM should be considered in infant suspected of parotid abscess, as smaller LMs frequently present during an infective episode

Image Interpretation Pearls
- Uncomplicated LMs are anechoic, commonly multiseptated with posterior acoustic enhancement
- When complicated with infection of hemorrhage, low-level internal echoes are often present

Reporting Tips
- MR should be performed in larger lesions to evaluate full anatomical extent

SELECTED REFERENCES

1. Adams MT et al: Head and neck lymphatic malformation treatment: a systematic review. Otolaryngol Head Neck Surg. 147(4):627-39, 2012
2. Ibrahim M et al: Congenital cystic lesions of the head and neck. Neuroimaging Clin N Am. 21(3):621-39, viii, 2011
3. Zhou Q et al: Treatment guidelines of lymphatic malformations of the head and neck. Oral Oncol. 47(12):1105-9, 2011
4. Wiegand S et al: Pathogenesis of lymphangiomas. Virchows Arch. 453(1):1-8, 2008
5. Mandel L: Parotid area lymphangioma in an adult: case report. J Oral Maxillofac Surg. 62(10):1320-3, 2004
6. Lille ST et al: The surgical management of giant cervicofacial lymphatic malformations. J Pediatr Surg. 31(12):1648-50, 1996
7. Borecky N et al: Imaging of cervico-thoracic lymphangiomas in children. Pediatr Radiol. 25(2):127-30, 1995
8. Goshen S et al: Cystic hygroma of the parotid gland. J Laryngol Otol. 107(9):855-7, 1993

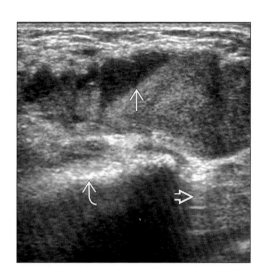

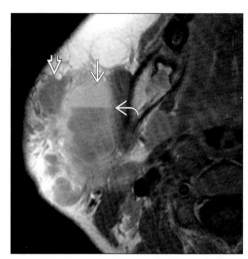

(Left) Transverse grayscale US of right parotid LM shows a multiseptated lesion with low-level internal echoes, fluid-sediment level ➡, & posterior enhancement ➡. Findings suggest recent hemorrhage in LM. The mandible ➡ is also shown. *(Right)* Corresponding axial T1WI MR defines extent of parotid LM, involving superficial lobe of right parotid gland ➡ and overlying subcutaneous layer ➡. Fluid-fluid level ➡ suggests previous hemorrhage. T2WI best provides lesion conspicuity & defines extent.

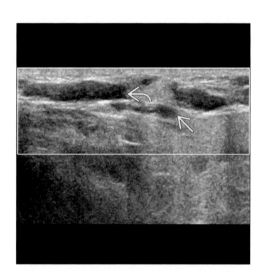

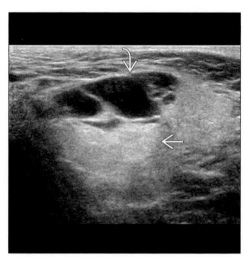

(Left) Power Doppler US shows a soft mass in the parotid region. Note cystic spaces in the superficial lobe of the parotid gland ➡ & in the subcutaneous layer ➡. No significant Doppler signal is demonstrated *(Right)* Corresponding longitudinal grayscale US shows larger, cystic, anechoic, septated LM ➡ with posterior enhancement ➡ in the superficial parotid. US with its high resolution readily evaluates superficial lobe & safely guides needle for sclerosant therapy if indicated.

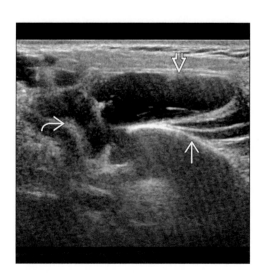

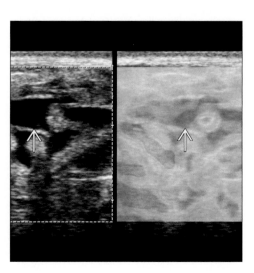

(Left) Transverse grayscale US shows a parotid LM. Note cystic locule ➡ in superficial parotid lobe while other locules ➡ appear serpiginous/sinusoidal & mimic parotid VVM. Absence of phlebolith & flow (grayscale & Doppler) identify LM. Note mandible ➡. *(Right)* US elastography of parotid LM shows side-by-side chromatic representation of tissue stiffness. Cystic spaces appear blue, corresponding to low stiffness ➡; surrounding parenchyma appears yellow, indicating intermediate stiffness.

PAROTID VENOUS VASCULAR MALFORMATION

Key Facts

Imaging

- More commonly occurs in superficial lobe
- Most (80%) appear heterogeneously hypoechoic
- Anechoic spaces are seen in < 50% and are serpiginous & sinusoidal
- Lesions with small vascular channels may appear echogenic (due to multiple acoustic interfaces reflecting sound)
- Intraluminal "to and fro" movement of echoes on real-time US, representing slow vascular flow
- Echogenic phleboliths with posterior acoustic shadowing are characteristic
- Occasionally involves entire parotid gland, mimicking diffuse or infiltrative pathology
- Monophasic low velocity flow may occasionally be detected within anechoic & hypoechoic spaces, representing patent vessels with significant flow
- Prominent color Doppler signal is present in areas where flow is significant
- Absent Doppler signal if slow flow or thrombosed
- Use low wall filter & pulse repetition frequency (PRF) to increase Doppler sensitivity
- Flow signal may occasionally be augmented by Valsalva maneuver or with distal compression, but latter is difficult to perform in facial region

Top Differential Diagnoses

- Hemangioma
- Arteriovenous malformation
- Sialolithiasis

Diagnostic Checklist

- VVM should be considered in a heterogeneous, trans-spatial lesion, ± phleboliths, ± slow flow
- T2WI FS MR recommended to evaluate full anatomical extent & relations of lesion

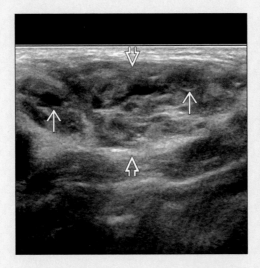
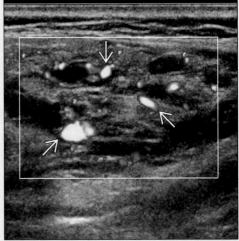

(Left) Longitudinal grayscale US in patient shows intraparotid VVM in superficial lobe ➡. Note multiple, cystic sinusoidal spaces within lesion ➡. "To and fro" motion is detected in these sinusoidal vascular spaces on real-time scans with the transducer held gently over the lesion. *(Right)* Corresponding longitudinal power Doppler US (low wall filter & pulse repetition frequency [PRF]) shows Doppler flow signal within the lesion ➡. VVM may appear avascular if vessels are thrombosed or if intravascular flow is very slow.

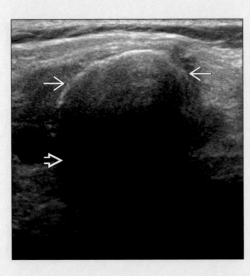
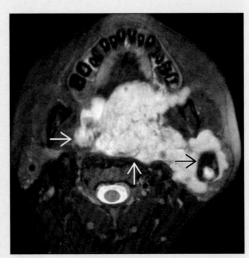

(Left) Transverse grayscale US in a patient with large intraparotid VVM shows a large curvilinear phlebolith ➡ with dense posterior shadowing ➡, obscuring visualization behind the phlebolith. *(Right)* Corresponding axial T2WI FS MR shows the transspatial nature of VVM extending into the oropharynx ➡. Note the large phlebolith ➡. Although US readily suggests diagnosis, T2WI MR best demonstrates multiplicity (if any), extent of lesion, & its anatomical relation to major adjacent structures.

PAROTID VENOUS VASCULAR MALFORMATION

TERMINOLOGY

Abbreviations
- Venous vascular malformation (VVM)

Synonyms
- Venous malformation

Definitions
- Benign vascular proliferation composed of a conglomerate of slow-flow, postcapillary endothelial-lined vascular sinusoids

IMAGING

General Features
- Best diagnostic clue
  - Heterogeneously hypoechoic lesion, sinusoidal vascular spaces, "to and fro" motion on real time, ± echogenic phleboliths
  - Prominent flow signal on color or power Doppler
  - Monophasic low velocity flow on pulsed Doppler
- Location
  - 40% of all VVMs occur in head and neck, with the most common site being in parotid gland, followed by masseter muscle
  - Can occur anywhere within parotid gland
    - More commonly occurs in superficial lobe
    - Entire parotid gland may be involved
  - Not uncommonly trans-spatial, extending to other cervical spaces; commonly the masticator space
- Size
  - Variable, may enlarge to > 10 cm
- Morphology
  - Lobulated, insinuating

Ultrasonographic Findings
- Grayscale ultrasound
  - Most (80%) appear heterogeneously hypoechoic
  - Anechoic spaces are seen in < 50% and are serpiginous & sinusoidal
  - Lesions with small vascular channels may appear echogenic (due to multiple acoustic interfaces reflecting sound)
  - Margins may be difficult to define since components of lesion may be isoechoic to parotid parenchyma & blend imperceptibly
  - Intraluminal "to and fro" movement of echoes on real-time US, representing slow vascular flow
  - Echogenic phleboliths with posterior acoustic shadowing are characteristic
    - Reported to be present in only 20% of VVMs
  - Occasionally involves entire parotid gland, mimicking diffuse or infiltrative pathology
- Pulsed Doppler
  - Monophasic low velocity flow may occasionally be detected within anechoic & hypoechoic spaces, representing patent vessels with significant flow
  - Absent Doppler signal if slow flow or thrombosed
- Color Doppler
  - Prominent color Doppler signal is present in areas where flow is significant
    - Use low wall filter & pulse repetition frequency (PRF) to increase Doppler sensitivity
  - Absent Doppler signal if slow-flow or thrombosed

- Doppler flow signal is altered by various maneuvers
  - In superficial areas of involvement, Doppler signal may be obliterated by direct transducer compression over lesion
  - Flow signal may occasionally be augmented by Valsalva maneuver or with distal compression, but latter is difficult to perform in facial region

CT Findings
- NECT
  - Hypo- to isoattenuating mass
  - High density phleboliths within lesion
- CECT
  - Slow, heterogeneous, mainly peripheral enhancement
  - Areas of nonenhancement representing thrombosed vessel lumen
  - Dysmorphic veins may be seen in the vicinity
  - Rarely, an enlarged draining vein is demonstrated

MR Findings
- T1WI
  - Intermediate signal
  - High signal in acutely thrombosed vessels
- T2WI
  - Heterogeneously hyperintense
    - Venous lakes appear as larger, cyst-like areas of homogeneous high T2W signal
    - Smaller vascular channels appear more solid & intermediate in signal intensity
- T2WI FS
  - Heterogeneously hyperintense
  - Best sequence for lesion conspicuity, assessing extent & adjacent relations
- T2* GRE
  - Phleboliths & areas of hemorrhage are seen as signal voids with blooming artifacts
- T1WI C+ FS
  - Heterogeneous enhancement
  - Areas of nonenhancement represent thrombosed vessel lumen
  - Dysmorphic veins may be seen in the vicinity
  - Rarely, an enlarged draining vein is demonstrated

Imaging Recommendations
- Best imaging tool
  - US is diagnostic when characteristic grayscale, Doppler signal, & phleboliths are visualized
  - MR is best imaging tool to evaluate multiplicity, extent, & anatomical relations
- Protocol advice
  - Ultrasound
    - Grayscale & color Doppler
  - MR
    - T1WI, T2WI FS, T1WI C+ FS

DIFFERENTIAL DIAGNOSIS

Hemangioma
- Occurs in infancy & early childhood
- Homogeneously hypoechoic
- Diffuse & marked hypervascularity on color Doppler & enhancement on CT/MR
- Absence of phleboliths

PAROTID VENOUS VASCULAR MALFORMATION

Arteriovenous Malformation
- High-flow conglomeration of vessels
  - Prominent color Doppler & power Doppler signal
  - Presence of arterial-type pulsed Doppler waveform
- Absence of phleboliths

Sialolithiasis
- Phleboliths may be misinterpreted as calculi
- ± salivary ductal dilatation, ± parotitis
- No significant contrast enhancement on CT & MR
- Associated with clinical history of intermittent pain

Non-Hodgkin Lymphoma
- Parenchymal: Lobulated, hypoechoic, heterogeneous with hypervascularity, ± involvement of entire gland
- Nodal: Discrete, hypoechoic, solid & homogeneous ± abnormal nodal vascularity
- Anechoic spaces are uncommon as lymphomas rarely undergo internal necrosis

PATHOLOGY

Staging, Grading, & Classification
- In 1982, Mulliken & Glowacki classified vascular anomalies based on endothelial characteristics
  - Hemangioma; rapid growth in early infancy & subsequent slow regression
    - Hemangioma shows endothelial hyperplasia in proliferating phase & fibrosis & fat deposition in involuting phase
  - Vascular malformation; grow proportionately with growth of the child & do not involute
    - Vascular malformations comprise abnormal combined vascular elements; divided into low flow (venous, capillary, lymphatic) & high flow (arterial & arteriovenous)

Gross Pathologic & Surgical Features
- Poorly defined conglomeration of post-capillary vessels
- Vessels are variable in size & wall thickness
- Lumen is commonly congested &/or thrombosed & sometimes calcified
- Vessel walls are lined by mitotically inactive endothelium & scant smooth muscle

CLINICAL ISSUES

Presentation
- Most common signs/symptoms
  - Slow-growing, soft, mobile masses
  - No associated facial nerve palsy or cervical lymph node enlargement
  - Usually asymptomatic but may present with a painless swelling
  - Bluish tinge of overlying skin is infrequently seen due to deep location
  - Pain & skin necrosis are rare & due to microthrombotic events & blood shunting, respectively
  - Sudden enlargement & hardening may be experienced after local trauma & secondary hemorrhage
- Other signs/symptoms
  - "Turkey wattle" sign has been described & reported to occur in 10% of patients

- Lesion volume increases with Valsalva maneuver or when head is tilted forward

Demographics
- Age
  - Develops at birth, seldom presents in childhood, proportionate growth with patient
  - Usually presents later in life (4th decade)
- Gender
  - Female predilection

Natural History & Prognosis
- Slow, gradual enlargement
- More rapid growth may be encountered after trauma, infection, or hormonal changes

Treatment
- Conservative management
  - Considered for small, asymptomatic lesions only
- Surgical excision is mainstay for curative therapy
  - Results vary according to size & extent; recurrence is more common with diffuse lesions due to incomplete removal
- Sclerotherapy with ethanol injection
  - Primary form of nonsurgical therapy & can be performed prior to surgery to "downstage" lesions
- Laser therapy is in development & can be considered for smaller lesions

DIAGNOSTIC CHECKLIST

Consider
- VVM should be considered in a heterogeneous, trans-spatial lesion, ± phleboliths, ± slow flow

Image Interpretation Pearls
- Mixed echogenicity lesion, multiple cystic vascular spaces with "to and fro" motion of debris on real time
- Margins may be difficult to define on ultrasound since components of lesion may be isoechoic to parotid parenchyma & merge imperceptibly
- Presence of phleboliths is diagnostic as they only form in slow-flow lesions
- Monophasic slow velocity Doppler signal is characteristic but absent in thrombosed vessels

Reporting Tips
- MR recommended to evaluate full anatomical extent & relations of lesion

SELECTED REFERENCES
1. Achache M et al: Management of vascular malformations of the parotid area. Eur Ann Otorhinolaryngol Head Neck Dis. 130(2):55-60, 2013
2. Lee BB: Venous malformation and haemangioma: differential diagnosis, diagnosis, natural history and consequences. Phlebology. 28 Suppl 1:176-87, 2013
3. Hamilton J et al: Avoiding misdiagnosis in venous malformation of the parotid. Ear Nose Throat J. 91(8):317-8, 2012
4. Groppo ER et al: Vascular malformation masquerading as sialolithiasis and parotid obstruction: a case report and review of the literature. Laryngoscope. 120 Suppl 4:S130, 2010
5. Dubois J et al: Soft-tissue venous malformations in adult patients: imaging and therapeutic issues. Radiographics. 21(6):1519-31, 2001

PAROTID VENOUS VASCULAR MALFORMATION

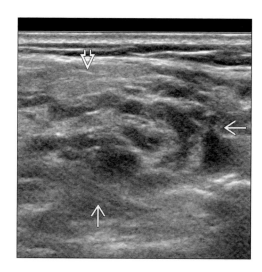
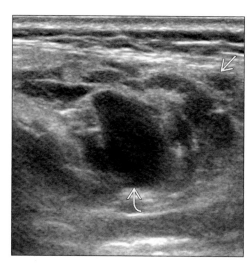

(Left) Longitudinal grayscale US shows a parotid venous vascular malformation (VVM) in the superficial lobe ➡. Note that its borders are not defined as it merges imperceptibly with adjacent salivary parenchyma ➡. *(Right)* Longitudinal grayscale US shows another VVM ➡ in superficial parotid, merging with adjacent salivary tissue. Large anechoic area represents a venous lake ➡. On real-time grayscale US, slow flow is often seen as "to and fro" motion of debris. Doppler may not demonstrate such flow if it is slow.

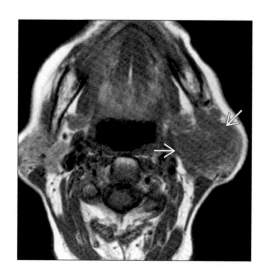
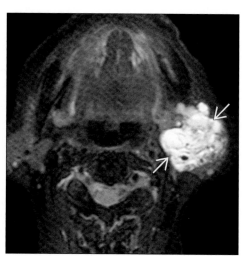

(Left) Axial T1WI MR shows VVM ➡ in the left parotid involving most of the gland. It is hypointense relative to normal contralateral parotid tissue. *(Right)* Corresponding axial T1WI C+ FS MR shows avid enhancement of a parotid VVM ➡. Note that MR clearly defines extent of entire lesion & its adjacent relations. T2WI FS MR is the best sequence to demonstrate extent of VVM, which appears heterogeneously hyperechoic, & T2W* GRE shows phleboliths & hemorrhage as signal voids with blooming artifacts.

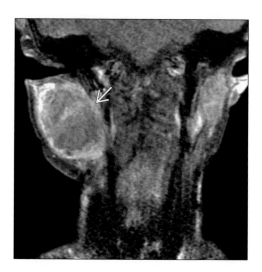
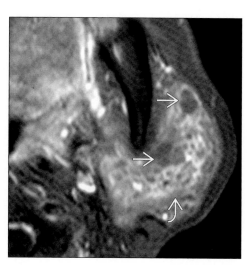

(Left) Coronal T1WI C+ FS MR shows a large right parotid VVM ➡. Note its predominantly peripheral enhancement following gadolinium injection. *(Right)* Axial T1WI C+ FS MR of a patient with a large left parotid VVM ➡ shows intense enhancement with focal nonenhancing areas within the lesion. These represent sites of thrombosed vessels ➡. Also note the edges of the VVM merge imperceptibly with salivary parenchymal tissue.

PAROTID INFANTILE HEMANGIOMA

Key Facts

Terminology
- Infantile hemangioma (IH)
- Benign vascular neoplasm
- Not a vascular malformation

Imaging
- Well-defined, homogeneous, solid, noncalcified soft tissue mass
- PP: Hypoechoic to parotid parenchyma; IP: Iso- to mildly hyperechoic
- Mean venous peak velocities not elevated (elevated in true arteriovenous malformation)
- Marked Doppler flow signal throughout, with intralesional vessels
- Ultrasound provides efficient and optimal characterization of superficial lesions
- MR/CECT to assess deep lesions, extent, and anatomic relations
- MRA to identify associated vascular abnormalities

Top Differential Diagnoses
- Congenital hemangioma
- Venous malformation (VM)
- Arteriovenous malformation (AVM)

Clinical Issues
- Growing soft tissue mass, typically with warm, reddish or strawberry-like cutaneous discoloration in infant (proliferating phase)
- Occasionally deep, present with bluish coloration of skin secondary to prominent draining veins
- Typically inapparent at birth; median age at presentation: 2 weeks; majority present by 1-3 months
- PP begins few weeks after birth, continues 1-2 years
- IP shows gradual regression over next several years
  ○ 90% resolve by 9 years
- Majority do not require treatment; expectant waiting

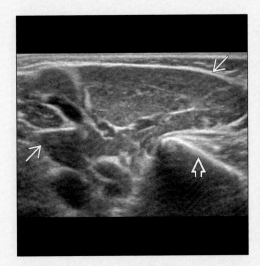 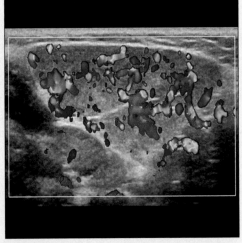

(Left) Transverse grayscale ultrasound of an infant with right parotid hemangioma shows a well-defined, solid, homogeneous mass occupying the entire superficial lobe ➡. The mandibular ramus with posterior acoustic shadowing ⇨ obscures visualization of the deep lobe. (Right) Corresponding longitudinal color Doppler ultrasound reveals marked hypervascularity throughout the lesion. Such profuse vascularity (of variable resistance) is often seen in parotid infantile hemangiomas.

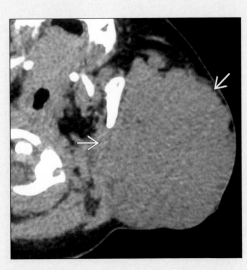 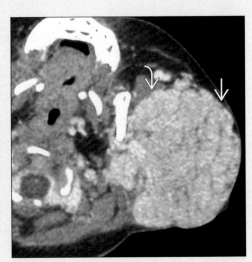

(Left) NECT of a baby with left parotid infantile hemangioma reveals a large, homogeneous mass of intermediate attenuation ➡ occupying most of the parotid gland. (Right) Corresponding CECT shows avid homogeneous enhancement. Anatomical extent and trans-spatial nature of the lesion is well depicted, involving the entire left parotid gland, subcutaneous layer ➡, and masseter muscle ➡. Although US readily identifies and characterizes such lesions, CECT/MR better delineate extent and anatomical relations.

PAROTID INFANTILE HEMANGIOMA

TERMINOLOGY

Abbreviations
- Infantile hemangioma (IH)

Synonyms
- Hemangioma of infancy
- Capillary hemangioma (older term)

Definitions
- Benign vascular neoplasm of proliferating endothelial cells
- Not a vascular malformation

Associated Syndromes
- PHACES association
  - **P**osterior fossa and supratentorial brain malformations (Dandy-Walker malformation/variant, migrational anomaly)
  - **H**emangioma of face and neck
  - **A**rterial stenosis, occlusion, aneurysm, hypoplasia, agenesis, aberrant origin
  - **C**ardiovascular defects (aortic coarctation/aneurysm/dysplasia, aberrant subclavian artery ± vascular ring, VSD)
  - **E**ye abnormalities (PHPV, coloboma, morning glory disc anomaly, optic nerve hypoplasia, peripapillary staphyloma, microphthalmia, cataract, sclerocornea)
  - **S**upraumbilical raphe and sternal clefts/defects
  - Recent reports of associated endocrine abnormalities (hypopituitarism, ectopic thyroid)
- Kasselbach-Merrit syndrome
  - Hemangioma associated with thrombocytopenia
  - Platelet consumption from large hemangiomas

IMAGING

General Features
- Best diagnostic clue
  - Well-defined mass with diffuse intralesional hypervascularity/intense enhancement
  - Vessels in and adjacent to mass during proliferative phase (PP)
  - Decrease size with fatty replacement during involuting phase (IP)
- Location
  - 60% occur in head and neck
    - Any space: Parotid space, orbit, nasal cavity, subglottic airway, face, neck, rarely intracranial
- Size
  - Depends on phase of growth and regression (ranges from few cm to large trans-spatial masses)
- Morphology
  - Majority are single lesions in subcutaneous tissues
  - Occasionally multiple, trans-spatial or deep

Ultrasonographic Findings
- Grayscale ultrasound
  - Well-defined, solid, noncalcified soft tissue mass
  - Homogeneous echo pattern
  - PP: Hypoechoic to parotid parenchyma; IP: Iso- to mildly hyperechoic
- Pulsed Doppler
  - Arterial and venous waveforms

- Mean venous peak velocities not elevated (elevated in true arteriovenous malformation)
- Resistive index variable, probably depending on phase (0.4-0.8)
- Power Doppler
  - Marked Doppler flow signal throughout, with intralesional vessels

CT Findings
- NECT
  - Intermediate attenuation
  - Rarely remodeling of adjacent osseous structures; no osseous erosion
  - Fatty infiltration during IP
- CECT
  - Diffuse and prominent contrast enhancement
  - Prominent vessels in and adjacent to mass in PP

MR Findings
- T1WI
  - PP: Isointense to muscle
  - IP: Hyperintense from fatty replacement
- T2WI: Mildly hyperintense relative to muscle
- T1WI C+: Intense contrast enhancement
  - Vessels in and adjacent to mass
- MRA: Stenosis, occlusion, agenesis, aneurysm (PHACES association)

Imaging Recommendations
- Best imaging tool
  - Ultrasound provides efficient and optimal characterization of superficial lesions
  - MR (or CT) C+ to assess deep lesions and show diffuse enhancement
  - MRA to identify associated vascular abnormalities
  - Imaging indications
    - Assessment of deep extension
    - Pretreatment if considering medical or surgical/laser treatment
    - Assessment of response to treatment
    - Suspect PHACES association
    - Atypical history, older patient

DIFFERENTIAL DIAGNOSIS

Congenital Hemangioma (RICH/NICH)
- Present at birth or on prenatal imaging
  - Rapidly involuting congenital hemangioma (RICH): Involutes by 8-14 months
  - Noninvoluting congenital hemangioma (NICH)

Parotid Venous Vascular Malformation
- Congenital vascular malformation composed of large venous lakes
- Phleboliths, serpiginous sinusoidal spaces, slow flow

Arteriovenous Malformation
- Congenital vascular malformation
- Ill-defined parenchymal mass, high-flow feeding arteries, arteriovenous shunting, and large draining veins

Rhabdomyosarcoma
- Suspect malignant neoplasm if age, appearance, growth history, or imaging are atypical for IH

PAROTID INFANTILE HEMANGIOMA

- Rhabdomyosarcoma, extraosseous Ewing sarcoma, undifferentiated sarcoma
  - Mild to moderate enhancement ± osseous erosion

Parotid Non-Hodgkin Lymphoma

- Uncommon in infants
- Parenchymal parotid NHL: Diffuse parotid infiltration with diffuse hypervascularity
- Heterogeneous echo pattern ± infiltrative margins
- May detect cervical lymphadenopathy

Parotid Lipoma (Angiolipoma)

- Difficult to differentiate from fatty involuting hemangioma on imaging; does not involute

PATHOLOGY

General Features

- Etiology
  - Proposed theory = clonal expansion of angioblasts with high expression of basic fibroblast growth factors and other angiogenesis markers
- Genetics
  - Majority sporadic
  - Rare association with chromosome 5q31-q33

Microscopic Features

- Prominent endothelial cells, pericytes, mast cells with mitotic figures, and multilaminated endothelial basement membrane
- GLUT1 immunohistochemical marker positive in all phases of growth and regression

CLINICAL ISSUES

Presentation

- Most common signs/symptoms
  - Growing soft tissue mass, typically with warm, reddish, or strawberry-like cutaneous discoloration in infant (proliferating phase)
    - Spontaneous involution over next several years
  - Occasionally deep, present with bluish coloration of skin secondary to prominent draining veins
- Other signs/symptoms
  - Ulceration of overlying skin
  - Airway obstruction from airway involvement
  - Proptosis from orbital lesion
  - Associated abnormalities in PHACES association

Demographics

- Age
  - Typically inapparent at birth; median age at presentation is 2 weeks, majority present by 1-3 months
    - Up to 1/3 nascent at birth, i.e., pale or erythematous macule, telangiectasia, pseudoecchymotic patch or red spot
- Gender
  - F:M = 2.5:1
- Epidemiology
  - Most common head and neck tumor in infants
  - Incidence is 1-2% of neonates, 12% by age 1 year
  - ↑ in preterm infants and low birth weight infants
    - Up to 30% of infants weighing < 1 kg
- Ethnicity
  - Most frequent in Caucasians

Natural History & Prognosis

- PP begins few weeks after birth and continues 1-2 years
- IP shows gradual regression over next several years
- IP usually completes by late childhood; 90% resolve by 9 years
- Large & segmental facial hemangiomas have higher incidence of complications and need for treatment

Treatment

- Majority do not require treatment; expectant waiting
- Treatment indications
  - Compromise vital structures, such as optic nerve compression or airway obstruction
  - Significant skin ulceration
- Medical therapy
  - Steroids (systemic or intralesional), propranolol, interferon
- Procedural therapy
  - Laser, rarely surgical excision and embolization

DIAGNOSTIC CHECKLIST

Consider

- Visible shortly after birth
- Radiological appearances change during phases of involution
- Diffuse intralesional vascularity in a homogeneous mass is characteristic
- Large vessels/vascular spaces suggest AVM or VVM
- If age, appearance, growth history, or imaging are atypical for IH, consider malignancy (rhabdomyosarcoma, NHL)

SELECTED REFERENCES

1. Dubois J et al: Vascular anomalies: what a radiologist needs to know. Pediatr Radiol. 40(6):895-905, 2010
2. Sinno H et al: Management of infantile parotid gland hemangiomas: a 40-year experience. Plast Reconstr Surg. 125(1):265-73, 2010
3. Storch CH et al: Propranolol for infantile haemangiomas: insights into the molecular mechanisms of action. Br J Dermatol. 163(2):269-74, 2010
4. Frieden IJ et al: Propranolol for infantile hemangiomas: promise, peril, pathogenesis. Pediatr Dermatol. 26(5):642-4, 2009
5. Judd CD et al: Intracranial infantile hemangiomas associated with PHACE syndrome. AJNR Am J Neuroradiol. 28(1):25-9, 2007
6. Mulliken JB et al: Vascular anomalies. Curr Probl Surg. 37(8):517-84, 2000
7. Robertson RL et al: Head and neck vascular anomalies of childhood. Neuroimaging Clin N Am. 9(1):115-32, 1999
8. Yang WT et al: Sonographic features of head and neck hemangiomas and vascular malformations: review of 23 patients. J Ultrasound Med. 16(1):39-44, 1997
9. Mulliken JB et al: Hemangiomas and vascular malformations in infants and children: a classification based on endothelial characteristics. Plast Reconstr Surg. 69(3):412-22, 1982

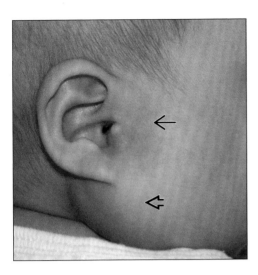

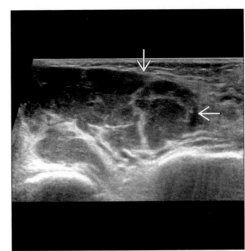

(Left) Clinical photograph shows an infant with a large right parotid infantile hemangioma. There is a large mass centered at the angle of the mandible ⮕, with reddish strawberry tinges of the overlying skin ⮕. *(Right)* Corresponding oblique transverse US shows a well-defined, solid, noncalcified, homogeneously hypoechoic mass ⮕ involving the parotid gland. US readily identifies the abnormality, suggests diagnosis, and evaluates temporal change in children on expectant treatment.

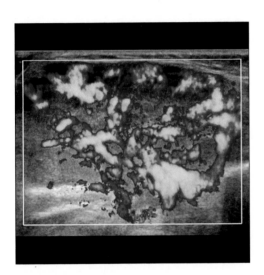

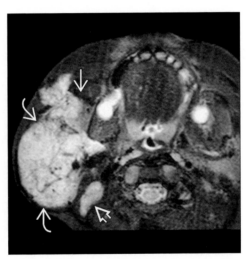

(Left) Power Doppler ultrasound of parotid IH (same child) reveals marked, diffuse vascularity scattered throughout the lesion. Such graphic vascularity often alarms accompanying parent(s). *(Right)* Corresponding axial T2WI FS MR (same patient) best demonstrates lesion conspicuity and anatomical extent on this sequence. Note this IH ⮕ extends to the masseter muscle ⮕. A separate IH is seen posteriorly ⮕ within paraspinal musculature.

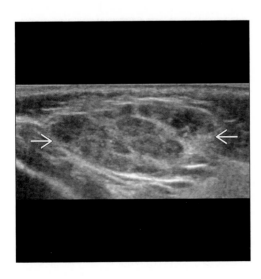

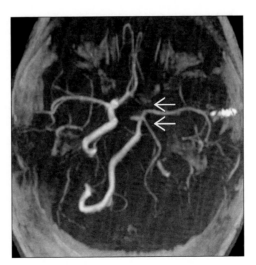

(Left) Another parotid IH is seen on ultrasound as a well-defined mass within the superficial lobe of the left parotid gland ⮕. This lesion has a heterogeneous echo pattern with internal areas of hyperechoic fat, typical for IH in involutional phase. *(Right)* Axial MRA shows absent left internal carotid artery ⮕ in a child with bilateral facial IHs and PHACES syndrome. An MRA of head and neck should be performed in patients with facial IH to exclude associated vascular abnormalities.

BENIGN LYMPHOEPITHELIAL LESIONS-HIV

Key Facts

Terminology
- Cystic lesions: Benign lymphoepithelial cysts
- Mixed solid and cystic lesions: Benign lymphoepithelial lesions
- Solid lesions: Persistent, generalized, parotid gland lymphadenopathy

Imaging
- Cysts: Usually multiple, avascular, anechoic to hypoechoic, ± mobile internal echoes, posterior acoustic enhancement
- Mixed lesions: Hypoechoic, no posterior acoustic enhancement, variable vascularity
- Solid lesions: Oval hypoechoic intraparotid nodes with hilar vascularity
- Other findings associated with HIV: Reactive cervical adenopathy, adenoid hypertrophy

Top Differential Diagnoses
- Parotid Sjögren syndrome
- 1st branchial cleft cyst
- Warthin tumor
- Non-Hodgkin lymphoma in parotid nodes

Clinical Issues
- Patient need only be HIV-positive to manifest BLEL
- BLEL may precede HIV seroconversion
- Historically, 5% of HIV-positive patients develop BLEL
- Left untreated, grow into chronic, mumps-like state with significant bilateral parotid enlargement

Diagnostic Checklist
- Bilateral, cystic, or solid masses within enlarged parotids in HIV-positive patient should be considered BLEL until proven otherwise

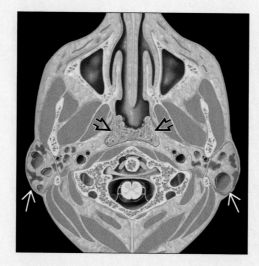
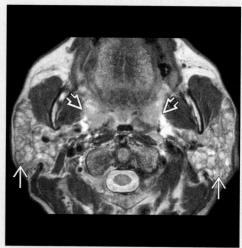

(Left) Axial graphic shows classic findings of benign lymphoepithelial lesions (BLEL) as bilateral, intraparotid cysts mixed with bilateral, solid, lymphoid aggregates ➡. Associated adenoidal hypertrophy ➡ is also characteristic. *(Right)* Axial T2WI FS MR through the oropharynx of a patient with BLEL shows typical findings of multiple hyperintense cysts in both parotid glands ➡. Appearances may be identical to parotid Sjögren syndrome. Symmetrical tonsillar hypertrophy, feature of BLEL-HIV, is also present ➡.

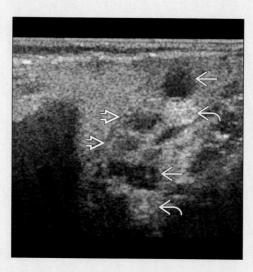
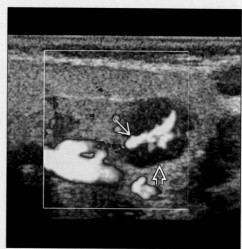

(Left) Transverse grayscale US of a patient with BLEL-HIV reveals both ill-defined, hypoechoic, lymphoid aggregates ➡ as well as cysts ➡ in the left parotid gland. Note posterior acoustic enhancement ➡. *(Right)* Longitudinal power Doppler US (same patient) reveals a hypoechoic, intraparotid node ➡ with hilar vascularity ➡. Note the round shape and nodal, cortical hypertrophy. (Courtesy A. Kulkarni, MD.)

BENIGN LYMPHOEPITHELIAL LESIONS-HIV

TERMINOLOGY

Abbreviations
- Benign lymphoepithelial lesions (BLEL)-HIV
- Benign lymphoepithelial (BLE) cysts

Synonyms
- AIDS-related parotid cysts (ARPC)
  - Avoid ARPC synonym
    - Patient need only be HIV-positive to manifest BLEL
    - May not have full-blown AIDS with BLEL

Definitions
- Multifocal mixed cystic and solid intraparotid masses found in HIV-infected patients
- 3-tiered classification
  - Cystic lesions: BLE cysts
  - Mixed solid and cystic lesions: BLEL
  - Solid lesions: Persistent, generalized parotid gland lymphadenopathy

IMAGING

General Features
- Best diagnostic clue
  - Multiple cystic and solid masses enlarging both parotid glands associated with tonsillar hyperplasia and reactive cervical adenopathy
- Location
  - Bilateral parotid spaces
  - Rarely seen in submandibular or sublingual salivary glands
    - Only parotid has intrinsic lymphoid tissue
- Size
  - Variable: Typically several mm, ≤ 3.5 cm
- Morphology
  - Cysts are well circumscribed, rounded
  - Solid lymphoid aggregates may be poorly defined
  - Often innumerable small masses; uncommonly solitary

Ultrasonographic Findings
- Grayscale ultrasound
  - Spectrum of sonographic findings ranging from simple cysts to mixed and solid masses
    - Cystic, mixed, and solid lesions can occur simultaneously in parotid glands
  - Cystic lesions (benign lymphoepithelial cysts)
    - Well defined, variable in size
    - Anechoic to hypoechoic
    - Posterior acoustic enhancement
    - Network of thin septa ± mural nodules
    - Internal echoes are common, which may be mobile
    - "Honeycomb" appearance of parotid parenchyma when innumerable and diffuse
  - Mixed lesions (benign lymphoepithelial lesions)
    - May be ill defined, variable in size
    - Predominantly hypoechoic, can be heterogeneous
    - No posterior acoustic enhancement
  - Solid lesions (parotid lymphadenopathy)
    - Oval/round, hypoechoic, intraparotid nodes, multiple
    - Prominent cortex, ± hilar architecture
  - Associated reactive cervical lymphadenopathy
- Color Doppler
  - Cystic lesions: Avascular to mild vascular flow in septa, intramural nodules, and periphery
  - Mixed lesions: Variable, mild to moderate vascularity
  - Solid lesions: Hilar vascularity in intraparotid nodes

CT Findings
- NECT
  - Multiple, bilateral, well-circumscribed cystic and solid masses within enlarged parotid glands
- CECT
  - Thin rim enhancement of cystic lesions with heterogeneous enhancement of solid lesions
  - Other CECT findings associated with HIV
    - Reactive cervical adenopathy
    - Adenoidal, palatine, and lingual tonsillar hypertrophy

MR Findings
- T1WI
  - Low signal intensity cystic lesions
  - Heterogeneous variable signal in solid lesions
    - Normal parotid fat provides good inherent contrast
- T2WI
  - Hyperintense, bilateral, well-circumscribed, round to ovoid intraparotid lesions
  - Hyperintense, bilateral, cervical lymphadenopathy
  - Waldeyer lymphatic ring enlargement with high signal
- T1WI C+
  - Thin rim enhancement in cystic lesions with variable heterogeneous enhancement of solid lesions
  - Solid lesions may be less conspicuous on C+ than unenhanced T1WI because of surrounding fat

DIFFERENTIAL DIAGNOSIS

Parotid Sjögren Syndrome
- Older women with Sicca syndrome (dry eyes, dry mouth, dry skin) and connective tissue disorder (rheumatoid arthritis); antinuclear antibodies
- Cystic lesions may be identical to BLEL cysts on imaging
- Heterogeneous background parotid parenchyma difficult to appreciate with innumerable cysts
- ± involvement of submandibular and lacrimal glands

1st Branchial Cleft Cyst (BCC)
- Solitary, unilateral, cystic, intraparotid mass
  - Work type 2
- Anechoic, ± fine debris, thin walls, pseudosolid appearance, posterior enhancement
- May see beaking towards bony external auditory canal (EAC)
- Lymphadenopathy when inflammation present

Warthin Tumor
- Solitary or multifocal parotid masses
  - Solid or mixed cystic-solid parotid masses with nodular walls
  - 20% are multifocal but never innumerable
  - Solid/cystic, thick walls, septi, internal debris, ± vascularity particularly hilar in small lesions
  - Lacks associated tonsillar hyperplasia and cervical adenopathy

BENIGN LYMPHOEPITHELIAL LESIONS-HIV

Non-Hodgkin Lymphoma in Parotid Nodes
- Bilateral, solid, intraparotid masses in systemic NHL
  - May be identical to persistent parotid gland lymphadenopathy
  - Lymphadenopathy elsewhere usually already apparent
  - Solid, round, noncalcified, hypoechoic, reticulated/ pseudocystic, hilar > peripheral vascularity
- Primary parotid NHL very uncommon
  - Unilateral, multifocal, solid intraparotid masses or diffuse parenchymal heterogeneity

Metastatic Disease to Parotid Nodes
- Unilateral, multifocal, solid parotid masses, ± central necrosis, abnormal vascularity
- Primary malignancy and other metastatic deposits already apparent

Parotid Sarcoidosis
- Cervical and mediastinal lymph nodes
  - May be identical to BLEL
- Intraparotid sarcoid is very rare

PATHOLOGY

General Features
- Etiology
  - Hypothesis 1: Periductal lymphoid aggregates cause ductal radicular obstruction, periductal atrophy, and distal cyst formation
  - Hypothesis 2: Cystification; cyst formation occurs in included glandular epithelium within intraparotid nodes
  - Does not arise directly from intraparotid lymph nodes
- Associated abnormalities
  - Cervical lymphadenopathy and nasopharyngeal lymphofollicular hyperplasia
- Cystic spaces lined by squamous epithelium accompanied by abundant lymphoid stroma
- Rare transformation to B-cell lymphoma reported

Gross Pathologic & Surgical Features
- Diffusely enlarged parotid glands with multiple well-delineated nodules with rubbery consistency and smooth, tan-white, fleshy appearance

Microscopic Features
- Thin, smooth-walled cysts measuring a few mm to 3-4 cm
- Aspiration of cyst fluid reveals foamy macrophages, lymphoid and epithelial cells, and multinucleated giant cells
  - Intense immunoexpression of S100 and p24 (HIV-1) protein in multinucleated giant cells

CLINICAL ISSUES

Presentation
- Most common signs/symptoms
  - Bilateral painless parotid gland enlargement
- Other signs/symptoms
  - Cervical lymphadenopathy
  - Tonsillar swelling
- Clinical profile
  - Bilateral parotid masses in HIV-positive patient

- Initially seen in HIV-positive patients prior to AIDS onset
  - BLEL may precede HIV seroconversion
  - BLEL not considered precursor to AIDS

Demographics
- Age
  - Any age infected with HIV
- Epidemiology
  - Historically, 5% of HIV-positive patients develop BLEL
  - BLEL seen less frequently since institution of combination antiviral therapy

Natural History & Prognosis
- Left untreated, grow into chronic, mumps-like state with significant bilateral parotid enlargement
- Rarely may transform into B-cell lymphoma
- Patient prognosis dependent on other HIV- and AIDS-related diseases, not on BLEL

Treatment
- Combination antiretroviral therapy for HIV will completely or partially treat BLEL of parotid glands
- Radiotherapy yields mixed, temporary regression
- BLE cysts: Intralesional doxycycline or alcohol sclerotherapy if painful or if not antiviral candidate
- Surgical excision not recommended in AIDS patients

DIAGNOSTIC CHECKLIST

Consider
- Bilateral cystic or solid masses within enlarged parotids in HIV-positive patient should be considered BLEL until proven otherwise
- BLE may be 1st sign of HIV infection; recommend HIV testing in characteristic cases

Image Interpretation Pearls
- Cystic, mixed, and solid lesions can occur simultaneously within the parotid glands
- Nonnecrotic cervical adenopathy with tonsillar hypertrophy can be important clue to BLEL diagnosis on CT or MR
- When BLE cysts present as unilateral, solitary, cystic intraparotid mass, may be mistaken for 1st branchial cleft cyst
- When BLEL presents as unilateral, solid, intraparotid mass, may be mistaken for parotid tumor

SELECTED REFERENCES

1. Kabenge C et al: Diagnostic ultrasound patterns of parotid glands in human immunodeficiency virus-positive patients in Mulago, Uganda. Dentomaxillofac Radiol. 39(7):389-99, 2010
2. Berg EE et al: Office-based sclerotherapy for benign parotid lymphoepithelial cysts in the HIV-positive patient. Laryngoscope. 119(5):868-70, 2009
3. Martinoli C et al: Benign lymphoepithelial parotid lesions in HIV-positive patients: spectrum of findings at gray-scale and Doppler sonography. AJR Am J Roentgenol. 165(4):975-9, 1995
4. Som PM et al: Nodal inclusion cysts of the parotid gland and parapharyngeal space: a discussion of lymphoepithelial, AIDS-related parotid, and branchial cysts, cystic Warthin's tumors, and cysts in Sjogren's syndrome. Laryngoscope. 105(10): 1122-8, 1995

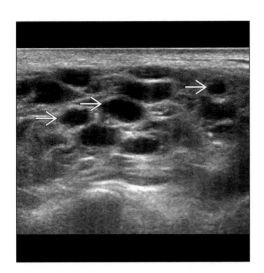

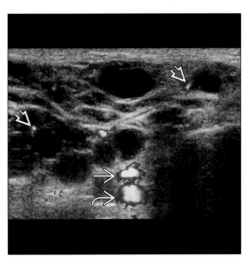

(Left) Longitudinal grayscale ultrasound of the right parotid gland in a patient in with BLEL shows innumerable anechoic to hypoechoic lymphoepithelial cysts throughout superficial lobe ➡. (Right) Corresponding axial power Doppler ultrasound reveals that lesions are essentially anechoic with some showing mild peripheral vascularity ➡. Retromandibular vein ➡ and external carotid artery ➡ are shown. Appearances are similar to macrocysts in Sjögren syndrome.

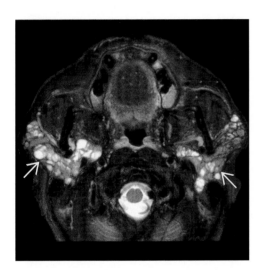

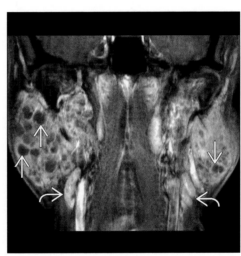

(Left) Axial T2WI FS MR (same patient) at level of oropharynx shows innumerable cystic lesions within enlarged parotid glands bilaterally ➡, giving the parotid glands a "honeycomb" appearance. (Right) Corresponding coronal T1WI C+ FS MR shows multiple nonenhancing lymphoepithelial cysts ➡ against an enhancing parotid parenchyma. Note bilateral, reactive, upper cervical lymphadenopathy ➡ associated with BLEL.

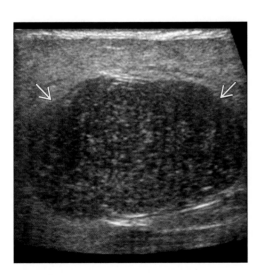

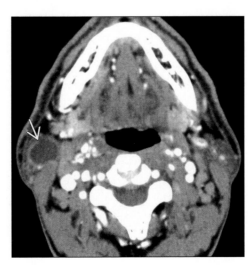

(Left) Longitudinal grayscale US shows BLEL-HIV cyst in the left parotid gland as a solitary, unilocular cystic lesion ➡, with low-level internal echoes consistent with debris. Features mimic 1st branchial cleft cyst. (Courtesy R. Sofferman, MD.) (Right) Axial CECT of a different patient through midoropharynx shows an isolated, rim-enhancing BLEL-HIV cyst of the right parotid gland ➡. When solitary, BLEL-HIV may be mistaken for 1st BCC.

ACUTE PAROTITIS

Key Facts

Terminology

- Acute inflammation of parotid gland (4 types)
  - Bacterial: Localized bacterial infection; ± abscess
  - Viral: Usually from systemic viral infection
  - Calculus-induced: Ductal obstruction by sialolith
  - Autoimmune: Acute episode of chronic disease

Imaging

- Parotid is most commonly inflamed salivary gland (absent bacteriostatic mucin in its serous secretions)
- Diffuse glandular enlargement, unilateral or bilateral, depending on underlying etiology
- Heterogeneous hypoechoic echo pattern, ± ↑ parenchymal vascularity
- Tiny hyperechoic foci within glandular parenchyma, represent air within intraglandular ducts
- Tender on transducer pressure
- Presence of reactive peri-/intraparotid lymph nodes

- Uncontrolled disease → abscess formation seen as ill-defined, hypoechoic necrotic mass ± air/gas
- Parotid ductal calculi: Echogenic filling defect within dilated parotid duct ± posterior acoustic shadowing
  - Dilatation of intraparenchymal ducts within affected parotid gland
- In absence of dilated duct, US may miss small parotid calculus; NECT is more sensitive
- US is imaging modality of choice for suspected bacterial acute parotitis
  - Detection of stone, which requires surgical removal
  - Detect any abscess and guide aspiration of pus

Top Differential Diagnoses

- Sjögren syndrome
- Parotid sialosis
- Benign lymphoepithelial lesion-HIV
- Parotid sarcoidosis

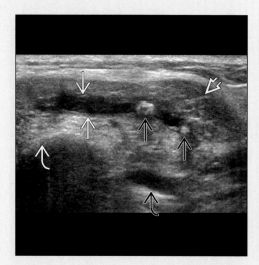
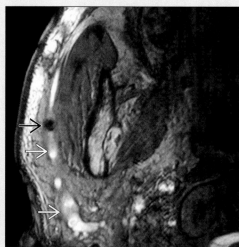

(Left) Longitudinal grayscale US of the parotid gland shows a dilated intraparotid duct ⬇ with multiple small calculi ⇨ within. Note parotid salivary parenchyma ⇨ is diffusely hypoechoic and heterogeneous (with ↑ vascularity, not shown), evidence of parotitis. Note the mandibular cortex ⇨ and retromandibular vein (RMV) ⇨. *(Right)* Corresponding MR sialogram also shows a dilated intraparotid duct ⇨ with ductal calculus ⇨, seen as signal void focus within the dilated duct.

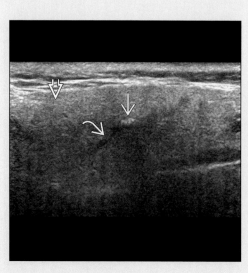
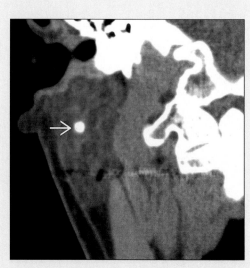

(Left) Longitudinal grayscale US shows subtle echogenicity ⇨ (calculus) in a parotid gland with minimal adjacent duct dilatation ⇨. Note adjacent parotid parenchyma ⇨ shows its normal fine, bright parenchymal echo pattern, suggesting that an acute episode of calculus parotitis has resolved. *(Right)* Corresponding coronal NECT clearly shows calculus ⇨ in the right parotid gland. In the absence of a dilated duct, US may miss small parotid calculus. NECT is more sensitive in detecting small parotid calculi.

ACUTE PAROTITIS

TERMINOLOGY

Definitions
- Acute inflammation of parotid gland (4 types)
  - Bacterial: Localized infection may become suppurative, with central abscess
  - Viral: Usually from systemic viral infection
  - Calculus-induced: Ductal obstruction by sialolith
  - Autoimmune: Acute episode of chronic disease

IMAGING

General Features
- Location
  - Bacterial: Usually unilateral
  - Viral: 75% bilateral; submandibular and sublingual glands may also be involved
  - Calculus-induced: Unilateral, with radiopaque stone in parotid duct
    - Most frequent locations for calculus: Hilum of gland, distal parotid duct
  - Autoimmune: Usually bilateral
- Morphology
  - Usually involves entire gland but can be focal

Ultrasonographic Findings
- Diffuse glandular enlargement
  - Unilateral or bilateral, depending on underlying etiology, ± ↑ parenchymal vascularity
- Heterogeneous hypoechoic echo pattern
- Tiny hyperechoic foci within glandular parenchyma
  - Represent air within intraglandular ducts
- Tender on probe pressure
- Presence of reactive periparotid and intraparotid lymph nodes
  - Mildly enlarged, elliptical, preserved echogenic hilum and hilar vascularity
- Uncontrolled disease may progress to abscess formation
  - Ill-defined, hypoechoic mass with liquefied component ± gas
- Detection of parotid ductal calculi
  - Trace along course of parotid duct
  - Echogenic focus within dilated parotid duct
  - ± posterior acoustic shadowing
  - Dilatation of intraparenchymal ducts within affected parotid gland

Imaging Recommendations
- Best imaging tool
  - Viral and autoimmune parotitis are clinical diagnosis
    - Imaging is usually not necessary
  - US is imaging modality of choice for suspected bacterial acute parotitis
    - Detection of stone that requires subsequent removal
      - Particularly for patient with recurrent episodes of infection
    - Detection of abscess formation: US can be used to guide aspiration of pus
    - In absence of dilated duct, US may be insensitive to presence of small parotid calculus; NECT is more sensitive

DIFFERENTIAL DIAGNOSIS

Sjögren Syndrome
- Dry eyes and mouth, arthritis
- Involvement of submandibular and lacrimal glands in addition to parotid glands
- Heterogeneous parenchyma with macro-/microcysts and reticulated appearance

Parotid Sialosis
- Bilateral, prolonged, painless, soft parotid (and occasionally submandibular gland) enlargement
- Associated with alcoholism, endocrinopathies (especially diabetes mellitus), malnutrition (including anorexia nervosa, bulimia)

Benign Lymphoepithelial Lesion-HIV
- Often with cystic and solid lesions
- Bilateral heterogeneous parotids

Parotid Sarcoidosis
- Uveitis and facial paralysis (Heerfordt disease)
- Diffuse hypoechoic enlargement of both parotid glands
- Nodal enlargement

PATHOLOGY

General Features
- Etiology
  - Bacterial: Usually due to ascending infection
    - May result from adjacent cellulitis
    - *Staphylococcus aureus* (50-90%) > *Streptococcus*, *Haemophilus*, *Escherichia coli*, anaerobes
  - Viral: Mumps paramyxovirus most common cause
  - Recurrent parotitis of childhood
    - Recurrent episodes mimic mumps
    - Usually begin by age 5; resolves by age 10-15
    - Etiology unknown

CLINICAL ISSUES

Presentation
- Most common signs/symptoms
  - Bacterial: Sudden-onset parotid pain and swelling
  - Viral: Prodromal symptoms of headaches, malaise, myalgia followed by parotid pain, earache, trismus
  - Calculus-induced: Recurrent episodes of swollen, painful gland, usually related to eating
  - Autoimmune: Recurrent episodes of tender gland swelling, accompanied by dry mouth

Demographics
- Age
  - Bacterial: > 50 years & neonates
  - Viral: Most < 15 years; peak age: 5-9 years
    - Frequently seen in children who have not received MMR vaccine
      - Adults usually immune from childhood exposure or MMR vaccine

SELECTED REFERENCES

1. Sodhi KS et al: Role of high resolution ultrasound in parotid lesions in children. Int J Pediatr Otorhinolaryngol. 75(11):1353-8, 2011

ACUTE PAROTITIS

(Left) Longitudinal grayscale US shows diffuse, smooth dilatation of a parotid duct ➡ as it passes over the masseter muscle ➡ toward its intraoral opening after piercing the buccinator muscle. Note the mandibular cortex ➡. *(Right)* Corresponding MR sialogram demonstrates the entire length of dilated intraparotid duct ➡ with no obvious focal intraductal calculus. This patient had a history of recent passage of parotid calculus.

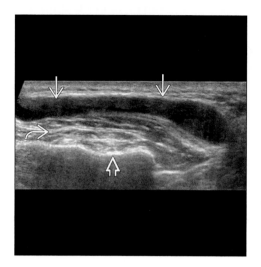
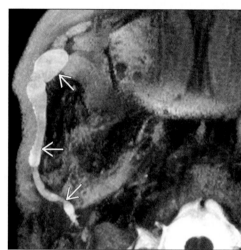

(Left) Transverse grayscale US in a patient with bacterial parotitis shows diffuse enlargement of the parotid gland ➡ with rounded contours. Note the diffuse, hypoechoic, heterogeneous parenchymal echo pattern typically seen with acute parotitis. Intraparotid duct ➡ is mildly dilated with debris within. No obvious calculus is seen. Note thickening of overlying subcutaneous tissue ➡. *(Right)* Corresponding power Doppler US shows ↑ vascularity in the salivary parenchyma, a feature of acute parotitis.

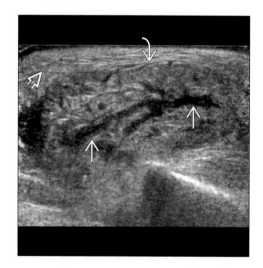
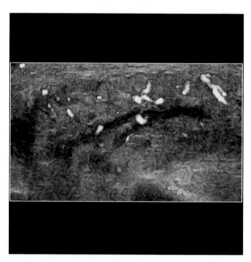

(Left) Transverse grayscale US shows acute parotitis in a patient receiving radiation therapy for H&N cancer. Note diffuse enlargement of parotid gland ➡, rounded contours, heterogeneous parenchymal echo pattern, and subcutaneous edema ➡. Multiple, hypoechoic bands ➡ (avascular on Doppler) are seen within parenchyma, representing interstitial edema. *(Right)* Corresponding longitudinal US shows extent of parotid involvement. Such glands are usually tender on transducer pressure.

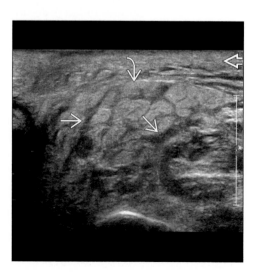
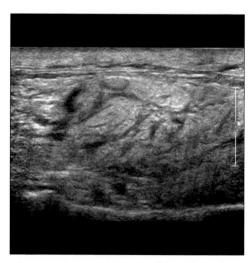

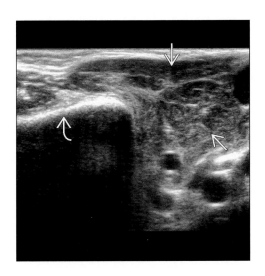

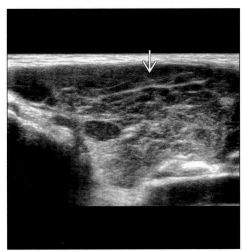

(Left) Transverse grayscale US in a child with mumps shows enlargement of the parotid gland ➔ and diffuse hypoechoic parenchymal echo pattern. No focal duct dilatation or calculus is seen. Note the mandibular cortex ➔. (Courtesy S. Vaid, MD.) *(Right)* Corresponding longitudinal grayscale US shows extent of involvement of the parotid gland ➔. Such parotitis is usually self-limiting and seen in children who have not received MMR vaccination, and usually no imaging is required. (Courtesy S. Vaid, MD.)

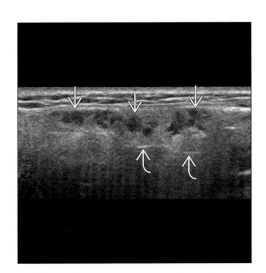

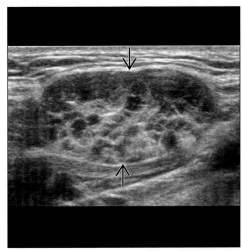

(Left) Longitudinal grayscale US shows focal, hypoechoic, heterogeneous areas ➔ within parotid gland, mimicking focal acute parotitis. Nondilated intraparotid duct ➔ is seen as an echogenic linear structure within parenchyma. *(Right)* Transverse grayscale US of the submandibular gland (SMG) (same patient) shows characteristic "cirrhotic" appearance ➔, a feature of chronic sclerosing sialadenitis. These patients have painless enlargement of multiple salivary glands, SMG > parotid.

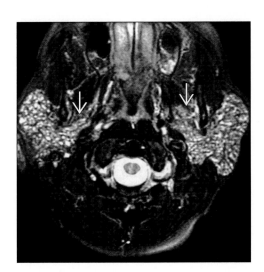

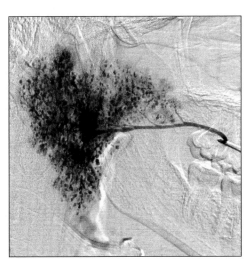

(Left) Axial T2WI FS MR in a patient with acute exacerbation of autoimmune sialadenitis shows diffuse enlargement of both parotid glands with numerous foci of increased signal. Note diffuse involvement includes deep parotid lobes ➔. (Courtesy B. Branstetter, MD.) *(Right)* Lateral sialogram in a young woman with Sjögren syndrome with parotid swelling and discomfort shows diffuse globular contrast collections in the right parotid and relatively normal ducts. (Courtesy B. Branstetter, MD.)

SUBMANDIBULAR GLAND BENIGN MIXED TUMOR

Key Facts

Imaging

- Well defined, solid & hypoechoic compared to adjacent salivary tissue
- Homogeneous internal echo pattern with posterior enhancement
- Larger tumors may have heterogeneous internal echoes due to hemorrhage and necrosis
- Heterogeneous BMT may have ill-defined margins simulating malignant mass
- Calcification unusual, seen in longstanding tumor
- Overlying skin & subcutaneous tissues are normal
- No obviously abnormal/metastatic adjacent node
- Color Doppler: Peripheral vessels, mainly venous
- Spectral Doppler: Low intranodular vascular resistance (RI < 0.8 & PI < 2.0)

Top Differential Diagnoses

- Malignant tumor, submandibular gland (ACCa or MECa)

- Chronic sclerosing sialadenitis, Kuttner tumor
- Adenopathy, SMS

Diagnostic Checklist

- If left untreated, benign mixed tumor (BMT) may undergo malignant change; risk ↑ with chronicity
- Presence of calcification in BMT, implies longstanding tumor and should raise suspicion
- In evaluating submandibular salivary masses, always carefully assess
  - Edge: Malignant tumors have ill-defined edges compared to benign lesions
  - Internal architecture: Malignant tumors have heterogeneous architecture; benign tumors usually have homogeneous architecture
- Malignant tumors more likely to show pronounced vascularity with RI > 0.8 & PI > 2.0
- Malignant tumors more likely associated with extraglandular infiltration & nodal involvement

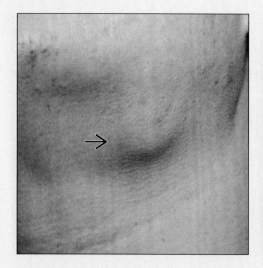
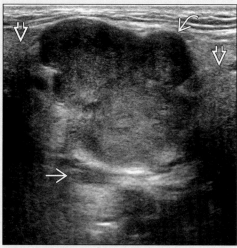

(Left) Clinical photo shows a patient presenting with a painless mass ⟶ in the left submandibular region. *(Right)* Corresponding transverse grayscale US shows a solid, hypoechoic, homogeneous, noncalcified mass ⟶ in the left submandibular gland. Note its lobulated, sharply defined outlines, posterior enhancement ⟶, and lack of involvement of overlying soft tissues. US features are suggestive of a nonaggressive salivary gland tumor such as BMT (confirmed at surgery). Note normal submandibular parenchyma ⟶.

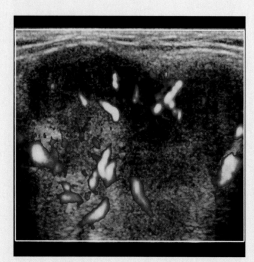
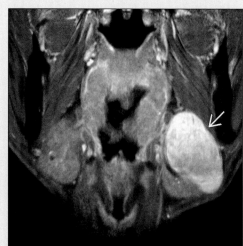

(Left) Transverse power Doppler US (same patient) shows intranodular vessels, which are relatively sparse compared to size of lesion. These vessels are usually of low resistance with RI < 0.8 and PI < 2.0. *(Right)* Coronal T1WI C+ FS shows avid homogeneous enhancement of a submandibular BMT ⟶. Larger tumors show heterogeneous enhancement with areas of intratumoral necrosis. MR/CT may be indicated for large tumors where US is unable to define the entire extent of the lesion.

SUBMANDIBULAR GLAND BENIGN MIXED TUMOR

TERMINOLOGY

Abbreviations
- Benign mixed tumor (BMT) of submandibular gland (SMG)

Definitions
- Benign mixed tumor of submandibular gland origin composed of epithelial, myoepithelial, and stromal components

IMAGING

Ultrasonographic Findings
- Grayscale ultrasound
  - Well defined, solid and hypoechoic compared to adjacent salivary tissue
  - Homogeneous internal echo pattern with posterior enhancement
    - Tumor offers few interfaces and allows sound to penetrate easily, producing posterior enhancement
  - Larger tumors may have heterogeneous internal echoes due to hemorrhage and necrosis
  - Heterogeneous BMT may have ill-defined margins, simulating malignant mass
  - Large tumors may be lobulated and appear pedunculated
  - Calcification unusual, seen in longstanding tumor
  - Overlying skin and subcutaneous tissues are normal
  - No obviously abnormal/metastatic adjacent node
- Color Doppler
  - Peripheral vessels, mainly venous; often sparse
  - Spectral Doppler: Low intranodular vascular resistance (resistive index [RI] < 0.8 and pulsatility index [PI] < 2.0)

MR Findings
- T1WI
  - Small BMT: Low-signal intensity mass
  - Large BMT: Inhomogeneous mixed-signal mass
- T2WI
  - Small BMT: Increased-signal SMG mass
  - Large BMT: Inhomogeneous, lobulated, mixed signal intensity SMG mass
- T1WI C+
  - Small BMT: Variable, mostly homogeneously enhancing mass
  - Large BMT: Heterogeneously enhancing mass
  - Low-intensity capsule surrounding BMT may be seen, especially with fat saturation

CT Findings
- NECT
  - Small BMT: Smoothly marginated, homogeneous, spherical mass; higher density than SMG
  - Large BMT: Nonhomogeneous, lobulated, mixed-density mass with areas of lower attenuation from foci of degenerative necrosis and old hemorrhage
- CECT
  - Mild to moderate enhancement
  - Adjacent inflammatory changes ± hemorrhage cause indistinct border, mimicking malignancy

Imaging Recommendations
- Best imaging tool

- US is ideal imaging tool for evaluating submandibular lesions, as it visualizes complete gland
  - US also evaluates adjacent nodes and soft tissues for tumor involvement, if any
  - US is readily combined with guided fine-needle aspiration cytology (FNAC), which has sensitivity of 83%, specificity of 86%, and accuracy of 85% for salivary gland tumors
- Protocol advice
  - BMT is most common tumor of submandibular gland
    - 55% of SMG tumors are benign; 45% malignant
  - In evaluating SMG masses, carefully assess
    - Edge: Malignant tumors have ill-defined edges compared to benign lesions
    - Internal architecture: Malignant tumors have heterogeneous architecture; benign tumors usually have homogeneous architecture
  - Malignant tumors more likely associated with extraglandular infiltration and nodal involvement
  - Malignant tumors more likely to show pronounced vascularity with RI > 0.8 and PI > 2.0

DIFFERENTIAL DIAGNOSIS

Malignant Tumor, SMG (ACCa or MECa)
- Ill-defined, heterogeneous mass with adjacent malignant lymphadenopathy, ± extraglandular extension and abnormal vascularity

Chronic Sclerosing Sialadenitis, Kuttner Tumor
- Bilateral involvement; multiple hypoechoic areas simulating salivary mass; no associated mass effect or vascular displacement; end-stage "cirrhotic" pattern

Adenopathy, SMS
- Solid, round, hypoechoic with echogenic hilus and normal hilar vascularity

CLINICAL ISSUES

Natural History & Prognosis
- Recurrent tumor tends to be multifocal
  - Recurrence rate < 50% and take years to develop because of slow growth rate
- If left untreated, BMT may undergo malignant change; risk ↑ with chronicity

DIAGNOSTIC CHECKLIST

Image Interpretation Pearls
- Differentiation of submandibular space masses
  - In masses of submandibular space, first decide if mass is within or outside submandibular gland
    - If within gland, smaller BMT is easily recognized by its well-demarcated, homogeneous appearance
  - Larger BMT may be difficult to tell from SMG malignancy because of its multilobular, heterogeneous nature, ± ill-defined edges

SELECTED REFERENCES
1. Lee YY et al: Imaging of salivary gland tumours. Eur J Radiol. 66(3):419-36, 2008

SUBMANDIBULAR GLAND BENIGN MIXED TUMOR

(Left) Transverse grayscale US shows a solid, hypoechoic, homogeneous, noncalcified, well-defined tumor ➡ with posterior enhancement ➡ arising from the right submandibular gland ➡. *(Right)* Transverse grayscale US shows another patient with a solid, well-defined, lobulated, hypoechoic, homogeneous, & noncalcified right submandibular mass ➡. In both cases, BMT was confirmed at surgery. For such small lesions, US is the ideal imaging modality as it demonstrates the entire extent and nature of the tumor.

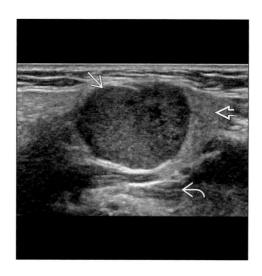
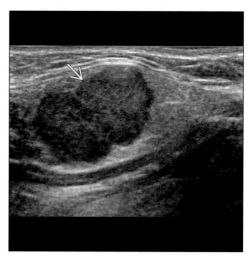

(Left) Transverse grayscale US shows a hypoechoic, heterogeneous, slightly lobulated, noncalcified BMT ➡ arising from the left submandibular gland ➡. US clearly shows that the BMT is restricted to the SMG with no extension into adjacent tissues. No further imaging is usually required for such a small tumor. US also readily guides needle biopsy for confirmation. *(Right)* Corresponding power Doppler US shows sparse peripheral vessels (mainly venous) within the SMG BMT.

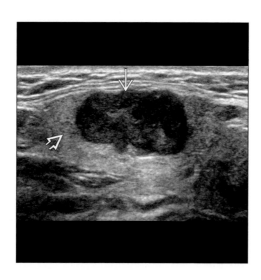
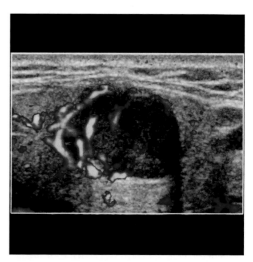

(Left) Longitudinal grayscale US at the angle of the mandible shows a large, well-defined homogeneous solid BMT ➡ arising from the right SMG. Note the rim of normal salivary tissue ➡. The entire edge of this tumor is not clearly defined, a limitation of US for large SMG tumors. The mandible ➡ is shown. *(Right)* Corresponding T1WI C+ FS shows the entire extent of this heterogeneously enhancing left SMG BMT ➡. Exact extent and anatomic relations of large BMTs are better demonstrated by MR/CT.

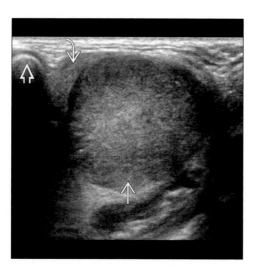
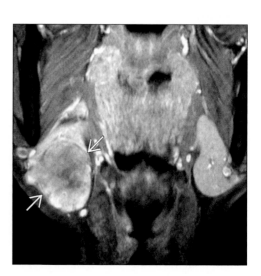

SUBMANDIBULAR GLAND BENIGN MIXED TUMOR

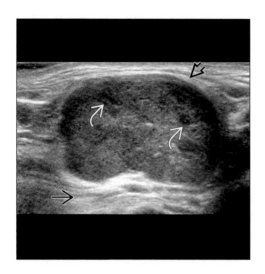

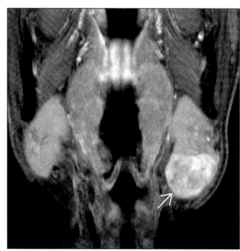

(Left) Transverse grayscale US shows a large left SMG BMT ➡. Note that it has well-defined outlines and is predominantly homogeneous but has areas of intratumoral necrosis ➡ and demonstrates posterior enhancement ➡. *(Right)* Corresponding T1WI C+ FS MR shows heterogeneous enhancement within left SMG BMT ➡. Larger lesions appear heterogeneous on MR with areas of necrosis, and a longstanding tumor may demonstrate signal void corresponding to calcification.

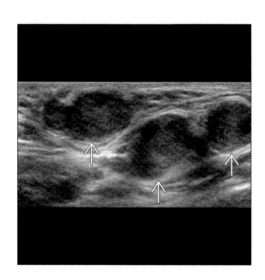

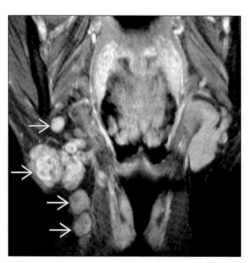

(Left) Grayscale US in a patient with previous history of excision of SMG BMT shows multiple solid, homogeneous, noncalcified nodules ➡ at the operative site. These were confirmed to be recurrent BMTs. Operative rupture of BMT capsule seeds the surgical bed, resulting in multifocal recurrence, which is surgically challenging. Recurrence usually takes years to develop because of slow growth rate. *(Right)* Corresponding T1WI C+ FS MR clearly demonstrates multifocal recurrence of BMT ➡ at the operative site.

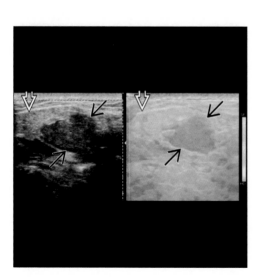

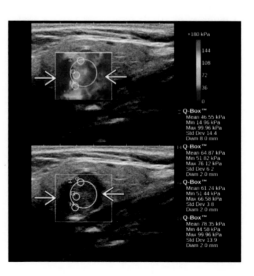

(Left) Transverse grayscale US and qualitative strain EI show a SMG BMT ➡. Strain color scale ranges from purple (elastic, soft) to red (inelastic, hard). It is inelastic compared with normal SMG ➡. *(Right)* Transverse grayscale US and SWE show SMG BMT ➡. SWE color scale ranges from blue (0 kPa, soft) to red (180 kPa, stiff). It is heterogeneous on SWE with a maximum SWE value of ~ 100 kPa. This suggests a relatively stiff lesion. BMTs may overlap in EI stiffness with malignant salivary tumor.

SUBMANDIBULAR GLAND CARCINOMA

Key Facts

Imaging

- Best imaging clue: Ill-defined, hypoechoic mass arising from SMG ± invasion of extraglandular soft tissues/perineural spread, ± nodal involvement
- Small tumors may be well defined and have homogeneous internal architecture
- Large tumors are ill defined and heterogeneous with invasive edges and areas of necrosis/hemorrhage
- ± extraglandular invasion of soft tissues
- ± metastatic skin/subcutaneous nodules
- ± adjacent nodal, disseminated metastases
- Pronounced intratumoral vascularity
- Spectral Doppler: Increased intravascular resistance

Top Differential Diagnoses

- Malignant node, submandibular space (SMS)
- Chronic sclerosing sialadenitis, Kuttner tumor
- Benign mixed tumor (BMT) of submandibular gland (SMG)

Clinical Issues

- 45% of SMG tumors are malignant; 55% benign
- Most common SMG carcinoma is ACCa (40%)
- 50% 5-year survival for all SMG cancers
- Metastatic disease accounts for 30% of deaths
- ACCa spreads via nerves, also to lungs
- MECa and AdCa: Nodal & hematogenous spread

Diagnostic Checklist

- US is useful in identifying tumor, suggesting its malignant nature and guiding biopsy
  - Evaluate tumor edge, extraglandular/nodal involvement, internal heterogeneity
- US cannot evaluate entire extent of large tumors or delineate perineural spread
  - MR ideally evaluates tumor, its local extent, perineural spread, and nodal involvement, if any
- Low FDG avidity on PET/CT, unless high grade

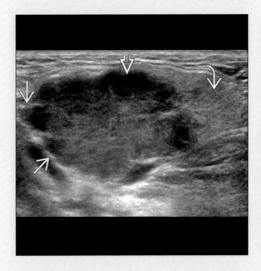
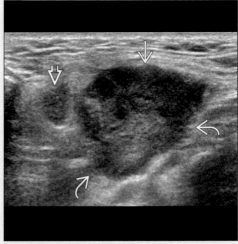

(Left) Transverse grayscale US shows left submandibular carcinoma ⮊ as a solid, ill-defined, noncalcified, hypoechoic tumor with spiculated edges at the periphery ➡ and extraglandular extension. Note its origin from SMG parenchyma ➡.
(Right) Corresponding longitudinal grayscale US again demonstrates ill-defined, spiculated edges ➡ and an extraglandular extension of SMG carcinoma ➡. Note the adjacent malignant-looking node ⮊ associated with SMG carcinoma.

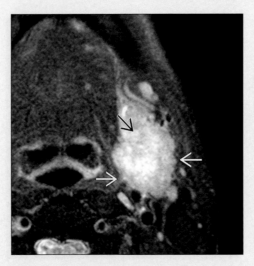
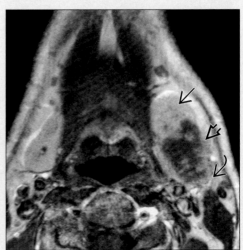

(Left) Axial T2WI MR (same patient) shows diffuse involvement of left SMG by hyperintense tumor ➡. Note its extraglandular extension into soft tissues ➡. *(Right)* Corresponding T1WI C+ MR shows a heterogeneously enhancing mass ⮊ emerging from the left SMG ➡ with extraglandular extension into soft tissues posteriorly ➡. MR ideally evaluates the anatomical extent and perineural involvement of malignant salivary tumors.

SUBMANDIBULAR GLAND CARCINOMA

TERMINOLOGY

Definitions
- Major carcinomas of submandibular gland (SMG)
  - Adenoid cystic carcinoma (ACCa), mucoepidermoid carcinoma (MECa), and adenocarcinoma (AdCa)

IMAGING

General Features
- Best diagnostic clue
  - Ill-defined, hypoechoic mass arising from SMG ± invasion of extraglandular soft tissues/perineural spread, ± nodal involvement
- Location
  - Most often superficial aspect of SMG in submandibular space (SMS)
    - Inferolateral to mylohyoid muscle

Ultrasonographic Findings
- Grayscale ultrasound
  - Unable to differentiate various malignant tumors
  - Small tumors may be well-defined and have homogeneous internal architecture
  - Large tumors are ill-defined, heterogeneous with invasive edges and areas of necrosis/hemorrhage
  - ± extraglandular invasion of soft tissues
  - ± metastatic skin/subcutaneous nodules
  - ± adjacent nodal, disseminated metastases
- Color Doppler
  - Pronounced intratumoral vascularity
  - Spectral Doppler: Increased intravascular resistance
    - Resistive index (RI) > 0.8, pulsatility index (PI) > 2.0

CT Findings
- NECT
  - Asymmetry of size and heterogeneous SMG
- CECT
  - Small tumor: Well-circumscribed, ovoid mass
  - Large tumor: Enhancing mass arising from SMG into SMS with invasive margins
  - Uncommon to have bone erosion unless locally advanced tumor

MR Findings
- T1WI
  - Isointense to muscle, hypointense to glandular tissue
- T2WI
  - Intermediate to high mixed signal intensity
  - High grade tends to be intermediate to low signal
- T1WI C+
  - Variable contrast enhancement
  - Small tumor: Ovoid, intraglandular enhancing mass with sharp borders
  - Large tumor: Enhancing mass emerging from SMG into SMS with poorly defined margins

Imaging Recommendations
- Best imaging tool
  - US is ideal imaging modality to evaluate SMG tumors due to their superficial location
  - US readily combines with fine-needle aspiration cytology, which has sensitivity of 83%, specificity of 86%, and accuracy of 85% for salivary gland tumors
- Protocol advice
  - Evaluate tumor edge, extraglandular/nodal involvement, internal heterogeneity
  - US cannot evaluate entire extent of large tumors and delineate perineural spread
    - US is useful in identifying tumor, suggesting its malignant nature and guiding biopsy
  - MR ideally evaluates tumor, its local extent, perineural spread, and nodal involvement, if any
  - Low FDG avidity on PET/CT, unless high grade

DIFFERENTIAL DIAGNOSIS

Malignant Node, Submandibular Space (SMS)
- Hypoechoic, well-defined
  - ± multiple, reticulated/pseudocystic echo pattern in NHL
- Abnormal vascularity, hilar > peripheral

Chronic Sclerosing Sialadenitis, Kuttner Tumor
- Bilateral involvement; multiple, hypoechoic areas in SMG with no mass effect or vascular displacement
- End stage: Cirrhotic pattern

Benign Mixed Tumor (BMT) of SMG
- Well defined, solid, hypoechoic, and homogeneous with posterior enhancement

PATHOLOGY

Staging, Grading, & Classification
- Adapted from American Joint Committee on Cancer (AJCC), 7th edition (2010)
  - T1: ≤ 2 cm without extraparenchymal extension
  - T2: > 2 and ≤ 4 cm, no extraparenchymal extension
  - T3: > 4 cm &/or extraparenchymal extension
  - T4a: Invades skin, mandible, ear canal, ± facial nerve
  - T4b: Invades skull base ± pterygoid plates ± encases carotid artery

CLINICAL ISSUES

Presentation
- Most common signs/symptoms
  - Painless submandibular swelling or focal mass

Demographics
- Age
  - 40-70 years
- Epidemiology
  - 45% of SMG tumors are malignant; 55% benign
  - Most common SMG carcinoma is ACCa (40%)

Natural History & Prognosis
- 50% 5-year survival for all cancers
- Metastatic disease accounts for 30% of deaths
- ACCa spreads via nerves, also to lungs
- MECa and AdCa: Nodal and hematogenous spread

Treatment
- Surgical removal, node dissection, postop radiotherapy

SELECTED REFERENCES
1. Lee YY et al: Imaging of salivary gland tumours. Eur J Radiol. 66(3):419-36, 2008

SUBMANDIBULAR GLAND CARCINOMA

(Left) Transverse grayscale US shows an ill-defined, isoechoic, noncalcified, heterogeneous tumor ⇨ arising from the superficial part of left SMG ⇨ with no extraglandular extension. Note intratumoral cystic necrosis ⇨ and the presence of thick walls/mural nodule ⇨, features suspicious of malignant salivary tumor. *(Right)* Corresponding T1WI C+ FS MR clearly defines origin, extent of tumor, and the presence of intratumoral necrosis →, confirmed to be a low-grade mucoepidermoid carcinoma (MECa).

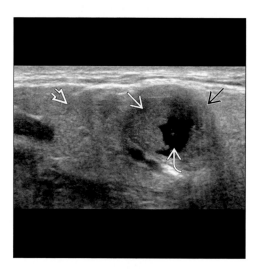 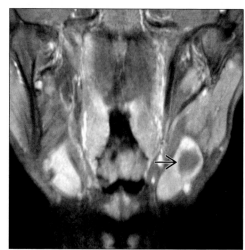

(Left) Axial grayscale US shows a large, ill-defined, hypoechoic mass with spiculated edges ⇨ arising from the left SMG ⇨. Note its extraglandular extension posteriorly ⇨. These are typical features of a malignant SMG tumor. *(Right)* Corresponding power Doppler US shows sparse intratumoral vascularity, which may be a reflection of an infiltrative tumor obliterating intratumoral vessels. Although malignant tumors have prominent vascularity, hypovascular tumors are also often seen.

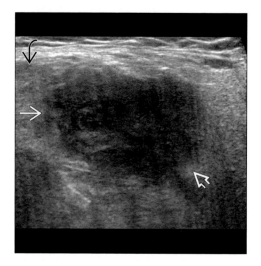 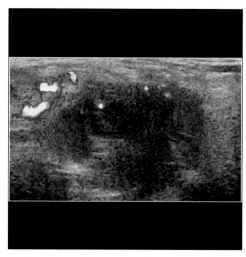

(Left) Transverse grayscale US (same patient) shows a round, solid, hypoechoic node ⇨ with absent hilum located in the left upper neck, adjacent to SMG tumor. US features are typical of malignant lymphadenopathy. *(Right)* Corresponding axial T1-weighted C+ MR shows infiltrative left SMG tumor ⇨ and adjacent lymphadenopathy ⇨. In the absence of perineural spread (more commonly seen with adenocarcinoma [ACCa]) imaging is unable to differentiate between various malignant SMG tumors.

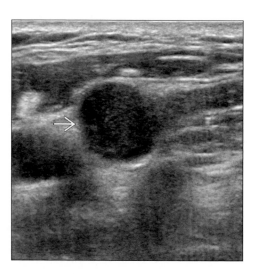 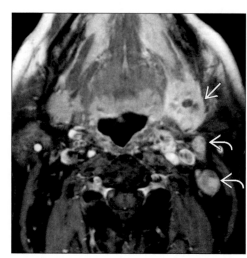

SUBMANDIBULAR GLAND CARCINOMA

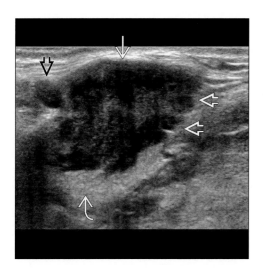

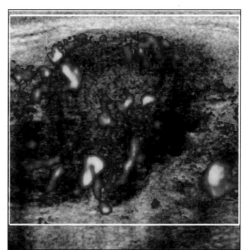

(Left) Longitudinal grayscale US shows a solid, hypoechoic, noncalcified tumor ➡ with spiculated margins ⇨ arising from the right SMG ➡. Note the presence of an adjacent malignant-looking lymph node ➡. *(Right)* Corresponding power Doppler US shows pronounced intratumoral vascularity. These vessels are usually of high resistance with RI > 0.8 and PI > 2.0. MECa & AdCa show nodal and hematogenous spread whereas ACCa usually spreads via nerves to lungs.

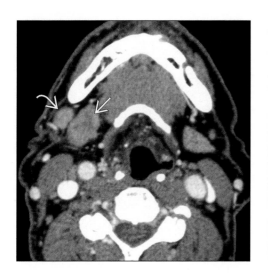

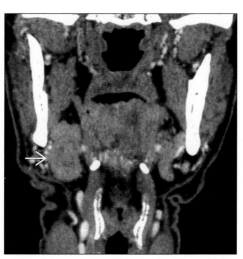

(Left) Axial CECT (same patient) shows a heterogeneous right SMG tumor ➡ with adjacent lymphadenopathy ➡. *(Right)* Corresponding coronal reformat CECT demonstrates the tumor ➡ arising from the right SMG. Note that 45% of all SMG tumors are malignant and 40% of malignant SMG tumors are ACCa.

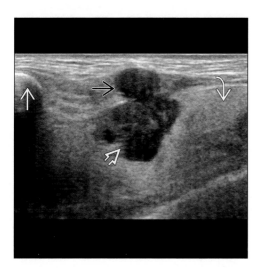

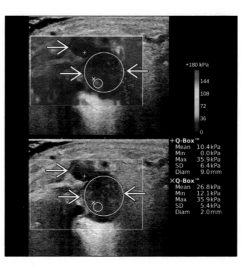

(Left) Longitudinal grayscale US clearly shows a myoepithelial carcinoma ➡ arising from the SMG ➡ with a mushroom-shaped extraglandular extension ➡ through the capsule of the SMG. Note the mandible ➡. *(Right)* Transverse grayscale US and SWE show a myoepithelial SMG carcinoma ➡. SWE color scale ranges from blue (0 kPa, soft) to red (180 kPa, stiff). It has a low SWE signal with maximum SWE of 36 kPa, which is only slightly higher than normal tissue.

SUBMANDIBULAR METASTASIS

Key Facts

Terminology

- Hematogenous spread of cancer cells to submandibular gland(s)

Imaging

- Imaging findings of submandibular gland metastasis are nonspecific, shared features with other submandibular gland malignancies
- Most commonly appears as an ill-defined, solid mass
- Hypoechoic relative to submandibular gland, isoechoic to mildly hyperechoic to muscle
- ± cystic component representing internal necrosis
- ± extraglandular spread, involvement of adjacent structures
- ± adjacent submandibular space lymph nodes
- Prominent intranodular hypervascularity
- Heterogeneously enhancing mass on CECT and MR

Top Differential Diagnoses

- Mucoepidermoid carcinoma
- Adenoid cystic carcinoma
- Submandibular gland carcinoma
- Non-Hodgkin lymphoma
- Chronic submandibular sialadenitis

Pathology

- Metastasis usually from distant sites (breast, lungs, genitourinary tract, colon)
- Locoregional primary is uncommon

Diagnostic Checklist

- Submandibular metastasis is rare and should only be considered if there is known primary cancer
- Ultrasound-guided fine-needle aspiration (FNA)/ biopsy recommended for pathological confirmation

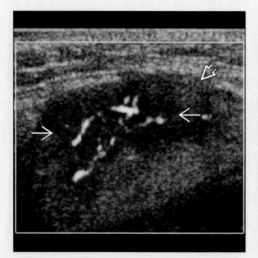
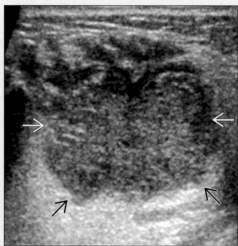

(Left) Power Doppler ultrasound in a patient with submandibular metastasis from breast carcinoma shows an ill-defined, hypoechoic mass ➡️ in the superficial portion of the submandibular gland ➡️. Note the irregular edge and pronounced intranodular vascularity. (Right) Transverse grayscale US in another patient with submandibular metastasis from neuroblastoma shows a large, solid, heterogeneous, irregular, hypoechoic mass within the right submandibular gland ➡️ with extraglandular extension ➡️.

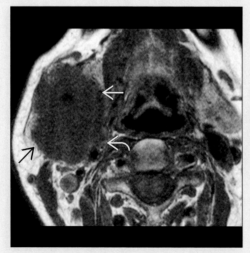
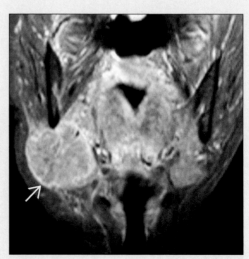

(Left) Axial T1WI MR of the same patient shows a large, ill-defined, solid mass almost entirely replacing the right submandibular gland ➡️. It infiltrates overlying subcutaneous tissue ➡️ and closely abuts the ipsilateral carotid sheath ➡️. (Right) Corresponding coronal T1WI C+ FS MR in the same patient shows intense heterogeneous enhancement within the mass ➡️. Imaging features are similar to other submandibular malignancies, which are more common than metastasis.

SUBMANDIBULAR METASTASIS

TERMINOLOGY

Definitions
- Hematogenous spread of cancer cells to submandibular gland(s)

IMAGING

General Features
- Best diagnostic clue
  - Imaging features are nonspecific
  - Most commonly appears as ill-defined, solid, hypoechoic mass ± internal necrosis
  - Intranodular vascularity/heterogeneous enhancement
- Location
  - Superficial/deep lobes of submandibular gland
  - Can be unilateral and solitary or bilateral
- Size
  - Usually < 5 cm
- Morphology
  - Irregular ± infiltrative margins

Ultrasonographic Findings
- Grayscale ultrasound
  - Ill-defined, solid mass
  - Hypoechoic relative to submandibular gland, isoechoic/mildly hyperechoic to muscle
  - ± cystic component representing internal necrosis
  - ± extraglandular spread, involvement of adjacent structures
    - Platysma muscle, subcutaneous tissue; mylohyoid, hyoglossus, digastric muscles; facial artery, retromandibular vein
  - ± ipsilateral submandibular space, cervical lymph nodes
- Power Doppler
  - Prominent intranodular hypervascularity

CT Findings
- CECT
  - Ill-defined, heterogeneously enhancing mass
  - Adjacent mandibular erosion best evaluated on CT

MR Findings
- T1WI
  - Hypointense relative to submandibular gland parenchyma, mildly hyperintense to muscle
- T2WI FS
  - Hyperintense ± internal necrosis
  - Most sensitive sequence for detecting perineural invasion (inferior alveolar nerve)
  - More conspicuous with fat saturation
- T1WI C+ FS
  - Heterogeneous enhancement

Imaging Recommendations
- Best imaging tool
  - MR for anatomical extent and perineural spread
  - Ultrasound guides fine-needle aspiration (FNA)/ biopsy for pathological diagnosis

DIFFERENTIAL DIAGNOSIS

Mucoepidermoid Carcinoma
- Well defined/ill defined, homogeneous/heterogeneous depending on grade
- Intranodular hypervascularity
- Infiltration of adjacent tissue in high-grade disease

Adenoid Cystic Carcinoma
- Well defined/ill defined, homogeneous/heterogeneous depending on grade
- Intranodular hypervascularity
- Tendency for perineural infiltration

Submandibular Gland Carcinoma
- Heterogeneous, ill-defined, hypoechoic mass with intranodular hypervascularity
- ± extraglandular spread, lymph nodes

Non-Hodgkin Lymphoma (NHL)
- Parenchymal NHL may affect submandibular glands
- Usually multiglandular with synchronous parotid involvement

Chronic Submandibular Sialadenitis
- Heterogeneous, hypoechoic "mass," prominent vascularity, cirrhotic gland (Kuttner tumor)
- ± dilated duct with stone
- Presents with pain ± salivary colic

PATHOLOGY

General Features
- Etiology
  - Hematogenous tumor spread
    - Not lymphatic spread as there are no lymph nodes within submandibular gland
  - Primary not known in ~ 20% of cases
  - From distant sites (more common)
    - Breast, lungs, genitourinary tract, colon
  - From head and neck (uncommon)
    - Oral cavity, tongue, oropharynx; some may be attributed to local invasion from primary tumor or adjacent lymph node

CLINICAL ISSUES

Presentation
- Most common signs/symptoms
  - Painless mass in submandibular region

SELECTED REFERENCES

1. Naidu TK et al: Oral cavity squamous cell carcinoma metastasis to the submandibular gland. J Laryngol Otol. 126(3):279-84, 2012
2. Serouya SM et al: Late solitary metastasis of renal cell carcinoma to the submandibular gland. J Oral Maxillofac Surg. 70(10):2356-9, 2012
3. Spiegel JH et al: Metastasis to the submandibular gland in head and neck carcinomas. Head Neck. 26(12):1064-8, 2004
4. Vessecchia G et al: Submandibular gland metastasis of breast carcinoma: a case report and review of the literature. Virchows Arch. 427(3):349-51, 1995
5. Ellis et al. Surgical Pathology of the Salivary Glands. Philadelphia: W.B. Saunders, 1991

SALIVARY GLAND LYMPHOEPITHELIOMA-LIKE CARCINOMA

Key Facts

Terminology

- Lymphoepithelioma-like carcinoma (LELC)
- Malignant tumor with morphologic features identical to nasopharyngeal carcinoma according WHO classification

Imaging

- Enhancing solid mass within parotid (~ 75%) or submandibular gland (~ 25%)
- Imaging features are nonspecific
- Ill-defined or well-defined borders
- Hypoechoic, homogeneous or heterogeneous
- Marked internal vascularity on color Doppler
- May see abnormal intraparotid, periparotid, cervical lymph nodes
- Heterogeneous enhancement on CECT and MR
- Scan from skull base to clavicles to look for cervical lymphadenopathy and exclude primary tumor in nasopharynx

- Advise nasopharyngeal endoscopy upon diagnosis of salivary gland LELC

Top Differential Diagnoses

- Warthin tumor
- Benign mixed tumor
- Mucoepidermoid carcinoma
- Adenoid cystic carcinoma
- Metastatic disease of parotid nodes
- Parotid non-Hodgkin lymphoma

Clinical Issues

- Most common in South East Asians and Inuit populations, rare in Caucasians
- Presenting symptoms: Neck lump/cervical lymphadenopathy, facial nerve palsy in parotid LELC
- Variable association with Epstein-Barr virus (EBV)
- Radiosensitive tumor, similar to its nasopharyngeal counterpart

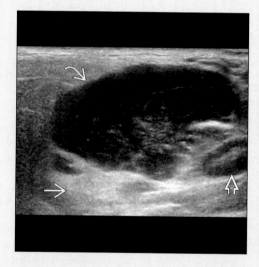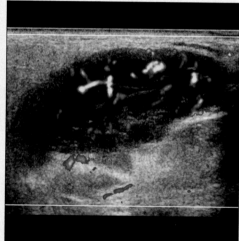

(Left) Longitudinal grayscale ultrasound of the left parotid in an elderly man shows a well-defined, heterogeneous, lobulated mass in the parotid tail ➔. Internal architecture is heterogeneous, and there is posterior acoustic enhancement ➔. Note the normal periparotid lymph node ➔. *(Right)* Corresponding power Doppler ultrasound reveals profuse internal vascularity. This was later confirmed to be LELC but sonographic features are nonspecific. The location and appearance mimic Warthin tumor.

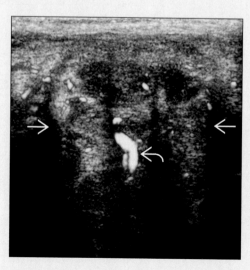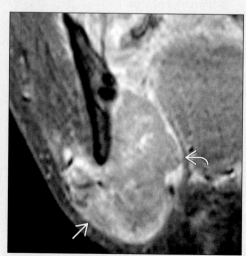

(Left) Transverse power Doppler US of submandibular region in another patient with biopsy-proven LELC shows an ill-defined, solid, hypoechoic, heterogeneous mass ➔ with prominent intratumoral vessels ➔. The normal submandibular gland and deep margin of the tumor are not well visualized. *(Right)* Corresponding coronal T1WI C+ FS MR shows a heterogeneously enhancing solid mass wrapping around the mandible ➔. There is replacement of submandibular glandular tissue and nodular extraglandular growth ➔.

SALIVARY GLAND LYMPHOEPITHELIOMA-LIKE CARCINOMA

TERMINOLOGY

Abbreviations
- Lymphoepithelioma-like carcinoma (LELC)

Synonyms
- Lymphoepithelial carcinoma
- Malignant lymphoepithelial lesion
- Undifferentiated carcinoma with lymphoid stroma
- Eskimoma (old term, no longer used)

Definitions
- Malignant tumor with morphologic features identical to nasopharyngeal carcinoma (NPC) according WHO classification

IMAGING

General Features
- Best diagnostic clue
  - Enhancing solid mass within parotid or submandibular gland
- Location
  - Parotid gland: ~ 75%
  - Submandibular gland: ~ 25%
  - Other locations in head and neck (rare)
    - Floor of mouth, tongue, tonsil, soft palate, hypopharynx, larynx
  - Rest of body (rare)
    - Lung, thymus, stomach and duodenum, breast, renal pelvis and urinary bladder, cervix, endometrium, ovary, vagina
- Size
  - 1-5 cm
- Morphology
  - Variable
    - Well-defined lobulated to infiltrative margins

Ultrasonographic Findings
- Grayscale ultrasound
  - Solitary solid mass within parotid or submandibular glandular parenchyma
  - Can have well-marginated, lobulated, or ill-defined/ infiltrative borders
  - Hypoechoic relative to salivary parenchyma
  - Posterior acoustic enhancement common
  - Occasionally central cystic component representing necrosis
  - May see associated abnormal intraparotid, periparotid, cervical lymph nodes
- Color Doppler
  - Moderate to marked intranodular vascularity

CT Findings
- NECT
  - Solid soft tissue mass within salivary gland
    - Hyperattenuating compared to parotid and submandibular parenchyma
    - Isoattenuating relative to muscle
- CECT
  - Homogeneous or heterogeneous enhancement

MR Findings
- T1WI
  - Iso- to hypointense signal relative to salivary gland
- T2WI FS
  - Mildly hyperintense tumor ± lymph node involvement
  - Occasionally hyperintense cystic center representing necrosis
  - Fat saturation improves lesion conspicuity
    - Best sequence to evaluate extent, local infiltration, and perineural invasion
- T1WI C+ FS
  - Homogeneous or heterogeneous enhancement

Imaging Recommendations
- Best imaging tool
  - Imaging features are nonspecific, simulating other salivary neoplasms
  - MR best modality to look for anatomical extent
  - Ultrasound guides FNA for cytological diagnosis
- Protocol advice
  - Scan from skull base to clavicles to look for cervical lymphadenopathy and exclude primary tumor in nasopharynx

DIFFERENTIAL DIAGNOSIS

Benign Mixed Tumor
- Well-defined, lobulated, homogeneous mass
- Posterior acoustic enhancement
- Sparse vascularity

Warthin Tumor
- Well-defined, hypoechoic intraglandular mass
- Heterogeneous internal architecture with solid and cystic components
- Commonly located in parotid tail
- 20% multicentric

Mucoepidermoid Carcinoma
- Well defined/ill defined, homogeneous/heterogeneous depending on tumor grade
- Prominent vascularity
- ± infiltration of adjacent tissue, metastatic lymph nodes

Adenoid Cystic Carcinoma
- Ill defined/well defined, homogeneous/heterogeneous depending on tumor grade
- Prominent vascularity
- Tendency for perineural infiltration

Metastatic Disease of Parotid Nodes
- Solitary/multiple, ill-defined, heterogeneous architecture
- Primary tumor known or apparent around ear, NPC

Parotid Non-Hodgkin Lymphoma (NHL)
- Parenchymal NHL: Infiltrative parotid lesion/diffuse parenchymal heterogeneity
- Nodal NHL: Solitary/multiple solid intraparotid lymph nodes, prominent hilar vascularity

PATHOLOGY

General Features
- Etiology
  - Most arise de-novo
    - Genetic and environmental risk factors

SALIVARY GLAND LYMPHOEPITHELIOMA-LIKE CARCINOMA

- ○ Minority develop in setting of benign lymphoepithelial lesion (BLEL)
- ○ Association with Epstein-Barr virus (EBV)
  - Variable, related to racial and geographical factors
  - Oncologic role of EBV is controversial

Gross Pathologic & Surgical Features

- Can be circumscribed, multilobulated or infiltrative
- Gray-tan to yellow-gray
- Necrosis and hemorrhage uncommon

Microscopic Features

- Tumor cells: Syncytial cytoplasm, large vesicular nuclei, and prominent nucleoli in a lymphoid stroma
- Immunohistochemistry: Cytokeratin antibody AE1, p63, and EMA positive
- EBER in situ hybridization: 100% positive in Chinese and Inuit patients, variable in Caucasians

Blood Tests

- Serum EBV-VCA IgA and EBV-EA IgA positive in many patients
- Elevated EBV DNA in ~ 40%
- Elevated neutrophil lymphocyte ration (NLR)
  - ○ Possible prognostic significance

CLINICAL ISSUES

Presentation

- Most common signs/symptoms
  - ○ Neck lump/cervical lymphadenopathy (40-70%)
  - ○ Facial nerve palsy in parotid LELC (20%)
  - ○ Uncommonly pain or tenderness

Demographics

- Age
  - ○ 20-70 years
- Gender
  - ○ No gender predilection
- Ethnicity
  - ○ Most common in South East Asians and Inuit populations
    - LELC represents the majority (92%) of all salivary gland carcinomas in Inuits
  - ○ Rare in Caucasians
- Epidemiology
  - ○ < 1% of all salivary gland malignancies in nonendemic regions

Natural History & Prognosis

- Better overall prognosis compared with other undifferentiated carcinomas of salivary glands and nasopharyngeal carcinoma
- Survival rates
  - ○ 5-year: 66-90%, 10-year: 29-75%
- Unencapsulated tumor with tendency to metastasize
  - ○ Intraparotid nodes → retroauricular → cervical → supraclavicular → paratracheal nodes
- 20% occult metastatic disease in lymph nodes of prophylactic neck dissection
- 20% distant metastasis within 3 years following therapy
  - ○ Most common sites: Lung, bone, liver

Treatment

- Surgical excision and postoperative radiotherapy ± therapeutic neck dissection
  - ○ Radiosensitive tumor, similar to its nasopharyngeal counterpart
- Role of routine/prophylactic neck dissection is controversial

DIAGNOSTIC CHECKLIST

Consider

- Coexisting nasopharyngeal carcinoma must be excluded
  - ○ Metastasis from nasopharyngeal primary is treated differently

Image Interpretation Pearls

- Imaging features for LELC are nonspecific and variable
  - ○ Shared features with both malignant and benign salivary gland neoplasms
- Diagnosis depends on cytology/histology

Reporting Tips

- Advise nasopharyngeal endoscopy upon diagnosis of salivary gland LELC

SELECTED REFERENCES

1. Ambrosio MR et al: Lymphoepithelial-like carcinoma of the parotid gland: a case report and a brief review of the western literature. Diagn Pathol. 8(1):115, 2013
2. Ma H et al: Primary lymphoepithelioma-like carcinoma of salivary gland: 69 cases with long-term follow-up. Head Neck. Epub ahead of print, 2013
3. Friborg J et al: A spectrum of basaloid morphology in a subset of EBV-associated "lymphoepithelial carcinomas" of major salivary glands. Head Neck Pathol. 6(4):445-50, 2012
4. Schneider M et al: Lymphoepithelial carcinoma of the parotid glands and its relationship with benign lymphoepithelial lesions. Arch Pathol Lab Med. 132(2):278-82, 2008
5. Hsiung CY et al: Lymphoepithelioma-like carcinoma of salivary glands: treatment results and failure patterns. Br J Radiol. 79(937):52-5, 2006
6. Wang CP et al: Lymphoepithelial carcinoma versus large cell undifferentiated carcinoma of the major salivary glands. Cancer. 101(9):2020-7, 2004
7. Wu DL et al: Malignant lymphoepithelial lesion of the parotid gland: a case report and review of the literature. Ear Nose Throat J. 80(11):803-6, 2001
8. Ahuja AT et al: Palatal lymphoepitheliomas and a review of head and neck lymphoepitheliomas. Clin Radiol. 54(5):289-93, 1999
9. Dubey P et al: Nonnasopharyngeal lymphoepithelioma of the head and neck. Cancer. 82(8):1556-62, 1998
10. Kuo T et al: Lymphoepithelioma-like salivary gland carcinoma in Taiwan: a clinicopathological study of nine cases demonstrating a strong association with Epstein-Barr virus. Histopathology. 31(1):75-82, 1997
11. Abdulla AK et al: Lymphoepithelial carcinoma of salivary glands. Head Neck. 18(6):577-81, 1996
12. Iezzoni JC et al: The role of Epstein-Barr virus in lymphoepithelioma-like carcinomas. Am J Clin Pathol. 103(3):308-15, 1995
13. Hamilton-Dutoit SJ et al: Undifferentiated carcinoma of the salivary gland in Greenlandic Eskimos: demonstration of Epstein-Barr virus DNA by in situ nucleic acid hybridization. Hum Pathol. 22(8):811-5, 1991

SALIVARY GLAND LYMPHOEPITHELIOMA-LIKE CARCINOMA

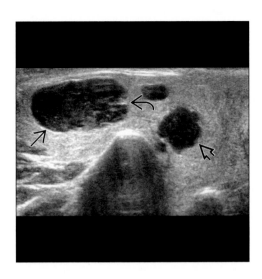
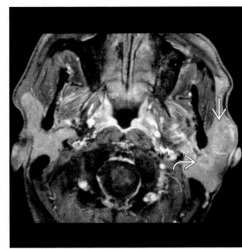

(Left) Transverse grayscale US of the left parotid gland shows a heterogeneous mass in the superficial lobe ➡. The lesion is partially ill defined ➡, and there are associated abnormal intraparotid nodes ➡. US-guided FNA of the larger lesion revealed LELC. *(Right)* Corresponding axial T1WI C+ FS MR (same patient) shows the LELC as a heterogeneously enhancing mass in the superficial lobe of the left parotid ➡, as well as a probable metastatic intraparotid node ➡. Note the nasopharynx appears unremarkable.

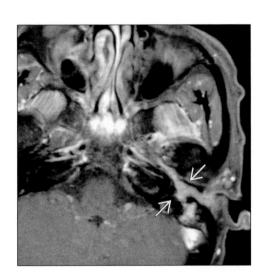
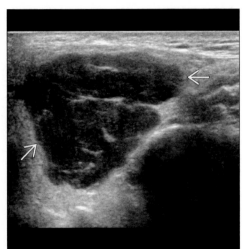

(Left) Axial T1WI C+ FS MR (same patient) in a more superior scan reveals enhancing soft tissue along the external auditory canal ➡. This was later found to be the primary tumor. A thorough search for the primary should be performed upon pathological diagnosis of salivary gland LELC. By far, the most common primary is nasopharyngeal carcinoma (NPC). *(Right)* Transverse grayscale US of the right parotid shows a well-defined heterogeneous mass with bosselated margins in the superficial lobe ➡.

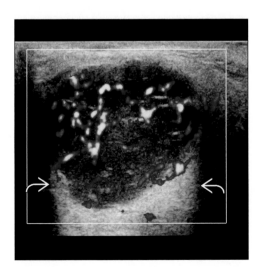
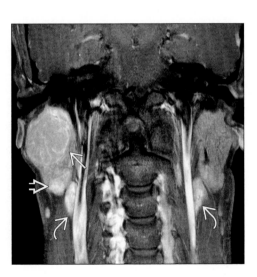

(Left) Corresponding power Doppler US (same patient) shows marked internal vascularity within the tumor and posterior enhancement ➡. *(Right)* Coronal T1WI C+ FS MR (same patient) shows a uniformly enhancing solid mass in the right parotid ➡. Reactive nodes are found in the parotid ➡, as well as in the bilateral upper cervical regions ➡. These features of LELC are nonspecific and are found in benign as well as low-grade malignant salivary gland neoplasms.

SUBMANDIBULAR SIALADENITIS

Key Facts

Imaging

- Acute sialadenitis, calculus
  - Unilateral, enlarged, hypoechoic, heterogeneous submandibular gland (SMG)
  - Intra-/extraglandular duct dilatation and calculus
  - Tender on transducer pressure, no obvious ↑ in vascularity
- Acute sialadenitis, acalculous
  - Unilateral, enlarged hypoechoic gland
  - No duct dilatation or calculi
  - Tender on transducer pressure, ↑ intraglandular vascularity
- Salivary gland abscess
  - Liquefied component with mobile internal debris and thick walls
  - Marked soft tissue swelling and edema
  - Enlarged, reactive-type regional lymph nodes
- Chronic sclerosing sialadenitis

  - Hypoechoic, heterogeneous nodules/cirrhotic appearance, bilateral involvement

Top Differential Diagnoses

- Enlarged submandibular lymph node
- Benign mixed tumor, submandibular gland
- SMG carcinoma

Diagnostic Checklist

- US is ideal imaging modality for SMG sialadenitis as it fully evaluates SMG, identifies calculus, duct dilatation, and complications (e.g., abscess formation)
- Always trace entire length of submandibular (SM) duct in multiple planes and compare with contralateral side
- Enlarged SM duct is often best clue to presence of calculus/stenosis
- Evaluate adjacent nodes as they may be enlarged during an acute episode

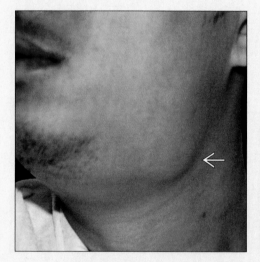
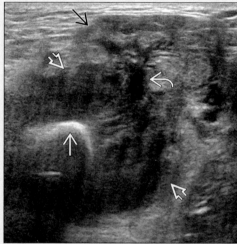

(Left) Clinical photograph shows a patient presenting with fever and painful submandibular swelling ➡. *(Right)* Corresponding transverse grayscale US shows a large, extraglandular, echogenic calculus ➡ within the associated abscess ⤀. Note the heterogeneous echo pattern of the submandibular gland (SMG) indicating sialadenitis ➡ and the dilated proximal Wharton duct ➡ as it exits the SMG. US is an ideal modality to investigate SMG calculus as it evaluates course of Wharton duct, adjacent tissues, and SMG.

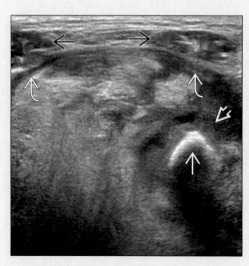
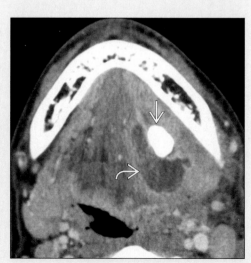

(Left) Transverse grayscale US at floor of mouth (FOM) of same patient clearly identifies a large calculus ➡ within an associated abscess ⤀. Note the clear depiction of adjacent anatomy; mylohyoid muscle ➡ and anterior belly of digastric muscle ➡. *(Right)* Corresponding axial CECT shows the large calculus ➡ and the associated rim-enhancing abscess ➡ at FOM but does not add any additional information compared to prior US in this case.

SUBMANDIBULAR SIALADENITIS

TERMINOLOGY

Abbreviations
- Submandibular gland (SMG) sialadenitis

Definitions
- SMG sialadenitis: SMG inflammation ± submandibular (SM) duct calculus or stenosis
- Acute sialadenitis (AS): Acute SMG inflammation; submandibular > > parotid involvement
  - Most common organism is *Staphylococcus aureus*
    - Others include *Streptococcus viridans*, *Haemophilus influenzae*, and *Escherichia coli*
- Chronic sialadenitis(CS): Chronic SMG inflammation
  - Associated with conditions linked to ↓ salivary flow, including calculi and salivary stasis
- Chronic sclerosing sialadenitis (CSS), Kuttner tumor
  - Tumor-like condition of salivary glands, submandibular > parotid involvement
  - Periductal sclerosis, lymphocytic infiltration, reduction of secretory gland parenchyma, fibrosis, associated sialolithiasis (30-83%)

IMAGING

General Features
- Best diagnostic clue
  - Acute: Unilateral enlarged, hypoechoic SMG, increased vascularity, ± ductal dilatation, ± calculus
  - Chronic: Unilateral atrophic, hypoechoic, heterogeneous, hypovascular, ± ductal dilatation, ± calculus
- Location
  - Submandibular space (SMS); SMG stones can be divided by location
    - Distal: Toward ductal opening in anterior sublingual space (SLS)
    - Proximal: Toward SMG hilum in SMS
  - SMG calculi are more likely to occur within duct than within SMG parenchyma

Ultrasonographic Findings
- Acute sialadenitis, calculus
  - Unilateral, enlarged, hypoechoic, heterogeneous SMG
  - Intra-/extraglandular duct dilatation and calculus
  - No obvious increase in vascularity
  - Tender on transducer pressure
- Acute sialadenitis, acalculous
  - Unilateral, enlarged hypoechoic gland
  - No duct dilatation or calculi
  - Tender on transducer pressure
  - Increased intraglandular vascularity
- Salivary gland abscess
  - Liquefied component with mobile internal debris and thick walls
  - Marked soft tissue swelling and edema
  - Enlarged, reactive-type regional lymph nodes
- Chronic sclerosing sialadenitis
  - Hypoechoic, heterogeneous nodules/cirrhotic appearance, bilateral involvement
  - Prominent intraglandular vessels running through nodules with no mass effect/displacement

Imaging Recommendations
- Best imaging tool
  - US is ideal imaging modality for SMG sialadenitis as it fully evaluates SMG, identifies calculus, duct dilatation, and complications (e.g., abscess formation)
    - For detection of salivary calculi, US has sensitivity of 94%, specificity of 100%, and accuracy of 96%
- Protocol advice
  - Use of high-resolution (≥ 7.5 MHz) transducer is mandatory
  - Always trace entire length of submandibular (SM) duct in multiple planes & compare with contralateral side
  - Enlarged SM duct is often best clue to presence of calculus/stenosis
  - Evaluate adjacent nodes as they may be enlarged during an acute episode

DIFFERENTIAL DIAGNOSIS

Enlarged Submandibular Lymph Node
- Reactive: Oval/round, hypoechoic with hilar architecture and vascularity
- Lymphoma: Round, solid, hypoechoic, reticulated node with hilar > peripheral vascularity
- Metastatic SCCa: Round, hypoechoic, cystic necrosis, peripheral vascularity and absence of hilum

Benign Mixed Tumor, Submandibular Gland
- Well-defined, solid, hypoechoic, homogeneous mass with posterior enhancement, may or may not be lobulated

Submandibular Gland Carcinoma
- Ill-defined, solid, hypoechoic, heterogeneous mass with extraglandular infiltration, ± adjacent abnormal node

CLINICAL ISSUES

Presentation
- Most common signs/symptoms
  - Unilateral, painful SMG swelling associated with eating or psychological gustatory stimulation (salivary colic)
  - Other signs/symptoms
    - 30% of cases with SMG duct stones present with painless SMS mass
    - 80% of cases presenting with painful SMG mass are secondary to calculus disease
    - Physical examination: If calculus in anterior duct, may be palpable to bimanual examination

DIAGNOSTIC CHECKLIST

Image Interpretation Pearls
- SMG sialadenitis imaging questions
  - If stone seen, is it in anterior or posterior SMG duct
    - Anterior stones are removed per oral route
    - Posterior stones removed with SMG and duct
  - Is SMG affected without ductal pathology
    - Consider Sjögren, AIDS, or primary SMG infection

SELECTED REFERENCES

1. Orlandi MA et al: Ultrasound in sialadenitis. J Ultrasound. 16(1):3-9, 2013

SUBMANDIBULAR SIALADENITIS

(Left) Oblique grayscale US at FOM shows entire course of dilated Wharton duct ➡ with a calculus at its tip ➡. This is the 1st site to be investigated in patients with suspected calculus SMG sialadenitis as calculi are lodged just proximal to papilla. Note the SMG ➡ itself still shows normal, bright parenchymal echoes with no obvious inflammation. *(Right)* Corresponding axial MR sialogram shows the course of the dilated Wharton duct ➡ exiting the SMG ➡ and obstructing the calculus at its tip ➡.

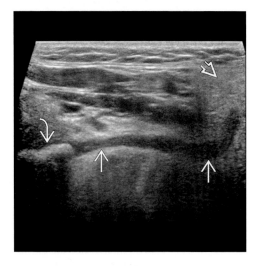
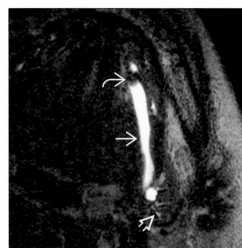

(Left) Oblique grayscale US shows the calculus ➡ impacted between mylohyoid ➡ & hyoglossus muscles ➡. This is the 2nd site to be investigated for localization of suspected calculus as Wharton duct is compressed between 2 muscles. *(Right)* Transverse grayscale US shows a hypoechoic, heterogeneous SMG ➡ with calculus ➡ impacted at exit of Wharton duct. This is the 3rd site to be investigated for SMG calculus as the exiting duct is curved like the end of a hockey stick & calculi are impacted at the bend.

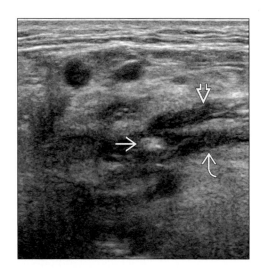
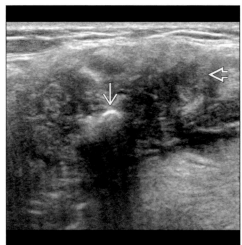

(Left) Transverse grayscale US in a patient with acute acalculous SMG sialadenitis shows multiple small, hypoechoic areas ➡ (lymphoid hypertrophy) diffusely scattered within the parenchyma of an enlarged SMG ➡. A similar appearance is also seen in MALToma of SMG and must be viewed with a high degree of suspicion. *(Right)* Transverse grayscale US in a patient with calculous SMG sialadenitis shows an enlarged SMG ➡ with a diffuse, homogeneous, hypoechoic parenchymal echo pattern.

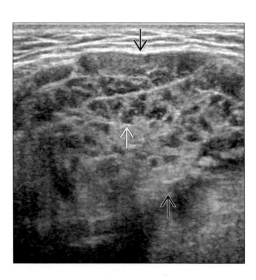
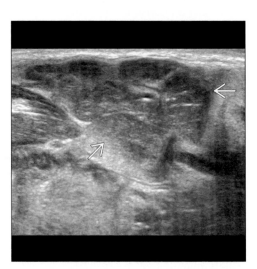

SUBMANDIBULAR SIALADENITIS

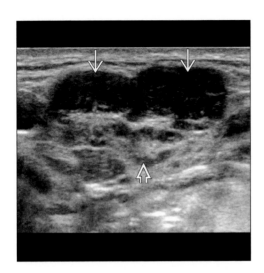

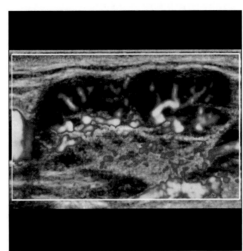

(Left) Transverse grayscale US shows typical appearance of chronic sclerosing sialadenitis (CSS). Note the cirrhotic appearance of SMG ➡️ and large focal hypoechoic areas ➡️ simulating SMG tumors. (Right) Corresponding power Doppler US shows intraglandular vessels running through hypoechoic areas with no displacement or mass effect. The combination of grayscale and Doppler features are characteristic of CSS, which is often bilateral and may involve multiple salivary glands (submandibular > parotid).

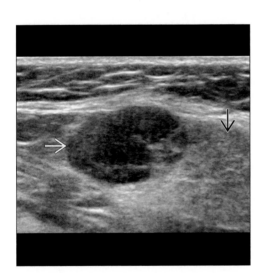

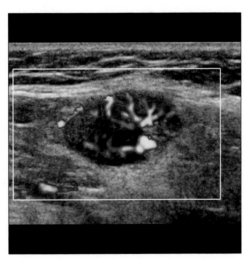

(Left) Transverse grayscale US shows a focal, hypoechoic, heterogeneous, noncalcified mass ➡️ in the SMG ➡️ with heterogeneous background parenchymal echoes. (Right) Corresponding power Doppler US shows radiating vascularity within the mass and no mass effect/vascular displacement. FNAC confirmed CSS, a tumor-like condition of salivary glands. Patients often present with bilateral, painless enlargement of the SMG, which may also be seen incidentally in elderly patients.

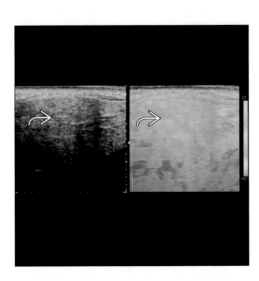

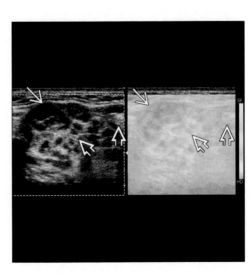

(Left) Transverse grayscale US and qualitative strain elastogram show a normal SMG. Strain color scale ranges from purple (elastic, soft) to red (inelastic, hard). The normal SMG appears relatively uniform and elastic ➡️. (Right) Transverse grayscale US and qualitative strain elastogram show SMG CSS. The abnormal SMG is heterogeneous and contains coalescent hypoechoic foci on grayscale US ➡️, which appear less elastic (stiffer) than areas of milder involvement within the same gland ➡️.

SALIVARY GLAND TUBERCULOSIS

Key Facts

Imaging

- Hypoechoic solid or cystic parenchymal mass(es) with irregular margins and parenchymal edema
- Parotid (70%), submandibular (27%), sublingual (3%)
- Uniglandular > > multiglandular/bilateral
- Solid nodal phase: Perisalivary TB lymphadenitis
  - Single or multiple hypoechoic round nodes ± periadenitis (nodal matting + edema)
- Necrotic phase: Necrotizing lymphadenitis with loss of normal nodal features progressing to frank abscess
  - Hypoechoic mass(es) with caseous necrosis
  - Abscess wall is thick, irregular; contents are heterogeneously hypoechoic
  - Linear hypoechoic bands in surrounding parenchyma (inflammation/edema)
  - ± extension of abscess into subcutaneous/cutaneous tissues (collar-stud abscess/discharging sinus)

- US allows initial characterization and image-guided aspiration for diagnosis and therapy

Top Differential Diagnoses

- Salivary neoplasm
- Acute suppurative parotitis (non-mycobacterial)
- Sarcoidosis

Diagnostic Checklist

- Usually presents as slowly enlarging, painless salivary mass, hence commonly mistaken for neoplasm
- Less commonly presents as acute sialadenitis
- Consider SG TB in patient with salivary abscess and relatively minimal erythema or systemic symptoms
- Specifically request TB tests in FNA specimens
- Perform chest radiograph to screen for pulmonary TB

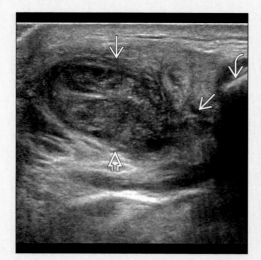
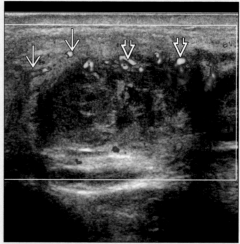

(Left) Transverse grayscale US shows a large, irregular, hypoechoic intraparotid abscess ➡. The abscess is thick walled, ill defined, and has heterogeneous contents. Note evidence of inflammatory change in the adjacent salivary parenchyma ➡. Ramus of the mandible ➡ is shown. (Right) Corresponding longitudinal power Doppler US (same patient) shows increased vascularity in the abscess wall ➡ and surrounding inflammatory parenchyma ➡. Absent vascularity within the abscess cavity is due to caseous necrosis within.

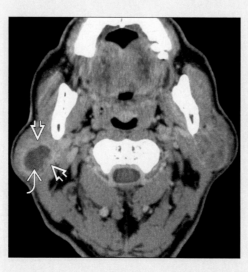
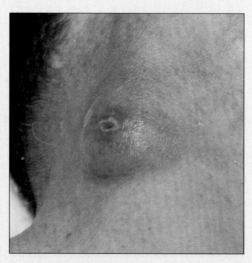

(Left) Axial CECT (same patient) shows a right parotid abscess ➡ with thick irregular enhancing walls and central fluid content ➡. (Right) Clinical photograph (same patient) shows parotid abscess tracks inferiorly, reaching the skin where there is a sinus. This abscess cultured Mycobacterium chelonae and the patient responded well to drainage & antimicrobial therapy. Open wounds render US examination difficult and due transducer care must be taken to prevent cross infection.

SALIVARY GLAND TUBERCULOSIS

TERMINOLOGY

Abbreviations
- Salivary gland tuberculosis (SG TB)

Definitions
- Salivary infection due to *Mycobacterium tuberculosis* (MTB) or atypical Mycobacteria (AMTB)

IMAGING

General Features
- Best diagnostic clue
  - Unilateral, irregular, thick-walled cystic salivary mass (abscess) with adjacent edema
    - ± subcutaneous extension (collar-stud abscess) or discharging skin sinus
- Location
  - Parotid (70%), submandibular (27%), sublingual (3%)
  - Usually unilateral (bilateral very rare)

Ultrasonographic Findings
- Grayscale ultrasound
  - Solid nodal phase: Perisalivary TB lymphadenitis
    - Single or multiple hypoechoic round nodes ± periadenitis (nodal matting + edema)
  - Necrotic phase: Necrotizing lymphadenitis with loss of normal nodal features progressing to frank abscess
    - Hypoechoic mass(es) with caseous necrosis
    - Abscess wall typically thick, irregular; contents are heterogeneously hypoechoic
    - ± extension of abscess into (sub)cutaneous tissues (collar-stud abscess/discharging sinus)
- Power Doppler
  - ↑ vascularity in abscess wall and adjacent soft tissues

CT Findings
- CECT
  - Solid phase: Single or multiple, smooth, round, homogeneously enhancing perisalivary nodes
  - Necrotic phase: Irregular, thick-walled abscess; edema and inflammatory enhancement in soft tissues & skin

Imaging Recommendations
- Best imaging tool
  - US allows initial characterization and image-guided aspiration for diagnosis and therapy

DIFFERENTIAL DIAGNOSIS

Salivary Neoplasm
- Includes primary tumors, metastases, lymphoma
- Diverse US appearances: Solid/cystic, smooth/irregular margins, variable echotexture & vascularity
- Often indistinguishable from chronic SG TB

Acute Suppurative Parotitis (Nonmycobacterial)
- Acute presentation: Rapidly enlarging, painful unilateral salivary swelling, skin erythema
- US: Irregular hypoechoic mass with central necrosis
- Indistinguishable from acute presentation of SG TB

Sarcoidosis
- Bilateral perisalivary hypoechoic nodes, multiple diffuse hypoechoic parenchymal infiltrates

- Necrosis is not a feature, usually has extrasalivary involvement (e.g., hilar lymphadenopathy)

PATHOLOGY

General Features
- Etiology
  - 2 mechanisms of mycobacterial spread to salivary parenchyma postulated
    - Retrograde via salivary duct or via lymphatics from contaminated sputum or oral infection
    - Hematogenous from distant infective source, especially pulmonary TB

Microscopic Features
- Chronic granulomatous inflammation, multinucleate giant cells, ± caseating necrosis
- Ziehl-Neelsen stain positive for MTB
  - Other tests required for ATB detection
- PCR tests for TB ↑ diagnostic sensitivity of fine-needle aspiration

CLINICAL ISSUES

Presentation
- Most common signs/symptoms
  - Painless, indolent, enlarging salivary mass(es) with minimal skin erythema
- Other signs/symptoms
  - Acute painful sialadenitis ± skin erythema

Demographics
- Age
  - Any age group
    - Young children more prone to infection by ATB, e.g., *Mycobacterium avium-intracellulare*
- Epidemiology
  - Higher incidence in developing countries within Asia and Africa with endemic TB and in specific groups in developed countries (e.g., HIV/AIDS, immigrants)
  - Although cervicofacial involvement in TB is common, salivary gland involvement is rare

Treatment
- Anti-TB chemotherapy ± abscess drainage ± gland resection

DIAGNOSTIC CHECKLIST

Consider
- Consider SG TB in patient with salivary abscess and relatively minimal erythema or systemic symptoms
- Specifically request TB tests in FNA/tissue specimens
- Perform chest radiograph to screen for pulmonary TB

SELECTED REFERENCES

1. Vaid S et al: Tuberculosis in the head and neck--a forgotten differential diagnosis. Clin Radiol. 65(1):73-81, 2010
2. Alyas F et al: Diseases of the submandibular gland as demonstrated using high resolution ultrasound. Br J Radiol. 78(928):362-9, 2005
3. Lee IK et al: Tuberculous parotitis: case report and literature review. Ann Otol Rhinol Laryngol. 114(7):547-51, 2005

SALIVARY GLAND TUBERCULOSIS

(Left) Transverse grayscale US shows a submandibular gland abscess ➡ due to MTB. It involves the gland parenchyma and penetrates through the gland capsule ➡ into the subcutaneous tissues, resulting in a waisted or collar-stud appearance. This is very suggestive of tuberculous infection. The abscess contents have mixed low-level echoes ➤. Note the normal salivary tissue ➤. *(Right)* Corresponding power Doppler US shows ↑ vascularity in the abscess walls ➤.

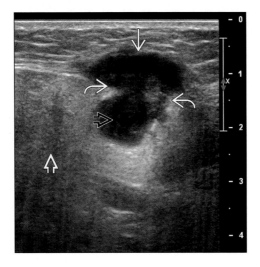
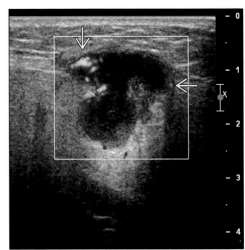

(Left) Transverse grayscale US of a parotid gland shows an partially liquefied abscess ➡ due to MTB. It is ill-defined and heterogeneous, with a small anechoic focus suggestive of abscess fluid ➤. Note the ramus of the mandible ➤. *(Right)* Transverse grayscale US in a patient with a slowly enlarging, painless parotid swelling and minimal systemic symptoms shows a large parotid abscess due to MTB ➡. Note the irregular abscess walls ➡ and mixed internal echoes ➤. *(Courtesy A. Momin, MD.)*

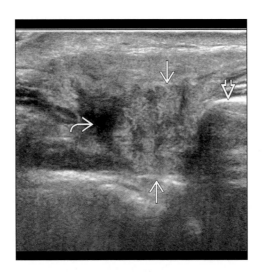
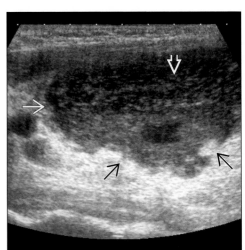

(Left) Transverse grayscale US of a submandibular gland shows an intraparenchymal abscess due to MTB. Note its markedly irregular, ill-defined walls ➡ and heterogeneous fluid content ➤. US allows initial characterization and guided aspiration for diagnosis. *(Right)* Corresponding coronal T1WI C+ FS MR shows a thick-walled, rim-enhancing abscess ➡ inseparable from the left submandibular gland ➤. The gland is enlarged and abnormally enhancing when compared to its normal counterpart ➤.

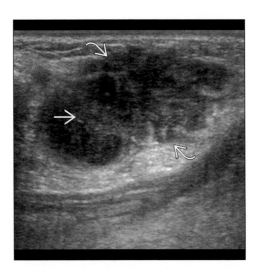
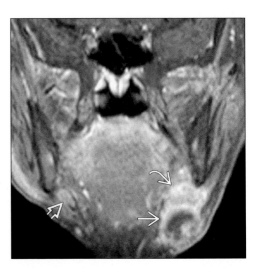

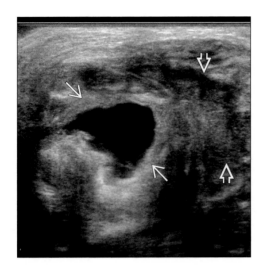

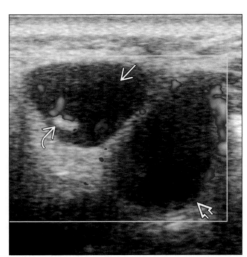

(Left) Transverse grayscale US shows a large intraparotid MTB abscess with thick walls ⇨ & anechoic fluid content. Note the striking inflammatory edema within the adjacent parotid parenchyma ⇨. *(Right)* Transverse color Doppler US shows 2 abnormal intraparotid lymph nodes, confirmed as TB lymphadenitis on FNAC. The node on the right has no echogenic hilum or hilar vascularity ⇨, whereas the node on the left has eccentric cortical thickening ⇨ that displaces the hilum ⇨.

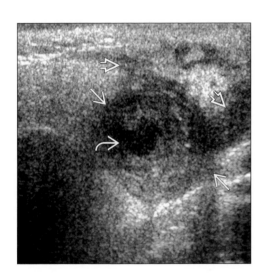

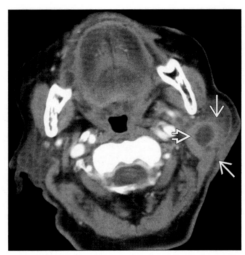

(Left) Transverse grayscale US of a parotid gland shows an MTB abscess with an irregular, thick wall ⇨ and small central fluid content ⇨. Hypoechoic regions indicative of marked inflammation extend into the surrounding tissues ⇨. *(Right)* Corresponding axial CECT shows an irregular, thick-walled, enhancing abscess in the left parotid gland ⇨. Note the ill-defined enhancement extending directly into the adjacent parotid tissue and overlying skin ⇨, which is thickened due to edema/inflammation.

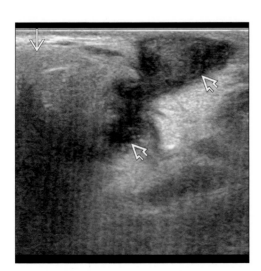

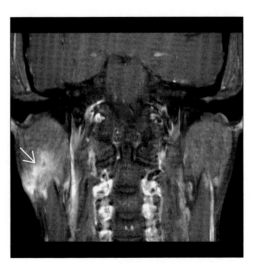

(Left) Longitudinal grayscale US of a parotid gland shows an irregular, hypoechoic TB abscess with internal debris, extending inferolaterally into subcutaneous tissues ⇨. Superior aspect of the parotid gland appears relatively spared ⇨. *(Right)* Corresponding coronal T1WI C+ FS MR shows irregular inflammatory change in the right parotid gland communicating with the overlying skin ⇨. The accompanying abscess had discharged spontaneously via skin in the time between US & MR examinations.

SJÖGREN SYNDROME

Key Facts

Imaging

- Imaging findings are combination of cystic and solid lesions ± calcification
- Although Sjögren syndrome (SjS) affects salivary and lacrimal glands, involvement may appear asymmetrical on imaging
- Early stage "miliary" cysts (≤ 1 mm punctate cystic changes) may be missed; later stages seen on US
- Diffuse hypoechogenicity of salivary and lacrimal glands may be the only clue in early SjS
- Heterogeneous parenchymal echoes in salivary and lacrimal glands
- Multiple discrete hypoechoic foci scattered throughout lacrimal and salivary glands
- Diffuse reticulated/"leopard skin" appearance of salivary and lacrimal glands with hypoechoic septa due to lymphoid aggregation, microcysts

- Lymphomatous change is seen as dominant, ill-defined, solid, hypoechoic mass in salivary glands ± nodal disease
- Increased parenchymal vascularity in SjS

Top Differential Diagnoses

- Chronic sclerosing sialadenitis, Kuttner tumor
- Sialadenitis
- BLEL-HIV

Diagnostic Checklist

- Diagnosis of SjS is based on clinical, serologic, and histologic evidence
- Primary role of imaging is to confirm or exclude salivary gland involvement and surveillance for lymphomatous change
- Large solid, hypoechoic lesions and cervical lymphadenopathy should raise concern for NHL or alternative diagnosis

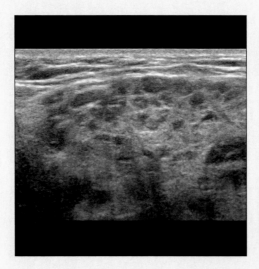
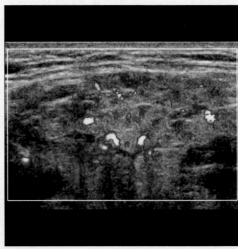

(Left) Transverse grayscale US of the submandibular gland (SMG) shows multiple, small hypoechoic areas scattered in the glandular parenchyma. These are a combination of cysts & lymphoid aggregates, giving the gland a "leopard skin" appearance. A similar appearance is also seen in sialadenitis and salivary MALToma. *(Right)* Corresponding power Doppler US (same patient) shows prominent vascularity within an involved SMG. Vascularity correlates well with the severity of gland involvement.

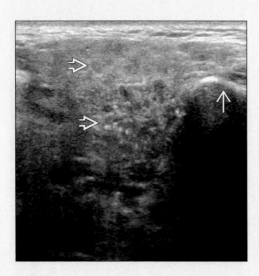
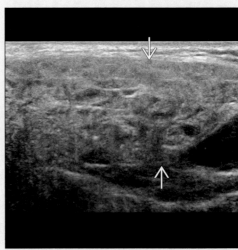

(Left) Transverse grayscale US of a parotid gland (same patient) shows a heterogeneous parenchymal echo pattern with hypoechoic areas ⮞ scattered within the gland. The mandibular ramus ➡ is also shown. *(Right)* Corresponding longitudinal grayscale US shows involvement of the entire parotid superficial lobe ➡. Note the heterogeneous parenchymal echo pattern with focal hypoechoic areas within the gland. Note that US is unable to evaluate deep lobe involvement as it is obscured by the mandible.

SJÖGREN SYNDROME

TERMINOLOGY

Abbreviations
- Sjögren syndrome (SjS)

Synonyms
- Sicca syndrome

Definitions
- Chronic systemic autoimmune exocrinopathy that causes salivary and lacrimal gland tissue destruction

IMAGING

General Features
- Best diagnostic clue
  - Bilateral enlarged parotids, ± submandibular glands (SMG) and lacrimal glands, multiple micro- and macrocystic intraparotid solid lesions, and intraglandular calcifications
- Location
  - Bilateral salivary and lacrimal glands
- Size
  - Range: < 1 mm microcysts to > 2 cm macrocysts (± mixed solid-cystic masses)
- Imaging appearance depends on stage of disease and presence or absence of lymphocyte aggregates within salivary and lacrimal glands
  - Early-stage SjS: May appear normal
  - Intermediate-stage SjS: "Miliary pattern" of small cysts diffusely throughout both parotid glands
  - Late-stage SjS: Larger cystic (parenchymal destruction) and solid masses (lymphocyte aggregates) in bilateral parotid, submandibular, and lacrimal glands
  - Any stage may have solid intraparotid masses due to lymphocytic accumulation mimicking tumor
  - Invasive salivary gland mass ± cervical adenopathy may signal lymphomatous transformation

Ultrasonographic Findings
- Grayscale ultrasound
  - Imaging findings are combination of cystic and solid lesions ± calcification
  - Although SjS affects salivary and lacrimal glands, involvement may appear asymmetrical on imaging
  - Early stage "miliary" (≤ 1 mm punctate cystic changes) may be missed; later stages readily seen on US
  - Diffuse hypoechogenicity of salivary and lacrimal glands may be only clue in early SjS
  - Heterogeneous parenchymal echoes in salivary and lacrimal glands
  - Multiple discrete hypoechoic foci scattered throughout lacrimal and salivary glands
    - If solid, represent lymphocytic aggregates
    - Microcysts due to acinar destruction or terminal duct dilatation due to compression by lymphoid aggregates
    - Macrocysts due to destruction of salivary tissue
  - Diffuse reticulated/"leopard skin" appearance of salivary and lacrimal glands with hypoechoic septa due to lymphoid aggregation, microcysts
  - Lymphomatous change is seen as dominant, ill-defined, solid, hypoechoic mass in salivary glands ± nodal disease
- Color Doppler
  - Increased parenchymal vascularity in SjS
    - Correlates with severity of disease

Imaging Recommendations
- Best imaging tool
  - Diagnosis is based on clinical, serologic, and histologic evidence
  - Primary role of imaging is to confirm or exclude salivary gland involvement and surveillance for lymphomatous change
  - Large, solid, hypoechoic lesions and cervical lymphadenopathy should raise concern for non-Hodgkin lymphoma (NHL) or alternative diagnosis
  - US is cost-effective in surveillance of SjS patients

DIFFERENTIAL DIAGNOSIS

Chronic Sclerosing Sialadenitis, Kuttner Tumor
- Submandibular > parotid, bilateral, hypoechoic heterogeneous nodules with no mass effect, cirrhotic-looking gland

Sialadenitis
- Hypoechoic, heterogeneous gland, ± ↑ vascularity, ± duct dilatation, ± calculus

BLEL-HIV
- Mixed cystic and solid lesions enlarging both parotid glands, therefore mimicking SjS
- Tonsillar hyperplasia and cervical reactive adenopathy

NHL, Parotid Nodes
- Bilateral, solid, hypoechoic, hilar > peripheral vascularity ± other evidence of NHL

Sarcoidosis
- Presence of cervical and mediastinal lymph nodes
- Diffuse hypoechogenicity of salivary glands; affect submandibular > parotid glands

CLINICAL ISSUES

Presentation
- Clinical profile
  - Patient complains of recurrent acute episodes of tender glandular swelling
  - Less common: Chronic glandular enlargement with superimposed acute attacks to nonpainful enlargement
  - Other signs/symptoms: Dry eyes, mouth, and skin
    - Rheumatoid arthritis >> systemic lupus erythematosus > progressive systemic sclerosis
- Laboratory
  - Positive labial biopsy or autoantibody against Sjögren-associated A or B antigen, Rh factor positive in 95% and ANA positive in 80%

Natural History & Prognosis
- Slowly progressive syndrome that evolves over years
- NHL may complicate this otherwise chronic illness
- Parotid or GI locations most common NHL sites

SELECTED REFERENCES

1. Ahuja AT et al: Ultrasound features of Sjögren's syndrome. Australas Radiol. 40(1):10-4, 1996

(Left) Transverse grayscale US shows the right SMG ⮱. Note diffuse parenchymal hypoechogenicity with focal cystic areas ➡ within the gland. *(Right)* Transverse grayscale US (same patient) of contralateral left SMG ➡ shows diffuse parenchymal hypoechogenicity with microcysts ➡ within. Subtle glandular hypoechogenicity ± microcysts may be the 1st sonographic evidence of Sjögren syndrome (SjS). Multiglandular involvement is common in SjS.

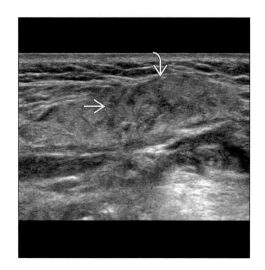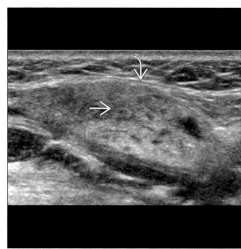

(Left) Longitudinal grayscale US in a patient with SjS shows multiple macrocysts ➡ scattered throughout the parotid parenchyma. This is the result of activated lymphocytes destroying salivary tissue and leaving large cysts. *(Right)* Longitudinal grayscale US (same patient) shows a large macrocyst ➡ in the parotid parenchyma of a patient with SjS. Note echogenic foci ➡ within the cyst signifying calcification, which is often seen in SjS and is better demonstrated on NECT than US.

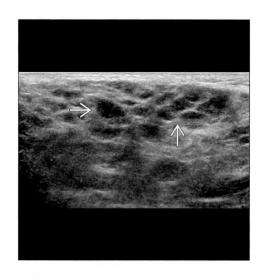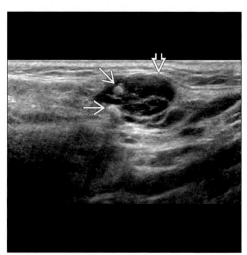

(Left) Coronal NECT shows diffuse enlargement of both parotid glands ➡ with multiple micro- and macrocysts scattered throughout the salivary parenchyma. NECT is also sensitive to detection of foci of intraglandular calcification in SjS. *(Right)* Corresponding coronal T2WI MR shows multiple high-signal areas within both parotid glands representing cystic dilatation ➡ of intraglandular ducts in SjS.

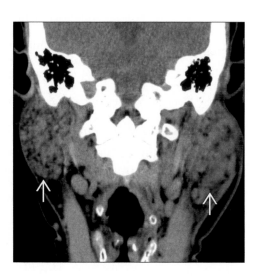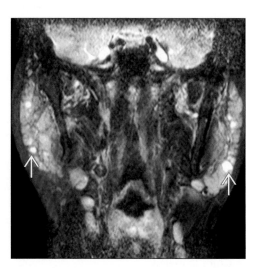

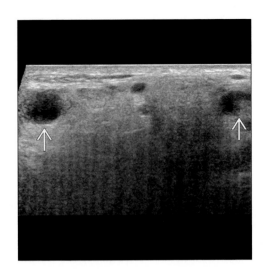

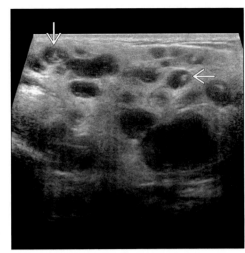

(Left) Longitudinal grayscale US of a parotid gland shows multiple large cysts ➡ scattered within salivary parenchyma. (Right) Corresponding grayscale US of the contralateral parotid (same patient) shows multiple cysts of varying sizes scattered throughout salivary parenchyma. Note some of the cysts have internal debris & septation ➡, and are not completely anechoic. The appearances suggest benign lymphoepithelial cysts. Note that they mimic macrocysts in SjS.

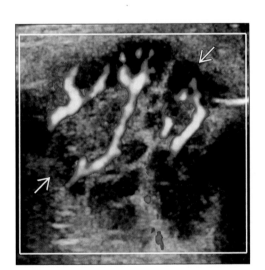

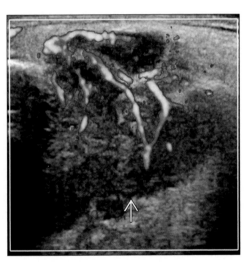

(Left) Transverse power Doppler US shows a lacrimal gland ➡ in a patient with SjS. Note it is markedly enlarged, solid, and hypoechoic with diffuse heterogeneous parenchymal architecture and prominent intralesional vascularity. (Right) Transverse power Doppler US of the contralateral lacrimal gland (same patient) ➡ shows a similar appearance. Although SjS involves salivary & lacrimal glands, the involvement may be asymmetrical. US readily evaluates lacrimal glands and guides confirmatory biopsy.

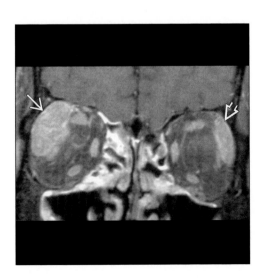

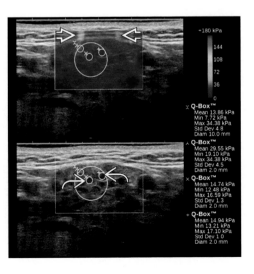

(Left) Coronal T1WI C+ FS MR in the same patient with SjS shows heterogeneous enhancement of the right ➡ and left ⇒ lacrimal glands, which appear enlarged, the right more so than the left. (Right) Longitudinal grayscale US & SWE show SMG SjS. SWE color scale ranges from blue (0 kPa, soft) to red (180 kPa, stiff). Hypoechoic foci ➡ have a maximum SWE of 17.1 kPa, which is low (normal SMG is ~ 11-15 kPa). Note the SWE artifacts ⇒.

IgG4-RELATED DISEASE IN HEAD & NECK

Key Facts

Terminology

- Recently recognized idiopathic systemic fibroinflammatory condition; tendency to form tumor-like lesion with dense lymphoplasmacytic infiltrate rich in IgG4-positive cells

Imaging

- Head and neck region commonly involved, especially orbits and salivary glands
- Bilateral chronic dacryoadenitis ± sialadenitis
  - Bilateral symmetrical > asymmetrical; affects lacrimal > submandibular > parotid glands
  - Involved glands enlarged; rounded contour with nodular or diffuse hypoechoic pattern and nondisplaced hypervascularity on USG
- Orbital involvement could be extraocular muscle myositis ± pseudotumor ± perineural disease
- Cervical lymph node and thyroid gland involvement less common

- Lesions typically T2 hypointense on MR due to high cellularity and fibrosis
- US more sensitive in detecting subclinical sialadenitis or dacryoadenitis
- MR comprehensively assesses head and neck involvement including retrobulbar and sinonasal spaces; T2W and T1W C+ sequences are helpful

Top Differential Diagnoses

- Sjögren disease
- MALToma
- Sarcoidosis
- Orbital inflammatory pseudotumor
- Thyroid orbitopathy

Clinical Issues

- Adult patients, male predominance
- Indolent disease course; patients feel relatively well despite multiorgan involvement

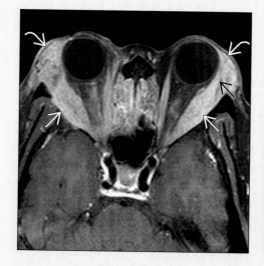
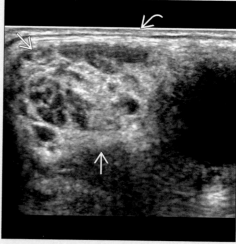

(Left) Axial T1WI C+ FS MR shows IgG4-related orbital myositis of lateral recti ➡ and mildly enlarged lacrimal glands ➡. Homogeneous enhancement is typical. Orbital myositis involves tendon insertion ➡, as opposed to thyroid ophthalmopathy. *(Right)* Transverse grayscale US (same patient) shows parenchymal chronic dacryoadenitis with diffusely enlarged right lacrimal gland ➡ and nodular hypoechoic pattern. There is no inflammatory change in adjacent tissue ➡ in contrast to acute dacryoadenitis.

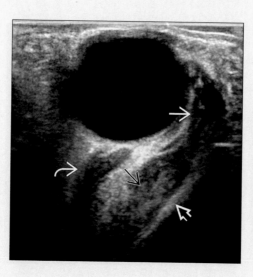
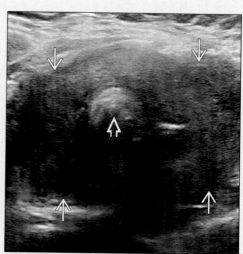

(Left) Transverse grayscale US of the left orbit (same patient) shows a markedly thickened left lateral rectus muscle ➡ with involvement of tendon insertion ➡. Note the lateral orbital wall ➡ and optic nerve ➡. *(Right)* Transverse grayscale US in a patient with Riedel thyroiditis shows that the thyroid ➡ is diffusely enlarged with a rounded contour and hypoechoic parenchyma. The thyroid parenchyma is often hypovascular and may encase major neck vessels. Note the trachea ➡. (Courtesy A. Momin, MD.)

IgG4-RELATED DISEASE IN HEAD & NECK

TERMINOLOGY

Abbreviations
- IgG4-related disease (IgG4-RD)

Synonyms
- Previously recognized head and neck conditions now acknowledged to fall within spectrum of IgG4-RD
  - Mikulicz syndrome
  - Kuttner tumor
  - Riedel thyroiditis
  - Inflammatory pseudotumor
  - Eosinophilic angiocentric fibrosis

Definitions
- Recently recognized idiopathic systemic fibroinflammatory condition characterized by tendency to form tumor-like lesion with dense lymphoplasmacytic infiltrate rich in IgG4-positive cells

IMAGING

General Features
- Best diagnostic clue
  - Bilateral chronic dacryoadenitis > submandibular sialadenitis > parotiditis &/or orbital inflammatory pseudotumor, myositis, perineural disease

Ultrasonographic Findings
- IgG4-related ophthalmic disease
  - Perhaps the most commonly affected organ system
  - IgG4-related dacryoadenitis
    - Most common lesion in orbits
    - Most cases described are accompanied by salivary gland disease, as seen in Mikulicz disease
    - Bilateral symmetrical > unilateral
    - Diffuse enlargement of lacrimal gland
    - Round or lobulated contour
    - Scattered hypoechoic nodular pattern (likely represents early disease)
    - Diffusely hypoechoic, coarse parenchyma (likely represents later more fibrotic disease)
    - Diffuse, nondisplaced hypervascularity
    - No inflammation of surrounding tissue
    - Unilateral lacrimal lesion may occur and may be difficult to differentiate from infectious dacryoadenitis or lacrimal tumors on imaging
  - IgG4-related orbital inflammation or IgG4-related orbital inflammatory pseudotumor
    - Irregular, hypoechoic, vascular soft tissue mass in retrobulbar &/or periorbital tissue
    - Retrobulbar lesion requires MR for full evaluation
  - IgG4-related orbital myositis
    - Extraocular muscle thickening is hypoechoic, avascular, and typically includes tendon insertion
  - IgG4-related perineural disease
    - Commonly affects branches of trigeminal nerve (e.g., frontal and infraorbital nerves) > optic nerve
    - Optic nerve lesion may be partially seen on US as diffuse thickening of nerve with lobular contour
    - Frontal and infraorbital nerve lesions are obscured by bone unless very large
- IgG4-related sialadenitis
  - Affects submandibular glands > parotid glands, superficial lobe > deep lobe
  - Bilateral symmetrical > asymmetrical
  - Sonographic pattern similar to that of lacrimal gland except it is usually less severe
  - Chronic, submandibular involvement similar to Kuttner tumor
  - Absence of sialolith
- IgG4-related thyroiditis
  - Less common than dacryoadenitis or sialadenitis
  - Several studies have observed high prevalence of hypothyroidism in patients with autoimmune pancreatitis (AIP)
  - Riedel thyroiditis and fibrosing variant of Hashimoto thyroiditis are suspected as being part of spectrum
    - Riedel thyroiditis: Diffuse hypoechoic, hypovascular thyroid glands ± vascular encasement (carotid artery or jugular vein)
  - Some believe an entity of IgG4-related thyroiditis may exist
    - Lower likelihood of diffuse goiter
    - Male predominance, comparatively older age
- IgG4-related lymphadenopathy
  - Localized disease adjacent to specific organ affected, or generalized lymphadenopathy as sole manifestation
  - Appearance is similar to reactive lymphadenopathy
    - Typically 1-2 cm, multiple and bilateral
  - Could be difficult to diagnose histologically due to less common storiform fibrosis
    - Often regarded as reactive follicular hyperplasia

CT Findings
- Homogeneous attenuation, enhancement of tumor-like lesions or enlarged lacrimal/salivary glands

MR Findings
- T1WI: Isointense to skeletal muscle
- T2WI: Typically low signal due to increased cellularity and fibrosis; high signal lesion is also possible
- T1WI C+: Homogeneously enhancing

Nuclear Medicine Findings
- FDG-18 PET
  - Most reported lesions are hypermetabolic; may be helpful tool in demonstrating multiorgan involvement

Imaging Recommendations
- Best imaging tool
  - MR allows comprehensive assessment of head & neck involvement including retrobulbar and sinonasal spaces
    - T2W and T1W C+ sequences are helpful
  - US may be more sensitive in detecting subclinical sialadenitis or dacryoadenitis

DIFFERENTIAL DIAGNOSIS

Sjögren Disease
- Affects parotid glands > submandibular glands > lacrimal glands (reverse order to IgG4-RD)
- Sicca syndrome is more common
- Can be differentiated clearly by clinical, serologic, and pathologic findings

Mucosal-Associated Lymphoid Tissue Lymphoma
- Unilateral > bilateral symmetrical

IgG4-RELATED DISEASE IN HEAD & NECK

- ± coarse, hypoechoic mass in lacrimal or salivary glands ± diffuse lymphoid hyperplasia

Sarcoidosis

- Imaging appearance can be similar to IgG4-RD
- Differentiated by serology

Orbital Inflammatory Pseudotumor

- Indistinguishable from IgG4-RD on USG if asymmetrical or unilateral involvement; T2W hyperintense

Thyroid Orbitopathy

- Extraocular muscle hypertrophy with tendon sparing ± hyperthyroidism

---

PATHOLOGY

General Features

- Etiology: Unknown
- Diagnosis based on histopathology and immunostaining characteristics of pathologic tissue

Microscopic Features

- Characteristic histopathologic features
  ○ Dense lymphoplasmacytic infiltrate that is rich in IgG4 plasma cells
  ○ Storiform fibrosis
    ▪ Pattern likened to cartwheel, with bands of fibrosis emanating from center
    ▪ Characteristic of IgG4-RD except being uncommon in IgG4-related lymphadenopathy
  ○ Mild to moderate eosinophil infiltrate
    ▪ Postulated association with allergic or atopic manifestation
  ○ ± obliterative phlebitis
    ▪ Always present in pancreas and submandibular gland; much less often in lacrimal gland

Immunohistochemical Features

- Semiquantitative analysis of IgG4 immunostaining may provide compelling features
  ○ > 30 IgG4-positive cells per high-power field
  ○ IgG4:IgG ratio > 50%
  ○ Lower cutoff point for IgG4-positive cells is acceptable in cases with characteristic morphologic features

Serum IgG4 Level

- Not sufficient in and of itself as a diagnostic test
  ○ Elevated in majority (can be ≥ 25x upper limit of normal) but also found normal in significant minority (20-40%)

CLINICAL ISSUES

Presentation

- Most common signs/symptoms
  ○ Head and neck region is commonly involved
    ▪ Ophthalmic disease > salivary glands > thyroid gland, lymph nodes, sinonasal cavities, laryngeal lesion
  ○ Typically presents as tumor-like lesion with indolent disease course (develops over months/years)
    ▪ Bilateral > unilateral proptosis ± visual disturbance due to optic nerve compression
    ▪ Bilateral firm submandibular > parotid swelling

- ▪ ± hypothyroidism &/or goiter
  ○ Constitutional symptoms subtle or absent
- Other signs/symptoms
  ○ Involvement outside head and neck
    ▪ Neurologic: Pituitary hypophysitis, hypertrophic pachymeningitis
    ▪ Chest: Lung involvement, mediastinitis, pleuritis
    ▪ Abdomen: Type 1 AIP, sclerosing cholangitis, cholecystitis, renal disease, retroperitoneal fibrosis
    ▪ Vascular: Aortitis/periaortitis, etc.
  ○ Longstanding allergic or atopic manifestations are common

Demographics

- Age
  ○ Adults; most > 50 years of age
- Gender
  ○ Male predominance (62-83%)
- Epidemiology
  ○ Limited data on global incidence and prevalence

Natural History & Prognosis

- Indolent disease course; patients often feel well even in setting of multiorgan disease
- Occasionally, aggressive disease course with systemic symptoms and rapid organ failure

Treatment

- Excellent response to glucocorticoid therapy
- Chronic, fibrotic lesions may be resistant to treatment

DIAGNOSTIC CHECKLIST

Consider

- Bilateral chronic dacryoadenitis > submandibular sialadenitis > parotiditis
- Orbital inflammatory disease ± dacryoadenitis

Image Interpretation Pearls

- Be aware of possible involvement of other sites inside/outside head and neck

---

SELECTED REFERENCES

1. Ferry JA et al: IgG4-related disease in the head and neck. Semin Diagn Pathol. 29(4):235-44, 2012
2. Fujita A et al: IgG4-related disease of the head and neck: CT and MR imaging manifestations. Radiographics. 32(7):1945-58, 2012
3. Inoue D et al: IgG4-Related Perineural Disease. Int J Rheumatol. 2012:401890, 2012
4. Stone JH et al: Mechanisms of Disease: IgG4-related disease. N Engl J Med. 36:539-51, 2012
5. Stone JH: IgG4-related disease: nomenclature, clinical features, and treatment. Semin Diagn Pathol. 29(4):177-90, 2012
6. Toyoda K et al: MR imaging of IgG4-related disease in the head and neck and brain. AJNR Am J Neuroradiol. 33(11):2136-9, 2012
7. Hennessey JV: Clinical review: Riedel's thyroiditis: a clinical review. J Clin Endocrinol Metab. 96(10):3031-41, 2011
8. Slman R et al: Ultrasound, elastography, and fluorodeoxyglucose positron emission tomography/computed tomography imaging in Riedel's thyroiditis: report of two cases. Thyroid. 21(7):799-804, 2011
9. Yamamoto M et al: A new conceptualization for Mikulicz's disease as an IgG4-related plasmacytic disease. Mod Rheumatol. 16(6):335-40, 2006

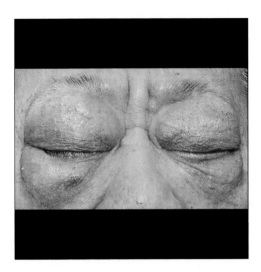

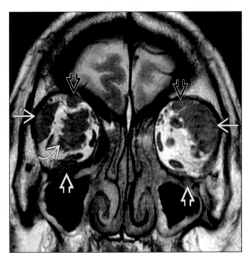

(Left) Clinical photo shows an adult male patient with bilateral, symmetrical floppy eyelids and known biopsy-proven IgG4-RD. *(Right)* Corresponding coronal T2WI MR shows bilateral dacryoadenitis ➡, right retrobulbar inflammatory pseudotumor ➡, and perineural disease involving frontal ⇥ and infraorbital ➡ nerves, a pattern typical of IgG4-related pan-orbital inflammation. Note that the lesions are characteristically hypointense on T2WI, typical for IgG4-RD due to high cellularity and fibrosis.

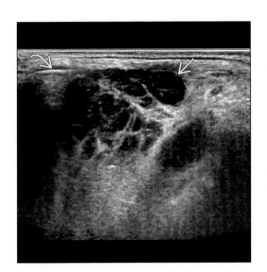

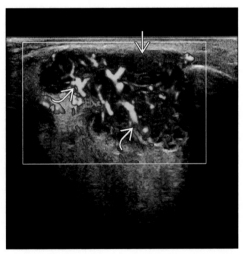

(Left) Transverse US of the right lacrimal gland (same patient) shows chronic dacryoadenitis ➡ (rounded contour, diffuse, coarse hypoechoic appearance) likely to represent late, fibrotic phase. Note the lateral orbital wall ➡. *(Right)* Transverse power Doppler US of the contralateral lacrimal gland shows symmetrical chronic dacryoadenitis ➡. Diffuse, nondisplaced hypervascularity ➡ is typical. Grayscale and Doppler US are reminiscent of a submandibular Kuttner tumor.

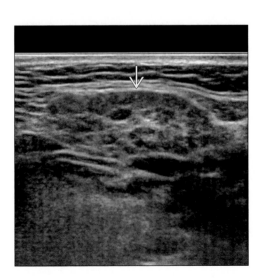

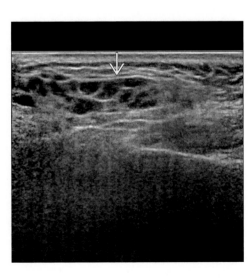

(Left) Transverse grayscale US (same patient) shows chronic sialadenitis of the left submandibular gland ➡ with diffuse nodular hypoechoic pattern. The right submandibular gland was similarly involved. *(Right)* Corresponding transverse grayscale US of the right parotid gland shows chronic parotiditis ➡, which is more severe in the superficial lobe. Note that in this patient, smaller glands are involved more severely, a common pattern in IgG4-RD and similar to Mikulicz disease.

SALIVARY GLAND MALToma

Key Facts

Terminology
- SG MALToma: Most common subtype of primary lymphoma of salivary gland parenchyma

Imaging
- Discrete mass(es)
  - Irregular/lobulated/ill-defined margins
  - Hypoechoic/pseudocystic, ± posterior enhancement, thin hyperechoic septations
- Multiple hypoechoic nodules; few mm to ~ 1-2 cm
  - Ill-defined/confluent or smooth margins
- Appearances likened to tortoiseshell or cobblestones
- ↑ vascularity in hypoechoic areas ± rest of gland

Top Differential Diagnoses
- Lymphoma (non-MALT)
- Sjögren syndrome (SjS)
- Chronic sclerosing sialadenitis
- Benign lymphoepithelial lesion (BLEL)-HIV

- Parotid nodal metastatic disease
- Warthin tumor

Pathology
- Derived from MALT, which is not normally present in salivary tissue but develops as result of chronic immune stimulation
- ↑ risk in SjS (up to 44x) and chronic sialadenitis

Diagnostic Checklist
- Imaging overlaps appreciably with benign conditions associated with intrasalivary lymphoid proliferation
- However, consider MALToma if
  - Hypoechoic/pseudocystic masses with septations, tortoiseshell or cobblestone appearance
  - Enlarging mass in SjS or chronic sialadenitis
- Consider core biopsy if MALToma is suspected

(Left) Longitudinal grayscale US of the left parotid gland in a 58-year-old woman with primary salivary MALToma who presented with gradual, painless swelling shows an irregular, multinodular, hypoechoic/pseudocystic "mass" with thin intervening hyperechoic septations ➡ resembling tortoiseshell or cobblestones. Some parenchyma in the deep lobe is spared ➡. Note the retromandibular vein ➡. (Right) Corresponding power Doppler US shows ↑ intralesional vascularity, mainly in hypoechoic areas ➡.

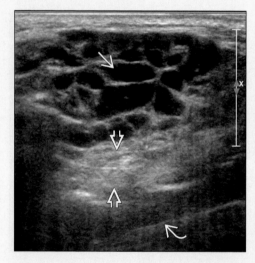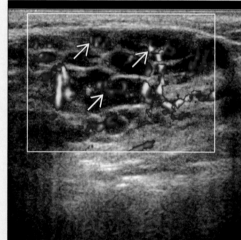

(Left) Coronal T2WI MR (same patient) reveals a left parotid lesion appearing as a solid hypointense mass ➡ with infiltrative margins medially ➡. The rest of both parotid glands appear heterogeneous due to chronic sialadenitis ➡. (Right) Corresponding axial T1WI MR shows the left parotid mass composed of multiple hypointense lobules interspersed by thin hyperintense septations ➡ resembling a tortoiseshell or cobblestone appearance on US, suggestive of parenchymal NHL.

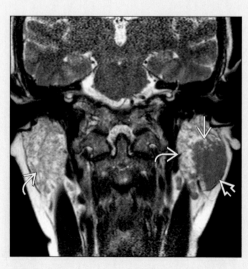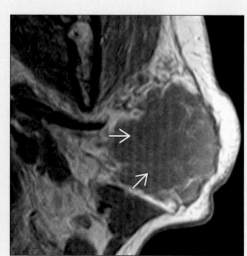

SALIVARY GLAND MALToma

TERMINOLOGY

Abbreviations
- Salivary gland (SG), mucosa-associated lymphoid tissue (MALT)

Synonyms
- MALT lymphoma

Definitions
- Extranodal marginal zone B-cell lymphoma of MALT within salivary parenchyma

IMAGING

General Features
- Best diagnostic clue
  - Irregular hypoechoic/pseudocystic parenchymal mass with thin hyperechoic septations
- Location
  - Parotid (80%), submandibular (20%)
  - Single gland ~ 90%, multiple glands ~ 10%
- Size
  - Variable: Few mm to several cm
- Morphology
  - Multiple nodules or single solid irregular mass

Ultrasonographic Findings
- Grayscale ultrasound
  - Discrete mass
    - Irregular/lobulated/ill-defined margins
    - Hypoechoic/pseudocystic, ± posterior enhancement, thin hyperechoic septations
  - Multiple hypoechoic nodules; few mm to ~ 1-2 cm
    - Ill-defined/confluent or smooth margins
  - Appearances likened to tortoiseshell or cobblestones
  - ± cystic spaces, calcifications (both are rare)
  - ± (peri)salivary lymphomatous nodes (uncommon)
- Power Doppler
  - ↑ vascularity in hypoechoic areas ± rest of gland

Imaging Recommendations
- Best imaging tool
  - US for initial characterization and image-guided Bx
  - MR/CT to assess deep lobe of parotid and for staging

DIFFERENTIAL DIAGNOSIS

Lymphoma (Non-MALT)
- Parenchymal NHL can be due to non-MALT subtypes
  - Irregular nodules/masses, hypoechoic/pseudocystic, posterior enhancement, ± septa, ↑ vascularity
- Cannot reliably separate NHL subtypes on US

Sjögren Syndrome (SjS)
- Involves salivary and lacrimal glands
- Diffuse micronodular/cystic ± dominant masses

Chronic Sclerosing Sialadenitis
- Focal hypoechoic areas/mass, "cirrhotic" gland, submandibular > parotid, undisplaced vessels

Benign Lymphoepithelial Lesion (BLEL)-HIV
- Hypoechoic solid/cystic mass, parotid > submandibular, irregular or smooth, often multifocal/bilateral in HIV patients

- If AIDS patient has NHL, imaging may be complex

Parotid Nodal Metastatic Disease
- Unilateral/bilateral nodal masses, invasive margins, ± necrosis, ± other cervical nodal metastases
- Usually known primary cancer in head and neck

Warthin Tumor
- Well-defined, hypoechoic, solid/partly cystic mass, ± septa, ± branching vascularity resembling a node
- Most are intra- or periparotid, 20% multicentric

PATHOLOGY

General Features
- Etiology
  - MALT is normally absent in SGs but can be acquired due to chronic immune stimulation, which occurs in SjS and chronic sialadenitis
  - MALToma risk ↑ in SjS (9-44x) and chronic sialadenitis
  - 5-10% of patients with SG MALToma have SjS
  - MALToma involves specific tissues: Stomach (2/3), lungs, thyroid, orbits, breast, salivary glands

Staging, Grading, & Classification
- Typically low grade and low stage
- Classified as 1° if no intrasalivary nodal or extrasalivary lymphoma is present, otherwise 2°

CLINICAL ISSUES

Presentation
- Most common signs/symptoms
  - Painless salivary swelling ± constitutional symptoms

Demographics
- Age: Mainly 6th-7th decades; median ~ 60 years
- Gender: Female > male (~ 1.7-3:1)

Natural History & Prognosis
- Usually indolent, remains localized for years
- If spreads, tends to involve other MALT sites (homing)
- < 10% convert to high-grade NHL; ↑ risk if young
- Typically good prognosis (80-95% 5-year survival)

Treatment
- Depends on grade and stage
  - Low: Surgical resection ± radiotherapy
  - High: Rituximab ± cytotoxic chemotherapy

Diagnosis
- By core/excision biopsy as FNAC is often inconclusive

DIAGNOSTIC CHECKLIST

Image Interpretation Pearls
- Hypoechoic/pseudocystic masses with septations, tortoiseshell or cobblestone appearance
- Enlarging mass in SjS or chronic sialadenitis

SELECTED REFERENCES
1. Lee YY et al: Imaging of salivary gland tumours. Eur J Radiol. 66(3):419-36, 2008

SALIVARY GLAND MALToma

(Left) Axial T1WI MR in a 73-year-old woman with progressive painless left parotid swelling shows bilateral, slightly irregular, hypointense intraparotid masses ➡ that were diagnosed histologically as MALTomas. Multicentric involvement can occur in MALToma. *(Right)* Corresponding US of the left parotid gland shows a large, lobulated hypoechoic MALToma ➡. Note multiple internal septations ➡ resulting in a tortoiseshell appearance and posterior acoustic enhancement ➡.

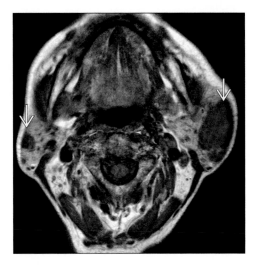

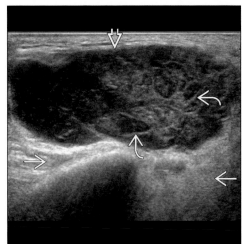

(Left) Longitudinal grayscale US of the right parotid gland (same patient) shows a smaller discrete MALToma ➡. Note again the irregular margins, pseudocystic appearance, subtle internal septa ➡, and posterior acoustic enhancement ➡. *(Right)* Corresponding power Doppler US shows moderate increased vascularity within MALToma, confirming its solid nature. Note posterior enhancement ➡ in the normal surrounding parenchyma.

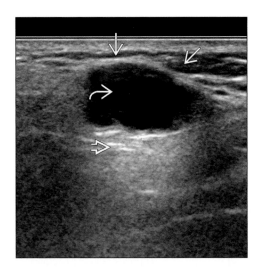

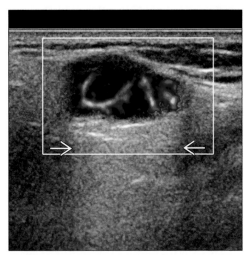

(Left) Longitudinal grayscale US of the right submandibular gland in a 63-year-old woman shows a hypoechoic mass distorting the gland ➡, which was a primary MALToma. Note the mylohyoid muscle ➡ and mandible ➡. *(Right)* Transverse grayscale US of the right submandibular gland ➡ in 66-year-old man shows a focal hypoechoic, irregular mass ➡, confirmed as chronic sclerosing sialadenitis (Kuttner tumor). Lack of mass effect favors this diagnosis, although it can mimic MALToma on imaging.

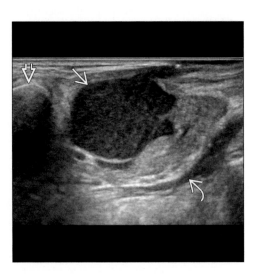

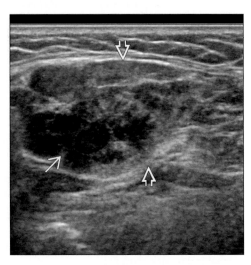

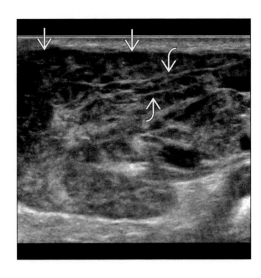

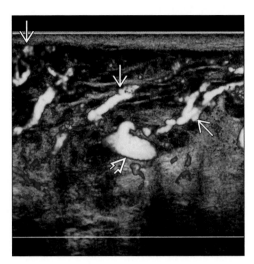

(Left) Transverse US shows a parotid gland in a 72-year-old man with cough and bilateral painless salivary swellings, diagnosed as low-grade MALToma, which involved both lungs, major salivary glands, and bone marrow. Note the gross glandular enlargement and heterogeneous hypoechoic echo pattern, with ill-defined hypoechoic foci ➡ & linear septations ➡. *(Right)* Corresponding power Doppler US shows ↑ vascularity distributed throughout gland ➡. Note retromandibular vein ➡.

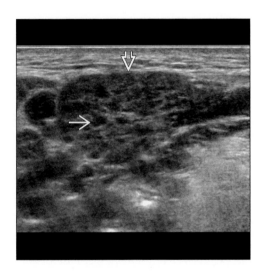

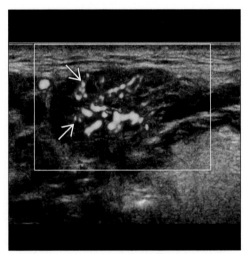

(Left) Transverse grayscale US of a submandibular gland ➡ (same patient) shows a heterogeneous appearance with multiple small, hypoechoic infiltrates ➡. *(Right)* Corresponding power Doppler US shows ↑ vascularity in the gland ➡. This is regarded as secondary MALToma of salivary glands since other extrasalivary sites were involved at diagnosis. Patient developed high-grade B-cell NHL after 3 years, reflecting MALToma transformation, to which he ultimately succumbed.

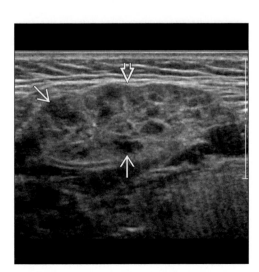

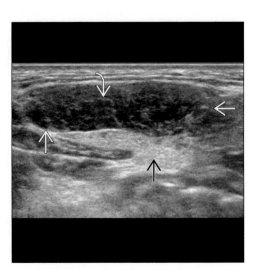

(Left) Transverse US of a submandibular gland ➡ in a 61-year-old woman with painless swelling shows multifocal ill-defined, hypoechoic infiltrates ➡, resembling MALToma. Histology showed chronic sialadenitis. *(Right)* Transverse US shows a submandibular gland in a 79-year-old man with painless swelling diagnosed as mantle cell NHL. Note the focal irregular, heterogeneous, hypoechoic mass ➡ with subtle septations ➡, mimicking MALToma, and normal deep lobe parenchyma ➡.

SALIVARY GLAND AMYLOIDOSIS

Key Facts

Terminology

- Salivary gland (SG) amyloidosis: Abnormal extracellular deposition of amyloid within salivary parenchyma

Imaging

- Amyloidosis is multifactorial with localized and systemic forms
- Although head and neck are commonly involved in amyloidosis, SG involvement is very rare
- Multifocal, irregular, heterogeneous, hypoechoic parenchymal nodules/masses
- Intranodular vascularity reduced/absent on power Doppler
- Hypoechoic stranding in adjacent parenchyma
- ± lymphadenopathy (reactive or neoplastic if due to underlying dyscrasia)

○ Round, hypoechoic/pseudocystic nodes, reticulated echo pattern, preserved/absent hila, variable vascularity

Top Differential Diagnoses

- Sjögren syndrome
- Salivary gland metastases
- Salivary gland non-Hodgkin lymphoma

Diagnostic Checklist

- Consider SG amyloidosis if irregular, hypoechoic, avascular parenchymal infiltrates are found in patient with known plasma cell dyscrasia or chronic inflammatory disease
- If systemic amyloidosis is suspected, perform CT/MR to identify conditions associated with amyloidosis and to evaluate other potential sites of systemic involvement

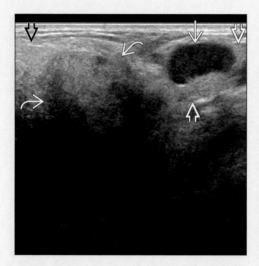
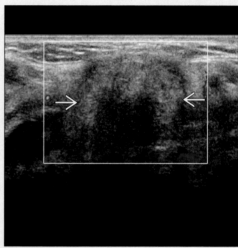

(Left) Transverse grayscale US shows the parotid tail and submandibular region in a patient with multiple myeloma and histologically confirmed salivary amyloidosis. Note the irregular, ill-defined hypoechoic parotid infiltrates ➡, mainly within the deep lobe, and an adjacent involved submandibular lymph node ➡. Some parotid ⬆ and submandibular ➡ tissue appears relatively spared. *(Right)* Corresponding power Doppler US shows minimal vascularity within and around a parotid amyloidosis infiltrate ➡.

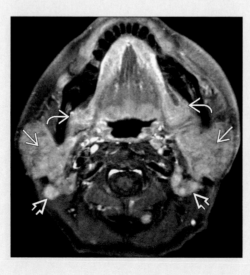
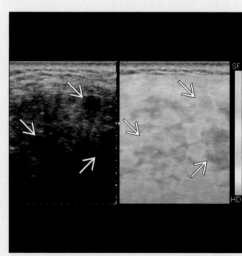

(Left) Axial T1WI C+ FS MR (same patient) shows multiple nodular enhancing amyloidosis infiltrates enlarging both parotid ➡ and submandibular ➡ glands. Note several adjacent matted lymph nodes ➡. *(Right)* Transverse grayscale US and qualitative strain elastogram in same patient shows that strain color scale ranges from purple (elastic, soft) to red (inelastic, hard). Ill-defined amyloidosis infiltrates ➡ show mosaic green & red pattern, suggesting intermediate to low elasticity (moderate to mostly high stiffness).

SALIVARY GLAND AMYLOIDOSIS

TERMINOLOGY

Abbreviations
- Salivary gland (SG)

Definitions
- Abnormal extracellular deposition of amyloid within salivary parenchyma
- Amyloid refers to variety of insoluble proteins with specific properties
  - β-pleated sheet structure on x-ray crystallography
  - Apple-green birefringence under polarized light with Congo red staining
  - Amorphous eosinophilic appearance on H&E stain

IMAGING

General Features
- Best diagnostic clue
  - Imaging appearances are variable and not well documented to date (c.f. limited to case reports)
- Location
  - Parotid > submandibular/sublingual
- Morphology
  - Diffuse/focal, glandular enlargement

Ultrasonographic Findings
- Grayscale ultrasound
  - Multifocal, irregular, heterogeneous, hypoechoic parenchymal infiltrates
  - Hypoechoic stranding in adjacent parenchyma
  - ± lymphadenopathy (reactive or neoplastic if due to an underlying dyscrasia)
    - Round, hypoechoic/pseudocystic nodes, reticulated echo pattern, preserved/absent hila
- Power Doppler
  - Reduced/absent vascularity within infiltrates

CT Findings
- CECT: Well- or ill-defined, iso- or hypodense, poorly enhancing nodules/masses, ± calcification

MR Findings
- T1-hypointense, T2-hypointense, poorly enhancing nodules/masses

Imaging Recommendations
- Best imaging tool
  - US: Initial salivary evaluation, image-guided biopsy
  - CT/MR: Evaluation of deep lobe of parotid and extrasalivary tissues

DIFFERENTIAL DIAGNOSIS

Sjögren Syndrome
- Hypoechoic, heterogeneous, reticulated, microcysts/macrocysts
- Multiple SGs ± lacrimal glands

Salivary Gland Metastases
- Solitary/multiple ill-defined, hypoechoic masses
- ± known head and neck primary malignancy

Salivary Gland Non-Hodgkin Lymphoma
- Especially MALToma: Solitary/multiple, hypoechoic/pseudocystic, tortoiseshell/cobblestone appearance

PATHOLOGY

General Features
- Etiology
  - Amyloidosis occurs in a wide variety of conditions, notably plasma cell dyscrasia including myeloma, chronic inflammatory conditions including autoimmune diseases and chronic infections, and certain types of cancer; has hereditary/familial forms
    - Can accumulate almost anywhere in the body
    - Involving SG is very rare

Staging, Grading, & Classification
- Divided clinically into localized (single site/organ involved) or systemic amyloidosis; also divided biochemically according to protein precursor (~ 25 types)
- 90% of patients with systemic amyloidosis develop deposits in head, neck, or respiratory tract

Gross Pathologic & Surgical Features
- Amyloid deposits can be microscopic or macroscopic
  - Macroscopic deposit is called amyloidoma

CLINICAL ISSUES

Presentation
- Most common signs/symptoms
  - Painless salivary gland mass or diffuse swelling, xerostomia
  - Multiple enlarged (peri)salivary lymph nodes or distant nodal enlargement
- Other signs/symptoms
  - Systemic amyloidosis: Constitutional (e.g., weight loss, edema), organ dysfunction (e.g., cardiac and renal failure)

Natural History & Prognosis
- Localized: Usually indolent with good prognosis
- Systemic: Usually fatal (1-2 years) due to progressive cardiac and renal infiltration causing severe organ failure

Treatment
- Localized: None or symptomatic resection
- Systemic: Multiple treatment options including of underlying condition, e.g., cytotoxic chemotherapy ± stem cell transplantation for myeloma

DIAGNOSTIC CHECKLIST

Consider
- If irregular, avascular SG parenchymal deposits are found in patient with known plasma cell dyscrasia or chronic inflammatory condition
- Perform CT/MR to identify diseases associated with amyloidosis and evaluate potential systemic involvement

SELECTED REFERENCES

1. Finkel KJ et al: Amyloid infiltration of the salivary glands in the setting of primary systemic amyloidosis without multiple myeloma. Otolaryngol Head Neck Surg. 135(3):471-2, 2006

KIMURA DISEASE

Key Facts

Terminology
- Triad of painless, unilateral, cervical adenopathy, subcutaneous nodules, and salivary gland lesions
- Blood & tissue eosinophilia; markedly ↑ serum IgE

Imaging
- Nodal involvement
  - Enlarged, well-defined, hypoechoic lymph nodes
  - Homogeneous internal architecture, nonnecrotic and preserved echogenic hilum
  - No nodal matting or adjacent soft tissue edema
  - Doppler: Hilar vascularity (87%), mixed hilar & peripheral (13%); low resistance, RI < 0.8, PI >1.6
- Subcutaneous/soft tissue involvement
  - Well-/ill-defined, hypoechoic masses or plaque-like lesions
  - Homogeneous or heterogeneous internal architecture

- Hypoechoic areas interspersed with hyperechoic areas; "wooly" appearance
- Color Doppler: Arterial & venous flow within lesions
- Spectral Doppler: Low resistance, RI < 0.8, PI < 1.6
- Salivary gland involvement
  - Focal/diffuse hypoechoic, heterogeneous parenchymal echo pattern
  - Enlarged intraparotid nodes; hypoechoic, heterogeneous, low-resistance vascularity

Top Differential Diagnoses
- Parotid primary malignancy
- Parotid nodal metastases
- Non-Hodgkin lymphoma nodes

Diagnostic Checklist
- Check combination of imaging findings, patient's ethnicity with chronicity of lesions, positive serology, confirmatory imaging-guided biopsy

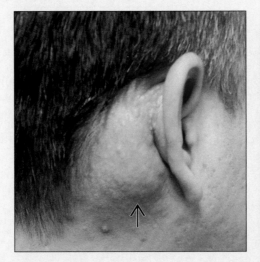
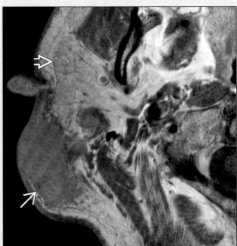

(Left) Clinical photograph shows a young Chinese male with a postauricular mass ⊟ that is painless and has been slowly growing over years. *(Right)* Axial T1WI C + MR shows an ill-defined mass ⊟ in postauricular soft tissues. Note that it is separate from the underlying superficial parotid gland ⊟, which otherwise appears normal. Minimal enhancement was seen in this mass, a feature of chronic fibrotic lesions. These masses are otherwise isointense/hypointense to parotid on T1WI and show solid enhancement.

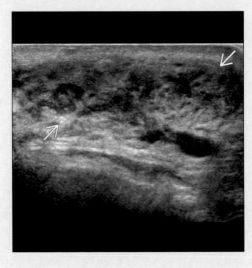
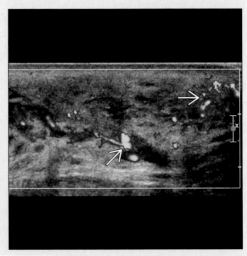

(Left) Longitudinal grayscale US (same patient) shows the ill-defined, solid, hypoechoic, heterogeneous nature of a postauricular soft tissue mass ⊟. *(Right)* Corresponding power Doppler US shows the presence of vessels ⊟ within the soft tissue lesion. Such vascularity is usually low resistance on spectral Doppler. The combination of location, US appearance, ethnicity of patient, and chronicity suggested Kimura disease (KD), which was confirmed by biopsy.

KIMURA DISEASE

TERMINOLOGY

Abbreviations
- Kimura disease (KD)

Definitions
- Chronic inflammatory disorder of head & neck, primarily in young Asian males
  - Triad of painless, unilateral, cervical adenopathy, subcutaneous nodules, and salivary gland lesions
  - Blood & tissue eosinophilia; markedly ↑ serum IgE

IMAGING

General Features
- Location
  - Most commonly involves unilateral lymph nodes, salivary glands, and subcutaneous tissues of head & neck
    - Most have involvement of parotid gland or submandibular gland; rarely lacrimal gland
    - Occasionally, axillary or inguinal lymph nodes or subcutaneous forearm lesions
- Morphology
  - Enlarged lymph nodes and ipsilateral subcutaneous mass lesions
  - Salivary gland involvement: Diffuse infiltration or ill-defined mass or focal intraparotid nodes

Ultrasonographic Findings
- Nodal involvement
  - Enlarged lymph nodes with well-defined border and hypoechoic appearance
  - Homogeneous internal architecture, nonnecrotic and preserved echogenic hilum
  - No nodal matting or adjacent soft tissue edema
  - Color Doppler: Hilar vascularity (87%), mixed hilar & peripheral (13%)
  - Spectral Doppler: Low-resistance vascularity, resistive index (RI) < 0.8, pulsatility index (PI) < 1.6
- Subcutaneous/soft tissue involvement
  - Well-/ill-defined, hypoechoic masses or plaque-like lesions
  - Homogeneous or heterogeneous internal architecture
  - Hypoechoic areas interspersed with hyperechoic areas; "wooly" appearance
  - Color Doppler: Arterial & venous flow within lesions
  - Spectral Doppler: Low resistance, RI < 0.8, PI < 1.6
- Salivary gland involvement
  - Focal/diffuse, hypoechoic, heterogeneous parenchymal echo pattern
  - Enlarged intraparotid nodes; hypoechoic, heterogeneous, low-resistance vascularity

Imaging Recommendations
- Best imaging tool
  - US is ideal initial modality of choice
    - Evaluates nodal, soft tissue, and salivary gland manifestations of KD
    - Readily combined with guided biopsy, which helps confirm diagnosis of KD
    - Cannot evaluate deep lobe parotid involvement; in such cases, MR is preferred over CT

DIFFERENTIAL DIAGNOSIS

Parotid Primary Malignancy
- Ill-defined, solid, hypoechoic mass with intranodal vascularity, ± extraglandular extension, ± facial nerve involvement, ± associated malignant nodes

Parotid Nodal Metastases
- Solitary/multiple, ill-defined, hypoechoic masses with abnormal vascularity and known associated primary (SCCa, NPC, adjacent melanoma)

Non-Hodgkin Lymphoma Nodes
- Multiple, solid, hypoechoic nodes, reticulated echo pattern, hilar > peripheral vascularity, ± posterior enhancement

Sarcoidosis, Head & Neck
- Primary manifestation is multiple enlarged nodes
- Can involve entire parotid gland or intraparotid nodes; diffuse hypoechoic gland, submandibular > parotid

Sjögren Syndrome
- Hypoechoic, heterogeneous gland; reticulated pattern, microcysts/macrocysts, multiple glands involved

CLINICAL ISSUES

Presentation
- Most common signs/symptoms
  - Insidious onset of solitary or multiple painless swellings of head and neck, predominantly in preauricular and submandibular regions
  - Marked lymphadenopathy (cervical [67-100%], axillary, inguinal)

Demographics
- Gender
  - M:F = 3:1
- Ethnicity
  - Endemic in Asians, particularly Chinese and Japanese

Natural History & Prognosis
- Chronic benign course with nodules present for years
- Slowly progressive over years
- Potentially disfiguring
  - Large (≥ 5 cm) subcutaneous lesions may ulcerate
- No malignant potential
- Spontaneous resolution reported

DIAGNOSTIC CHECKLIST

Image Interpretation Pearls
- Look for combination of imaging findings, particularly in Asian males with chronicity of lesions and positive serology
  - Unilateral cervical adenopathy
  - Subcutaneous, well-/ill-defined masses
  - Salivary gland abnormality: Intraparotid nodes or ill-defined or infiltrative mass

SELECTED REFERENCES

1. Takeishi M et al: Kimura disease: diagnostic imaging findings and surgical treatment. J Craniofac Surg. 18(5):1062-7, 2007

(Left) Clinical photograph shows a Chinese man with a longstanding, slowly growing painless mass ⊟ in the right parotid region. *(Right)* Transverse grayscale US shows an ill-defined, solid, hypoechoic, heterogeneous mass ➡ in the right superficial parotid gland. Note its ill-defined, infiltrating edges ⊟. Compare its echogenicity to normal hyperechoic, fine, bright parenchymal echoes ➡. Sonographically, the mass simulates a malignant salivary mass. Biopsy confirmed KD. Note mandibular cortex ➡.

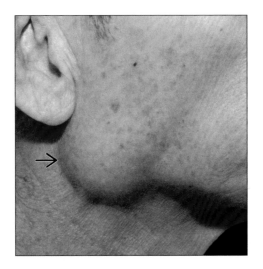
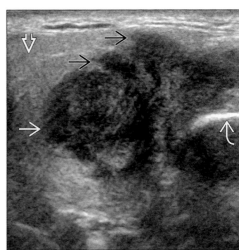

(Left) Longitudinal grayscale US *(same patient)* shows an ill-defined mass ➡ with infiltrative margins ➡ in the right superficial parotid. *(Right)* Corresponding power Doppler US shows focal, large, intratumoral vessels. Such US appearances of KD closely simulate a malignant salivary tumor. However, the patient's ethnicity, chronicity of lesion, slow growth over years ± other subcutaneous masses, and enlarged nodes in the vicinity of salivary glands, (+/-) serology should raise suspicion of KD.

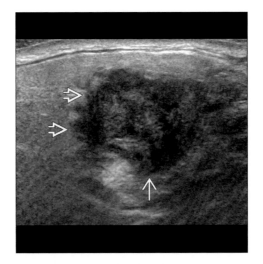
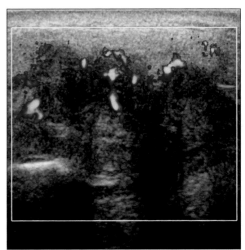

(Left) Axial T1WI MR *(same patient)* shows an ill-defined, hypointense (to parotid) mass ➡ in the right superficial parotid. Note its ill-defined, infiltrative edges. *(Right)* Corresponding coronal T1WI C+ FS MR shows diffuse enhancement of the parotid mass ➡ with no focal necrotic areas. In such cases, US identifies the location of the lesion, suggests probable diagnoses, and guides biopsy for confirmation. MR better delineates extent of abnormality and its relationship to adjacent structures.

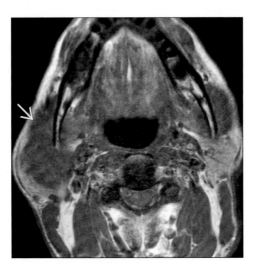
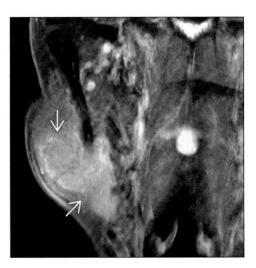

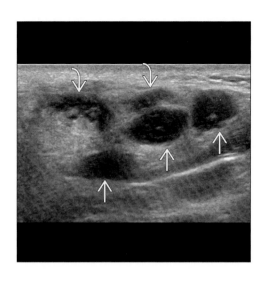

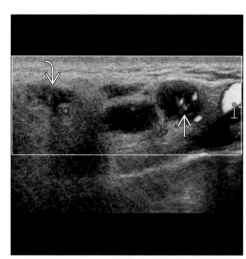

(Left) Longitudinal grayscale US in KD shows multiple enlarged intraparotid nodes ➡ and focal, hypoechoic, heterogeneous parenchymal echogenicity ➡. *(Right)* Corresponding power Doppler US shows hilar type of intranodal vascularity ➡. KD nodes invariably show hilar vascularity and a small percentage have mixed hilar and peripheral vascularity. Intranodal vessels show low resistance on spectral Doppler, RI < 0.8 and PI < 1.6. No significant vascularity is seen in the parenchymal lesion ➡.

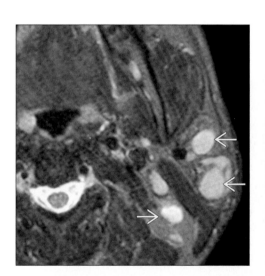

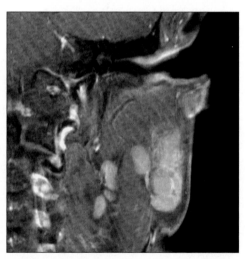

(Left) Axial T2WI MR shows multiple hyperintense, enlarged intraparotid nodes ➡. *(Right)* Coronal fat-suppressed T1WI C+ MR (same patient) shows solid, intense enhancement within intraparotid nodes, characteristic of KD. Multiple intranodal enlargements in KD simulate lymphoma and metastatic disease. Combination of ethnicity, chronicity, serology, and associated lesions help in suggesting diagnosis of KD.

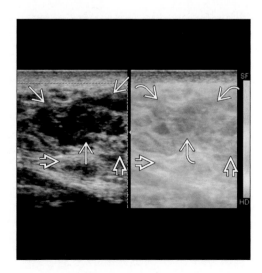

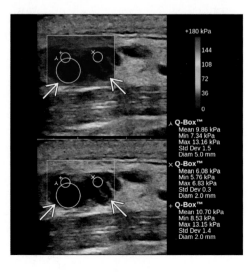

(Left) Transverse grayscale US and qualitative strain elastogram show KD ➡ in a parotid gland. Strain color scale ranges from purple (elastic, soft) to red (inelastic, hard). Infiltrate ➡ appears purple and green (elastic), similar to, or more elastic than, adjacent parotid tissue ➡. *(Right)* Transverse grayscale US and SWE show KD in parotid lymph nodes ➡. SWE color scale ranges from blue (0 kPa, soft) to red (180 kPa, stiff). Nodes appear blue with a maximum SWE value of 13.2 kPa, which is low.

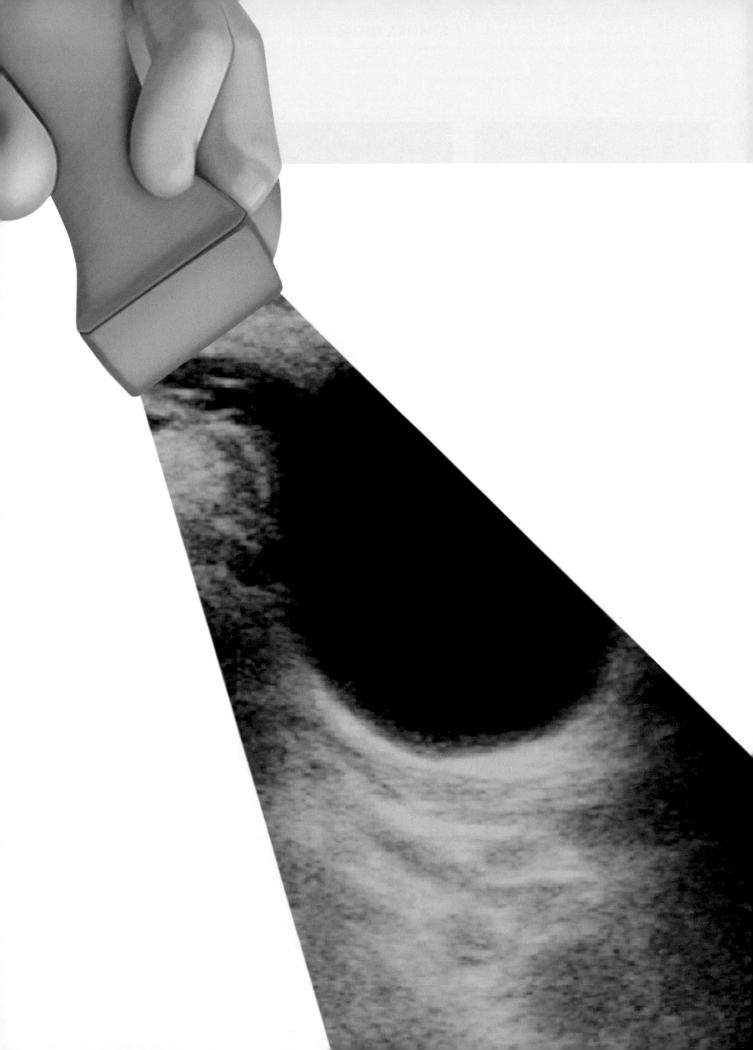

SECTION 5
Lumps and Bumps

Cystic

Solid

Miscellaneous

RANULA

Key Facts

Terminology

- Simple ranula (SR): Post-inflammatory retention cyst of sublingual gland (SLG) or minor salivary glands in sublingual space (SLS) with epithelial lining
- Diving ranula (DR): Extravasation pseudocyst; term used when SR becomes large and ruptures out of posterior SLS into submandibular space (SMS), creating pseudocyst lacking epithelial lining

Imaging

- Uncomplicated SR: Anechoic, well-defined, thin-walled, unilocular cystic mass ± fine internal echoes/debris, ± posterior acoustic enhancement
  - Restricted to SLS
- Uncomplicated DR: Unilocular or multilocular, thick-walled, cystic mass ± internal echoes/debris
  - Involves SLS and SMS
  - Located anterior or posterior to SMG, depending on mode of passage in relation to mylohyoid muscle

- Infected SR/DR: Thick internal debris, irregular thick walls, and soft tissue inflammation
- Color Doppler: SR and DR are avascular, but if infected, vascularity is seen in thick wall and surrounding soft tissue
- SLS is best scanned with transducer placed transverse under chin, midline and off midline
- Transducer is angled cranially under chin to evaluate mylohyoid muscle and its relation to ranula
- Identify relation of lesion to SLG, mylohyoid muscle, and extension into SMS
- US is ideal initial imaging modality for confirming diagnosis and extent of ranula
- MR is best for defining extent of large lesions

Top Differential Diagnoses

- Lymphatic malformation
- Dermoid/epidermoid, SLS or SMS
- 2nd branchial cleft cyst

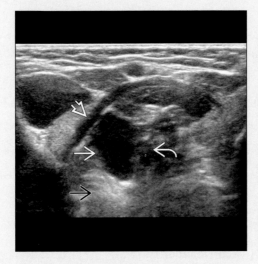
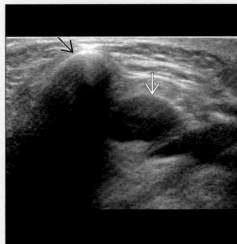

(Left) Transverse grayscale US shows a simple ranula (SR) ➡ in the right sublingual space. Note its relation to the right mylohyoid ⮞ and genioglossus ➡ muscles. The SR is well defined and anechoic with thin walls and posterior enhancement ➡. (Right) Corresponding longitudinal grayscale US shows an SR ➡ confined to the sublingual space. Common differential diagnoses include dermoid/epidermoid and lymphatic malformation. Note the mandible ➡.

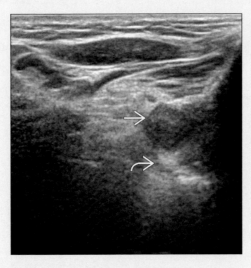
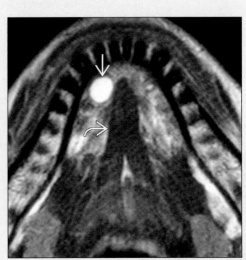

(Left) Oblique grayscale US shows small a SR ➡ restricted to the sublingual space (SLS). Note that it has internal debris and mimics a solid lesion. Note posterior enhancement ➡, which suggests its cystic nature. (Right) Corresponding axial T2WI MR confirms the location of SR ➡ in the SLS. Note its relation to the ipsilateral genioglossus muscle ➡. US is an ideal imaging modality for evaluation of SR as it defines its location and extent (vs. diving ranula [DR]).

RANULA

TERMINOLOGY

Abbreviations
- Simple ranula (SR), diving ranula (DR)

Definitions
- Retention cyst resulting from trauma or inflammation of sublingual gland (SLG) or minor salivary glands in sublingual space (SLS)
  - SR: Post-inflammatory retention cyst of SLG or SLS minor salivary glands with epithelial lining
    - Located above mylohyoid muscle near SLG
  - DR: Extravasation pseudocyst; term used when SR becomes large and ruptures out of posterior SLS into submandibular space (SMS), creating pseudocyst lacking epithelial lining

IMAGING

General Features
- Best diagnostic clue
  - SR: Well-defined, cystic, thin-walled SLS mass
  - DR: SLS + SMS cyst extension
- Location
  - SR: SLS
  - DR: SLS + SMS
- Size
  - SR: < 3 cm
  - DR: < 6 cm; may be giant
- Morphology
  - SR: Oval to lenticular, unilocular SLS mass
  - DR: Unilocular mass with 1 component in SLS with extension into SMS
    - When large, will involve inferior parapharyngeal space (PPS)
    - If plunging through mylohyoid vascular cleft, may end up anterior to submandibular gland (SMG)

Ultrasonographic Findings
- Uncomplicated SR (USR)
  - Anechoic, well-defined, thin-walled, unilocular cystic mass ± fine internal echoes/debris, ± posterior acoustic enhancement
  - Restricted to SLS
- Uncomplicated DR (UDR)
  - Unilocular or multilocular, thick-walled, cystic mass ± internal echoes/debris
  - Involves SLS and SMS
  - Located anterior or posterior to SMG, depending on mode of passage in relation to mylohyoid muscle
  - SR ruptures and leads to pseudocyst/DR
    - Posterior rupture over posterior margin of mylohyoid to posterior SMS
    - Rupture laterally through boutonnière defect, anterior to SMG
    - Extension to PPS, occurs in < 10% of all ranulas
- Infected SR/DR: Thick internal debris, irregular thick walls, and soft tissue inflammation
- Color Doppler: SR and DR are avascular, but if infected, vascularity is seen in thick wall and surrounding soft tissue

Imaging Recommendations
- Best imaging tool
  - Diagnosis is often made clinically, and imaging is used to evaluate extent of lesion
  - US is ideal initial imaging modality for confirming diagnosis and extent of ranula
    - May not be able to evaluate entire extent of large ranulas and extension into PPS
  - MR is best for defining extent of large lesions
- Protocol advice
  - SLS is best scanned with transducer placed transverse under chin, midline and off midline
  - Transducer is angled cranially under chin to evaluate mylohyoid muscle and its relation to ranula
  - Identify relation of lesion to SLG, mylohyoid muscle, and extension into SMS
  - SLG is identified by its fine, bright parenchymal echo pattern and relationship to lingual artery
  - Compare with contralateral side

DIFFERENTIAL DIAGNOSIS

Lymphatic Malformation
- Multilocular, trans-spatial cystic mass
- Mimics ranula on imaging; often does not involve SLS
- Multiloculated, septate, ± fine internal echoes
- Avascular on Doppler

Dermoid/Epidermoid, SLS or SMS
- Anechoic/pseudosolid, paramedian mass in SLS or SMS, ± soft tissue and fat within its matrix
- Hetero-/homogeneous echo pattern, ± calcification
- Avascular on Doppler

2nd Branchial Cleft Cyst
- Ovoid unilocular mass in posterior SMS, anechoic or pseudosolid echo pattern on US

Suppurative Submandibular Lymph Node
- Multiple SMS nodes with intranodal cystic necrosis
- Thick walls in clinical setting of infection

Abscess, Oral Cavity
- Patient is usually septic with tender oral cavity
- Single or multiple heterogeneous fluid collection, thick walls, ± rim vascularity on Doppler

DIAGNOSTIC CHECKLIST

Consider
- Lymphatic malformation and epidermoid/dermoid cyst of SLS can be clinical and imaging mimics

Image Interpretation Pearls
- DR is suspected based on presence of cystic mass in SLS and SMS closely related to mylohyoid muscle
  - Define anatomy of ranula rupture
    - If behind posterior margin of mylohyoid muscle, SMS cyst component will be posterior to SMG
    - If anterior through mylohyoid vascular cleft, SMS cystic component will be anterior to SMG

SELECTED REFERENCES
1. Harnsberger HR et al: Diagnostic Imaging: Head & Neck. 2nd ed. Salt Lake City: Amirsys, Inc. 1-14, 20-23, 2011
2. Ahuja AT et al: Practical Head & Neck Ultrasound. London: Greenwich Medical Media. 85-104, 2000

RANULA

(Left) Transverse grayscale US shows an SR ➡ restricted to the right sublingual space. It is anechoic, with ill-defined walls and posterior enhancement ➡. Note its adjacent anatomic relation to the genioglossus ➡ and mylohyoid ➡ muscles. *(Right)* Corresponding power Doppler US (same patient) shows no significant vascularity in the walls of SR ➡ or soft tissues around it. Note normal lingual vessel ➡.

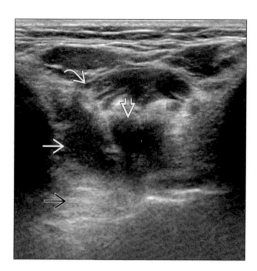 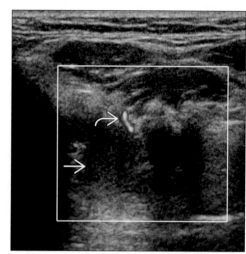

(Left) Corresponding axial T2WI MR (same patient) shows a right SR ➡ as a lesion with markedly high (fluid/cerebrospinal fluid) intensity and its relation to the ipsilateral genioglossus muscle ➡. *(Right)* Corresponding coronal T2WI MR further demonstrates the location of SR ➡, which is restricted to the SLS.

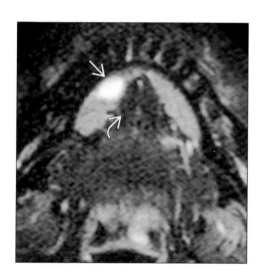 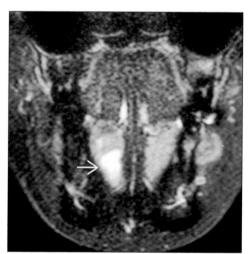

(Left) Transverse grayscale US in a patient with submandibular region swelling shows predominantly cystic mass in the left SLS ➡ extending into the left submandibular space (SMS) ➡. It is mostly anechoic with faint internal debris and posterior enhancement ➡. *(Right)* Corresponding power Doppler US clearly shows debris ➡ within the mass and posterior enhancement ➡. No obvious vascularity is seen in the walls of the cystic mass or in adjacent soft tissues. Note normal lingual vessels ➡.

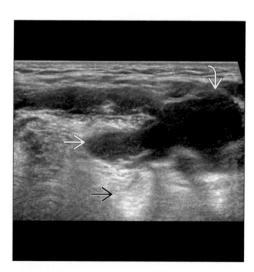 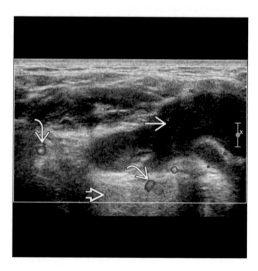

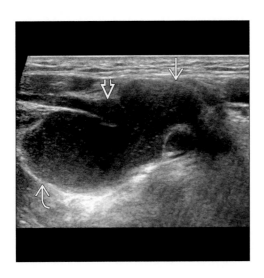

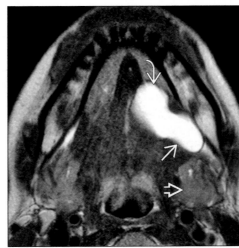

(Left) Transverse grayscale US (same patient) shows the relation of a cystic mass in SLS ➡ extending to the SMS ➡ behind the free edge of the left mylohyoid muscle ➡, suggesting a diagnosis of DR. *(Right)* Corresponding axial T2WI MR confirms a DR involving the left SLS ➡ and SMS ➡. Note submandibular gland (SMG) ➡. Rupture of SR leads to a pseudocyst (DR), which extends in posterior SMS over posterior margin of the mylohyoid (as in this patient) or laterally through boutonnière defect anterior to SMG.

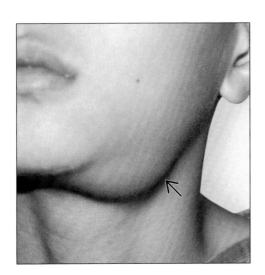

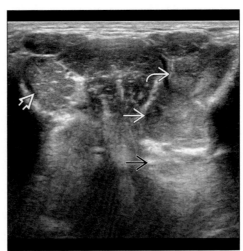

(Left) Clinical photograph of a young boy shows a soft, painless left submandibular region mass ➡. *(Right)* Transverse grayscale US of the left SLS demonstrates a well-defined mass ➡ with uniform internal debris closely related to the left SLG ➡. Note posterior enhancement ➡ providing a clue to the cystic nature of the mass. Uniform internal debris gives it a pseudosolid appearance. Note a normal right SLG ➡.

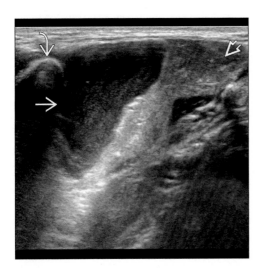

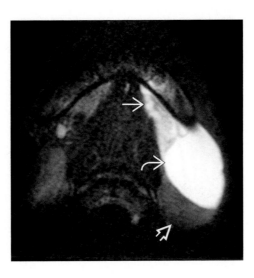

(Left) Corresponding grayscale US of SMS (same patient) shows an extension of the sublingual cystic mass ➡ (with internal debris and posterior enhancement) into the ipsilateral SMS, suggesting a diagnosis of DR. Note the relation of the mass to the SMG ➡ and mandible ➡. *(Right)* Corresponding axial T2WI FS MR shows fluid tracking from the left SLS ➡ into the left SMS ➡ and its relation to the SMG ➡, compatible with DR. Differential diagnosis at this site includes lymphatic malformation.

DERMOID AND EPIDERMOID

Key Facts

Imaging

- Dermoid: Cystic, well-demarcated mass with fatty, fluid, or mixed content
- Epidermoid: Cystic, well-demarcated mass with fluid content only
- Dermoid: Mixed internal echoes from fat, ± echogenic foci with shadowing indicating calcification, osseo-dental elements
- Fat within lesion produces sound attenuation and distal portion of lesion maybe obscured
- Epidermoid: Well-defined, anechoic cyst with thin walls and posterior acoustic enhancement
- Pseudosolid appearance with uniform internal echoes due to cellular material within
- Posterior acoustic enhancement is clue to cystic nature of lesion
- Intermittent transducer pressure causes swirling motion of debris, seen on real-time scans

- In absence of fat &/or osseo-dental structures, dermoid cannot be reliably differentiated from epidermoid on US
- Color Doppler: Both dermoid and epidermoid show no significant vascularity within lesion or its walls
- By increasing Doppler power, swirling motion of debris/artifacts in pseudosolid lesions may be seen

Top Differential Diagnoses

- Thyroglossal duct cyst
- Lymphatic malformation, oral cavity
- Simple ranula

Diagnostic Checklist

- MR/CT indicated for large, deep lesions that cannot be fully evaluated by US or lesions with large fat content that attenuates sound
- US features may overlap with ranula/diving ranula, lymphangioma, thyroglossal duct cyst

(Left) Transverse grayscale US shows an ill-defined, heterogeneous, hyperechoic mass ⇒ at the floor of mouth (FOM), where normal genioglossus muscle should be seen. Note the normal location of the geniohyoid ⇒, anterior belly digastric ⇒, and mylohyoid muscles ⇒. (Right) Corresponding longitudinal grayscale US shows the inferior edge ⇒ of the mass ⇒. The hyoid bone ⇒ is shown. Note that posterior parts of the mass cannot be evaluated. Fat attenuates sound transmission and is hyperechoic on US.

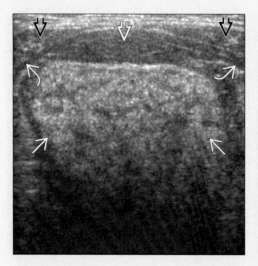
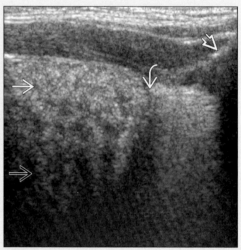

(Left) Corresponding axial T2WI MR (same patient) shows a "sack of marbles" appearance, suggesting that the mass is a dermoid ⇒. Note the fluid content appears hyperintense whereas coalescent fat globules ⇒ ("marbles") appear hypointense against a fluid background. (Right) Sagittal T1WI C+ MR shows the full extent of the dermoid ⇒, its relation to the tongue ⇒, FOM ⇒, and a rim of contrast enhancement ⇒. Compared with US, MR better delineates its location, extent, and anatomical relations.

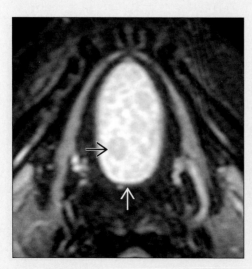
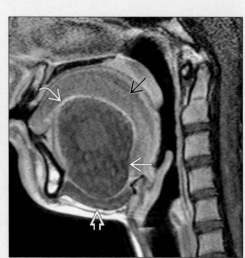

DERMOID AND EPIDERMOID

TERMINOLOGY

Definitions
- Cystic lesion resulting from congenital epithelial inclusion or rest
  - Dermoid: Epithelial elements plus dermal substructure including dermal appendages
  - Epidermoid: Epithelial elements only

IMAGING

General Features
- Best diagnostic clue
  - Dermoid: Cystic, well-demarcated mass with fatty, fluid, or mixed content
  - Epidermoid: Cystic, well-demarcated mass with fluid content only
- Location
  - Dermoid and epidermoid lesions most commonly involve floor of mouth
    - Submandibular space (SMS), sublingual space (SLS), or root of tongue (ROT)
  - Sternal notch
- Size
  - Typically < 4 cm and clinically evident early on
- Morphology
  - Ovoid or tubular
    - Most show thin, definable wall (75%)
    - No nodular soft tissue in wall or outside cyst (80%)

Ultrasonographic Findings
- As many dermoids/epidermoids are superficial in location, US is ideal initial imaging modality
- Dermoid: Mixed internal echoes from fat, ± echogenic foci with shadowing indicating calcification, osseo-dental elements
  - Fat within lesion produces sound attenuation and distal portion of lesion may be obscured
- Epidermoid: Well-defined, anechoic cyst with thin walls and posterior acoustic enhancement
  - Pseudosolid appearance with uniform internal echoes due to cellular material within
    - Posterior acoustic enhancement is due to cystic nature of lesion
    - Intermittent transducer pressure causes swirling motion of debris, seen on real-time scans
- In absence of fat &/or osseo-dental structures, US cannot reliably differentiate dermoid from epidermoid
- Color Doppler: Both dermoid and epidermoid show no significant vascularity within lesion or its walls
  - By increasing Doppler power, swirling motion of debris/artifacts in pseudosolid lesions may be seen

Imaging Recommendations
- Best imaging tool
  - US is ideal imaging modality for superficial lesions
  - MR/CT indicated for large, deep lesions that cannot be fully evaluated by US
  - MR/CT indicated for lesions with large fat content that attenuates sound and obscures evaluation by US
- Protocol advice
  - On grayscale US, look for posterior acoustic enhancement (clue to cystic nature of pseudosolid lesions)
  - Look for swirling motion/artifact in pseudosolid lesions on intermittent transducer pressure or if Doppler power is ↑

DIFFERENTIAL DIAGNOSIS

Thyroglossal Duct Cyst
- Anechoic, pseudosolid, or heterogeneous cystic mass
- No complex elements (no fat or calcifications)

Lymphatic Malformation, Oral Cavity
- Multilocular, anechoic, avascular, trans-spatial cystic septate mass with no significant adjacent mass effect

Simple Ranula
- Anechoic, thin wall, faint internal debris, avascular and not crossing mylohyoid; exactly mimics epidermoid

Diving Ranula
- Simple ranula that ruptures from SLS into SMS, internal debris, hypoechoic, avascular mass

CLINICAL ISSUES

Natural History & Prognosis
- Benign lesion; usually cosmetic considerations
- Very slow growth; dormant for years
  - Present, but small and dormant, during childhood
  - Becomes symptomatic during rapid growth phase in young adults

DIAGNOSTIC CHECKLIST

Image Interpretation Pearls
- If mass is superficial in location between mylohyoid and platysma (i.e., submental space)
  - Epidermoid/dermoid: Anechoic, cystic, thin wall, internal debris, pseudosolid, avascular, ± osseo-dental structures
  - Submental lymph node: Elliptical, solid, hypoechoic with hilar architecture and vascularity
- If mass in SLS, SMS
  - Epidermoid/dermoid: Anechoic, cystic, thin wall, internal debris, pseudosolid, avascular, ± osseo-dental structures
  - Thyroglossal duct cyst: Suprahyoid, anechoic, heterogeneous, pseudosolid, avascular
  - Ranula/diving ranula: Anechoic, faint internal debris, thin wall, posterior enhancement, avascular, ± extension across mylohyoid
- If mass in sternal notch
  - Epidermoid/dermoid: Anechoic, cystic, thin wall, internal debris, pseudosolid, avascular, ± osseo-dental structures
  - Multinodular goiter: Heterogeneous nodules, multiple, cystic, septa, "comet tail" artifact, dense calcification, perinodular vascularity
  - Hypertrophied node following neck radiotherapy: Hypoechoic, hypertrophied cortex, hilar vascularity and architecture

SELECTED REFERENCES

1. Harnsberger HR et al: Diagnostic Imaging: Head & Neck. 2nd ed. Salt Lake City: Amirsys, Inc. I-14,12-15, 2011

DERMOID AND EPIDERMOID

(Left) Clinical photograph shows a young girl with a smooth anterior neck mass ➡, immobile on tongue protrusion. Differential diagnosis at this site includes thyroglossal duct cyst and dermoid/epidermoid. *(Right)* Corresponding power Doppler US shows a well-defined mass ➡ with heterogeneous internal echoes, anterior to strap muscles ➡, which appear compressed by mass. No significant vascularity is seen within or around the mass. Note the right lobe of the thyroid ➡ and trachea ➡.

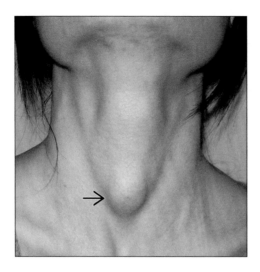
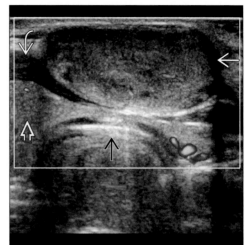

(Left) Longitudinal US (same case) shows the mass ➡ compresses strap muscles ➡ but is not embedded in them, suggesting epidermoid/dermoid vs. thyroglossal duct cyst (TGDC). Note the thyroid ➡. In the absence of fat/osseo-dental elements, US cannot differentiate between dermoid and epidermoid. *(Right)* Longitudinal US and qualitative strain elastogram show dermoid ➡. Strain color scale ranges from purple (soft) to red (hard). It appears mostly purple/green, suggestive of a soft lesion.

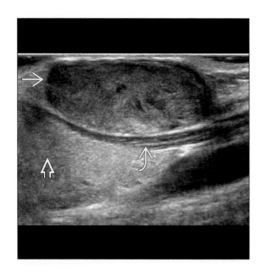
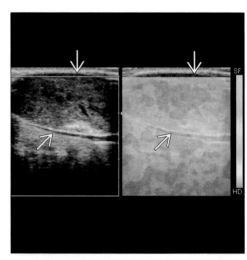

(Left) Clinical photograph shows a child with a small, soft, painless lump ➡ at the lateral edge of the right eyebrow. *(Right)* Corresponding grayscale US shows a well-defined nodule ➡ with homogeneous internal echoes, subtle posterior enhancement ➡, and a pseudosolid appearance. Location and US features are characteristic of an external angular dermoid. Epidermoids usually contain fluid, whereas dermoids are composed of fluid, fat, and mixed content.

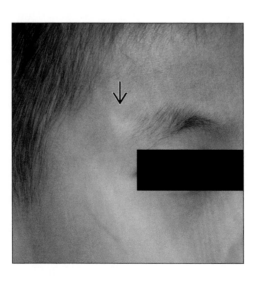
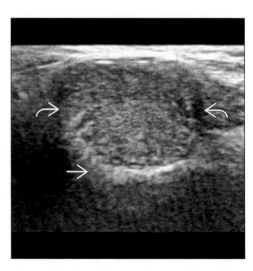

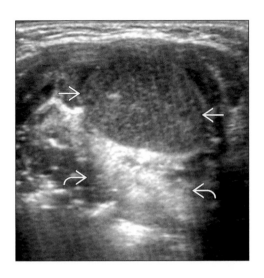

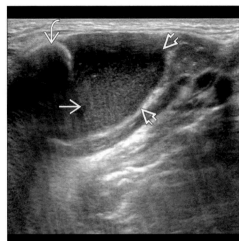

(Left) Transverse grayscale US at the FOM shows a well-defined, hypoechoic, heterogeneous mass ➡ with internal echoes and intense posterior enhancement ➡. Epidermoids appear anechoic/pseudosolid vs. dermoid with mixed echoes. *(Right)* Longitudinal grayscale US shows a lymphatic malformation (LM) ➡ with fine internal debris ➡ in the submandibular region. Note the mandible ➡. Compared with epidermoid, LMs are frequently multilocular, trans-spatial cystic lesions with debris and septi.

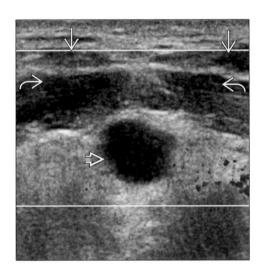

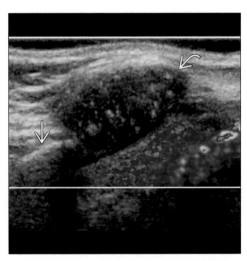

(Left) Transverse grayscale US shows an incidental FOM ➡ anechoic TGDC, a common differential of epidermoid/dermoid at this site. These are often seen as incidental lesions on a high-resolution US. Note anterior belly of digastric muscles ➡, mylohyoid muscles ➡. *(Right)* Longitudinal power Doppler US shows an infrahyoid TGDC ➡ with internal "comet tail" artifacts. Note its relation to the hyoid bone ➡. TGDCs are embedded in strap muscles vs. dermoid/epidermoid cysts.

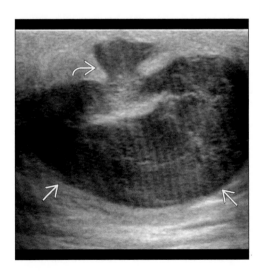

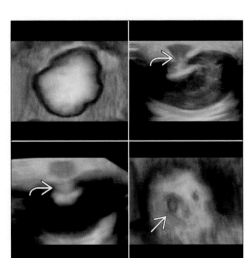

(Left) Transverse grayscale US shows a well-defined, hypoechoic, heterogeneous subcutaneous mass ➡ with a small tract ➡ extending to the skin. Features suggest a sebaceous cyst, and internal echoes are due to keratin, sebum, and debris within. *(Courtesy R. Kadasne, MD.)* *(Right)* Corresponding 3D rendering clearly defines the tract ➡ and punctum ➡ often seen in subcutaneous sebaceous cysts. *(Courtesy R. Kadasne, MD.)*

LYMPHATIC MALFORMATION

Key Facts

Imaging

- Best imaging clue: Uni-/multiloculated cystic neck mass, ± trans-spatial, no mass effect
- Appearances depend on whether there was previous hemorrhage/infection
- Nonhemorrhagic/uninfected lymphatic malformation (LM)
  - Uni-/multilocular, anechoic compressible cysts with thin walls and intervening septa
  - Despite large size they do not cause mass effect, in fact, adjacent muscles and vessels indent the lesion
  - Color Doppler: No vascularity seen if uninfected
- Hemorrhagic/infected LM
  - Uni- or multilocular heterogeneous cysts with irregular walls, internal debris
  - Noncompressible, hypoechoic, heterogeneous mass with thick walls, thick septa, & mass effect

- Fluid-fluid levels due to sedimentation & separation of different fluids (suggests prior hemorrhage)
  - Color Doppler: If infected, vascularity may be seen in soft tissues around lesion and in septa & walls
- Infiltrate between and around neurovascular structures

Top Differential Diagnoses

- 2nd branchial cleft cyst, thymic cyst, neck abscess, thyroglossal duct cyst

Diagnostic Checklist

- While US can diagnose LMs, MR or CT are necessary to map their entire extent
- US is ideal modality to guide injection of sclerosing agent and follow-up after treatment
- In large neck lesions, if lower extent of LM is not defined, evaluate axilla and mediastinum as they may be involved

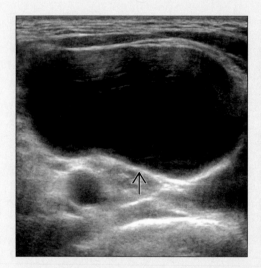
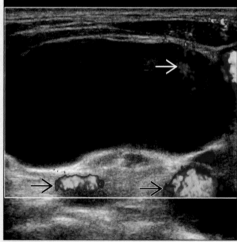

(Left) Transverse grayscale US shows large, unilocular lymphatic malformation (LM) ➡ in lower neck. Note that it is anechoic with thin walls. There is no evidence of septation, internal debris, solid component, or adjacent soft tissue inflammation. Such lesions are readily amenable to sclerotherapy under US guidance. *(Right)* Corresponding power Doppler US shows no vascularity within unilocular LM. Color signal seen within LM is artifactual ➡. Despite its size, note the absence of mass effect on vessels ➡ in its proximity.

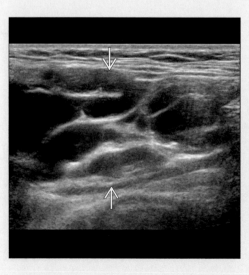
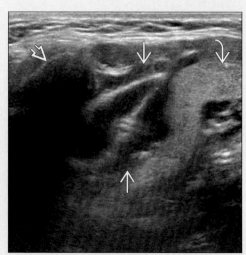

(Left) Transverse grayscale US in the submandibular region shows a large, multiloculated, cystic, septate LM ➡. *(Right)* Corresponding longitudinal grayscale US shows LM ➡ insinuating between the mandible ➡ and submandibular gland ➡. Note that although US readily identifies the lesion and makes diagnosis of LM possible, it is unable to clearly define anatomical extent and relationship with normal adjacent structures. MR and CT are often indicated to map extent, particularly prior to treatment.

LYMPHATIC MALFORMATION

TERMINOLOGY

Synonyms
- Vascular malformation, lymphatic type
- Lymphangioma & cystic hygroma (old terms)
- Venolymphatic malformation (VLM), combined elements of venous malformation & LM in same mass

Definitions
- Congenital vascular malformation composed of embryonic sacs

IMAGING

General Features
- Best diagnostic clue
  - Uni- or multiloculated cystic neck mass (with imperceptible walls) that insinuates itself between vessels and other normal structures
- Location
  - Often found in multiple contiguous spaces
  - Infrahyoid neck
    - Posterior cervical space most common space
  - Suprahyoid neck
    - Masticator & submandibular spaces most common
- Size
  - Varies from several cm to huge neck mass
- Morphology
  - May be unilocular or multilocular
  - Tends to invaginate between normal structures without mass effect

Ultrasonographic Findings
- May be detected on prenatal US
- Appearances depend on whether there was previous hemorrhage/infection
- Nonhemorrhagic/uninfected LM
  - Uni-/multilocular, anechoic compressible cysts with thin walls and intervening septa
  - Despite large size they do not cause mass effect, in fact, adjacent muscles and vessels indent the lesion
  - Color Doppler: No vascularity seen if uninfected
- Hemorrhagic/infected LM
  - Uni- or multilocular heterogeneous cysts with irregular walls, internal debris
  - Noncompressible hypoechoic, heterogeneous mass with thick walls, thick septa and mass effect
  - Fluid-fluid levels due to sedimentation and separation of different fluids (suggests prior hemorrhage)
  - Color Doppler: If infected, vascularity may be seen in soft tissues around lesion and in septa and walls
- Infiltrate between and around neurovascular structures

Imaging Recommendations
- Best imaging tool
  - While US can diagnose LMs, MR or CT are necessary to map entire extent
  - Larger lesions are best evaluated with MR
    - T2 high signal improves definition of local extension and relationship to normal adjacent structures, including vessels
- Protocol advice
  - In large neck lesions, if lower extent of LM is not defined, evaluate axilla and mediastinum as they may be involved
  - Lesions are superficial and compressible; avoid applying transducer pressure as this may compress the lesion
  - Prior to treating with sclerosing agent always perform preprocedure baseline imaging (US and MR)
  - US is ideal modality to guide injection of sclerosing agent and follow-up after treatment
  - For small superficial lesions, US safely guides injection of sclerosant following sedation in children
    - Reduces procedure time and increases safety of procedure

DIFFERENTIAL DIAGNOSIS

2nd Branchial Cleft Cyst
- Ovoid, unilocular mass at angle of mandible with characteristic displacement pattern
- Anechoic cyst, heterogeneous thick-walled cyst, or cyst with pseudosolid echo pattern

Thymic Cyst
- Unilocular, anechoic, well-defined infrahyoid lateral neck cyst with thin walls

Neck Abscess
- Thick, ill-defined, heterogeneous content with debris, ± air within, and rim vascularity on Doppler
- Adjacent soft tissues have cellulitis, myositis fasciitis

Thyroglossal Duct Cyst
- Unilocular, midline cystic mass in vicinity of hyoid
- Embedded in infrahyoid strap muscles
- Anechoic cyst, heterogeneous thick-walled cyst, or cyst with pseudosolid echo pattern

CLINICAL ISSUES

Presentation
- Most common signs/symptoms
  - Soft, doughy neck mass found in first 2 years of life
- Other signs/symptoms
  - Large LMs can present with airway obstruction

Demographics
- Age
  - Most commonly present at birth or within first 2 years of life (> 80%); small early adult group
  - Adult presentation unusual and suggests LM in adult may be acquired, probably post traumatic

DIAGNOSTIC CHECKLIST

Image Interpretation Pearls
- Trans-spatial multicystic neck mass with septation, debris, fluid level most likely indicates LM

SELECTED REFERENCES
1. Harnsberger HR et al: Diagnostic Imaging: Head & Neck. 2nd ed. Salt Lake City: Amirsys, Inc. III-1-6-9, 2011
2. Ahuja AT et al: Diagnostic Imaging: Ultrasound. 1st ed. Salt Lake City: Amirsys, Inc. 11-92-97, 2007

(Left) Transverse grayscale US shows a large, well-defined, unilocular LM ➡. Note the absence of internal echoes, thin walls, and posterior enhancement ⮞. *(Right)* Corresponding axial T2WI FS MR shows uniform hyperintensity within the LM ➡. Note that the MR clearly defines the extent of the abnormality and its relationship with adjacent structures.

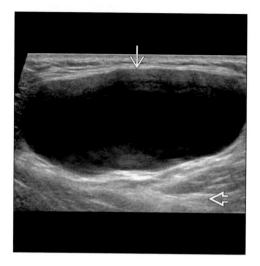
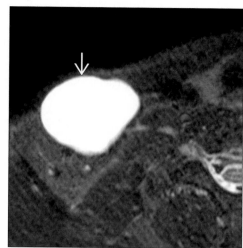

(Left) Longitudinal grayscale US of the right upper neck shows a large LM ➡ abutting the parotid gland ⮞. Note the thin internal septa ➡ and diffuse fine debris throughout the LM, suggesting a previous episode of intralesional hemorrhage. *(Right)* Corresponding transverse grayscale US shows a large LM ➡ wrapped around the mandible ➡. Note that its exact distribution and deeper extent are not mapped by US. This is one of the major limitations of US in evaluating head and neck LMs.

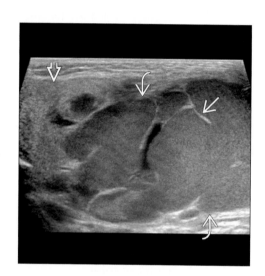
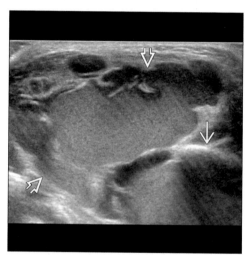

(Left) Axial T2WI FS MR of the same patient defines the location and extent of a large LM ➡ with intralesional fluid-fluid levels ⮞ reflecting hemorrhage within. T2WI best maps large LMs as it is hyperintense throughout. Large, trans-spatial lesions may be poorly marginated. On CECT and T1WI C+, enhancement in the lesion suggests a component of venous malformation. *(Right)* Transverse grayscale US in a patient with LM shows a large, curvilinear calcification ➔, an uncommon feature. Note the CCA ⮞.

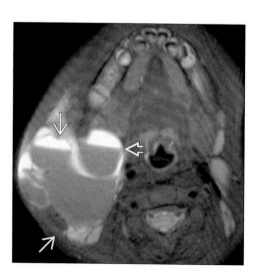
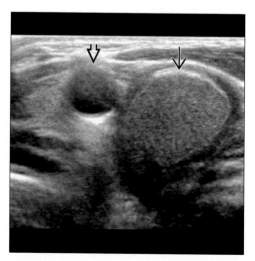

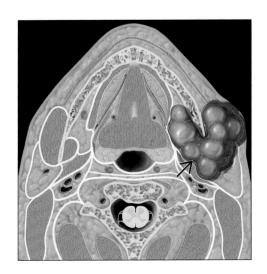

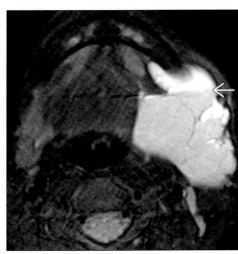

(Left) Axial graphic shows a well-defined, multiloculated, lobulated LM ➔ at the angle of the mandible. LM is a congenital vascular malformation composed of embryonic lymphatic sacs. VLM have combined elements of venous malformation and LM in the same lesion. *(Right)* Axial T2WI FS MR clearly defines the location and extent of LM and its anatomical relationship with adjacent structures. Note the fluid-fluid level ➔ suggesting previous intralesional hemorrhage.

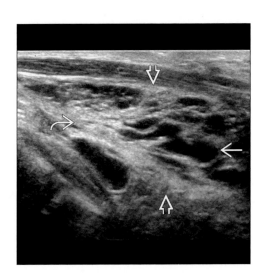

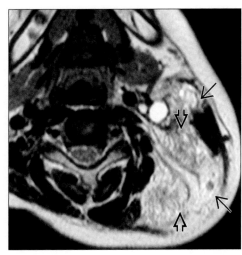

(Left) Longitudinal grayscale US shows a child who underwent 2 treatments of US-guided sclerotherapy for a large, multiloculated LM ➔. Note that small cystic locules ➔ persist; however, much of the LM has been replaced by fatty tissue ➔. US safely guides intralesional sclerosant and readily monitors post-treatment change in size and appearance. *(Right)* Corresponding axial T2WI MR after a 2nd injection of sclerosant shows reduction of cystic spaces and replacement by fatty tissue ➔ in the LM ➔.

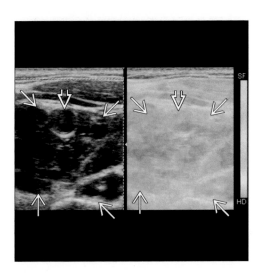

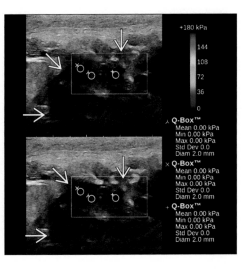

(Left) Transverse grayscale US and qualitative stain elastogram show a septate lymphangioma ➔ abutting the common carotid artery ➔. Strain color scale ranges from purple (elastic, soft) to red (inelastic, hard). It appears mostly purple and green (elastic) compared with surrounding tissues. *(Right)* Transverse grayscale US and SWE show cervical lymphangioma ➔. SWE color scale ranges from blue (0 kPa, soft) to red (180 kPa, stiff). It lacks SWE signal as shear waves do not travel in physical liquids.

1ST BRANCHIAL CLEFT CYST

Key Facts

Imaging

- Unilocular; thin walled; round, elliptical, or lobulated
- Anechoic or pseudosolid (fine internal debris)
- Movement of debris is seen (in real time) on gentle transducer pressure or on power Doppler
- Posterior acoustic enhancement
- Thick-walled, internal septa, and adjacent soft tissue induration if superimposed infection
- No internal vascularity; if infected, ± vascularity in thick wall or adjacent soft tissue
- Ultrasound is ideal for initial imaging, especially in children, as it is nonionizing and requires no sedation
- MR (particularly T2WI) is better for evaluating extent of tract and parapharyngeal space involvement

Top Differential Diagnoses

- Benign lymphoepithelial cysts
- Parotid sialocele
- Suppurative adenopathy/abscess

Pathology

- Remnant of 1st branchial apparatus; most common anomalies are cysts (2/3) >> sinuses or fistulas
- Most common terminal location for 1st BCC is between cartilaginous and bony portions of EAC

Clinical Issues

- Soft, painless, compressible periauricular or periparotid mass, particularly in children
- May enlarge with upper respiratory tract infection
- Prognosis is excellent if 1st BCC is completely resected
- May recur if residual cyst wall remains

Diagnostic Checklist

- Consider 1st BCC if chronic, unexplained otorrhea or recurrent parotid gland abscess
- Look for cyst in or adjacent to parotid gland, EAC, pinna, or (rarely) parapharyngeal space

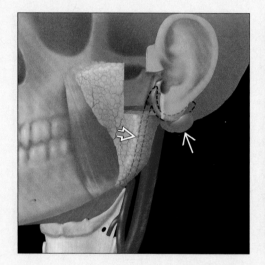
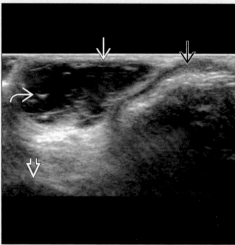

(Left) Oblique graphic of the ear and cheek reveals a Work type I 1st branchial cleft cyst (BCC) ➡ along the tract from the bony-cartilaginous junction of the external auditory canal (EAC) situated just posteroinferior to auricle. The tract of type II BCC ➡ would project inferiorly to angle of mandible. *(Right)* Transverse US of the right postauricular region shows a type I 1st BCC ➡ in the subcutaneous layer posterior to the pinna ➡. Thick, ill-defined walls and debris ➡ suggest previous infection. Note the mastoid process ➡.

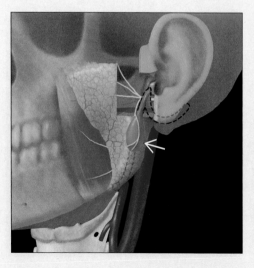
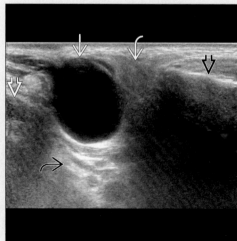

(Left) Oblique graphic of the ear and cheek shows an example of Work type II 1st BCC ➡ along the tract from the bony-cartilaginous junction of EAC to the angle of the mandible. Note the intimate relation of the BCC and the facial nerve. *(Right)* Transverse grayscale US shows a Work type II 1st BCC ➡ in the periparotid region, abutting the tail of the right parotid gland ➡. It is unilocular, thin walled, and anechoic with posterior enhancement ➡, suggesting an uncomplicated cyst. Note the mandibular ramus ➡ and mastoid process ➡.

1ST BRANCHIAL CLEFT CYST

TERMINOLOGY

Synonyms
- Branchial apparatus cyst

Definitions
- Most common 1st branchial cleft anomalies (BCAs) are branchial cleft cysts (BCC) or sinuses
- 1st BCC: Benign, congenital cyst in or adjacent to parotid gland, external auditory canal (EAC), or pinna
  - Remnant of 1st branchial apparatus: Most commonly used classification
    - Work type I: Duplication of membranous EAC; ectodermal (cleft) origin
    - Work type II: Duplication of membranous EAC and cartilaginous pinna
      - Skin (ectodermal cleft) and cartilage (mesodermal arch) origin
      - May also have contribution from 2nd arch
- 1st branchial cleft sinus tract opens near parotid gland, EAC, parapharyngeal space (PPS), or anterior triangle of neck

IMAGING

Ultrasonographic Findings
- Unilocular, thin-walled, and round, elliptical, or lobulated cyst
- May be anechoic or pseudosolid (homogeneous internal debris)
  - Movement of debris is seen (in real time) on gentle transducer pressure or on power Doppler
- Posterior acoustic enhancement
- Thick-walled, internal septa and adjacent soft tissue induration if superimposed infection is present
- No internal vascularity; if infected, ± vascularity in thick wall or adjacent soft tissue
- Work type I
  - Cyst anterior, inferior, or posterior to EAC
  - Often runs parallel to EAC
  - Lesion may "beak" toward bony-cartilaginous junction of EAC
- Work type II
  - Cyst in superficial or parotid space; extension to PPS requires MR for evaluation
  - May be as low as submandibular space
  - Deep projection may "beak" to bony-cartilaginous junction of EAC

CT Findings
- NECT
  - Low-density cyst
  - If previously infected, can be isodense
- CECT
  - Well-circumscribed, nonenhancing or rim-enhancing, low-density mass
  - If infected, may have thick enhancing rim

MR Findings
- T1WI
  - Low signal intensity unilocular cyst
- T2WI
  - High signal intensity unilocular cyst
  - May see sinus tract to skin, EAC, or (rarely) PPS
  - Absence of edema in surrounding soft tissues unless superinfection
- T1WI C+
  - Cyst wall normally does not enhance
  - Previous or concurrent infection may result in thick enhancing rim

General Features
- Best diagnostic clue
  - Cystic mass near pinna and EAC (Work type I) or extending from EAC to angle of mandible (Work type II)
- Location
  - Work type I: Periauricular cyst or sinus tract
    - Anterior, inferior, or posterior to pinna and concha
  - Work type II: Periparotid cyst or sinus tract
    - More intimately associated with parotid gland, medial or lateral to facial nerve
    - Superficial, parotid, and parapharyngeal spaces
- Size
  - Variable, but usually < 3 cm
- Morphology
  - Well-circumscribed cyst

Imaging Recommendations
- Best imaging tool
  - Ultrasound is ideal for initial imaging, especially in children, as it is nonionizing and requires no sedation
  - MR (particularly T2WI) is better for evaluating extent of tract and PPS involvement

DIFFERENTIAL DIAGNOSIS

Benign Lymphoepithelial Lesions
- Single or multiple
- When multiple and bilateral, suspect HIV
  - Rare in children
  - Usually associated with cervical adenopathy

Parotid Sialocele
- Focally distended salivary gland duct
  - Secondary to chronic inflammation or after parotid duct ligation

Suppurative Adenopathy/Abscess
- Presents with marked tenderness and fever
- Thick-walled, ovoid, cystic/necrotic mass within parotid

Lymphatic Malformation
- Unilocular or multilocular and trans-spatial
- Rarely shows pseudosolid appearance unless recently infected
- Insinuating border
- May involve multiple sites in head and neck region

Mycobacterium Adenitis
- Can be TB or non-TB
- *Mycobacterium avium-intracellulare* is most common agent if non-TB
- Thick-walled cystic lesion with internal debris
- Associated cervical lymphadenopathy
- ± surrounding inflammatory change
- ± signs and symptoms of acute infection

1ST BRANCHIAL CLEFT CYST

Sjögren Syndrome in Parotid Gland

- Collagen vascular disease with dry eyes/mouth
- Bilateral involvement; unilateral involvement is rare
- Submandibular glands and lacrimal glands may be involved
- Features of chronic sialadenitis in early phase; multicystic appearance in later phase

PATHOLOGY

General Features

- Associated abnormalities
  ○ May be seen in association with other 1st branchial apparatus anomalies
- Embryology/anatomy
  ○ Remnant of 1st branchial apparatus
    ▪ Cleft (ectoderm) of 1st apparatus gives rise to external auditory canal
    ▪ Arch (mesoderm) gives rise to mandible, muscles of mastication, trigeminal nerve, incus body, and malleus head
    ▪ Pouch (endoderm) gives rise to eustachian tube, middle ear cavity, and mastoid air cells
  ○ Branchial remnant occurs with incomplete obliteration of 1st branchial apparatus
  ○ Isolated BCC has no internal (pharyngeal) or external (cutaneous) communication
  ○ Branchial cleft fistula has both internal and external connections, from EAC lumen to skin
  ○ Branchial cleft sinus opens externally or (rarely) internally
    ▪ Closed portion ends as blind pouch
  ○ 2/3 of 1st branchial cleft remnants are isolated cysts

Gross Pathologic & Surgical Features

- Cystic neck mass
  ○ Easily dissected unless repeated infection
- Cyst content is usually thick mucus
- Facial nerve (CN7) may be medial or lateral to 1st BCC
- Cystic remnant may split CN7 trunk
- Close proximity to CN7 makes surgery more difficult
- Most common terminal location for 1st BAC is in EAC, between cartilaginous and bony portions

Microscopic Features

- Thin outer layer: Fibrous pseudocapsule
- Inner layer: Flat squamoid epithelium
- ± germinal centers and lymphocytes in cyst wall

CLINICAL ISSUES

Presentation

- Most common signs/symptoms
  ○ Soft, painless, compressible periauricular or periparotid suprahyoid neck mass
- Other signs/symptoms
  ○ Recurrent preauricular or periparotid swelling
  ○ Tender neck mass
  ○ Fever if infected
  ○ Present with EAC or skin sinus tract are rare
  ○ Chronic purulent ear drainage if there is ear sinus tract

Demographics

- Age
  ○ Majority of patients are < 10 years old
  ○ Presents earlier if there is sinus
  ○ When cyst only, may present later, even in adults
- Epidemiology
  ○ Accounts for 8% of all branchial apparatus remnants
  ○ Work type II > > Work type I 1st BCC

Natural History & Prognosis

- May enlarge with upper respiratory tract infection
  ○ Lymph follicles in wall react with secretion produced
- Often incised and drained as "abscess" with recurrence
- Prognosis is excellent if completely resected
- May recur if residual cyst wall remains

Treatment

- Complete surgical resection
- Proximity to facial nerve puts nerve at risk during surgery
  ○ Work type I: ↑ risk to proximal CN7
  ○ Work type II: ↑ risk to more distal CN7 branches

DIAGNOSTIC CHECKLIST

Consider

- 1st BCC in patient with chronic, unexplained otorrhea or recurrent parotid gland abscess
  ○ Look for cyst in or adjacent to parotid gland, EAC, pinna, or (rarely) PPS

SELECTED REFERENCES

1. Ankur G et al: First branchial cleft cyst (type II). Ear Nose Throat J. 88(11):1194-5, 2009
2. Martinez Del Pero M et al: Presentation of first branchial cleft anomalies: the Sheffield experience. J Laryngol Otol. 121(5):455-9, 2007
3. Schroeder JW Jr et al: Branchial anomalies in the pediatric population. Otolaryngol Head Neck Surg. 137(2):289-95, 2007
4. Koch BL: Cystic malformations of the neck in children. Pediatr Radiol. 35(5):463-77, 2005
5. Gritzmann N et al: Sonography of soft tissue masses of the neck. J Clin Ultrasound. 30(6):356-73, 2002
6. Nicollas R et al: Congenital cysts and fistulas of the neck. Int J Pediatr Otorhinolaryngol. 55(2):117-24, 2000
7. Robson CD et al: Nontuberculous mycobacterial infection of the head and neck in immunocompetent children: CT and MR findings. AJNR Am J Neuroradiol. 20(10):1829-35, 1999
8. Triglia JM et al: First branchial cleft anomalies: a study of 39 cases and a review of the literature. Arch Otolaryngol Head Neck Surg. 124(3):291-5, 1998
9. Nofsinger YC et al: Periauricular cysts and sinuses. Laryngoscope. 107(7):883-7, 1997
10. Arndal H et al: First branchial cleft anomaly. Clin Otolaryngol. 21(3):203-7, 1996
11. Benson MT et al: Congenital anomalies of the branchial apparatus: embryology and pathologic anatomy. Radiographics. 12(5):943-60, 1992
12. Doi O et al: Branchial remnants: a review of 58 cases. J Pediatr Surg. 23(9):789-92, 1988
13. Sherman NH et al: Ultrasound evaluation of neck masses in children. J Ultrasound Med. 4(3):127-34, 1985
14. Harnsberger HR et al: Branchial cleft anomalies and their mimics: computed tomographic evaluation. Radiology. 152(3):739-48, 1984
15. Olsen KD et al: First branchial cleft anomalies. Laryngoscope. 90(3):423-36, 1980

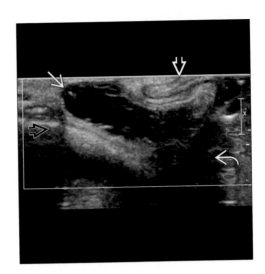

(Left) Clinical photo shows a type I BCC ➡ in the postauricular region, which had enlarged during an episode of upper respiratory tract infection, commonly seen with branchial cleft anomalies due to ↑ cyst wall secretion. *(Right)* Transverse power Doppler US (same patient) shows 1st BCC ➡ as an avascular, subcutaneous cyst with thick walls & internal debris. Deep extension ➡ between the mastoid process ➡ & pinna ➡ points in direction of EAC. MR was required to evaluate any sinus tract and its extent.

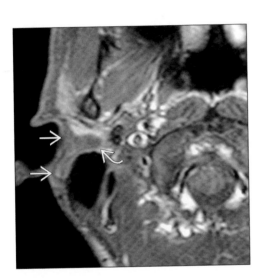
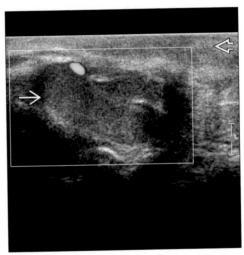

(Left) Axial T1WI C+ FS MR of 1st BCC ➡ (same patient) shows homogeneous, hypointense T1 signal and no enhancement of the cyst wall. Note the deep extension of the cyst to the parotid space ➡. *(Right)* Transverse power Doppler US shows a postauricular type I 1st BCC ➡ that appears pseudosolid with induration of overlying subcutaneous tissue ➡, suggesting superimposed infection. Movement of debris in real time and absence of intranodular vascularity on Doppler confirms its cystic nature.

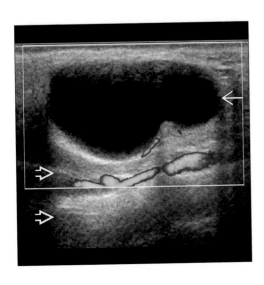
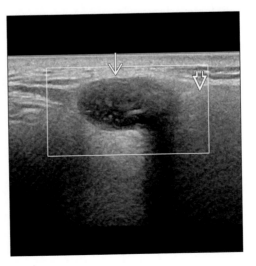

(Left) Transverse US of left parotid gland shows type II uncomplicated anechoic 1st BCC ➡ in superficial lobe. Note intense posterior acoustic enhancement ➡ and absence of vascularity *(Right)* Transverse power Doppler US shows type II BCC ➡ in superficial lobe of left parotid gland ➡. Thick walls and scattered internal debris suggest an infective episode. Differentials include benign lymphoepithelial lesion, sialocele, and infected/necrotic preauricular lymph node. FNAC helps establish the diagnosis.

2ND BRANCHIAL CLEFT CYST

Key Facts

Imaging

- Typical location of cyst in relation to carotid sheath, submandibular gland, and sternocleidomastoid muscle (SCM) is 1st clue
- Nonhemorrhagic/uninfected 2nd branchial cleft cyst (BCC)
  - Unilocular, anechoic cyst with thin walls, posterior enhancement, faint internal debris
  - "Pseudosolid": Well-defined, uniform homogeneous internal echoes due to mucus, debris, cholesterol crystals, and epithelial cells within cyst
  - Posterior acoustic enhancement; swirling motion of debris in cyst after applying intermittent transducer pressure or increasing power on Doppler (seen only in real-time scans)
  - Color Doppler: No vascularity seen within the cyst if uninfected; relationship with carotid artery defined
- Hemorrhagic/infected 2nd BCC

- Ill-defined thick walls, septa, internal debris, and inflammatory changes in adjacent soft tissue
- Color Doppler: If infected, vascularity may be seen within thick walls, septa, and adjacent soft tissues
- Hemorrhagic/infected 2nd BCC completely simulates necrotic nodal metastases from squamous cell carcinoma (SCCa) or papillary carcinoma of thyroid; in such cases FNAC essential for diagnosis
- US may show focal extension of cyst between ICA-ECA bifurcation; pathognomonic of 2nd BCC

Top Differential Diagnoses

- Cystic malignant adenopathy, neck abscess, lymphatic malformation

Diagnostic Checklist

- Beware adult with 1st presentation of "2nd BCC"
  - Mass may be metastatic node from H&N SCCa primary tumor or papillary thyroid cancer

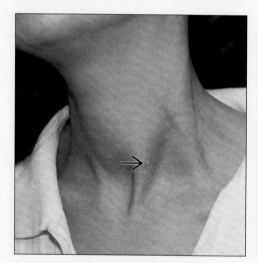
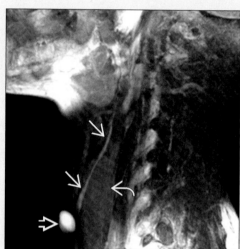

(Left) Clinical photograph of a young girl shows discharging cutaneous opening ⇨ over the lower sternomastoid, raising suspicion for 2nd branchial apparatus cyst/anomaly. (Right) Corresponding sagittal oblique MR shows the length of the tract ⇨ over the sternomastoid muscle ⇨, extending to low in the anterior neck. Surface marker ⇨ marking the fistula opening is noted. Anatomically, the tract may extend from the faucial tonsil to the low anterior neck.

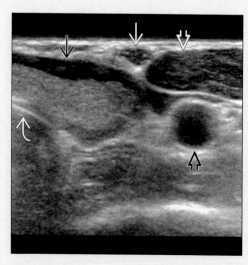
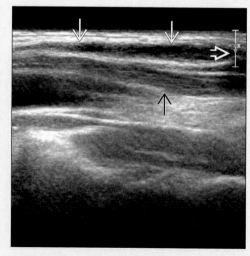

(Left) Transverse grayscale US in the same patient shows the subcutaneous location of the tract ⇨. Note its relationship to the medial edge of the left sternomastoid muscle ⇨. The left CCA ⇨, trachea ⇨, and strap muscle ⇨ are shown. (Right) Corresponding longitudinal grayscale US demonstrates a tract ⇨ running along the length of the subcutaneous tissue in left neck. Direction of the lower end/cutaneous opening of the tract ⇨ and strap muscle ⇨ are noted.

2ND BRANCHIAL CLEFT CYST

TERMINOLOGY

Abbreviations
- 2nd branchial cleft cyst (2nd BCC)

Synonyms
- 2nd branchial cleft remnant or branchial cleft anomaly

Definitions
- Cystic remnant related to developmental alterations of 2nd branchial apparatus
  - 2nd branchial remnants may be fistula, sinus, or cyst, or any combination of these

IMAGING

Ultrasonographic Findings
- Typical location of cyst in relation to carotid sheath, submandibular gland, and sternocleidomastoid muscle (SCM) is 1st clue
- Nonhemorrhagic/uninfected 2nd BCC
  - Unilocular, anechoic cyst with thin walls, posterior enhancement, faint internal debris
  - "Pseudosolid": Well-defined, uniform homogeneous internal echoes due to mucus, debris, cholesterol crystals, and epithelial cells within cyst
  - Clue to cystic nature of a "pseudosolid" cyst
    - Posterior acoustic enhancement, swirling motion of debris in cyst after applying intermittent transducer pressure or increasing power on Doppler; this swirling motion is seen only in real-time scans
  - Color Doppler: No vascularity seen within the cyst if uninfected; relationship with carotid artery is defined
- Hemorrhagic/infected 2nd BCC
  - Ill-defined thick walls, septa, internal debris, and inflammatory changes in adjacent soft tissue
  - Color Doppler: If infected, vascularity may be seen within thick walls, septa, and adjacent soft tissues
  - Completely simulates a necrotic nodal metastasis from squamous cell carcinoma (SCCa) or papillary carcinoma of thyroid and in such cases FNAC is essential for diagnosis
- Cranial, parapharyngeal extension may not be completely demonstrated by US and require CT/MR
- US may show focal extension of cyst between internal carotid artery (ICA) and external carotid artery (ECA) bifurcation; pathognomonic of 2nd BCC
- US may demonstrate presence of track or fistula associated with cyst

General Features
- Location
  - Characteristic location (most at or caudal to angle of mandible)
    - Posterolateral to submandibular gland
    - Lateral to carotid space (CS)
    - Anteromedial to SCM
  - Other (unusual) locations of 2nd BCC
    - Superiorly: Parapharyngeal space or carotid space
    - Inferiorly: Anterior surface of infrahyoid CS
    - Fistulous track may extend between ECAs & ICAs to palatine tonsil
  - Can occur anywhere along line from tonsillar fossa to supraclavicular region
- Size
  - Variable, may range from several cm to > 5 cm
- Morphology
  - Ovoid or rounded well-circumscribed cyst
  - Focal rim of cyst extending to carotid bifurcation: "Notch" sign pathognomonic for 2nd BCC

Imaging Recommendations
- Best imaging tool
  - US with FNAC is ideal for diagnosis of 2nd BCC and differentiating it from metastatic lymph node
  - Preoperative uS adequately evaluates adjacent anatomical relations; CT or MR may be necessary for larger cysts
- Protocol advice
  - Bear in mind the "pseudosolid" nature of these cysts; intermittent application of transducer pressure and increasing power on Doppler will demonstrate swirling motion within cyst on real-time examination

DIFFERENTIAL DIAGNOSIS

Cystic Malignant Adenopathy
- Necrotic mass with thick, ill-defined walls, hypoechoic, heterogeneous architecture, and abnormal vascularity
- Metastases from SCCa and papillary carcinoma of thyroid may have cystic appearance similar to 2nd BCC

Neck Abscess
- Ill-defined, hypoechoic, heterogeneous echo pattern with debris, gas, and vascularity in abscess wall

Lymphatic Malformation
- Multilocular, trans-spatial, fills available spaces; may appear anechoic or "pseudosolid," internal septation
- If unilocular, may be difficult to differentiate from 2nd BCC if it occurs in location typical for 2nd BCC

Thymic Cyst
- Cyst is inferior in cervical neck, centered in lateral visceral space and anechoic with thin walls

Vagus Schwannoma, Infrahyoid Carotid Space
- Continuity with vagus nerve clearly seen on US, fusiform with tapering edges
- Well-defined, hypoechoic, predominantly solid, sharp focal cystic areas and vascularity, which may "disappear" on US with increasing transducer pressure

DIAGNOSTIC CHECKLIST

Consider
- Is cyst thick walled, ill defined, and heterogeneous with septa and vascularity, suggesting infection?
- Could "cyst" be cystic nodal metastasis?

Image Interpretation Pearls
- Beware adult with 1st presentation of "2nd BCC"
  - Mass may be metastatic node from head and neck SCCa primary tumor
  - US-guided FNAC necessary to confirm diagnosis

SELECTED REFERENCES

1. Ahuja AT et al: Diagnostic Imaging: Ultrasound. 1st ed. Salt Lake City: Amirsys, Inc. 11-98-101, 2007

2ND BRANCHIAL CLEFT CYST

(Left) Transverse grayscale US shows a typical 2nd BCC ➡. It is anechoic and well-defined with thin walls. Note its relation to the sternomastoid muscle ➡, submandibular gland ➡, and carotid vessels ➡. *(Right)* Power Doppler US shows "pseudosolid" 2nd BCC ➡. Note uniform internal echoes mimicking solid nodule, but presence of posterior enhancement ➡. Intracystic swirling motion of debris is seen on real-time Doppler scan. Submandibular gland ➡, carotid ➡, sternomastoid ➡ are noted.

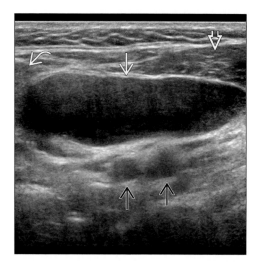
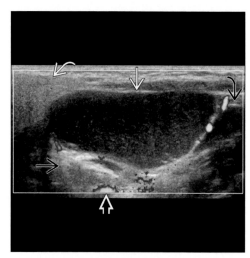

(Left) Transverse grayscale US shows typical, common "pseudosolid" appearance of 2nd BCC ➡. Note posterior enhancement ➡. Homogeneous intracystic echoes are due to mucus, debris, cholesterol crystals, & epithelial cells within cyst. Swirling motion of debris is seen (on real time) on transducer pressure & Doppler. Submandibular gland ➡, carotid ➡, sternomastoid ➡ are noted. *(Right)* Corresponding axial T2WI FS MR confirms cystic nature of "pseudosolid" mass ➡ & anatomic relations.

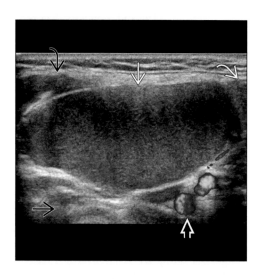
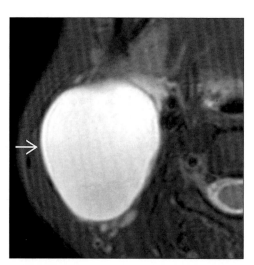

(Left) Transverse grayscale US shows a 2nd BCC, mainly anechoic with faint internal debris. Shear waves do not travel in fluid, limiting the role of SWE in cystic masses. *(Right)* Transverse US and SWE show a 2nd BCC ➡, mostly lacking SWE color signal ➡, which may reflect insufficient acoustic signal detection in anechoic areas and that shear waves do not travel in true liquids. The superficial aspect of the lesion appears blue, where an ROI measures up to 25.1 kPa, suggesting a soft lesion.

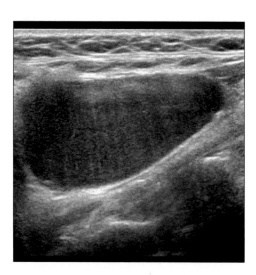
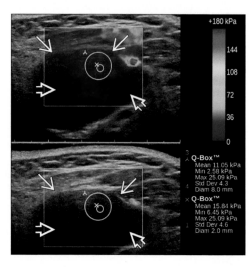

2ND BRANCHIAL CLEFT CYST

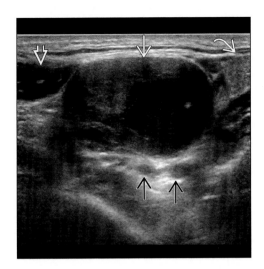
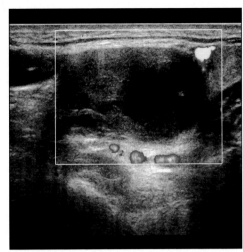

(Left) Transverse grayscale US shows a well-defined cystic mass with mural, solid nodule ➡ & septa in typical location of 2nd BCC. Sternomastoid ➡, submandibular gland ➡, and carotid vessels ➡ are noted. *(Right)* Corresponding power Doppler US shows no vascularity in solid mural portion. However, ill-defined jagged edges of solid component (± vascularity), septation, and in location of JD node should raise suspicion of metastases (from SCCa, papillary thyroid carcinoma). FNAC confirmed SCCa metastatic LN.

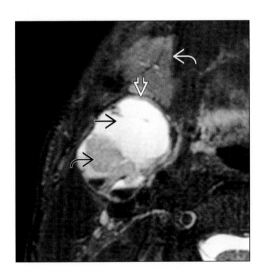
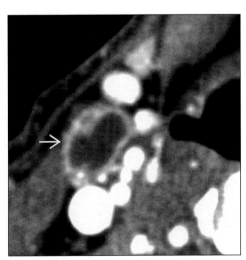

(Left) Axial T2WI FS MR in the same patient shows cystic ➡ and solid ➡ component within a metastatic node ➡, located at typical site of 2nd BCC. The submandibular gland ➡ is noted. *(Right)* Corresponding axial CECT shows enhancing thick walls and cystic center of metastatic SCCa node ➡. Such appearances (on US, CECT, MR) should raise suspicion for LN metastases (despite no known history of primary head & neck cancer) rather than infected 2nd BCC. Confirmatory FNAC is mandatory.

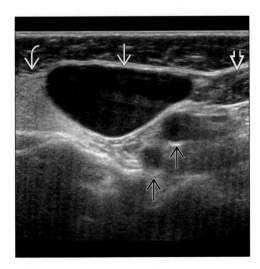
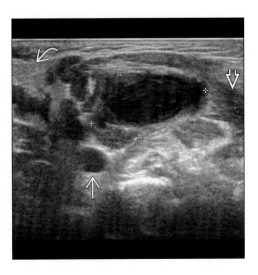

(Left) Transverse grayscale US shows an anechoic, thin-walled 2nd BCC ➡ at its typical location. Submandibular gland ➡, carotid vessels ➡, and sternomastoid ➡ are noted. *(Right)* Transverse grayscale US at similar location (same patient) shows thick-walled cystic mass (calipers) with internal debris at site of 2nd BCC. Thick walls and debris raise suspicion for nodal metastases, infected necrotic LN/abscess. FNAC confirmed abscess. Submandibular gland ➡, carotid ➡, and sternomastoid ➡ are noted.

THYROGLOSSAL DUCT CYST

Key Facts

Imaging

- Relationship of cyst to hyoid bone and its location along expected course from foramen cecum to thyroid bed is 1st clue to diagnosis
- Nonhemorrhagic/uninfected TGDC
  - Unilocular, well-defined, anechoic cyst with posterior enhancement and faint internal debris
  - No evidence of mural nodule/mass or calcification
  - "Pseudosolid" appearance: Well-defined cyst with uniform, homogeneous internal echoes due to proteinaceous content secreted by lining
  - Color Doppler: No vascularity seen within cyst
- Hemorrhagic/infected TGDC
  - Ill-defined thick walls, internal debris, septa, and inflammatory changes in soft tissues
  - Color Doppler shows no vascularity within intracystic blood clots; infected walls and septa may show vascularity

- Thyroid carcinoma can develop in a TGDC (1% in adults) and these appear as vascular solid nodules within cyst, ± calcification
  - US-guided FNAC is recommended

Top Differential Diagnoses

- Lingual or sublingual thyroid
- Dermoid or epidermoid at floor of mouth
- Malignant delphian chain necrotic node

Clinical Issues

- Complete surgical resection, Sistrunk procedure: ↓ recurrence rate from 50% to < 4%

Diagnostic Checklist

- TGDCs are diagnosed clinically; role of imaging is to
  - Confirm diagnosis and relation to hyoid bone
  - Identify any suspicious thyroid carcinoma and presence of normal thyroid tissue in thyroid bed

(Left) Longitudinal grayscale US shows a well-defined, suprahyoid thyroglossal duct cyst (TGDC) ➡ with uniform internal echoes & posterior enhancement ➡ ("pseudosolid" appearance). This homogeneous appearance of TGDC is due to intracystic proteinaceous content. Note the hyoid bone ➡. (Right) Corresponding power Doppler US shows no obvious vascularity within the TGDC ➡. Swirling motion of internal debris may be seen in real time on Doppler or by applying intermittent transducer pressure.

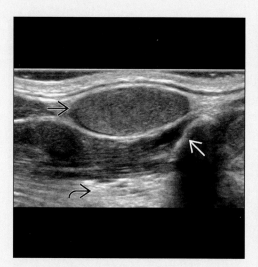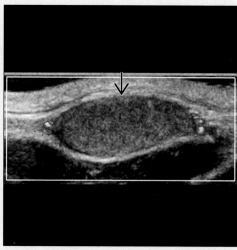

(Left) Transverse grayscale US shows a well-defined, anechoic TGDC ➡ at the floor of the mouth. Note the thin wall, absence of internal debris, and posterior enhancement ➡. TGDCs at this site are often detected incidentally. TGDC is the most common congenital neck cyst (3x more common than branchial cleft cyst). At autopsy, > 7% of the general population have TGDC along course of tract. (Right) Corresponding longitudinal grayscale US shows the relationship of TGDC ➡ to the hyoid bone ➡.

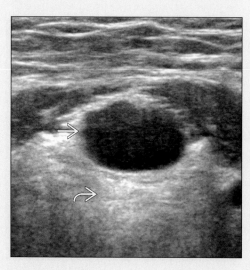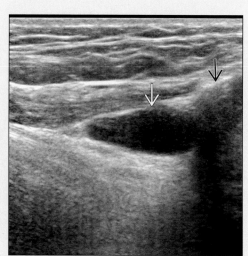

THYROGLOSSAL DUCT CYST

TERMINOLOGY

Synonyms
- Thyroglossal duct remnant

Definitions
- Remnant of thyroglossal duct (TGD) found between foramen cecum of tongue base and thyroid bed in infrahyoid neck

IMAGING

General Features
- Best diagnostic clue
  - Midline cystic neck mass embedded in infrahyoid strap muscles ("claw" sign)
- Location
  - 20-25% in suprahyoid neck, ~ 50% at hyoid bone, and 25% in infrahyoid neck
  - Most in suprahyoid neck are midline
  - May be paramedian in infrahyoid neck

Ultrasonographic Findings
- Relationship of cyst to hyoid bone and its location along expected course from foramen cecum to thyroid bed is 1st clue to diagnosis
- Nonhemorrhagic/uninfected TGDC
  - Unilocular, well-defined, anechoic cyst with posterior enhancement and faint internal debris
  - No evidence of mural nodule/mass or calcification
  - "Pseudosolid" appearance: Well-defined cyst with uniform, homogeneous internal echoes due to proteinaceous content secreted by lining
  - Clue to cystic nature of a "pseudosolid" TGDC
    - Posterior acoustic enhancement; swirling motion of debris within cyst after applying intermittent transducer pressure or increasing power on Doppler, evaluated only in real time and not on static images
  - Color Doppler: No vascularity seen in uninfected cyst
- Hemorrhagic/infected TGDC
  - Ill-defined thick walls, internal debris, septa, and inflammatory changes in soft tissues
  - Color Doppler shows no vascularity within intracystic blood clots; infected walls and septa may show vascularity
- Thyroid carcinoma can develop in TGDC (1% in adults) and these appear as vascular solid nodules within cyst, ± calcification
  - US-guided FNAC is recommended in presence of solid nodule within TGDC

Imaging Recommendations
- Best imaging tool
  - TGDCs are diagnosed clinically; role of imaging is to
    - Confirm diagnosis and relation to hyoid bone
    - Identify any suspicious thyroid carcinoma
    - Evaluate presence of normal thyroid tissue in thyroid bed
  - US is ideal imaging modality as it readily provides appropriate preoperative information
- Protocol advice
  - Scans in longitudinal plane clearly evaluate relation of TGDC to hyoid bone
  - Scans in transverse plane identify cyst embedded within strap muscles, any pre-epiglottic component and presence of normal thyroid tissue in thyroid bed
- Nuclear scintigraphy only if unable to identify normal thyroid gland

DIFFERENTIAL DIAGNOSIS

Lingual or Sublingual Thyroid
- Identify normal thyroid tissue in ectopic location; empty thyroid bed
- Well-defined nodule with fine bright parenchymal echo pattern with vascularity within, ± changes of nodular hyperplasia

Dermoid or Epidermoid at Floor of Mouth
- Neither directly involves hyoid bone; well-defined cystic mass, anechoic, ± pseudosolid pattern, moves independently of tongue

Malignant Delphian Chain Necrotic Node
- Without FNAC it may be difficult to differentiate necrotic node from infected TGDC, not embedded in strap muscle

Submandibular or Sublingual Space or Subcutaneous Abscess
- Not embedded in strap muscles; ill-defined, thick walls with septa, internal debris, vascularity in inflamed walls and adjacent soft tissues

PATHOLOGY

General Features
- Etiology
  - Failure of involution of TGD and persistent secretion of epithelial cells lining duct result in TGDC
  - TGDC and ectopic thyroid tissue can occur anywhere along route of descent of TGD

CLINICAL ISSUES

Natural History & Prognosis
- Recurrent, intermittent swelling of mass, usually following minor upper respiratory infection
- Rapid enlarging mass suggests either infection or associated differentiated thyroid carcinoma
  - Carcinoma is associated with TGDC (< 1%)
  - Differentiated thyroid carcinoma (85% papillary carcinoma)

Treatment
- Complete surgical resection, Sistrunk procedure
  - Cyst and midline portion of hyoid bone is resected
  - Tract to foramen cecum dissected free to prevent recurrence
- Sistrunk procedure decreases recurrence rate from 50% to < 4%

SELECTED REFERENCES

1. Sofferman RA et al: Ultrasound of the Thyroid and Parathyroid Glands. New York: Springer. 229-262, 2012
2. Ahuja AT et al: Sonographic evaluation of thyroglossal duct cysts in children. Clin Radiol. 55(10):770-4, 2000

THYROGLOSSAL DUCT CYST

(Left) Longitudinal grayscale US shows a large suprahyoid TGDC ➔. It is predominantly anechoic with posterior enhancement ➔ and has fine internal debris ➔ in its dependent portion. Note the hyoid bone ➔. *(Right)* Longitudinal grayscale US shows an infrahyoid TGDC ➔ paramedian in location. Note the internal debris & fairly thick walls ➔ suggesting previous infection/ hemorrhage. Patient had history of prior FNAC of this cyst. Note the hyoid bone ➔ and thyroid lamina ➔.

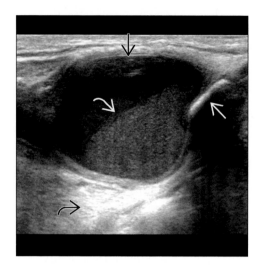
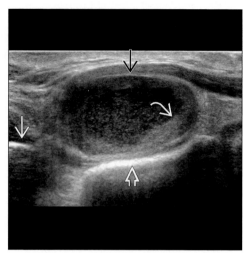

(Left) Longitudinal grayscale US shows infected infrahyoid TGDC ➔, paramedian in location. It is ill defined and appears solid and hypoechoic with heterogeneous internal echoes. Note hyoid bone ➔ and thyroid lamina ➔. *(Right)* Corresponding power Doppler US shows vascularity ➔ within the solid-appearing portion. Infected TGDC may also have vascularity in its wall & septa. Appearances mimic malignant component in TGDC and FNAC is indicated to rule out differentiated thyroid carcinoma.

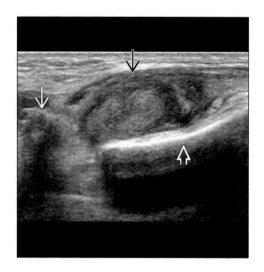
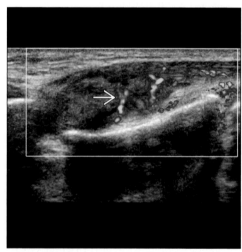

(Left) Axial T2WI MR in the same patient shows a paramedian TGDC ➔ with thick walls overlying the left thyroid lamina ➔. *(Right)* Corresponding axial T1WI C+ MR shows a thick enhancing wall ➔ and internal septa ➔ within the infected paramedian TGDC.

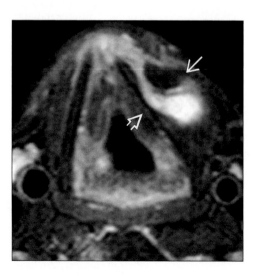
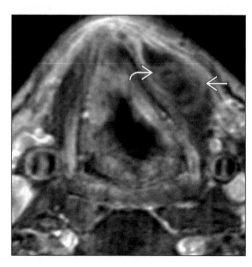

THYROGLOSSAL DUCT CYST

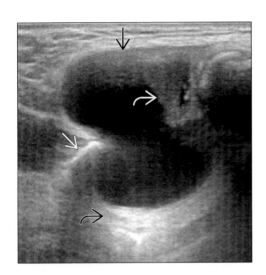

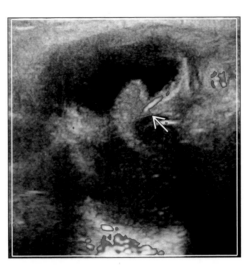

(Left) Longitudinal grayscale US shows a large, bilobed hyoid/infrahyoid TGDC ➡, predominantly anechoic with posterior enhancement ➡. Note the solid-looking component/septa ➡ in a nondependent position. The hyoid bone ➡ is shown. *(Right)* Corresponding power Doppler US in the same patient shows vascularity ➡ in septa within the TGDC. The patient had a history of previous infection within the cyst & US appearances corroborate history.

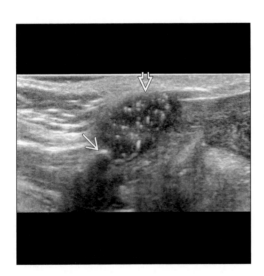

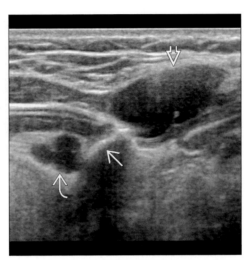

(Left) Longitudinal grayscale US shows TGDC ➡ at level of hyoid bone ➡. Note its predominant anechoic nature with multiple internal nonshadowing "comet tail" artifacts due to inspissated proteinaceous crystals. *(Right)* Longitudinal grayscale US shows multiple anechoic TGDCs and their relationship to both suprahyoid ➡ & infrahyoid ➡ components of hyoid bone ➡. These may be found midline/paramidline between foramen cecum at the tongue base and the thyroid bed in infrahyoid neck.

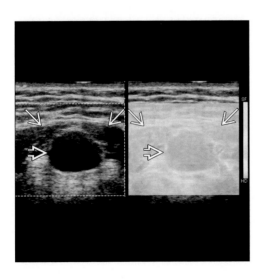

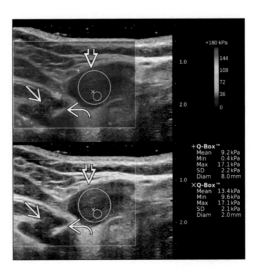

(Left) Transverse grayscale US & qualitative strain EI show a TGDC ➡. Strain color scale ranges from purple (elastic, soft) to red (inelastic, hard). TGDC has similar elasticity to the adjacent strap muscles ➡. *(Right)* Longitudinal grayscale US & SWE show TGDC. SWE color scale ranges from blue (0 kPa, soft) to red (180 kPa, stiff). The infrahyoid is blue with a maximum SWE of 17 kPa (soft) ➡. The suprahyoid lacks SWE color signal ➡, possibly because fluid within this part does not transmit shear waves. Note hyoid ➡.

CERVICAL THYMIC CYST

Key Facts

Imaging

- Along thymopharyngeal duct: Infrahyoid neck mass in lateral visceral space, closely related to carotid sheath from level of pyriform fossa to anterior mediastinum
- Almost always on left side, at level of thyroid gland
- Round, oval, or dumbbell-shaped if it crosses cervicothoracic junction
- Thin walled, unilocular
- Anechoic with posterior acoustic enhancement
- Internal debris due to proteinaceous content or previous hemorrhage
- No vascularity except in solid component (if any)
- USG-guided FNAC distinguishes cervical thymic cyst from other cystic neck masses

Top Differential Diagnoses

- Thyroid cyst
- Parathyroid cyst
- 2nd branchial cleft cyst

Pathology

- Hassall corpuscles in cyst wall confirm diagnosis
  ○ May not be identifiable if prior hemorrhage/infection

Clinical Issues

- Rare compared with other congenital neck masses
- Asymptomatic or soft, compressible neck mass
- When large, may cause dysphagia, respiratory distress, or vocal cord paralysis
- Large infantile cervicothoracic thymic cyst may present with respiratory compromise

Diagnostic Checklist

- Not to be confused with acquired thymic cyst, which is associated with inflammatory or neoplastic conditions

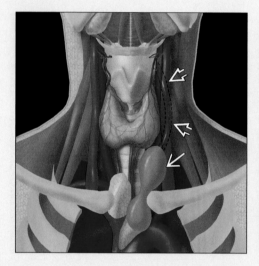
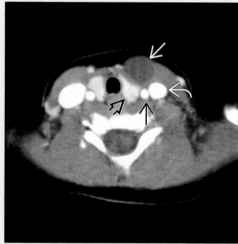

(Left) Coronal graphic shows typical bilobed cervical thymic cyst ➡ extending from the anterior mediastinum into the lower neck along the course of the thymopharyngeal duct ⮊. Note its close association with the carotid space. *(Right)* Axial CECT shows a well-defined cystic mass ➡ located near the anterior aspect of the carotid sheath and anterolateral to the left lobe of the thyroid ⮊. Note the relationship with the common carotid artery (CCA) ➡ and internal jugular vein (IJV) ➡.

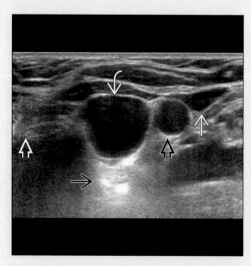
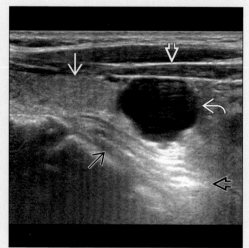

(Left) Transverse grayscale US shows a thin-walled unilocular cyst ➡ in the left lateral visceral space, immediately medial to the CCA ⮊. Note the posterior acoustic enhancement ➡, IJV ➡, and location of the trachea ⮊. *(Right)* Corresponding longitudinal US shows an oval-shaped cyst ➡ inferior to the left lobe of the thyroid ⮊. It is anechoic with posterior acoustic enhancement ⮊. Note the cervical esophagus ➡ & strap muscles ⮊.

CERVICAL THYMIC CYST

TERMINOLOGY

Abbreviations
- Cervical thymic cyst (CTC)

Synonyms
- Thymopharyngeal duct cyst, congenital thymic cyst

IMAGING

General Features
- Location
  - Along thymopharyngeal duct
    - Infrahyoid neck mass in lateral visceral space, closely related to carotid sheath from level of pyriform fossa to anterior mediastinum
  - Almost always on left side, usually at level of thyroid gland
- Morphology
  - Large dominant cyst, from few cm to very long
  - Round or oblong
  - Dumbbell-shaped if it crosses cervicothoracic junction
  - Unilocular or multiloculated
  - Rare solid components (aberrant thymic, lymphoid, or parathyroid tissue)
  - May be connected to mediastinal thymus directly or by fibrous cord

Ultrasonographic Findings
- Round, oval, or dumbbell-shaped if it crosses cervicothoracic junction
- Thin walled, unilocular
- Anechoic with posterior acoustic enhancement
- Internal debris due to proteinaceous content or previous hemorrhage
- No vascularity except in solid component (if any)

CT Findings
- CECT
  - Nonenhancing low-attenuation left lateral neck cyst

MR Findings
- T1WI
  - Homogeneous hypointense cyst (most common)
  - Iso- to hyperintense if filled with blood products, proteinaceous fluid, or cholesterol
- T2WI
  - Homogeneously hyperintense fluid content
- T1WI C+
  - Cyst wall or solid nodules may enhance slightly

Imaging Recommendations
- CECT or MR of neck including upper mediastinum
- USG-guided FNAC distinguishes CTC from other cystic neck masses

DIFFERENTIAL DIAGNOSIS

Thyroid Cyst
- Pedunculated thyroid cyst
- Often background multinodular thyroid

Parathyroid Cyst
- > 70% nonfunctional
- Presence of oxyphilic parathyroid cells in cyst fluid or cyst wall is diagnostic

2nd Branchial Cleft Cyst
- Anterior to carotid space when infrahyoid
- May mimic CTC when found in left lower neck

4th Branchial Anomaly
- Primary location: Cyst or abscess anterior to left thyroid lobe
- Often presents with acute suppurative thyroiditis

Lymphatic Malformation
- Transcompartmental
- May affect any space in head and neck
- Internal septa and fine internal debris (in patients with intracystic hemorrhage)

Abscess
- Presents with signs and symptoms of infection
- Thick walls, internal debris
- ± gas, adjacent soft tissue edema

PATHOLOGY

General Features
- Failure to obliterate thymopharyngeal duct (a remnant of 3rd pharyngeal pouch)
- Smooth, thin-walled cervical cyst often with caudal fibrous strand extending to mediastinal thymus
- Rarely may extend through thyrohyoid membrane into pyriform sinus
- Thymoma developed in CTC has been reported

Microscopic Features
- Presence of Hassall corpuscles in cyst wall confirms diagnosis
  - May not be identifiable if prior hemorrhage/infection
- May contain lymphoid, parathyroid, thyroid, or thymic tissue

CLINICAL ISSUES

Presentation
- Rare compared with other congenital neck masses
- Most present at 2-15 years of age; M > F
- Asymptomatic or soft, compressible neck mass
- When large, may cause dysphagia, respiratory distress, or vocal cord paralysis
- Large infantile cervicothoracic thymic cyst may present with respiratory compromise
- Rarely, may be associated with disordered calcium metabolism, if parathyroid component is functioning

DIAGNOSTIC CHECKLIST

Consider
- Cystic mass in lateral infrahyoid visceral space, closely related to carotid space
- Not to be confused with acquired thymic cyst, which is associated with inflammatory or neoplastic conditions

SELECTED REFERENCES

1. Sturm-O'Brien AK et al: Cervical thymic anomalies--the Texas Children's Hospital experience. Laryngoscope. 119(10):1988-93, 2009

CAROTID BODY PARAGANGLIOMA

Key Facts

Imaging

- Location of tumor at carotid bifurcation is 1st clue to its diagnosis
- Usually solid, noncalcified, well defined, and hypoechoic, splaying ICA & ECA
- Parenchymal echo pattern is homogeneous, ± serpiginous vessels within
- Large tumors may show heterogeneous architecture due to necrosis or hemorrhage within
- Large tumors may completely encase bifurcation
- Color Doppler: Confirms relationship of tumor to carotid bifurcation & splaying of ICA & ECA
- Commonly hypervascular with tortuous vessels within, indicating arteriovenous shunting
- Low-resistance waveform on spectral Doppler
- May appear avascular in deeper components, which are not well interrogated by Doppler

- Color power angiogram demonstrates vascular tumor in "Y" of carotid bifurcation
- Always evaluate contralateral side, as tumors may be bilateral in 5-10%
- During real-time scanning, use gentle transducer pressure to prevent compression of vessels within

Top Differential Diagnoses

- Vagal schwannoma/neurofibroma
- Metastatic node
- Sympathetic schwannoma

Diagnostic Checklist

- US is an ideal initial diagnostic modality; presence of other paragangliomas and associated syndromes are best evaluated by CT/MR
- Recommend surveillance in familial disease beginning at 20 years of age (preferably MR)

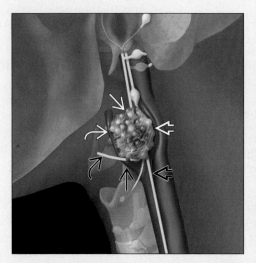
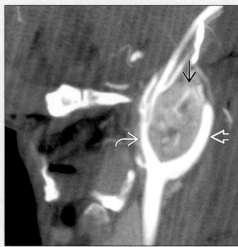

(Left) Lateral graphic shows the typical location of carotid body paraganglioma (CBP) ⮞ *at the carotid bifurcation splaying the ICA* ⮞ *and ECA* ⮞. *Note the ascending pharyngeal artery* ⮞, *vagus* ⮞, *and hypoglossal* ⮞ *nerves. (Right) CTA, oblique sagittal reconstruction, demonstrates the characteristic location of an intensely enhancing CBP* ⮞ *in the "Y" of the carotid bifurcation, splaying the ICA* ⮞ *and ECA* ⮞. *(Courtesy Dr. S. Vaid.)*

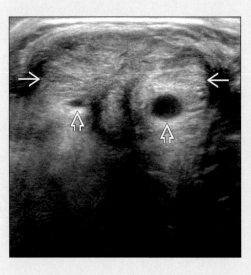
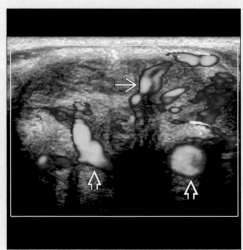

(Left) Transverse grayscale US at carotid bifurcation shows a large, solid, hypoechoic, noncalcified mass ⮞ *encasing the carotid bifurcation* ⮞. *(Right) Corresponding transverse power Doppler US clearly demonstrates the bifurcation* ⮞ *and large intratumoral vessels* ⮞. *The location of the tumor, its relationship to the carotid bifurcation, and its vascularity readily suggest diagnosis of CBP and differentiate it from other lesions at this site, such as vagal, sympathetic schwannomas, and lymphadenopathy.*

CAROTID BODY PARAGANGLIOMA

TERMINOLOGY

Synonyms
- Carotid body tumor, chemodectoma, nonchromaffin paraganglioma

Definitions
- Benign vascular tumor arising in glomus bodies in carotid body found in crotch of external carotid artery (ECA) and internal carotid artery (ICA) at carotid bifurcation

IMAGING

General Features
- Best diagnostic clue
  - Vascular mass splaying ECA and ICA
- Location
  - Carotid space just above hyoid bone
  - Mass centered in crotch of carotid bifurcation
- Size
  - Variable
  - 1-6 cm typical
- Morphology
  - Ovoid mass with broad lobular surface contour

Ultrasonographic Findings
- Location of tumor at carotid bifurcation is 1st clue
- Usually solid, noncalcified, well defined, and hypoechoic, splaying ICA and ECA
- Parenchymal echo pattern is homogeneous, ± serpiginous vessels within
- Large tumors may show heterogeneous architecture due to necrosis or hemorrhage within
- Large tumors may completely encase bifurcation
- Color Doppler: Confirms relationship of tumor to carotid bifurcation and splaying of ICA and ECA
  - CBPs are commonly hypervascular with tortuous vessels within, indicating arteriovenous shunting
  - Low-resistance waveform on spectral Doppler
  - CBPs may appear avascular in deeper components, which are not well interrogated by Doppler
  - Color power angiogram demonstrates vascular tumor in "Y" of carotid bifurcation
- Circumferential contact of tumor to ICA predicts surgical classification: Type I: < 180°; type II: 180-270°; type III: > 270°
- Angle of bifurcation predicts resectability; splaying > 90° indicates more difficult resection

Imaging Recommendations
- Best imaging tool
  - US is ideal initial modality to identify and diagnose
  - US readily examines opposite side for CBP but is unable to adequately evaluate other paragangliomas in neck
  - CECT or MR plus angiography done before surgery, coverage from temporal bones to lower neck
  - Preoperative angiography useful to provide roadmap and embolization for prophylactic hemostasis
- Always evaluate contralateral side, as tumors may be bilateral/multicentric in both sporadic and familial forms
- In familial patient group, screening CECT or MR beginning at 20 years old (preferably MR)

DIFFERENTIAL DIAGNOSIS

Vagal Schwannoma/Neurofibroma
- Clinical: Sporadic or NF2 or NF1 associated
- Fusiform, hypoechoic mass in carotid space (± separation of carotid vessels from internal jugular vein) in continuity with vagus nerve
- May demonstrate well-defined cystic areas within tumor and posterior enhancement
- Less prominent vascularity within mass, may disappear with transducer pressure

Metastatic Node
- Clinical: Asymptomatic "pulsatile mass," ± known head and neck primary tumor
- On US: Hypoechoic/hyperechoic mass, ± cystic necrosis, ± punctate calcification, abnormal vascularity, ± multiple, round with absent hilum

Sympathetic Schwannoma
- Location: Arises from cervical sympathetic chain in posterior carotid space, displaces carotid artery and internal jugular vein anteriorly
- On US: Usually solid, hypoechoic, posteriorly located mass with paucity of vessels, ± fusiform, ± cystic areas within

2nd Brachial Cleft Cyst (BCC)
- Cystic mass closely related to carotid artery, submandibular gland, sternomastoid muscle
- Noninfected: Anechoic/"pseudosolid" pattern, posterior enhancement
- Infected/hemorrhagic: Thin/thick walls, internal debris, septa, posterior enhancement, avascular/vascularity in wall

CLINICAL ISSUES

Presentation
- Most common signs/symptoms
  - Pulsatile, painless angle of mandible mass

Demographics
- Epidemiology
  - CBP is most common location for head and neck paragangliomas (60-67% of total)
  - 2-10% of paragangliomas are multicentric in nonfamilial group
  - Familial incidence of multiple tumors: 25-75%

DIAGNOSTIC CHECKLIST

Image Interpretation Pearls
- When imaging diagnosis of CBP made, radiologist must look for other paragangliomas, MEN type 2, and VHL syndromes
  - US is an ideal initial diagnostic modality; presence of other paragangliomas and associated syndromes are best evaluated by CT/MR

SELECTED REFERENCES

1. Ahuja AT et al: Diagnostic Imaging: Ultrasound. 1st ed. Salt Lake City: Amirsys, Inc. 11-102-105, 2007

CAROTID BODY PARAGANGLIOMA

(Left) Transverse grayscale US shows a large CBP ➡ at its typical location in the upper neck at the carotid bifurcation, splaying the ICA ⬈ and ECA ➡. *(Right)* Corresponding color Doppler US shows profuse vascularity within the tumor and large and tortuous intratumoral vessels ➡. This profuse vascularity is a reflection of intratumoral arteriovenous shunting. Note ICA ⬈, ECA ➡. Ascending pharyngeal artery is the main arterial feeder, and preoperative embolization offers prophylactic hemostasis.

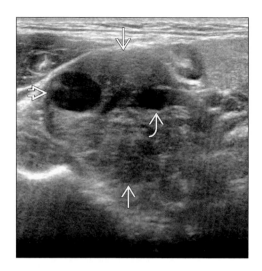
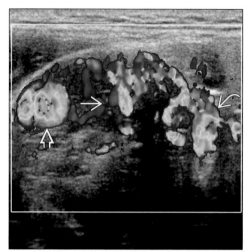

(Left) Transverse grayscale US of the contralateral side (same patient) shows another smaller CBP ➡ at the carotid bifurcation, splaying the ICA ⬈ & ECA ➡. *(Right)* Corresponding power Doppler US shows prominent intratumoral vessels ➡ within the CBP ➡. Note the ICA ⬈ & ECA ➡. In sporadic form, multicentric tumors are found in 2-10%, and multiple tumors are seen in 25-75% with familial type. US cannot evaluate paragangliomas such as glomus jugulare and vagale.

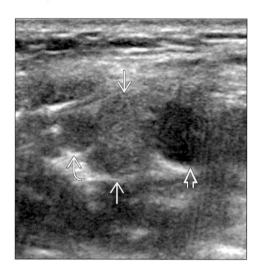
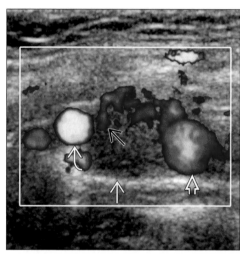

(Left) Axial T1WI MR in the same patient identifies bilateral CBPs ➡ in their typical location. Characteristic "salt & pepper" appearance is described on T1WI; "salt" (hyperintense foci) represents subacute hemorrhage, and "pepper" (flow voids) represents intratumoral vessels ➡. This appearances is expected finding in tumors > 2 cm. *(Right)* Corresponding T1 C+ FS MR shows intense enhancement of tumors ➡. MR also screens for glomus jugulare & glomus vagale.

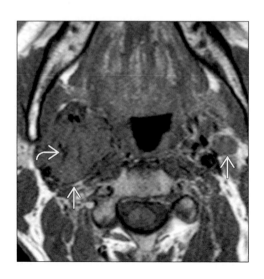
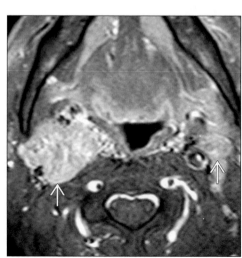

CAROTID BODY PARAGANGLIOMA

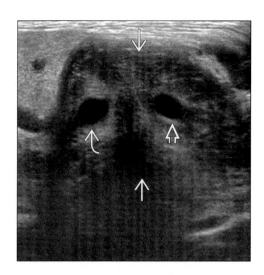

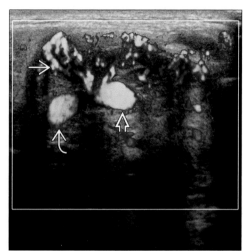

(Left) *Transverse grayscale US shows a large, solid, hypoechoic, noncalcified CBP ⮕ at its typical location at carotid bifurcation. Note ICA ⮕ & ECA ⮕. Posterior parts of such large tumors cannot be adequately assessed by US due to attenuation of sound. CECT and MR better delineate entire extent of large tumors and their adjacent anatomical relationship.* *(Right)* *Corresponding power Doppler US shows characteristic profuse intratumoral vascularity ⮕ and encased ICA ⮕ & ECA ⮕.*

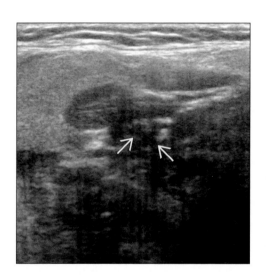

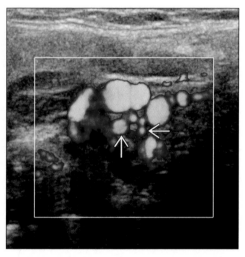

(Left) *Transverse grayscale US shows a patient with resection of contralateral CBP. On follow-up US, there was a cluster of vessels ⮕ on the nonoperated side, in the vicinity of the carotid bifurcation, but no obvious soft tissue mass could be seen.* *(Right)* *Power Doppler US confirmed the presence of multiple, prominent vessels ⮕ at the carotid bifurcation, and small CBP was suspected. The patient had a subsequent MR, which demonstrated small tumor at the suspected site. This was confirmed at surgery.*

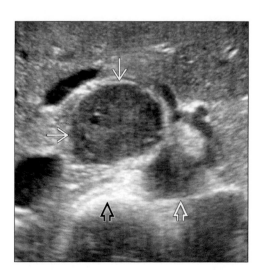

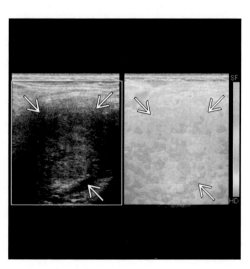

(Left) *Transverse grayscale abdominal US shows adrenal pheochromocytoma ⮕ in a patient with known CBP. Note the aorta ⮕ & vertebral body ⮕. Associated adrenal pheochromocytomas are seen in paraganglioma and MEN type 2 syndromes.* *(Right)* *Longitudinal grayscale US and qualitative strain elastogram of the upper neck shows CBP ⮕. Strain color scale ranges from purple (soft) to red (hard). The eterogeneous mass appears predominantly purple and green, suggestive of soft lesion.*

INFRAHYOID CAROTID SPACE VAGUS SCHWANNOMA

Key Facts

Terminology

- Benign tumor of Schwann cells that wrap around vagus nerve in carotid space (CS)

Imaging

- Ultrasound is able to evaluate/visualize nerve sheath tumors only in infrahyoid neck, vagal nerve schwannoma being most common
- Solid hypoechoic, heterogeneous mass
  - Well-demarcated tumor margin
  - Fusiform/oval in shape with tapering ends
  - ± show posterior enhancement (despite being solid)
- Sharply defined focal cystic areas may be seen
- Continuity with nerve/thickening of adjacent nerve (diagnostic)
- Color Doppler shows increased vascularity within tumor, prominent tortuous vessels
- Vascularity is sensitive to pressure and may "disappear" with increasing transducer pressure

- Mass effect with flattening/occlusion of jugular vein
- Separates carotid artery from internal jugular vein

Top Differential Diagnoses

- Carotid body paraganglioma
- Malignant lymph node
- Sympathetic schwannoma
- Internal jugular vein thrombosis

Diagnostic Checklist

- US is ideal imaging modality for infrahyoid schwannomas; adequately demonstrates tumor and adjacent relations
- FNAC/biopsy may trigger excruciating pain (considered diagnostic by some); important to recognize nature of these lesions to prevent biopsy
- CECT or MR can be used to confirm this diagnosis and evaluate anatomical extent of large tumors

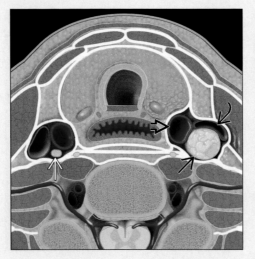
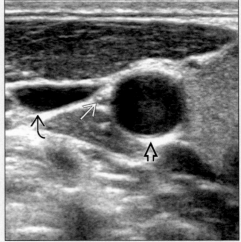

(Left) Transverse graphic shows relationship of vagal schwannoma ⟶ to CCA ⟩ & internal jugular vein (IJV) ⟶. Compare normal vagus nerve ⟶ on contralateral side. *(Right)* Transverse grayscale US shows normal vagus nerve ⟶ located in CS, CCA ⟩, and IJV ⟶. On transverse scans, vagus nerve often shows bright center (nerve signature), and "fibrillar" pattern on longitudinal scans. With modern high-resolution transducers, normal vagus nerve is always identified on transverse and longitudinal scans.

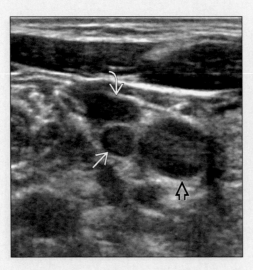
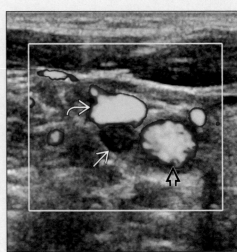

(Left) Transverse grayscale US in a patient with previous radiation to the neck shows a prominent, thickened vagus nerve ⟶ and its relationship to the CCA ⟩ & IJV ⟶. *(Right)* Corresponding power Doppler US helps to explain the relationship and mass effect of vagal schwannomas, which tend to flatten the IJV ⟶, displace the CCA ⟩ medially, and separate the IJV from the CCA. The location of schwannomas in the CS and continuity with the vagus nerve are clues to their diagnosis. Note the vagus nerve ⟶.

INFRAHYOID CAROTID SPACE VAGUS SCHWANNOMA

TERMINOLOGY

Synonyms
- Neuroma, neurilemmoma

Definitions
- Benign tumor of Schwann cells that wrap around vagus nerve in carotid space (CS)

IMAGING

General Features
- Size
  - Lesions are usually large when clinically detected
  - 2-8 cm range
- Morphology
  - Ovoid to fusiform
  - Tumor margins are smooth, sharply circumscribed
- In infrahyoid neck, mass displaces thyroid and trachea to contralateral side, common carotid artery (CCA) anteromedially, and separates carotid artery and internal jugular vein (IJV)

Ultrasonographic Findings
- Ultrasound is able to evaluate/visualize nerve sheath tumors only in infrahyoid neck, vagal nerve schwannoma being most common
- Solid hypoechoic, heterogeneous mass
  - Well-demarcated tumor margin
  - Fusiform/oval in shape with tapering ends
  - ± posterior enhancement (despite being solid)
- Sharply defined focal cystic areas may be seen
- Continuity with nerve/thickening of adjacent nerve (diagnostic)
- Color Doppler shows increased vascularity within tumor, prominent tortuous vessels
- Vascularity is sensitive to pressure and may "disappear" with increasing transducer pressure
- Mass effect with flattening/occlusion of jugular vein

Imaging Recommendations
- Best imaging tool
  - Ultrasound is ideal imaging modality for infrahyoid schwannomas as it adequately demonstrates tumor and adjacent relations
  - Ultrasound is unable to distinguish schwannomas from neurofibromas
    - Neurofibromas may be lobulated, do not show posterior enhancement, and show less vascularity than schwannomas
  - FNAC/biopsy may trigger excruciating pain (considered diagnostic by some); important to recognize nature of these lesions to prevent biopsy
- Protocol advice
  - Location of tumor in close proximity of carotid & IJV is clue to diagnosis
  - Separates carotid artery from IJV
  - Vagus nerve typically shows "fibrillar" pattern on high-resolution US with bright streaks within
  - Transverse scans identify tumor and longitudinal scans evaluate nerve continuity
- CECT or MR can be used to confirm this diagnosis and evaluate anatomical extent of large tumors

DIFFERENTIAL DIAGNOSIS

Carotid Body Paraganglioma
- Mass center: Nestled in CCA bifurcation with splaying of ICA, ECA
- Bilateral with prominent intratumoral vessels; solid, hypoechoic, and well defined with no posterior enhancement

Malignant Lymph Node
- History of known head and neck primary tumor
- Hypoechoic, heterogeneous, well-defined mass with peripheral vascularity, ± intranodal necrosis, ± multiple

Sympathetic Schwannoma
- Posterior to both vessels in carotid space and displaces them anteriorly as one
- No continuity with vagus nerve, hypoechoic, fusiform, ± cystic spaces within

2nd Branchial Cleft Cyst
- Location in relation to carotid, submandibular gland, and sternomastoid is key
- Anechoic, thin walled with posterior enhancement/pseudosolid/heterogeneous mass; avascular ± vessels in wall if infected

Internal Jugular Vein Thrombosis
- History of IJV instrumentation usually present
- Noncompressible IJV with heterogeneous echoes within; vascularity in thrombus if tumor thrombus

Carotid Artery Pseudoaneurysm, Neck
- Ovoid outpouching of carotid artery; Doppler identifies connection with carotid artery and demonstrates abnormal flow
- Well-defined, thin-walled anechoic structure ± flow within

CLINICAL ISSUES

Presentation
- Most common signs/symptoms
  - Asymptomatic palpable mass
    - Vagus nerve schwannoma: Anterolateral neck mass
  - Vagus nerve schwannomas may present with
    - Dysphagia, dysphonia
    - Hoarseness, arrhythmia
    - Pain occurs with large tumors

DIAGNOSTIC CHECKLIST

Image Interpretation Pearls
- Fusiform, sharply circumscribed, solid CS mass with posterior enhancement, sharp cystic spaces, and vascularity within, in continuity with vagus nerve suggests vagus nerve schwannoma
- Located in infrahyoid carotid space, separates carotid artery from IJV

SELECTED REFERENCES

1. Ahuja AT et al: Diagnostic Imaging: Ultrasound. 1st ed. Salt Lake City: Amirsys, Inc. 11-102-105, 2007

INFRAHYOID CAROTID SPACE VAGUS SCHWANNOMA

(Left) Longitudinal grayscale US in this patient with a large, painless, left upper neck mass shows the edge of the mass ⊅, tapering into and continuous with the vagus nerve ➡. Note the IJV ➡ and CCA ➥. This continuity with the vagus nerve made for quick diagnosis of vagal schwannoma, and easily differentiated it from other tumors at this site. (Right) Corresponding axial T1WI C+ MR shows diffuse enhancement of the vagus nerve schwannoma ➡. Note its displacement of CS vessels ➡ medially & anteriorly.

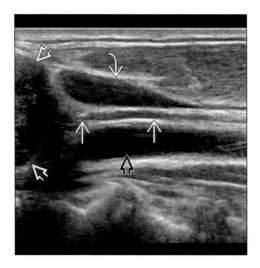
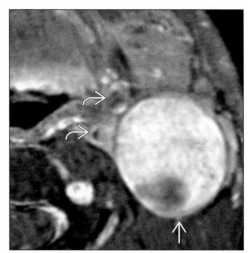

(Left) Transverse grayscale US shows the infrahyoid carotid space in a patient with no previous radiation to the neck. Note the prominent, hypoechoic vagus nerve ➡ and its relation to the CCA ➥ and IJV ➡. (Right) Corresponding longitudinal grayscale US (same patient) shows a focal, hypoechoic "mass" in continuity with the vagus nerve, suggesting a small vagus nerve schwannoma ➡. Note the bright central echoes in the vagus nerve ➡.

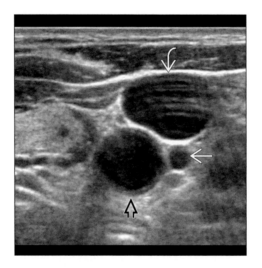
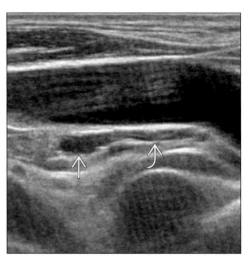

(Left) Longitudinal grayscale US shows multiple vagus schwannomas ➡ in continuity with the vagus nerve ➡. Sonographic visualization of the vagus nerve, with modern high-resolution transducers, makes such diagnoses possible without need for cytology/biopsy. (Right) Corresponding coronal fat-suppressed T2WI MR confirms multiple vagus nerve schwannomas ➡. US, to delineate continuity with nerve + MR to demonstrate the anatomic relationship of large schwannomas, is useful preoperatively.

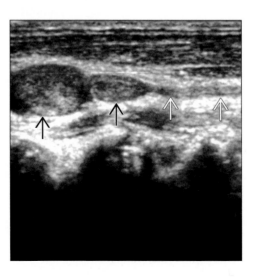
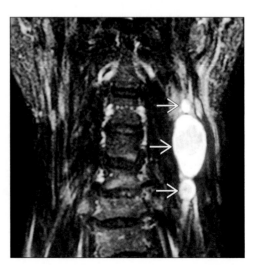

INFRAHYOID CAROTID SPACE VAGUS SCHWANNOMA

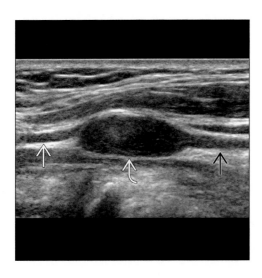
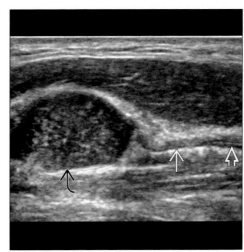

(Left) Longitudinal grayscale US of a small peripheral NST ⇗ shows continuity of the tumor with its originating nerve, proximally ➡ and distally ➡. *(Right)* Longitudinal grayscale US of an NST ⇗ in the posterior neck shows continuity with nerve ➡ distally, and bright linear echogenicity within nerve ⇥ ("nerve signature"). The ability of modern high-resolution US transducers to clearly demonstrate tumors, and their continuity with originating nerves, makes diagnoses of NSTs routinely possible.

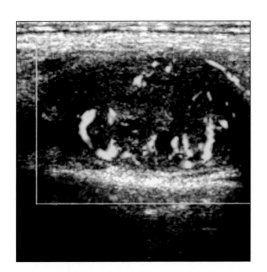
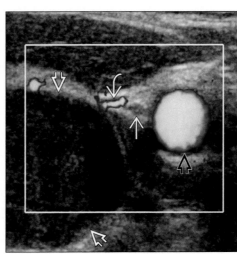

(Left) Power Doppler US of vagal schwannoma shows prominent vessels within tumor. These vessels are pressure sensitive and may disappear with ↑ transducer pressure. Neurofibromas are usually less vascular than schwannomas. *(Right)* Transverse power Doppler US shows large NST ⇥ and its relationship to vagus nerve ➡, CCA ⇥, & IJV ➡. It is separate from the vagus nerve and was NST of an exiting nerve root. This anatomical depiction is routinely possible with modern high-resolution transducers.

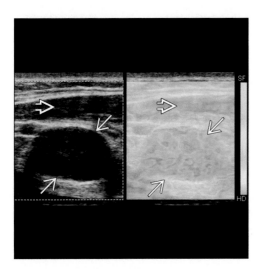
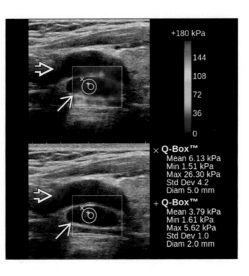

(Left) Longitudinal grayscale US and qualitative strain elastogram show a schwannoma ➡. Strain color scale ranges from purple (elastic, soft) to red (inelastic, hard). It has mixed strain pattern with green, purple, and a few red foci, appearing more elastic than adjacent muscle ⇥. *(Right)* Longitudinal grayscale US and SWE shows a vagal schwannoma ➡ abutting the CCA ⇥. SWE color scale ranges from blue (0 kPa, soft) to red (180 kPa, stiff). It appears blue with a max SWE value of 26.3 kPa (low).

SYMPATHETIC SCHWANNOMA

Key Facts

Terminology
- Benign, slow-growing tumor of Schwann cells investing cervical sympathetic chain

Imaging
- 3 types of displacement caused by cervical sympathetic chain schwannoma (CSCS)
  - Most common: Anterior ± lateral displacement of common carotid artery (CCA) and internal jugular vein (IJV) as one
  - Less common: Splaying of internal and external carotid arteries
  - Rare: Tumor splaying of IJV and CCA; renders differentiation from vagal schwannoma (VS) impossible unless definite separation from vagus nerve is demonstrated
- CSCS and VS are the 2 most common types of schwannoma in extracranial head and neck region
- Ultrasound findings

- Well-defined oval, round, or lobulated heterogeneously hypoechoic mass ± posterior enhancement
  - Cystic change in larger lesions
  - Long axis in craniocaudal direction
  - < 180° of circumference abuts carotid arteries & IJV
  - Ultrasound accurately identifies vagus nerve, helping to differentiate CSCS from VS
- CECT or enhanced MR findings
  - Heterogeneously enhancing ± cystic space
  - Small lesion may show homogeneous enhancement
- Low diagnostic yield of FNA cytology for nerve sheath tumor (reported rate: 20-25%)

Top Differential Diagnoses
- Vagal schwannoma
- Neurofibroma, carotid space
- Extracranial schwannoma from small nerve roots
- Carotid body paraganglioma

(Left) Transverse grayscale US shows the typical appearance of cervical sympathetic chain schwannoma (CSCS) ➡ seen as a well-defined, hypoechoic, heterogeneous neck mass displacing the internal ➡ and external ➡ carotid arteries anteriorly and medially. (Right) Corresponding power Doppler US shows sparse peripheral vascularity ➡ in CSCS. Schwannomas are typically hypovascular. US adequately identifies and characterizes CSCS. Despite their solid nature, posterior acoustic enhancement may also be seen in such lesions.

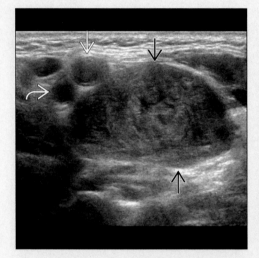
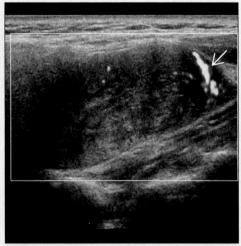

(Left) Axial T2WI FS MR (same patient) clearly demonstrates a hyperintense CSCS ➡ and its relation to the internal ➡ and external ➡ carotid arteries. (Right) Axial T1WI C + MR (same patient) shows heterogeneous enhancement of the CSCS ➡. The rim of hypointense signal ➡ may represent encapsulation. Note the anterior displacement of carotid vessels. Although US identifies and characterizes CSCS, CECT/MR better demonstrate the extent and adjacent anatomical relations.

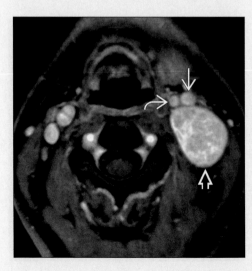
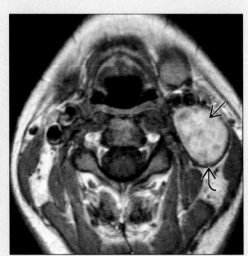

SYMPATHETIC SCHWANNOMA

TERMINOLOGY

Abbreviations
- Vagal schwannoma (VS)
- Cervical sympathetic chain schwannoma (CSCS)

Synonyms
- Sympathetic neurilemmoma or neuroma

Definitions
- Benign, slow-growing tumor of Schwann cells investing cervical sympathetic chain (CSC)

IMAGING

General Features
- Best diagnostic clue
  - Well-defined, oval, round/lobulated, heterogeneously enhancing mass along CSC course
- Location
  - CSC
    - Descends anterior to longus muscles, underneath prevertebral fascia, and posteromedial to carotid space
    - Converges medially from upper to lower cervical levels
    - Anatomical variant with CSC passing within posterior wall of carotid space
  - Can involve suprahyoid or infrahyoid neck
    - Center of lesion most commonly lies above carotid bifurcation
- Size
  - Range: 1.5-6 cm (mean: 3.5 cm) in reported series
- Morphology
  - Well-defined oval, round, or lobulated mass
  - Long axis in craniocaudal direction
  - Less than 180° circumference abuts common carotid artery (CCA) and internal jugular vein (IJV)
  - 3 types of displacement caused by CSCS in relation to carotid space vessels
    - Most common: Anterior ± lateral displacement of CCA and IJV as one unit
    - Less common: Splaying of internal and external carotid arteries
      - Internal carotid artery is often displaced posteriorly ± laterally
    - Rare: Tumor splaying of IJV and CCA; renders differentiation from VS impossible unless definite separation from vagus nerve is demonstrated

Imaging Recommendations
- Best imaging tool
  - Both CT and MR provide sufficient information for diagnosis, with MR slightly superior in tissue differentiation
  - Ultrasound is an ideal initial imaging tool for neck masses
    - Accurately identifies vagus nerve, helping to differentiate CSCS from VS

Ultrasonographic Findings
- Grayscale ultrasound
  - Vagus nerve runs separately from CSC
  - Well-defined oval, round, or lobulated mass along CSC course
  - Heterogeneously hypoechoic ± posterior acoustic enhancement
  - Cystic change often seen in larger lesions
  - Typically displaces IJV and CCA anteriorly as one unit
  - Direct connection with CSC is uncommonly demonstrated
- Power Doppler
  - Schwannomas are typically hypovascular
  - Scanty peripheral vascularity
    - Diminishes on light pressure
- US-guided FNAC
  - Low diagnostic yield for nerve sheath tumor
    - Reported rate: 20-25%
  - Needle tip should be targeted toward solid component under ultrasound guidance

CT Findings
- NECT: Hypoattenuating > isoattenuating to muscle
- CECT: Heterogeneously hypoenhancing in > 2/3
  - Avid, heterogeneous enhancement pattern reported, but uncommon
  - Cystic change in larger lesion is common

MR Findings
- T1WI
  - Hypointense to isointense to muscle
- T2WI
  - Heterogeneously hyperintense > homogeneously hyperintense
  - Target sign: Hypointense center = hypercellular region with Antoni A cells
  - ± discrete T2-hyperintense areas = cystic change
- T1WI C+
  - Inhomogeneous > homogeneous enhancement
  - Homogeneous enhancement in small lesions
  - Cystic change demonstrated as well-defined intratumoral nonenhancing areas
- No flow void in any sequence (unlike paraganglioma)

Nuclear Medicine Findings
- PET/CT
  - Wide range of FDG uptake value
  - High FDG avidity is a recognized pattern and is mistaken for malignant lymphadenopathy

DIFFERENTIAL DIAGNOSIS

Vagal Schwannoma
- Same morphological appearance, except VS tends to separate IJV and CCA
- Continuation with vagus nerve, which may be thickened

Neurofibroma, Carotid Space
- Similar to carotid space schwannoma
- Low density on CECT
- Connecting nerve fibers tend to enter/exit lesion centrically

Extracranial Head and Neck Schwannoma From Smaller Nerve Roots
- Simulates CSCS, particularly when connection with parent nerve cannot be established
- Less common than CSCS
- Location or axis may deviate from expected CSC course

SYMPATHETIC SCHWANNOMA

Carotid Body Paraganglioma

- Highly vascular, avidly enhancing, well-defined nodule at carotid bifurcation
  - Could be bilateral
- Completely fills carotid bifurcation crotch
- Splays and encases internal and external carotid arteries
- Marked intratumoral vascularity on Doppler
- Arteriovenous shunting seen

Glomus Vagale Paraganglioma

- Profuse vascularity
- Cystic change is uncommon
- Avid, heterogeneous enhancement with flow voids on MR
- Cannot be evaluated by ultrasound due to its location

PATHOLOGY

General Features

- Etiology
  - Benign tumor that originates from Schwann cells of neural sheath of CSC
- Associated abnormalities
  - Neurofibromatosis type 2 association
    - Schwannomas, meningiomas, and ependymomas

Gross Pathologic & Surgical Features

- Solitary, well-encapsulated tumor arising from peripheral nerve

Microscopic Features

- Spindle-shaped cells with elongated nuclei
  - Organized, compact cellular regions (Antoni A) and loose, relatively acellular tissue (Antoni B)
  - Both areas are invariably present in tumors

CLINICAL ISSUES

Presentation

- Most common signs/symptoms
  - Asymptomatic palpable neck mass
- Other signs/symptoms
  - Incidental finding on imaging study
  - Obstructive symptom, e.g., dysphagia, sore throat
  - Horner syndrome (rare)
    - May be related to the fact that most neuroprogenitor cells do not run through schwannoma but pass over tumor capsule
      - Also, CSCS lies in a relatively loose fascial compartment

Demographics

- Age
  - Adult patients
    - Wide age range (mean: 40-50 years)
- Gender
  - No gender predominance
- Epidemiology
  - CSCS and VS are the 2 most common types of schwannoma in extracranial head and neck region

Natural History & Prognosis

- Slow but constant tumor growth until treatment

Treatment

- Traditionally, radical excision to prevent tumor recurrence, but postoperative Horner syndrome is inevitable
- Currently, intracapsular enucleation is advocated for better (30-86%) preservation of CSC function with extremely low recurrence rate

DIAGNOSTIC CHECKLIST

Image Interpretation Pearls

- Evaluation of anatomical relationships with CCA, IJV, and vagus nerve is critical
- Diagnostic yield of FNAC is low
  - Definitive diagnosis may be made only after surgical excision
- Normal superior and middle cervical sympathetic ganglia measure about 5-6 mm and may be seen on MR in normal individuals
  - These are hypointense on T2WI and should not be confused with CSC
  - Superior sympathetic ganglion is most constant in location: Found at C2-C4 levels
  - Middle sympathetic ganglion is variable in location: May be present at C5-C7 levels and is not seen in up to 60% of patients

SELECTED REFERENCES

1. Yasumatsu R et al: Diagnosis and management of extracranial head and neck schwannomas: a review of 27 cases. Int J Otolaryngol. 2013:973045, 2013
2. Hsieh TC et al: Lower neck neurilemmoma can masquerade as lymph node metastasis on FDG PET/CT in patient with nasopharyngeal carcinoma. Clin Nucl Med. 36(12):e217-9, 2011
3. Liu HL et al: Extracranial head and neck Schwannomas: a study of the nerve of origin. Eur Arch Otorhinolaryngol. 268(9):1343-7, 2011
4. Anil G et al: Imaging characteristics of schwannoma of the cervical sympathetic chain: a review of 12 cases. AJNR Am J Neuroradiol. 31(8):1408-12, 2010
5. Kim SH et al: Schwannoma in head and neck: preoperative imaging study and intracapsular enucleation for functional nerve preservation. Yonsei Med J. 51(6):938-42, 2010
6. Saylam CY et al: Neuroanatomy of cervical sympathetic trunk: a cadaveric study. Clin Anat. 22(3):324-30, 2009
7. Tomita T et al: Diagnosis and management of cervical sympathetic chain schwannoma: a review of 9 cases. Acta Otolaryngol. 129(3):324-9, 2009
8. Civelek E et al: Surgical anatomy of the cervical sympathetic trunk during anterolateral approach to cervical spine. Eur Spine J. 17(8):991-5, 2008
9. Cheshire WP et al: Cervical sympathetic neuralgia arising from a schwannoma. Headache. 47(3):444-6, 2007
10. Langner E et al: Schwannomas in the head and neck: retrospective analysis of 21 patients and review of the literature. Sao Paulo Med J. 125(4):220-2, 2007
11. Saito DM et al: Parapharyngeal space schwannomas: preoperative imaging determination of the nerve of origin. Arch Otolaryngol Head Neck Surg. 133(7):662-7, 2007
12. Kiray A et al: Surgical anatomy of the cervical sympathetic trunk. Clin Anat. 18(3):179-85, 2005
13. Furukawa M et al: Differentiation between schwannoma of the vagus nerve and schwannoma of the cervical sympathetic chain by imaging diagnosis. Laryngoscope. 106(12 Pt 1):1548-52, 1996

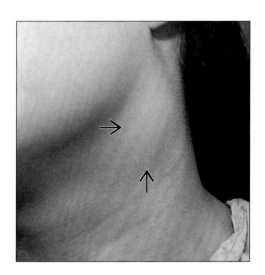

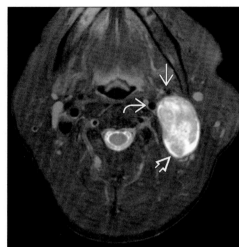

(Left) Clinical photograph shows a young female presenting with a painless left upper neck mass ➡. *(Right)* Corresponding axial T2WI FS MR shows a heterogeneous T2-hyperintense mass ➡. A rim of T2-hyperintense signal is frequently seen with schwannoma as opposed to neurofibroma. Note that the internal ➡ and external ➡ carotid arteries are splayed and anteriorly displaced. The location and appearances are consistent with CSCS. Vagus schwannoma (VS) is a differential diagnosis.

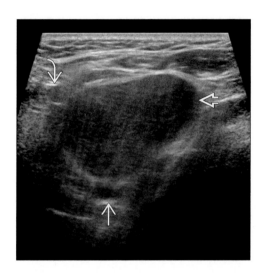

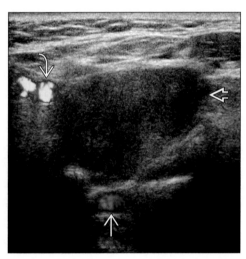

(Left) Transverse grayscale US shows a less common appearance of CSCS ➡. The internal ➡ and external ➡ carotid arteries are splayed and anteriorly displaced. Note that the mass abuts these arteries by < 180° of its circumference, unlike carotid body paraganglioma. *(Right)* Corresponding transverse power Doppler US shows that the internal ➡ and external ➡ carotid arteries are splayed and anteriorly displaced by CSCS ➡.

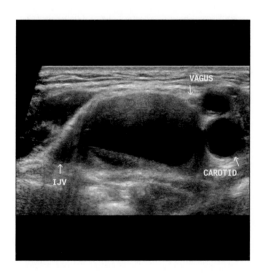

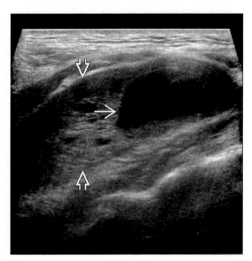

(Left) Transverse grayscale US shows a less common displacement of vessels by CSCS. Note the CSCS separating the internal jugular vein (IJV) and carotid arteries. VS is a close differential, but US clearly shows the vagus nerve as separate from the lesion. Separation of the IJV and common carotid artery is a rare but documented appearance of CSCS. *(Right)* Corresponding longitudinal grayscale US of CSCS ➡ shows a large cystic area ➡ in the schwannoma, a feature often seen in larger lesions.

BRACHIAL PLEXUS SCHWANNOMA

Key Facts

Imaging

- Lesions within PVS are situated between anterior and middle scalene muscles
- Ultrasound is best able to fully evaluate lesions in perivertebral space/lateral neck
- Solid mass with well-defined margin, hypoechoic and heterogeneous echo pattern
- Fusiform/oval shape, ± tapering ends in continuity with brachial plexus
- ± sharply defined cystic/hemorrhagic areas within
- May have pseudocystic appearance with posterior enhancement (despite being solid)
- Color Doppler shows vascularity within, which may disappear upon excessive transducer pressure
- US identifies nature of lesion in lateral neck but may be unable to delineate proximal and distal extent of large lesions

- MR confirms extent, multiplicity (if any) of large lesions after US has made diagnosis
- Pressure/manipulating mass with transducer or needle biopsy may cause symptoms of radiculopathy
- Development of pain in BP schwannoma raises suspicion of malignancy

Top Differential Diagnoses

- Neurofibroma
- Metastatic nodes
- Tuberculous nodes
- Lymphangioma

Clinical Issues

- Painless, slow-growing mass in lateral neck ± radiculopathy

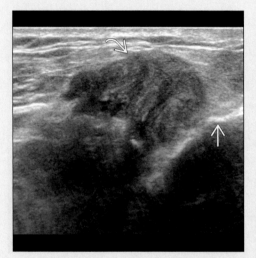
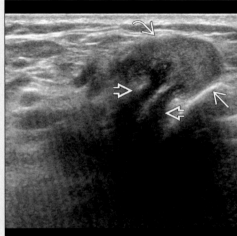

(Left) Transverse grayscale US in a patient with upper limb amputation for osteosarcoma shows a solid, hypoechoic, heterogeneous mass ➡, supraclavicular in location. Note the clavicle ➡. *(Right)* Transverse grayscale US (same patient) in a different plane shows continuation of the mass ➡ with emerging brachial plexus (BP) roots/rami ➡. Diagnosis of postoperative stump neuroma was made. US, with its high resolution, clearly identifies the mass and its continuation with the BP. Note the clavicle ➡.

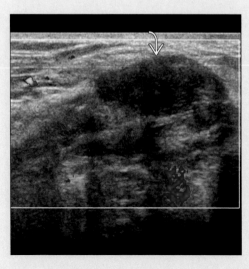
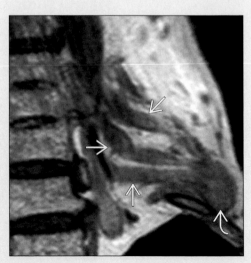

(Left) Corresponding longitudinal power Doppler US (same patient) shows no significant vascularity in the neuroma ➡. Intratumoral vascularity is sensitive to pressure and the transducer must be held gently. *(Right)* Coronal T1WI MR defines the extent of the mass ➡ and its continuity with BP roots/rami ➡. US is ideal initial imaging modality as it quickly establishes location and nature of such lesion. However, MR better defines its entire extent and relationship to adjacent structures.

BRACHIAL PLEXUS SCHWANNOMA

TERMINOLOGY

Definitions
- Benign neoplasm of Schwann cells that wrap brachial plexus (BP) nerves in perivertebral space (PVS)

IMAGING

General Features
- Best diagnostic clue
  - Well-circumscribed, fusiform, hypoechoic mass, ± intratumoral cystic spaces, vascularity, and in continuity with BP roots between anterior and middle scalene muscles
- Location
  - May arise anywhere along course of BP roots including intra- and extradural spaces, neural foramen, PVS
  - Lesions within PVS are situated between anterior and middle scalene muscles
  - Ultrasound is best able to fully evaluate lesions in perivertebral space/lateral neck

Ultrasonographic Findings
- Solid mass with well-defined margin, hypoechoic and heterogeneous echo pattern
- Fusiform/oval shape, ± tapering ends in continuity with brachial plexus
- Often has sharply defined cystic/hemorrhagic areas within
- May have pseudocystic appearance with posterior enhancement (despite being solid)
- Color Doppler shows vascularity within, which may disappear upon excessive transducer pressure
  - ± mass effect on adjacent vessels

CT Findings
- NECT
  - Typically isodense to muscle
  - Calcification is uncommon
- CECT
  - Moderate to strong enhancement

MR Findings
- T1WI
  - Isointense to muscle
- T2WI
  - Hyperintense, approaching signal of regional vessels
  - "Target" sign: Central hypo-, peripheral hyperintense signal commonly seen in benign peripheral nerve sheath tumor (PNST)
  - "Fascicular" sign: Multiple, irregular, central hypointense foci typical of benign PNST
- T1WI C+
  - "Reverse target" sign: Central enhancement > peripheral enhancement

Imaging Recommendations
- Best imaging tool
  - US identifies nature of lesion in lateral neck but may be unable to delineate proximal and distal extent of large lesions
  - MR confirms extent, multiplicity (if any) of large lesions after US has made diagnosis
- Protocol advice
  - Transverse scans identify normal BP roots/rami as 3 round, hypoechoic structures between anterior and middle scalene
  - Longitudinal scans identify roots/rami along their course
  - Transverse scans help to quickly identify tumor, and longitudinal scans continuity with brachial plexus
  - Intratumoral vascularity is sensitive to pressure, therefore, transducer must be held gently
  - Pressure/manipulating mass with transducer or needle biopsy may cause symptoms of radiculopathy

DIFFERENTIAL DIAGNOSIS

Neurofibroma
- May be indistinguishable from schwannoma
- Cystic degeneration, hemorrhage uncommon
- Less vascular and shows no posterior enhancement

Metastatic Nodes
- Multiple, heterogeneous, hypoechoic, round nodes with necrosis, peripheral vascularity, known primary

Tuberculous Nodes
- Multiple, matted, necrotic nodes with adjacent soft tissue edema; avascular/displaced vascularity within

Lymphangioma
- Trans-spatial, cystic, septate, avascular mass with negligible mass effect

CLINICAL ISSUES

Presentation
- Most common signs/symptoms
  - Painless, slow-growing mass in lateral neck ± radiculopathy
  - Malignant degeneration rare
  - Development of pain should raise suspicion for malignancy

Treatment
- Surgical excision
- Good prognosis with low risk of recurrence

DIAGNOSTIC CHECKLIST

Image Interpretation Pearls
- Fusiform solid mass, well-defined margin, ± intratumoral cystic spaces and vascularity in continuity with brachial plexus

Reporting Tips
- When describing any low neck lesion, always indicate its relationship to brachial plexus

SELECTED REFERENCES

1. Ahuja AT et al: Diagnostic Imaging: Ultrasound. 1st ed. Salt Lake City: Amirsys, Inc. 11-102-105, 2007
2. Harnsberger HR et al: Diagnostic Imaging: Head & Neck. 1st ed. Salt Lake City: Amirsys, Inc. III-10-14-15, 2004
3. Ahuja AT et al. Practical Head and Neck Ultrasound. London: Greenwich Medical Media. 85-104, 2000

BRACHIAL PLEXUS SCHWANNOMA

(Left) Longitudinal grayscale US shows a posterior triangle mass ➡ with intratumoral cystic degeneration/hemorrhage ➡. Note its proximal continuity with emerging BP root/rami ➡, suggesting BP schwannoma. *(Right)* Longitudinal grayscale US (same patient) shows cystic degeneration/hemorrhage ➡ within a BP schwannoma ➡. Note continuity with the BP distally ➡. US readily establishes a diagnosis of BP schwannoma and obviates the need for confirmatory FNAC.

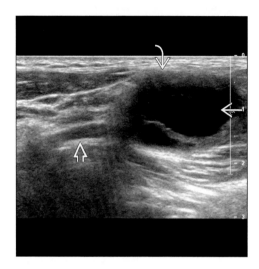
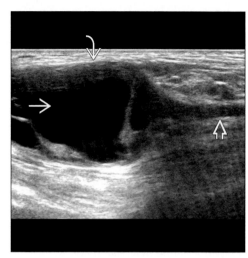

(Left) Corresponding power Doppler US of cystic BP schwannoma shows no significant vascularity within the lesion ➡. *(Right)* Coronal T1WI C+ MR clearly identifies BP schwannoma ➡, its location, and relationship to adjacent structures. Note its fusiform shape, moderate heterogeneous contrast enhancement, intratumoral cystic change, and continuity with brachial plexus. Cystic degeneration/hemorrhage is uncommon in neurofibroma vs. schwannoma.

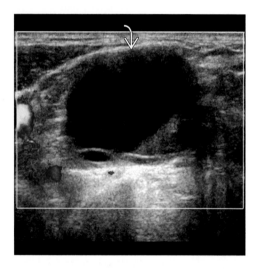
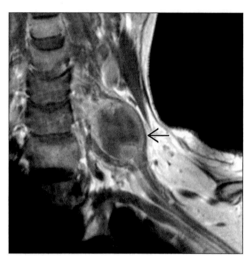

(Left) Transverse grayscale US shows a well-defined, solid, hypoechoic mass ➡ in the supraclavicular fossa. Note the proximal continuation with emerging BP root/rami ➡ suggesting BP schwannoma. Modern high-resolution transducers allow US to readily identify lesion and illustrate its continuity with BP, making biopsy unnecessary. Note clavicle ➡. *(Right)* Corresponding coronal T1WI MR shows the BP schwannoma ➡. Note its fusiform shape, isointensity to muscle, and continuity with BP.

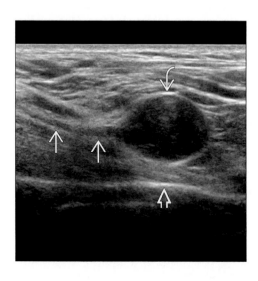
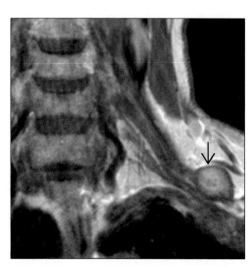

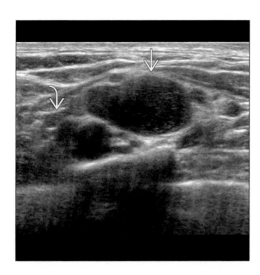

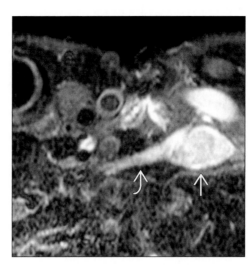

(Left) Transverse grayscale US shows a fusiform, hypoechoic mass ➡ low in left neck, in known location of BP. Note its continuity with emerging BP root/rami ➡. Longitudinal scan (not shown) also demonstrated this continuity & a diagnosis of BP schwannoma was suggested. *(Right)* Axial fat-suppressed T2WI MR demonstrates BP schwannoma ➡ and its continuity with an emerging root ➡. US quickly identifies the lesion and differentiates it from lymph nodes (which are more common) at the site.

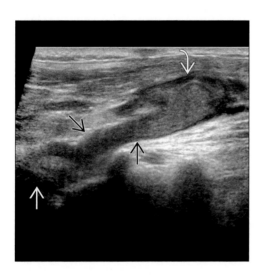

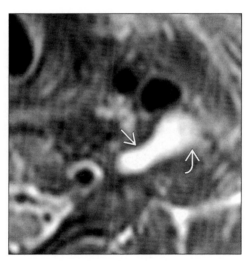

(Left) Longitudinal grayscale US shows diffusely enlarged nerve root ➡ emerging from the neural foramen ➡ and extending into the schwannoma ➡. *(Right)* Axial T2WI MR confirms fusiform enlargement of nerve root ➡ and schwannoma ➡. The ability of high-resolution US to delineate normal nerves, such as BP rami/roots and infrahyoid vagus nerve, makes it possible to suggest a definitive diagnosis of NST using US. MR further defines its extent and anatomical relations, making biopsy unnecessary.

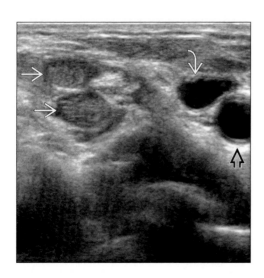

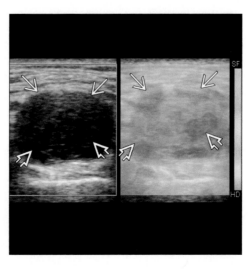

(Left) Transverse grayscale US of right lower posterior triangle in patient with previous RT to neck shows prominent roots/rami ➡ of BP between scalene muscles, not to be mistaken for enlarged lymph nodes. Note CCA ➡, IJV ➡. *(Right)* Longitudinal grayscale US and qualitative strain elastogram show PNST from BP. Strain color scale ranges from purple (soft) to red (hard). The mass is heterogeneous on strain image with areas displaying red ➡ and purple ➡, suggesting intermediate or mixed stiffness.

LIPOMA

Key Facts

Imaging

- 15% of lipomas occur in head and neck region and 5% are multiple
- Most common sites in neck: Posterior cervical and submandibular spaces
- Other locations: Anterior cervical and parotid spaces
- Well-defined, compressible, elliptical; hyperechoic (75%) or isoechoic/hypoechoic (25%) (relative to muscle)
- Internal multiple echogenic lines oriented parallel to transducer; feathered or striped appearance
- No calcification, nodularity or necrosis
- Displacement but no infiltration of structures
- Doppler: No significant vascularity in/around mass
- BSL: Diffuse, lobulated, isoechoic "mass" with echogenic lines within but no vascularity on Doppler
  - As the fat is unencapsulated, US cannot define degree of involvement
- CT/MR better define distribution of fat and compression of vital structures
  - May mask underlying neck malignancy; MR/CT evaluate it better than US
- HNL: Echogenic lines within lesion remain parallel to transducer irrespective of scanning plane

Top Differential Diagnoses

- Lymphatic malformation, venous vascular malformation, dermoid, liposarcoma

Diagnostic Checklist

- Liposarcoma if internal stranding, nodularity or heterogeneity, calcification, necrosis, and vascularity
- Define extent of large lipoma; inform surgeon if trans-spatial
- US readily identifies lipoma and BSL; however, it cannot define extent of large lesions and compression of vital structures

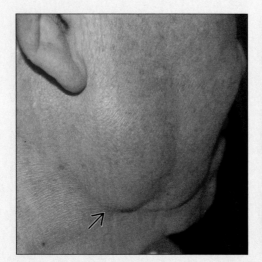
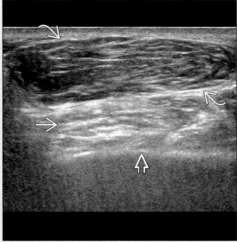

(Left) Clinical photograph shows a middle-aged man with a smooth, soft, palpable mass ➡ over the right mandible merging imperceptibly with adjacent soft issues. (Right) Corresponding transverse grayscale US shows a well-defined, heterogeneous mass ➡ with typical striped or feathered appearance in subcutaneous tissues over the right masseter ➡. US features are typical of lipoma & warrant no further imaging or biopsy. MR + FS may be indicated if entire extent of mass cannot be evaluated by US. Note the mandible ➡.

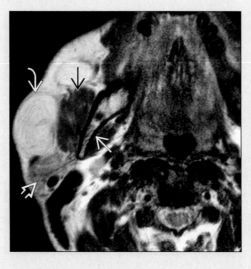
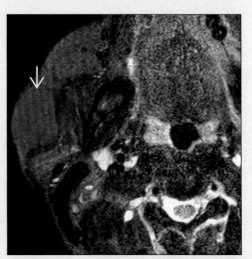

(Left) Axial T2WI MR in the same patient shows a hyperintense lipoma ➡ overlying the right masseter muscle ➡. Note the mandible ➡ and superficial parotid gland ➡. (Right) Corresponding T2WI FS MR shows complete suppression of signal intensity within the mass ➡, confirming diagnosis, location, and anatomic relations of lipoma, obviating the need for biopsy. Compared to US, MR better confirms location, extent, and relations of large lipomas, particularly intramuscular and at nape of the neck.

LIPOMA

TERMINOLOGY

Definitions
- Head and neck lipoma (HNL): Benign neoplasm composed entirely of mature fat

IMAGING

General Features
- Best diagnostic clue
  - Well-circumscribed, homogeneous mass composed entirely of fat
- Location
  - 15% of lipomas occur in head and neck and 5% are multiple
    - Most common sites in neck: Posterior cervical and submandibular spaces
    - Other common locations: Anterior cervical and parotid spaces
  - Can occur in every space in extracranial head and neck and involve multiple contiguous spaces
- Size
  - Highly variable; may become massive

Ultrasonographic Findings
- Well-defined, compressible, elliptical; hyperechoic (75%) or isoechoic/hypoechoic (25%) (relative to muscle)
- Internal multiple echogenic lines oriented parallel to transducer; feathered or striped appearance
- No calcification, nodularity, or necrosis
- No deep acoustic enhancement or attenuation
- Displacement without infiltration of adjacent structures
- Doppler: No significant vascularity in/around mass
- Liposarcoma suggested by several findings
  - Presence of adjacent soft tissue stranding
  - Nodular mass with septation and vascularity within lesion
  - Cystic/necrotic areas and calcification within lesion
- Benign symmetrical lipomatosis (BSL) = Madelung disease
  - Diffuse, lobulated, isoechoic "mass" with echogenic lines within but no vascularity on Doppler
  - As the fat is unencapsulated, US cannot define degree of involvement; CT/MR better define distribution of fat and compression of vital structures
  - May mask underlying neck malignancy; MR/CT evaluate it better than US

Imaging Recommendations
- Best imaging tool
  - US readily identifies lipoma and BSL, however, it cannot define extent of large lesions and compression of vital structures
  - CT and MR both clearly demonstrate extent of lesion and any underlying neck malignancy
  - Imaging required only if diagnosis is uncertain, or to demonstrate deep tissue extent
- Protocol advice
  - Echogenic lines within lesion remain parallel to transducer irrespective of scanning plane

DIFFERENTIAL DIAGNOSIS

Lymphatic Malformation
- Lipoma often clinically diagnosed as a lymphangioma
- Unilocular/multiloculated, septate, ± fine internal echoes, trans-spatial, avascular on Doppler

Venous Vascular Malformation
- Soft, compressible, multiple serpigeneous structures with slow flow, phleboliths, and vascularity on Doppler

Dermoid
- Most common cervical location is floor of mouth
  - Less commonly submandibular space
- Heterogeneous echo pattern, ± calcified foci with posterior shadowing, avascular on Doppler

Liposarcoma
- Well-differentiated liposarcoma may exactly mimic lipoma with stranding
- Internal nodules, calcification, necrosis, vascularity, infiltration/stranding of adjacent soft tissues

PATHOLOGY

General Features
- Associated syndromes
  - Benign symmetric lipomatosis = Madelung disease
    - Diffuse, symmetric, unencapsulated fatty deposition in cervical and upper dorsal region
    - Most common sites are posterior superficial, posterior and anterior cervical, and perivertebral spaces
    - Middle-aged males of Mediterranean descent with history of alcohol abuse
  - Familial multiple lipomatosis
    - Multiple small, well-demarcated, encapsulated lipomas; strong familial component
    - Commonly involve extremities with neck and shoulders usually spared (unlike BSL)
  - Dercum disease
    - Multiple, painful lipomas are hallmarks
    - Typically occur on extremities of obese postmenopausal women
  - Gardner syndrome
    - Characterized by osteomas, soft tissue tumors, and colonic adenomatous polyps
    - Soft tissue tumors include sebaceous inclusion cysts, lipoma, fibroma, leiomyoma, neurofibroma, and desmoid tumors

DIAGNOSTIC CHECKLIST

Consider
- All lipomas should be scrutinized for presence of internal nodularity, stranding, vascularity, calcification
- Liposarcoma if internal stranding, nodularity or heterogeneity, calcification, necrosis, and vascularity present
- Define extent of large lipoma

SELECTED REFERENCES
1. Harnsberger HR et al: Diagnostic Imaging: Head & Neck. 2nd ed. Salt Lake City: Amirsys, Inc. I-13, 6-9, 2011

LIPOMA

(Left) Grayscale US of left posterior triangle shows a large, well-defined, heterogeneous solid mass ➡ with linear echogenic streaks ➡ parallel to transducer (striped or feathered appearance of lipoma), inseparable from the levator scapulae muscle ➡. These linear streaks always remain parallel to the transducer irrespective of scanning longitudinally or in transverse plane. Note the trapezius ➡. *(Right)* Coronal T1WI MR confirms location & extent of lipoma ➡ in the levator scapulae muscle.

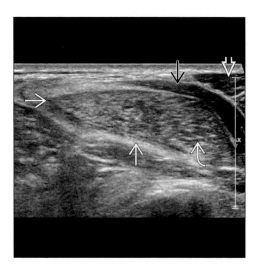
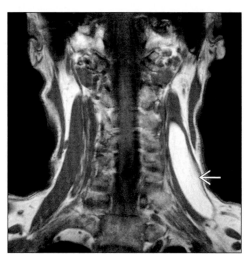

(Left) Longitudinal grayscale US at the nape of neck shows a large, solid, heterogeneous mass ➡. Linear echogenic streaks ➡ within suggest a lipomatous origin. Posterior parts of the mass cannot be clearly seen due to fat. Note the transverse process ➡. *(Right)* Axial T2WI FS MR shows complete suppression of signal within the mass (but for normal vessels) confirmed lipoma. Due to musculature, high-resolution US cannot fully evaluate nape lipomas, which are usually heterogeneous, not striped/feathered.

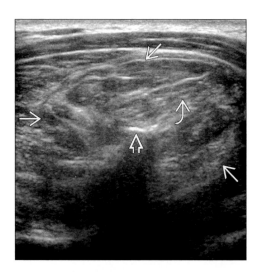
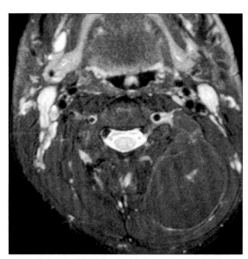

(Left) Coronal T1WI MR shows diffuse, symmetric, unencapsulated fatty accumulation ➡ in the cervical & upper dorsal regions in benign symmetric lipomatosis (BSL). *(Right)* Corresponding grayscale US shows lobular, diffuse infiltration of fat ➡ in soft tissues of neck. As fat deposition in BSL is diffuse and unencapsulated, US is unable to define the exact extent. In addition, BSL may mask an underlying neck malignancy & CT/MR evaluate it better than US.

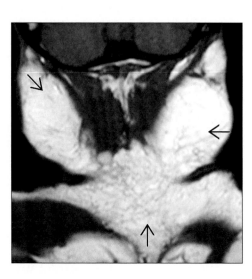
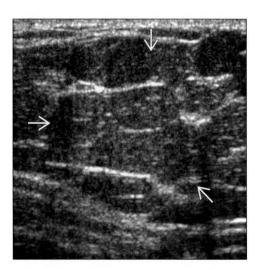

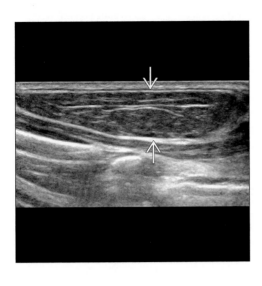
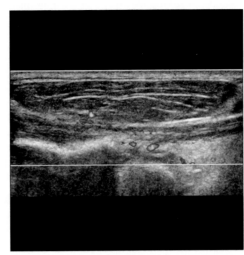

(Left) Longitudinal grayscale US shows a typical, well-defined lipoma ➡ with a striped or feathered appearance. *(Right)* Corresponding power Doppler US shows no obvious vascularity within the lipoma. The presence of hypoechoic heterogeneity on grayscale US & prominent vessels in a lipomatous lesion should raise possibility of sarcomatous change & warrant further imaging & biopsy. Well-differentiated liposarcoma may exactly mimic lipoma, but with stranding.

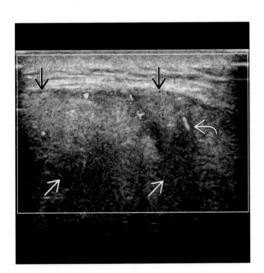
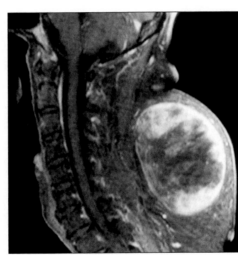

(Left) Longitudinal grayscale US shows a large mass ➡ over the nape of the neck in a middle-aged man. Note that the extent of the mass is not defined, but it shows hypoechoic heterogeneity ➡ & vascularity ➡ within. US appearances raise suspicion for sarcomatous change. *(Right)* Corresponding sagittal T1WI C+ FS MR shows tumor heterogeneity with areas of significant enhancement. Appearances remain suspicious for sarcomatous change.

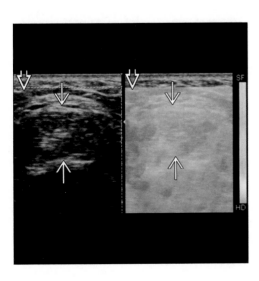
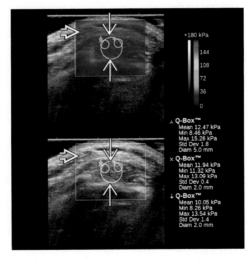

(Left) Transverse grayscale US & qualitative strain elastogram show a submental lipoma ➡. Strain color scale ranges from purple (elastic, soft) to red (inelastic, hard). It appears purple & green, similar to the surrounding tissue ➡, suggesting an elastic lesion. *(Right)* Transverse grayscale US & SWE show a submental lipoma ➡. SWE color scale ranges from blue (0 kPa, soft) to red (180 kPa, stiff). It appears blue, similar to subcutaneous tissues ➡, with a maximum SWE value of 15.3 kPa, which is low.

PILOMATRIXOMA

Key Facts

Imaging

- Subcutaneous nodule ± thinning overlying dermis
- Typically calcified
- Completely calcified: Irregular or arch-like echogenic interface with strong posterior acoustic shadow; obscured intralesional characteristics
- Partially calcified lesion: Well-circumscribed, oval nodule with scattered echogenic foci and variable degree of posterior shadow
  - Perilesional ± intralesional vascularity may be seen
- Noncalcified: Well-defined, hypoechoic nodule that mimics other benign skin lesion

Top Differential Diagnoses

- Foreign body granuloma/organized hematoma
- Venous vascular malformation
- Epidermoid or dermoid cyst
- Sebaceous cyst, calcified lymph node

Clinical Issues

- Benign appendage tumor related to hair cells matrix
- Wide age range; typically (45%) < 20 years
- Predilection for cervicomaxillofacial region (> 50%)
- Asymptomatic, firm to hard, well-circumscribed, mobile, slow-growing subcutaneous nodule
- Healthy-looking overlying skin; occasionally, change in color or ulcer
- Majority (75%) are < 15 mm; > 95% are solitary
- Multiple pilomatrixoma associated with Gardner syndrome, myotonic dystrophy, and sarcoidosis
- Frequently treated without imaging because of superficial location and benign clinical features
- Complete surgical excision

Diagnostic Checklist

- Densely calcified subcutaneous nodule in maxillofacial area of asymptomatic, young patient

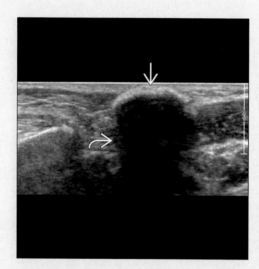
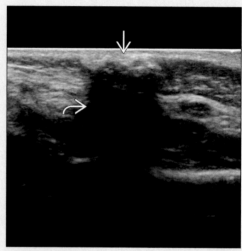

(Left) Grayscale US in a 6-year-old child with pilomatrixoma at left angle of the mandible shows dense, curvilinear calcification ➡ with marked posterior shadowing ➡. Dense calcification obscures the internal characteristics of lesion. (Right) Grayscale US in a 2-year-old child with a pilomatrixoma shows dense, heterogeneous calcification ➡ under the skin. Differential diagnosis includes calcified node (phlebolith) in venous vascular malformation. Shadowing from calcification ➡ prevents internal evaluation of the lesion.

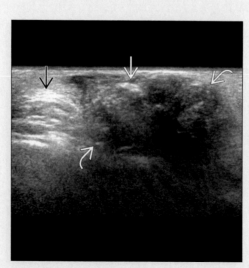
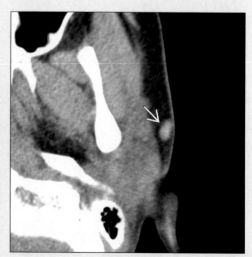

(Left) Grayscale US in a young male shows a pilomatrixoma ➡, pretragal in location, just below the skin surface with multiple areas of dense, shadowing calcification ➡ and heterogeneous internal echoes. Note tragal calcification ➡. (Right) Axial NECT shows a small pilomatrixoma ➡, just beneath the skin surface and overlying the parotid region. It is well-defined with no infiltrative edge. CT is normally restricted to larger lesions to define extent. Treatment is usually complete surgical excision.

PILOMATRIXOMA

TERMINOLOGY

Synonyms
- Calcified epithelioma, epithelioma of Malherbe, tricomatricoma, pilomatricoma

IMAGING

General Features
- Location
  - Subcutaneous; abuts overlying dermis
  - Anywhere in body except palm and sole
  - Predilection for cervicomaxillofacial region (> 50%)
    - Preauricular region > nasogenian region
- Size
  - Range: 2-50 mm; majority (75%) < 15 mm

Ultrasonographic Findings
- Subcutaneous nodule abuts ± thinning overlying dermis, typically calcified
- Completely calcified lesion
  - Irregular or arch-like echogenic interface with strong posterior acoustic shadow
  - Calcification completely obscures intralesional characteristics
- Partially calcified lesion
  - Well-circumscribed, oval nodule with scattered echogenic foci
  - Variable posterior acoustic shadow related to degree of calcification
  - Perilesional ± intralesional vascularity
- Noncalcified lesion
  - Well-defined, hypoechoic nodule that mimics other benign skin lesion
- Pseudocystic appearance and oval hypoechoic nodule with profuse vascularity have been described
  - Mimics other skin tumor

CT Findings
- Well-defined, subcutaneous nodule with variable degree of scattered calcification
- Helpful for assessment of large lesion

Imaging Recommendations
- Best imaging tool
  - High-resolution ultrasound
    - Superficial lesion in pediatric age group

DIFFERENTIAL DIAGNOSIS

Foreign Body Granuloma/Organized Hematoma
- History of foreign body injury/ trauma

Venous Vascular Malformation
- Phleboliths within cystic, serpiginous vascular spaces with slow flow on grayscale and Doppler ultrasound

Epidermoid or Dermoid Cyst
- Well-circumscribed, hypoechoic, ± homogeneous internal echoes/pseudosolid appearance
- ± calcification

Sebaceous Cyst
- Rarely calcified well-defined, hypoechoic, heterogeneous nodule ± punctum

Calcified Lymph Node
- Post-treatment tuberculous node
- ± displaced hilar vascularity/avascularity

Parotid Gland Tumor
- Deep-seated beneath superficial fascia

PATHOLOGY

General Features
- Benign skin appendage tumor belonging to group of suborganoid tumors with hair differentiation

Microscopic Features
- Circumscribed, subepidermal, nodular tumor of basal cell origin
- Variable keratinization and calcification
- Foreign body reaction surrounding keratinized zones

CLINICAL ISSUES

Presentation
- Most common signs/symptoms
  - Asymptomatic, firm to hard, well-circumscribed, mobile, slow-growing skin nodule
  - Healthy-looking overlying skin
- Other signs/symptoms
  - Change in skin color or ulceration secondary to epithelial thinning
  - Tenderness and itchiness

Demographics
- Age
  - Wide range; typically (45%) < 20 years
- Epidemiology
  - Relatively uncommon
  - ≤ 1% of all benign skin tumors
  - Majority (> 95%) are solitary lesions
  - Multiple pilomatrixoma
    - Associated with Gardner syndrome, myotonic dystrophy, and sarcoidosis

Natural History & Prognosis
- Benign, slow-growing lesion
- Relapse rate after surgical excision: 0.5-6%
- Malignant variety with distant metastasis reported

Treatment
- Complete surgical excision
- Frequently treated without imaging because of superficial location and benign clinical features

DIAGNOSTIC CHECKLIST

Consider
- Densely calcified subcutaneous nodule in maxillofacial area of asymptomatic, young patient

SELECTED REFERENCES
1. Abdeldayem M et al: Patient profile and outcome of pilomatrixoma in district general hospital in United kingdom. J Cutan Aesthet Surg. 6(2):107-10, 2013
2. Guinot-Moya R et al: Pilomatrixoma. Review of 205 cases. Med Oral Patol Oral Cir Bucal. 16(4):e552-5, 2011

SINUS HISTIOCYTOSIS (ROSAI-DORFMAN)

Key Facts

Terminology

- Rare, benign disorder characterized histologically by lymphatic sinus dilatation due to histiocyte proliferation

Imaging

- Typically massive bilateral cervical lymphadenopathy
- Tends to involve multiple sites with varying imaging manifestations, synchronous or metachronous
- Ultrasound
  - Round, solid, well-defined, hypoechoic lymph nodes with loss of echogenic hilum
  - Peripheral or mixed vascular pattern
  - Enlarged parotid glands with multiple hypoechoic intraparotid lymph nodes, ± parenchymal involvement
  - Enlarged submandibular glands with heterogeneous hypoechoic appearance
  - Unilateral lacrimal gland enlargement ± retrobulbar mass
  - Imaging appearance similar to a range of benign and malignant disease; requires histology for diagnosis
- If diagnosed in 1 site, screening and follow-up for other body parts are clinically useful

Top Differential Diagnoses

- Non-Hodgkin lymphoma
- Reactive lymph nodes
- Tuberculous adenopathy
- Castleman disease

Clinical Issues

- Most commonly diagnosed in children and adolescents with massive cervical lymphadenopathy
- Long-term clinical course characterized by exacerbations and remission
- Worse prognosis in patients with extranodal disease

(Left) Transverse grayscale US of an enlarged node ➡ in a patient with Rosai-Dorfman disease (RD) shows that the nodes are well defined, noncalcified, solid, and homogeneously hypoechoic with displacement of echogenic hilum ➡.
(Right) Corresponding power Doppler US shows a mixed vascular pattern with prominent hilar ➡ and peripheral ➡ vascularity. Such nodes are often mistaken for lymphomatous nodes. Diagnosis is made on histology.

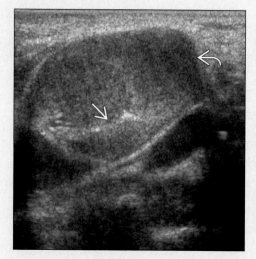
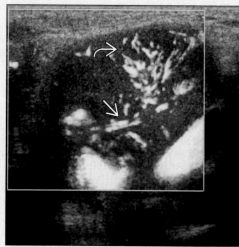

(Left) Axial T1WI shows multiple massively enlarged bilateral cervical lymph nodes ➡. These nodes are solid and typically homogeneously hypointense on T1WI.
(Right) Corresponding axial T2WI FS MR shows multiple hyperintense nodes ➡. These nodes may be hypointense to hyperintense relative to muscle. Note the associated enlarged submandibular glands ➡, which are also known to be involved in RD.

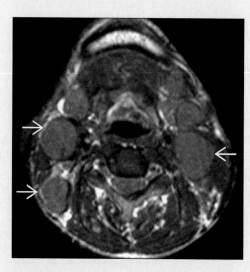
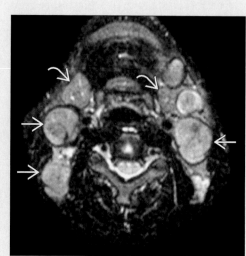

SINUS HISTIOCYTOSIS (ROSAI-DORFMAN)

TERMINOLOGY

Abbreviations
- Rosai-Dorfman disease (RD)

Synonyms
- Sinus histiocytosis with massive lymphadenopathy

Definitions
- Rare, benign disorder characterized histologically by lymphatic sinus dilatation due to histiocyte proliferation

IMAGING

General Features
- Best diagnostic clue
  - Massive, painless cervical lymphadenopathy in children or young adults
  - Tends to involve multiple nodal and extranodal sites with a variety of imaging manifestations, most commonly affecting head and neck region
  - When multiple sites are involved, disease can be synchronous or metachronous
- Location
  - Both nodal and extranodal involvement > isolated nodal or extranodal disease
  - Nodal sites (in up to 62%)
    - Bilateral cervical lymph nodes
    - Submandibular, deep cervical, retropharyngeal > mediastinal region
  - Extranodal sites (in up to 77%)
    - Cutaneous lesion is the most common type
      - Usually a manifestation of systemic disease
    - Head and neck is the most commonly affected region (in up to 75%)
      - Skin > sinonasal > orbits, salivary glands, and bone
    - Others: Central nervous system (CNS); rarely breast, lung, gastrointestinal, primary osseous, and primary subcutaneous lesions

Imaging Recommendations
- Contrast-enhanced MR or CT

Ultrasonographic Findings
- Cervical lymphadenopathy
  - Multiple, large, round, hypoechoic nodes
  - Solid, well-defined, noncalcified nodes with loss of echogenic hilum
  - Intranodal cystic change is uncommon; septate avascular cystic appearance described in pretracheal RD lymphadenopathy
  - Despite multiplicity, no periadenitis or nodal matting and soft tissue edema
  - Power Doppler: Peripheral or mixed hilar and peripheral vascularity
    - Similar to malignant lymphadenopathy; needs histopathology for diagnosis
- Cutaneous lesion
  - Ill-defined hypoechoic cutaneous and subcutaneous masses on face
  - Likely an extension of adjacent osseous or sinus lesion
- Salivary gland involvement
  - Multiple well-defined hypoechoic solid nodules in severely enlarged parotid glands with minimal intervening normal parenchyma = intraparotid lymphoid hyperplasia
  - Diffusely enlarged, hypoechoic, and heterogeneous
    - Typically affect submandibular glands
    - No local invasion (unlike malignant submandibular tumor)
  - Cystic change of parotid glands: Reported but uncommon; may represent a feature of coexisting disease or RD
- Orbits
  - Unilateral diffuse lacrimal gland enlargement and retrobulbar mass may be seen
- Ultrasound-guided biopsy helps in obtaining histological diagnosis
  - Ultrasound also helps in serial follow-up to evaluate any temporal change

CT Findings
- CECT
  - Large, homogeneously enhancing cervical lymph nodes; rarely, hypodense area (cystic change)
  - Enhancing extranodal infiltrates
    - Skin, sinuses, nose, orbit, eyelids, bone, salivary glands, and dura; may be associated with lytic bone change or periosteal reaction

MR Findings
- T1WI
  - Homogeneously hypointense signal
- T2WI
  - Hypointense to hyperintense relative to muscle
  - Hypointense signal reported with lymph nodes, sinuses, and dural lesions
- T1WI C+
  - Large, homogeneously enhancing neck nodes or infiltrating masses
- Site-specific appearance
  - Lymph node disease: Bilateral massive, solid, enhancing cervical lymphadenopathy, rarely with intranodal cystic areas
  - Sinuses: Maxillary > ethmoid sinus polypoid masses, mucosal thickening, &/or soft tissue opacification, ± osseous erosion and soft tissue extension
  - Salivary glands: Multiple lymphoid hyperplasia in the parotid gland; diffusely enlarged, enhancing submandibular glands
  - Orbits: Unilateral > bilateral lacrimal gland enlargement; enhancing extraconal soft tissue mass; eyelid/extraocular muscle infiltration
  - CNS: Intracranial > intraspinal dural-based masses with imaging appearances and signal intensity similar to that of meningiomas on all sequences; dural tail sign is common

Nuclear Medicine Findings
- Tc-99m pertechnetate salivary scans
  - Cold nodules with normal background parenchymal function in parotids = intraparotid lymphadenopathy
  - Involved submandibular gland would show markedly diminished uptake and secretion
- Gallium scan and FDG-18 PET
  - High uptake/hypermetabolic

SINUS HISTIOCYTOSIS (ROSAI-DORFMAN)

DIFFERENTIAL DIAGNOSIS

Non-Hodgkin Lymphoma
- May exactly mimic RD
- Multiple solid, round nodes
- Pseudocystic or reticulated appearance
- Hilar vascularity > peripheral vascularity

Reactive Lymph Nodes
- Large, elliptical, diffuse adenopathy common in children
- Preserved echogenic hilar architecture
- No peripheral vascularity

Tuberculous Adenopathy
- Posterior triangle lymphadenopathy
- Necrosis, matting, collar stud abscess, ± calcification (after treatment)

Langerhans Histiocytosis
- Nodal disease (rare)

Castleman Disease
- Lymphadenopathy may show signal void area due to hypervascular nature
- Retropharyngeal and parapharyngeal lymphadenopathy most commonly affected in neck
- Greater thoracic and abdominal manifestation

Kaposi Sarcoma
- In patients with advanced HIV infection or immunosuppressive therapy
- Lymphadenopathic form occurs in African children

Skull Base Meningioma
- Imaging appearance highly similar to RD with dural lesions of RD except for hypervascularity on angiogram

PATHOLOGY

General Features
- Etiology
  - Unknown
  - Postulated causes: Infection (e.g., Epstein-Barr virus, parvovirus B19, and human herpesvirus 6), immunodeficiency, autoimmune disease, neoplastic process

Microscopic Features
- Characterized by dilated lymph node sinuses filled with lymphocytes, plasma cells, and histiocytes
- Histiocytes classically exhibit emperipolesis
  - Histiocytes phagocytize lymphocytes, plasma cells, erythrocytes, or polymorphonuclear leukocytes
- Intracytoplasmic eosinophilic globules (Russell bodies) in plasma cells

Immunohistochemical Features
- Histiocytes show characteristic RD immunophenotype
  - Strong expression of S100 protein, positivity for histiocytic marker CD68, no reactivity for Langerhans cell marker CD1a

CLINICAL ISSUES

Presentation
- Most common signs/symptoms
  - Painless massive cervical lymphadenopathy
- Other signs/symptoms
  - Related to sites of disease involvement
    - Facial swelling and pain
    - Progressive nasal obstruction, epistaxis
    - Visual disturbance/proptosis, eyelid swelling
    - Salivary gland swelling, xerostomia
    - Headache, ataxia

Natural History & Prognosis
- Long-term clinical course characterized by exacerbations and remission
  - Worse prognosis in patients with extranodal disease
- Progressive course with fatal outcome reported

Treatment
- Clinical observation without treatment is preferred
- Surgical debulking in cases of vital structure compression

DIAGNOSTIC CHECKLIST

Consider
- RD is a rare disease with a variety of imaging manifestations and usually requires histology for diagnosis
- Although most commonly diagnosed in children and adolescents presenting with cervical lymphadenopathy, RD is a well-established diagnosis in all age groups with imaging manifestations throughout head and neck region
- If RD is diagnosed in 1 site, screening and follow-up for other body parts are clinically useful

SELECTED REFERENCES

1. Raslan OA et al: Rosai-Dorfman disease in neuroradiology: imaging findings in a series of 10 patients. AJR Am J Roentgenol. 196(2):W187-93, 2011
2. La Barge DV 3rd et al: Sinus histiocytosis with massive lymphadenopathy (Rosai-Dorfman disease): imaging manifestations in the head and neck. AJR Am J Roentgenol. 191(6):W299-306, 2008
3. Guven G et al: Rosai Dorfman disease of the parotid and submandibular glands: salivary gland scintigraphy and oral findings in two siblings. Dentomaxillofac Radiol. 36(7):428-33, 2007
4. Ahuja AT et al: Sonographic evaluation of cervical lymph nodes. AJR Am J Roentgenol. 184(5):1691-9, 2005
5. Lim R et al: FDG PET of Rosai-Dorfman disease of the thymus. AJR Am J Roentgenol. 182(2):514, 2004
6. Ying M et al: Grey-scale and power Doppler sonography of unusual cervical lymphadenopathy. Ultrasound Med Biol. 30(4):449-54, 2004
7. Yu JQ et al: Demonstration of increased FDG activity in Rosai-Dorfman disease on positron emission tomography. Clin Nucl Med. 29(3):209-10, 2004
8. McAlister WH et al: Sinus histiocytosis with massive lymphadenopathy (Rosai-Dorfman disease). Pediatr Radiol. 20(6):425-32, 1990

SINUS HISTIOCYTOSIS (ROSAI-DORFMAN)

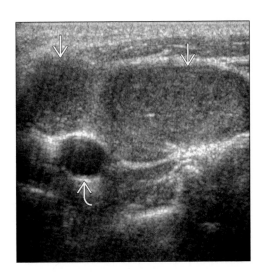
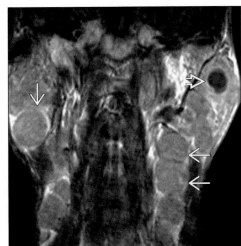

(Left) Transverse grayscale US of a patient with RD shows enlarged submandibular nodes ➡, which are markedly enlarged, solid, and uniformly hypoechoic with no echogenic hilus. There is no intranodal necrosis, associated periadenitis/adjacent soft tissue edema, or abscess formation. The internal carotid artery ➡ is shown. *(Right)* Coronal T1WI MR shows avid enhancement within large nodes ➡ bilaterally. Note the uncommon cystic change, probably within an intraparotid node ➡.

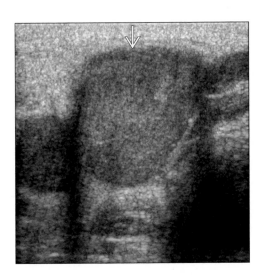
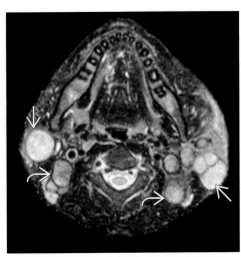

(Left) Transverse grayscale US shows parotid involvement in a patient with RD. Involvement may be in the form of enlarged nodes ➡, as in this case. These nodes are solid, homogeneously hypoechoic, and well-defined with loss of echogenic hilus and no intranodal necrosis. *(Right)* Corresponding axial T2WI FS MR shows multiple nodes, intraparotid ➡ and extraparotid ➡ in location. These are solid, well defined, and hyperintense relative to muscle.

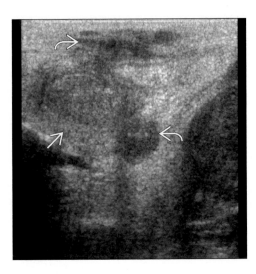
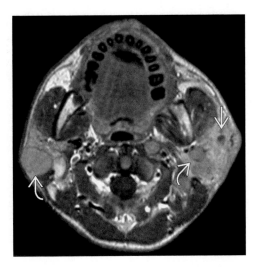

(Left) Transverse grayscale US of a parotid gland shows another form of involvement by RD. The parotid is enlarged with an area of ill-defined hypoechogenicity ➡ and areas of necrosis ➡. Salivary glands may be diffusely enlarged, hypoechoic, and heterogeneous, and contain multiple nodules with no normal intervening parenchyma. *(Right)* Corresponding T1WI C+ shows a necrotic ➡ area within the left parotid, and multiple nodules ➡ in both parotid glands.

BENIGN MASSETER MUSCLE HYPERTROPHY

Key Facts

Terminology

- Benign enlargement of muscles of mastication, most commonly involving masseter muscle

Imaging

- As masseter is superficial in location, US is ideal for diagnosis and for monitoring of treatment
- Smooth, diffuse enlargement of masseter muscle
- Enlarged masseter muscle with normal echogenicity and smooth outline
- No focal mass lesion, heterogeneity, calcification, cystic area within muscle
- Underlying mandibular cortex may be irregular, suggesting bony hyperostosis
- Color Doppler: No abnormal vessels seen in muscle
- Always evaluate underlying salivary glands to rule out salivary lesion simulating benign masseteric hypertrophy (BMH)
- Compare both sides to evaluate masseter muscle

- ○ 50% bilateral, usually asymmetric
- ○ If bilateral, may be difficult to appreciate hypertrophy; evaluate with known US measurements (< 13.5 mm on transverse scans)
- ○ Always compare at fixed landmarks: Angle of mandible, level of ear lobule, point between these 2 locations
- Muscles enlarge up to 3x normal size
- Other masticator muscles (medial and lateral pterygoids, temporalis) may also be involved
  - ○ Due to their location, they are not evaluated by US
- US ideally guides needle position for injection of botulinum toxin A to treat BMH & for follow-up

Top Differential Diagnoses

- Masseter muscle inflammation
- Masseter muscle abscess
- Masseter muscle metastases
- Mandibular metastases

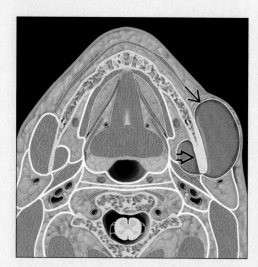
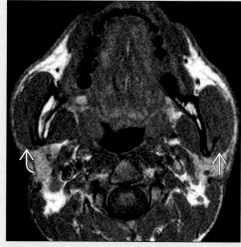

(Left) Axial graphic shows unilateral enlargement of the left masseter muscle ➡. Note underlying mandibular cortical thickening ➢. Compare with the normal contralateral masseter and mandible.
(Right) Corresponding axial T1WI MR shows diffuse enlargement of the left masseter muscle ➡ compared with the right ➢.

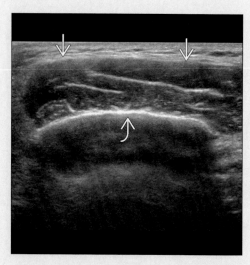
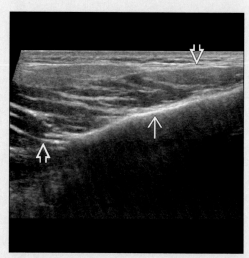

(Left) Transverse grayscale US shows diffuse enlargement of the masseter muscle ➡. Normal transverse diameter of the masseter muscle is < 13.5 mm on US. Note the normal internal architecture and smooth underlying mandibular cortex ➢. In addition to establishing diagnosis, US helps to safely guide intramuscular botulinum toxin A injection for treatment and for monitoring of response.
(Right) Grayscale US shows the normal contralateral masseter muscle ➢ and smooth underlying mandibular cortex ➡.

BENIGN MASSETER MUSCLE HYPERTROPHY

TERMINOLOGY

Synonyms
- Benign masticator muscle hypertrophy (BMMH)
- Benign masseteric hypertrophy (BMH)

Definitions
- Benign enlargement of muscles of mastication, most commonly involving masseter muscle

IMAGING

General Features
- Best diagnostic clue
  - Smooth, diffuse enlargement of masseter muscle
- Location
  - Masticator space; masseter most obviously affected
  - 50% bilateral, usually asymmetric
- Size
  - Muscles enlarge up to 3x normal size
  - Normal transverse diameter of masseter muscle on ultrasound is < 13.5 mm

Ultrasonographic Findings
- Enlarged masseter muscle, normal echogenicity, and smooth outline
- No focal mass lesion, heterogeneity, calcification, or cystic area within muscle
- Underlying mandibular cortex may be irregular, suggesting bony hyperostosis
- Color Doppler: No abnormal vessels are seen in muscle

CT Findings
- NECT
  - Enlarged masticator muscles with normal attenuation; cortical thickening affecting mandible and zygomatic arch
- CECT
  - Enlarged masticator muscles enhance normally

MR Findings
- T1WI
  - Enlarged masticator muscles isointense to normal muscle; decreased marrow signal in areas of cortical thickening (mandible, zygomatic arch)
- T2WI
  - Enlarged masticator muscles isointense to normal muscle
- T1WI C+
  - Enlarged masticator muscles enhance normally

Imaging Recommendations
- Best imaging tool
  - As masseter is superficial in location, US is ideal for diagnosis and for monitoring of treatment
  - Always compare at fixed landmarks: Angle of mandible, level of ear lobule, point between these locations
  - US ideally guides needle position for injection of botulinum toxin A to treat BMH & for follow-up
- Protocol advice
  - Always compare both sides to evaluate masseter muscle
  - If bilateral BMH, may be difficult to appreciate hypertrophy; evaluate with known US measurements (< 13.5 mm on transverse scans)
  - Always evaluate underlying salivary glands to rule out salivary lesion simulating BMH
  - Other masticator muscles (medial and lateral pterygoids, temporalis) may also be involved; due to their location, they are not evaluated by US

DIFFERENTIAL DIAGNOSIS

Masseter Muscle Inflammation
- Edematous, enlarged, hypoechoic masseter ± vascularity

Masseter Muscle Abscess
- Edematous hypoechoic masseter muscle enlargement
- Cystic/hypoechoic fluid collection

Masseter Muscle Metastases
- Solitary/multiple hypoechoic mass along long axis of muscle
- Clinical evidence of disseminated disease

Mandibular Metastases
- Focal bone destruction with mass infiltrating masseter

PATHOLOGY

General Features
- Etiology
  - Bruxism (nocturnal teeth grinding), gum chewing, temporomandibular joint dysfunction
  - Anabolic steroids ± unilateral chewing

Gross Pathologic & Surgical Features
- Normal skeletal muscle
- Process may involve hyperplasia (↑ number of fibers) rather than true hypertrophy

CLINICAL ISSUES

Presentation
- Most common signs/symptoms
  - Nontender lateral facial mass that enlarges with jaw clenching

Demographics
- Age
  - Usually begins in adolescence
- Gender
  - M:F = 2:1

Natural History & Prognosis
- Slowly progressive masticator muscle enlargement

Treatment
- Botulinum toxin A injection
- Surgery only for cosmetic reasons
- Treat temporomandibular joint (TMJ) dysfunction

SELECTED REFERENCES
1. Ahuja AT et al: Diagnostic Imaging: Ultrasound. 1st ed. Salt Lake City: Amirsys, Inc. 11-102-5, 2007
2. To EW et al: A prospective study of the effect of botulinum toxin A on masseteric muscle hypertrophy with ultrasonographic and electromyographic measurement. Br J Plast Surg. 54(3):197-200, 2001

MASSETER MUSCLE MASSES

Key Facts

Terminology
- Mass lesions within masseter muscle

Imaging
- Mass lesion centered in masseter muscle; differentials peculiar to this location
  - Abscess: Complication of odontogenic infection
  - Myositis ossificans: Post-traumatic hypertrophic bone formation within masseter muscle
  - Vascular malformation (VVM); masseter is common location of intramuscular VVM in head and neck
  - Metastasis from carcinoma of breast, colon, lung
  - Soft tissue tumor: Benign, intermediate, or malignant

Top Differential Diagnoses
- Masseter muscle hypertrophy
- Parotid gland tumors
- Subcutaneous lipoma

- Intraparotid lymphadenopathy
- Lymphatic malformation in buccal space
- Mandibular mass

Clinical Issues
- Angle of jaw swelling ± pain, tenderness
- Decrease mobility on clenching of teeth

Diagnostic Checklist
- Identify epicenter of lesion: Masseter vs. parotid, mandible or subcutaneous tissue
- Pertinent clinical data crucial in determining differential diagnosis
- US is ideal for initial investigation due to superficial location of masseter lesion
  - US is able to characterize range of extramasseteric/ benign lesions and guide needle biopsy
- MR for deep tissue or trans-spatial extension

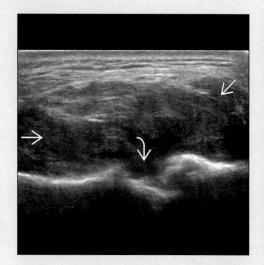
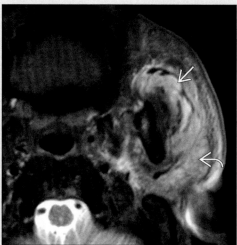

(Left) Longitudinal grayscale US in a patient with acute on chronic dental infection and cheek swelling shows diffuse enlargement of the masseter muscle ➡, which is hypoechoic and ill defined, and break in mandibular cortex due to chronic dental infection ➡. There is no evidence of abscess formation. Visualized superficial parotid gland also showed evidence of acute parotitis (not shown). *(Right)* Corresponding axial T2WI MR shows diffuse inflammation of the masseter muscle ➡ and superficial parotid gland ➡.

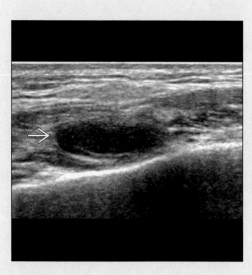
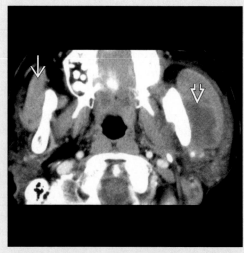

(Left) US shows a focal, hypoechoic intramasseteric "nodule" ➡ with thick walls and necrotic center in a patient with overlying tenderness, fever, and raised white cell count. US features suggest a masseter muscle abscess. Guided aspiration yielded pus and confirmed an abscess. *(Right)* Corresponding axial CECT confirms the intramasseteric location of the abscess ➡ with diffuse enlargement of left masseter muscle due to inflammation/ infection. Compare with normal contralateral masseter muscle ➡.

MASSETER MUSCLE MASSES

TERMINOLOGY

Definitions
- Mass lesions within masseter muscle

IMAGING

Masseter Muscle Abscess
- Rare complication of severe odontogenic infection
- Ill-defined, thick-walled, cystic mass within masseter muscle
- Edema/inflammation of remaining masseter, overlying skin/subcutaneous tissue
- MR indicated to exclude upward extension (in up to 50%) to temporalis &/or lateral pterygoid muscle

Myositis Ossificans
- History of trauma and severe limitation of jaw opening
- Well-defined mass with curvilinear echogenic interface and strong posterior acoustic shadow represents benign hypertrophic bone formation

Venous Vascular Malformation
- Well-defined, hypoechoic, heterogeneous mass with sinusoidal vascular space ± phleboliths (in 20%)
- Slow flow within vascular space may be seen better on grayscale ultrasound than on Doppler

Masseter Muscle Metastasis
- Uncommon; primary from breast, colon, lung, etc.
- Most cases associated with widespread metastasis
- Well-circumscribed, hypoechoic, heterogeneous mass ± necrosis (often along long axis of muscle); diffuse form is rare and mimics masseter muscle hypertrophy
- Does not involve mandibular cortex

Soft Tissue Tumor (STT)
- Benign, intermediate (potential for local invasion or metastasis), or malignant by World Health Organization (WHO) classification
  - Malignant: Rhabdomyosarcoma (children), Ewing sarcoma (adolescents), and liposarcoma and malignant fibrous histiocytoma (older adults)
- Differentiating the many types of STTs or even distinguishing between benign and malignant is often difficult with imaging alone
  - Pertinent clinical data must be taken into account (age, rapidity of onset, duration, pain, history of irradiation, predisposing or concomitant condition)
- US features that may suggest malignant tumor
  - Ill-defined margin, large size (> 5 cm), extracompartmental extension, broad interface with underlying fascia, internal necrosis &/or hemorrhage, local invasion

DIFFERENTIAL DIAGNOSIS

Masseter Muscle Hypertrophy
- Can be symmetrical or asymmetrical, unilateral or bilateral
- Normal echogenicity and muscular architecture
- Intact mandibular cortex

Parotid Gland Tumors
- Superficial parotid tumor ± invasion of masseter

- Benign/slow-growing tumors are well defined ± cystic change; malignant tumors tend to be ill defined ± local invasion and regional lymphadenopathy
  - Sonography cannot differentiate between different types of malignant salivary lesions

Subcutaneous Lipoma
- "Double masseter muscle" appearance
- Echogenic lines parallel to skin on both transverse and longitudinal planes (feathered appearance)

Intraparotid Lymphadenopathy
- Confined by parotid capsule; hypoechoic to parotid gland, well defined, round/oval + echogenic hilum if reactive; ill defined + loss of hilum if malignant

Lymphatic Malformation in Buccal Space
- Well defined, multicystic, septated, with fine debris, trans-spatial with insinuating border

Mandibular Mass
- Encompass developmental asymmetry, osteomyelitis, benign and primary or secondary malignant tumors
- 1 of the most common sites of metastasis in H&N: Irregular mandibular cortex ± cortical disruption

CLINICAL ISSUES

Presentation
- Often present to head and neck surgeon due to angle of jaw swelling ± pain, tenderness
  - Clinically mimic parotid or mandibular mass
- May decrease in mobility on clenching of teeth
- Age and clinical course important information in determining differential diagnosis

DIAGNOSTIC CHECKLIST

Image Interpretation Pearls
- Identify epicenter of lesion: Differential list of masseter muscle pathology very different from list of parotid/mandibular lesion; both are more common
- US is ideal for initial investigation due to superficial location of masseter lesion,
  - Able to characterize range of extramasseteric/benign lesions and guide needle biopsy

SELECTED REFERENCES

1. Razek AA et al: Soft tissue tumors of the head and neck: imaging-based review of the WHO classification. Radiographics. 31(7):1923-54, 2011
2. Schuknecht B et al: Masticator space abscess derived from odontogenic infection: imaging manifestation and pathways of extension depicted by CT and MR in 30 patients. Eur Radiol. 18(9):1972-9, 2008
3. Ahuja AT et al: Sonographic findings in masseter-muscle metastases. J Clin Ultrasound. 28(6):299-302, 2000
4. Eskey CJ et al: Imaging of benign and malignant soft tissue tumors of the neck. Radiol Clin North Am. 38(5):1091-104, xi, 2000
5. Yang WT et al: Sonographic features of head and neck hemangiomas and vascular malformations: review of 23 patients. J Ultrasound Med. 16(1):39-44, 1997
6. Kransdorf MJ: Malignant soft-tissue tumors in a large referral population: distribution of diagnoses by age, sex, and location. AJR Am J Roentgenol. 164(1):129-34, 1995

(Left) Grayscale US shows diffuse masseter muscle enlargement. Note multiple hypoechoic, septate, cystic spaces ➡ within muscle and focal area of curvilinear calcification ➡, features of VVM. Superficial parotid ➡ is shown. On grayscale, slow "to and fro" movement is seen within these cystic spaces. Heavy transducer pressure may compress these vascular channels. *(Right)* Corresponding power Doppler confirms presence of slow vascular flow within VVM. Grayscale US often better shows this slow flow.

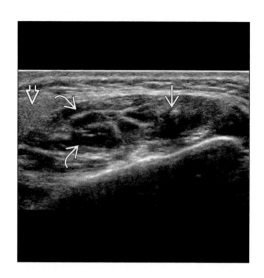
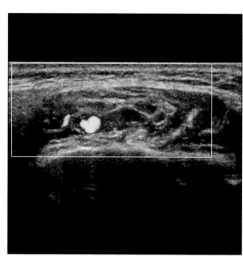

(Left) Longitudinal grayscale US shows focal enlargement of masseter muscle ➡ with subtle, hypoechoic nodule ➡ with borders merging imperceptibly with muscle fibers. Note focal area of curvilinear calcification (phlebolith) within ➡. Features are typical of VVM. In H&N, masseter, digastric, and temporalis are common sites of intramuscular VVM. *(Right)* Corresponding axial T2WI FS MR clearly shows masseter muscle VVM as hyperintense mass ➡ with focal areas of signal void (phleboliths).

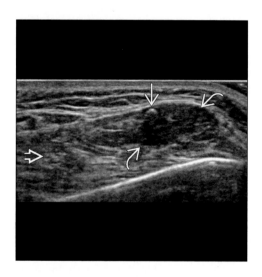
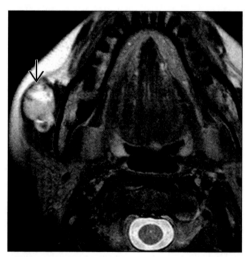

(Left) Transverse grayscale US shows "double masseter." Note normal masseter muscle ➡ and a mass ➡ with striped internal echo pattern superficial to it. This mass lesion demonstrated a similar appearance on longitudinal scan and no significant vascularity on Doppler. US features are consistent with lipoma. *(Right)* Corresponding axial T1W MR confirms location of lipoma ➡ and its relation to masseter muscle ➡. High signal within lipoma was suppressed on fat-suppression sequences.

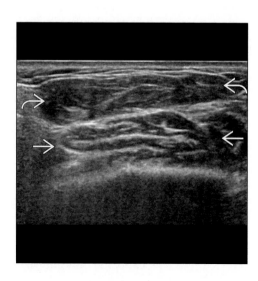
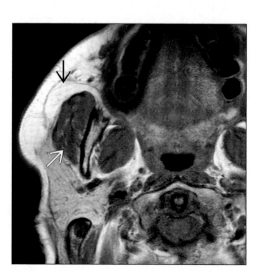

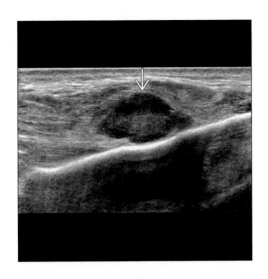

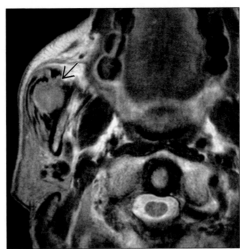

(Left) Longitudinal grayscale US from patient with lung cancer shows masseter muscle metastases ➡ that is solid, well defined, hypoechoic, intramasseteric, & aligned along long axis of muscle. Masseter muscle metastases are invariably accompanied by other sites of involvement (muscle, node, lung, etc.) as part of disseminated disease. *(Right)* Corresponding axial T1-weighted C+ MR shows well-defined, enhancing mets ➡ in right masseter muscle. MR often shows other sites of involvement.

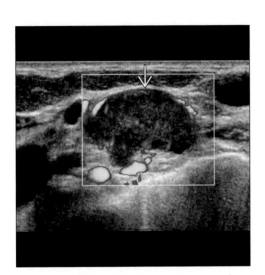

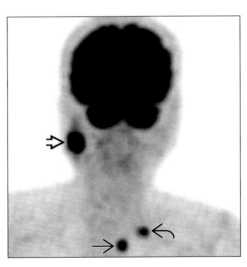

(Left) Transverse power Doppler US (same patient) shows left supraclavicular nodal metastases ➡ with abnormal intranodal vascularity. In addition to nodes, in patients with masseter metastases, other muscles such as digastric, pterygoid, temporalis, sternomastoid may also be involved. *(Right)* Corresponding FDG-18 PET shows hypermetabolic masseter muscle metastases ➡, SCF ➡ and mediastinal ➡ lymphadenopathy in this patient with carcinoma of lung.

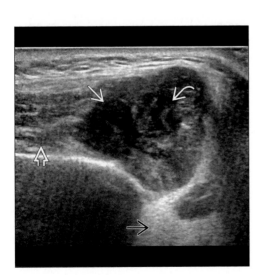

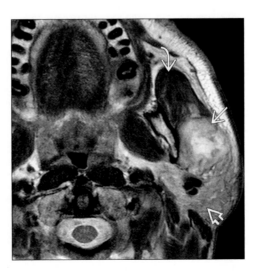

(Left) Transverse grayscale US shows low-grade myxoid fibrosarcoma ➡ in masseter muscle ➡ of a 53-year-old man presenting with rapid-onset, painful angle of jaw swelling. Note irregular, heterogeneous hypoechoic mass with cystic necrosis ➡. US appearances suspicious for soft tissue tumor. Parotid gland ➡ is shown. *(Right)* Corresponding T2WI MR shows heterogeneous, hyperintense signal ➡ within the masseter tumor. Note difficulty in differentiating between masseter ➡ and parotid ➡ origins.

FIBROMATOSIS COLLI

Key Facts

Terminology

- Synonym: Sternocleidomastoid tumor of infancy (SCMTI)
- Definition: Nonneoplastic sternocleidomastoid (SCM) muscle enlargement in early infancy

Imaging

- Nontender SCM muscle enlargement in infant
  - Right > left, rarely bilateral
- Diagnosis often based on clinical exam alone
- Ultrasound confirms clinical suspicion; modality of choice when imaging required (nonionizing, no sedation required)
- Ill-defined, heterogeneous, hyperechoic to hypoechoic mass within SCM in early phase
- Usually large and appears to involve entire SCM on axial plane
- Intact muscle fibers seen on longitudinal plane
- Later fusiform enlargement of SCM muscle

- No extramuscular mass or adenopathy
- Color Doppler: Variable hyperemia in acute phase, ↓ blood flow in fibrotic phase
- FNAC unnecessary and poorly tolerated by infants
- Follow-up US to exclude other neoplasm if lesion is unresolved (usually regresses by 8 months of age)

Top Differential Diagnoses

- Myositis related to neck infection
- Systemic nodal metastases
- Primary cervical neuroblastoma
- Rhabdomyosarcoma
- Teratoma

Clinical Issues

- Mass appears within 2 weeks of delivery
- Mass may increase in size for days to weeks
- 70% present by 2 months of age

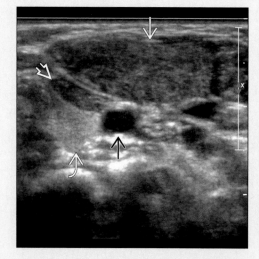
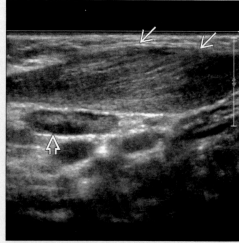

(Left) Transverse grayscale US shows a heterogeneously hyperechoic mass ➡ in the left sternocleidomastoid muscle (SCM). Heterogeneous appearance is believed to represent edema & muscle degeneration of different age. Strap muscle ➡, left lobe of thyroid ➡, and CCA ➡ are also shown. *(Right)* Corresponding longitudinal grayscale US shows marked focal thickening of the lower left SCM ➡. Note intact muscle fibers seen within the SCM. Reactive node ➡ deep to the SCM shows normal architecture.

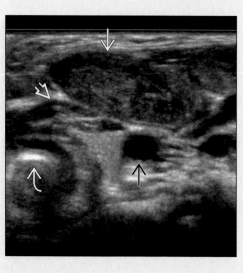
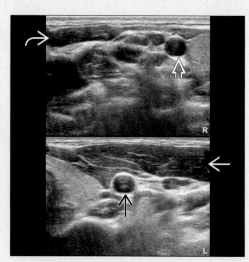

(Left) Axial grayscale US of an infant shows a heterogeneously iso- to hypoechoic mass ➡ within the left SCM. Mass was noticed by the parents a few weeks after delivery. There is no evidence of local invasion or associated lymphadenopathy. Trachea ➡, strap muscle ➡, and CCA ➡ are also shown. *(Right)* Axial US of a baby with torticollis and resolving neck mass shows asymmetrical enlargement of the left SCM ➡. Right SCM at similar level is shown for comparison ➡. Note right ➡ & left ➡ CCA.

FIBROMATOSIS COLLI

TERMINOLOGY

Synonyms
- Sternocleidomastoid tumor of infancy (SCMTI)
- Congenital muscular torticollis

Definitions
- Nonneoplastic sternocleidomastoid (SCM) muscle enlargement in early infancy

IMAGING

General Features
- Best diagnostic clue
  - Nontender SCM muscle enlargement in infant
    - Right > left, rarely bilateral
  - Diagnosis often based on clinical exam alone, without imaging
- Location
  - Mid to lower 1/3 of SCM muscle
    - Rarely, similar process involves trapezius muscle

Ultrasonographic Findings
- Grayscale ultrasound
  - Modality of choice when imaging is required (nonionizing, no sedation required)
  - Ill-defined heterogeneous hyperechoic to hypoechoic mass within SCM in early phase
    - Usually large and appears to involve entire SCM on axial plane
    - Intact muscle fibers seen on longitudinal plane
  - Later fusiform enlargement of SCM muscle
  - No extramuscular mass or adenopathy
- Color Doppler
  - Variable hyperemia in acute phase, ↓ blood flow in fibrotic phase
- FNAC unnecessary and poorly tolerated by infants

CT Findings
- CECT
  - Focal or fusiform enlargement of SCM muscle
  - Isodense compared to normal contralateral muscle
  - Usually not indicated/recommended due to ionizing radiation

MR Findings
- Fusiform enlargement of affected SCM
- Variable signal intensity
  - Usually iso- to hypointense to normal muscle on T1W and diffusely enhances on MR
- Better alternate compared to CT, but does require child to be sedated

Imaging Recommendations
- Best imaging tool
  - Ultrasound confirms clinical suspicion
  - Follow-up scan to exclude other neoplasm if lesion is unresolved (usually regresses by 8 months of age)
- Protocol advice
  - Real-time ultrasound mixed with solid dose of clinical knowledge produces correct diagnosis

DIFFERENTIAL DIAGNOSIS

Myositis Related to Neck Infection
- Tenderness, cellulitis evident clinically
- + inflammatory change and adenopathy

Systemic Nodal Metastases
- Adenopathy deep to normal SCM muscle
- Non-Hodgkin lymphoma/leukemia
- Metastatic neuroblastoma

Primary Cervical Neuroblastoma
- Close association with carotid sheath

Rhabdomyosarcoma
- Rare in newborns
- More discrete mass with aggressive margins

Teratoma
- Complex density (CT) or signal (MR) neck mass
- Often with fat, calcifications

CLINICAL ISSUES

Presentation
- Infant with nontender neck mass following breech or forceps delivery
- Unilateral longitudinal cervical neck mass
- Torticollis in up to 30%; ↓ range of movement
- ± associated plagiocephaly and facial asymmetry

Demographics
- No sex predominance
- 70% present by 2 months of age

Natural History & Prognosis
- Mass appears within 2 weeks of delivery
- Mass may ↑ in size for days to weeks
  - Usually regresses by 8 months of age
- Up to 20% progress to muscular torticollis despite conservative therapy

Treatment
- Most resolve spontaneously ± passive range of motion exercise by parents
- Muscle release or tenotomy for infants with torticollis that fail conservative therapy

DIAGNOSTIC CHECKLIST

Consider
- History of traumatic birth? Mass confined to SCM muscle?
  - If answer yes to both: Diagnosis = fibromatosis colli

SELECTED REFERENCES

1. Murphey MD et al: From the archives of the AFIP: musculoskeletal fibromatoses: radiologic-pathologic correlation. Radiographics. 29(7):2143-73, 2009
2. Wei JL et al: Pseudotumor of infancy and congenital muscular torticollis: 170 cases. Laryngoscope. 111(4 Pt 1):688-95, 2001
3. Cheng JC et al: Sternocleidomastoid pseudotumor and congenital muscular torticollis in infants: a prospective study of 510 cases. J Pediatr. 134(6):712-6, 1999

ESOPHAGOPHARYNGEAL DIVERTICULUM (ZENKER)

Key Facts

Terminology
- Pulsion diverticulum through Killian dehiscence

Imaging
- Oval-shaped or rounded nodule
- Contours may appear irregular if not fully distended
- Well-defined, hypoechoic rim
- Internal echotexture depends on content of diverticula
- Most commonly heterogeneous with multiple small echogenic foci
  - Swallowing leads to change in pattern of echogenic foci ± change in shape of sac
  - Represents debris intermixed with gas
- Arch-like echogenic interface with dirty posterior shadow
  - Less common, represents predominant gas content or gas-fluid level

- Isoechoic or hypoechoic nodule with occasional echogenic foci
  - Less common, represents predominant fluid content

Top Differential Diagnoses
- Killian-Jamieson diverticulum (KJD)
- Paratracheal air cyst
- Papillary carcinoma of thyroid
- Parathyroid adenoma/carcinoma
- Achalasia

Diagnostic Checklist
- Barium swallow or videofluoroscopic study differentiates Zenker diverticulum (ZD) from KJD
- Ultrasound helps to exclude other causes of neck mass if ZD presents as neck lump
- May need NECT if ultrasound is unable to differentiate between gas-containing sac and calcified mass

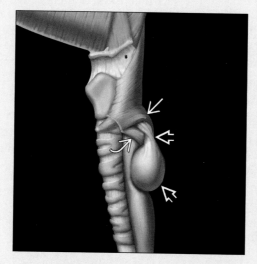
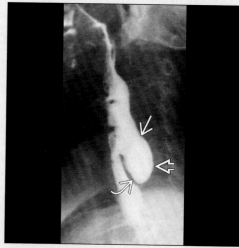

(Left) Graphic depicts a Zenker diverticulum (ZD) ➡ with herniation at the Killian dehiscence between the thyropharyngeal ➡ and cricopharyngeal ➡ fibers of the inferior constrictor muscle. *(Right)* Lateral fluoroscopic spot radiograph during barium swallow shows a ZD ➡ and diverticular neck ➡ protruding from the left posterior wall of the hypopharynx. Note the mass effect on the upper esophagus ➡.

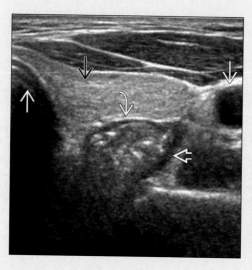
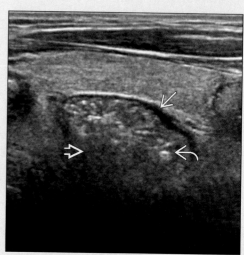

(Left) Transverse grayscale US shows a ZD ➡ as a heterogeneous mass behind left thyroid lobe ➡ in the expected location of the esophagus. Echogenic thyroid capsule ➡ depicts an extrathyroid location. Note the trachea ➡ & CCA. *(Right)* Corresponding longitudinal grayscale US shows a hypoechoic esophageal wall ➡, heterogeneous content in ZD with small echogenic foci ➡, & dirty posterior shadow ➡ representing intraluminal air. The posterior border is obscured due to attenuation by air.

ESOPHAGOPHARYNGEAL DIVERTICULUM (ZENKER)

TERMINOLOGY

Synonyms
- Zenker diverticulum (ZD)
- Pharyngeal pouch, pharyngoesophageal diverticulum, posterior hypopharyngeal diverticulum

Definitions
- Pulsion diverticulum through Killian dehiscence

IMAGING

General Features
- Location
  - Sac in paraesophageal or retroesophageal region, posterior to thyroid lobes
  - Diverticular neck from posterior wall of esophagus
  - Typically left sided
  - May form in midline if large
- Size
  - Variable
  - May be many centimeters in maximum length

Ultrasonographic Findings
- Oval-shaped or rounded nodule
- Contours may appear irregular if not fully distended
- Well-defined, hypoechoic rim
  - Represents muscularis layer
  - Normal layered wall structures are not visualized, may be due to similar echogenicity with sac content
- Medial border obscured by tracheal or esophageal gas
- Posterior border obscured by gas in sac content
- Internal echotexture depends on content of diverticula
  - Most commonly heterogeneous with multiple small echogenic foci
    - Represents debris intermixed with gas
    - Echogenic foci with dirty shadows and mobile content
    - Swallowing leads to change in pattern of echogenic foci ± change in shape of sac
    - Often, no emptying of content after swallowing
    - May mimic papillary thyroid carcinoma with punctate calcification or calcified parathyroid carcinoma/adenoma
  - Arch-like echogenic interface with dirty posterior shadow
    - Less common, represents predominant gas content or gas-fluid level
    - May mimic ring-like calcification or coarse calcification in longstanding thyroid adenoma
  - Isoechoic or hypoechoic nodule with occasional echogenic foci
    - Less common, represents predominant fluid content
- Power/color Doppler
  - Avascular
  - Movement of gas locule may cause scattered false-positive Doppler signal/artifacts

Fluoroscopic Findings
- Barium swallow or videofluoroscopic study (VFSS) for definitive diagnosis
  - Sac-like outpouching arising from posterior wall of hypopharynx, more from left side
  - Diverticular neck arises above cricopharyngeal bar
  - Lateral or oblique lateral view best shows diverticular neck
  - May show associated hiatal hernia and gastroesophageal reflux
  - Irregularity of diverticular mucosa suggests inflammation or neoplasia

CT Findings
- NECT
  - Paraesophageal sac containing debris, fluid, air, or air-fluid level
- CECT
  - Rim enhancement of esophageal wall
  - Diverticulum opens to posterior pharyngeal wall just above level of cricopharyngeus, C5-6 level

MR Findings
- Signal intensity depends on sac content
  - Signal void if contains air
  - Heterogeneous signal if sac contains debris and gas
  - Air-fluid level common
- Enhancement of diverticular wall

Imaging Recommendations
- Best imaging tool
  - Barium swallow or VFSS
    - Establish diagnosis of pharyngoesophageal diverticulum
    - Differentiate ZD from Killian-Jamieson diverticulum (KJD)
      - ZD neck arises above cricopharyngeus from posterior pharyngeal wall
      - KJD neck arises below cricopharyngeus from anterolateral wall
  - Ultrasound helps to exclude other causes of neck mass if ZD presents as neck lump
  - May need NECT if ultrasound is unable to differentiate between gas-containing sac and calcified mass

DIFFERENTIAL DIAGNOSIS

Killian-Jamieson Diverticulum
- Esophageal diverticulum herniated through the Killian-Jamieson space
  - Killian-Jamieson space: Anterolateral wall of the proximal cervical esophagus between cricopharyngeus and insertional fibers of longitudinal esophageal muscles
- Less common than ZD, most are asymptomatic
- 75% are left sided, may be bilateral
- Diverticular neck arises below cricopharyngeal bar

Paratracheal Air Cyst
- Common incidental finding on CT; occurs in 3-4% of population
- Seen in children and adults; cause unknown
- Appearance similar to gas-filled esophageal diverticulum on ultrasound except
  - All are right sided with thinner lesion wall
  - Obscured internal architecture from attenuation by air
  - Size and shape constant on swallowing

Papillary Carcinoma of Thyroid
- Echogenic foci (gas locule) in diverticulum may be difficult to differentiate from punctate calcification

ESOPHAGOPHARYNGEAL DIVERTICULUM (ZENKER)

- May need NECT to differentiate from calcified parathyroid/thyroid nodule
- Differentiation of intrathyroid vs. extrathyroid location important

Parathyroid Adenoma/Carcinoma

- Both are extrathyroidal and can be asymptomatic
- Intralesional vascularity
- Immobile calcification &/or its shadowing
- May require CT to confirm diagnosis

Achalasia

- Dilated esophagus cephalad to gastroesophageal junction
- Usually intrathoracic esophagus only

PATHOLOGY

General Features

- Etiology
  - Multiple causes proposed, likely multifactorial
    - Impaired relaxation of cricopharyngeus (cricopharyngeal dysfunction) and increased intraluminal pressure of hypopharynx
    - Constant increased upper sphincter muscle tone or scarring from esophageal reflux
    - Familial anatomical predisposition to large Killian dehiscence
- Associated abnormalities
  - Almost all have hiatal hernia
  - Many have reflux esophagitis

Gross Pathologic & Surgical Features

- Pulsion diverticulum through Killian dehiscence
  - Full-thickness herniation of esophageal wall
  - Involves mucosa, submucosa, and muscularis layers
- Killian dehiscence
  - Potential area of muscle weakness at dorsal pharyngeal-esophageal wall wall bounded by oblique inferior pharyngeal constrictor muscle and transverse fibers of cricopharyngeal muscle
  - Not to be confused with Killian-Jamieson space where KJD herniates

CLINICAL ISSUES

Presentation

- Most common signs/symptoms
  - Suprasternal dysphagia
  - May report regurgitation of contents or halitosis
  - Aspiration pneumonia common
  - Heartburn due to gastroesophageal reflux
- Other signs/symptoms
  - Occasionally presents as lower neck swelling or goiter
  - Boyce sign (neck swelling that gurgles on palpation)
  - May be incidentally detected on ultrasound if asymptomatic

Demographics

- Age
  - Middle age and elderly
  - Usually > 60 years of age; rarely < 40 years of age
- Gender
  - M > F
- Ethnicity

- Rare in Japan and Indonesia
- Epidemiology
  - 0.01–0.11% of population

Natural History & Prognosis

- Symptoms increase as diverticulum enlarges
- Complications mostly related to aspiration of retained ingested material
- Squamous cell carcinoma is rare complication (0.3%)
  - Uniformly poor prognosis
  - Progressive dysphagia, aphagia ± hemoptysis
  - Usually found in distal 2/3 of pouch
  - May be found only at histology

Treatment

- Less invasive treatment as mainstay since most affect frail elderly patients
- No randomized studies comparing different surgical and endoscopic approaches although general indications have emerged
  - Conservative treatment if patient asymptomatic or unfit for surgery
  - Small to medium-sized (< 5 cm) diverticula treated endoscopically: Laser or electrocoagulation (Dohlman technique), stapling
  - Very large diverticula may benefit from surgical excision, inversion, or suspension, especially in younger patients fit for surgery

DIAGNOSTIC CHECKLIST

Consider

- Intrathyroid vs. extrathyroid location
- Gas locule vs. microcalcification
- Barium swallow or VFSS for definitive diagnosis
- Exclude hiatus hernia, gastroesophageal reflux, and SCCa

SELECTED REFERENCES

1. Bizzotto A et al: Zenker's diverticulum: exploring treatment options. Acta Otorhinolaryngol Ital. 33(4):219-229, 2013
2. Herbella FA et al: Esophageal diverticula and cancer. Dis Esophagus. 25(2):153-8, 2012
3. Kim HK et al: Characteristics of Killian-Jamieson diverticula mimicking a thyroid nodule. Head Neck. 34(4):599-603, 2012
4. Lixin J et al: Sonographic diagnosis features of Zenker diverticulum. Eur J Radiol. 80(2):e13-9, 2011
5. Singaporewalla RM et al: Pharyngoesophageal diverticulum resembling a thyroid nodule on ultrasound. Head Neck. 33(12):1800-3, 2011
6. Grant PD et al: Pharyngeal dysphagia: what the radiologist needs to know. Curr Probl Diagn Radiol. 38(1):17-32, 2009
7. Buterbaugh JE et al: Paratracheal air cysts: a common finding on routine CT examinations of the cervical spine and neck that may mimic pneumomediastinum in patients with traumatic injuries. AJNR Am J Neuroradiol. 29(6):1218-21, 2008
8. Ferreira LE et al: Zenker's diverticula: pathophysiology, clinical presentation, and flexible endoscopic management. Dis Esophagus. 21(1):1-8, 2008
9. Rubesin SE et al: Killian-Jamieson diverticula: radiographic findings in 16 patients. AJR Am J Roentgenol. 177(1):85-9, 2001

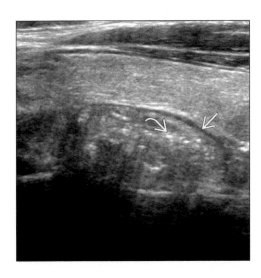

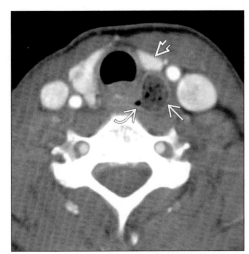

(Left) After swallowing, the "nodule" has slightly changed in contour ➡ and arrangement of internal echogenic foci ➡, suggesting communication with the upper digestive tract. Note that the contents of ZD have not emptied despite swallowing. (Right) Axial CECT shows a heterogeneous mass ➡ containing floccules of air posterior to the left thyroid lobe ➡. The medial aspect of the mass ➡ communicates with the posterolateral wall of the cervical esophagus.

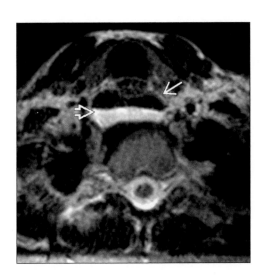

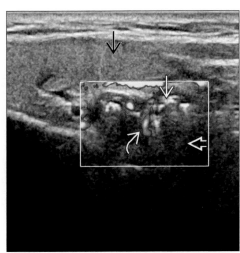

(Left) Axial T2WI MR demonstrates a large ZD in the retroesophageal region ➡. Air-fluid level ➡ is another common appearance on CT and MR and may not be clearly appreciated on US. (Right) Longitudinal power Doppler US shows a right-sided retrothyroid nodule with multiple echogenic gas foci ➡. Note the dirty posterior shadow ➡ and Doppler signal artifact ➡. Differential diagnoses include paratracheal air cyst and pharyngoesophageal diverticulum. The thyroid ➡ is also shown.

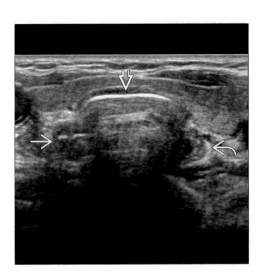

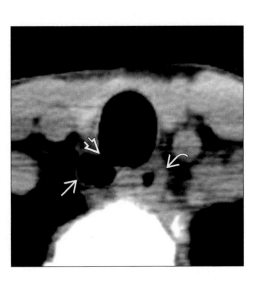

(Left) Transverse grayscale ultrasound of the same patient shows the "nodule" in the right paratracheal region ➡ whereas the esophagus ➡ is seen on the left side. The trachea ➡ is also shown. (Right) Corresponding axial CECT confirms a paratracheal air cyst ➡ communicating with the trachea ➡. No obvious connection with the esophagus ➡ is evident.

LARYNGOCELE

Key Facts

Terminology

- Synonyms
  - Internal laryngocele = simple laryngocele
  - Mixed (combined, external) laryngocele = laryngocele with extralaryngeal extension

Imaging

- **External laryngocele**
  - Outpouching in lateral/anterior neck with isthmus/waist through thyrohyoid membrane
  - Strong curvilinear echogenic line with mobile posterior shadow if gas filled
  - Anechoic cystic or containing debris if fluid filled
- **Internal laryngocele**
  - Inconspicuous on sonography if small or obscured by airway gas or thyroid cartilage calcification
  - If air filled, appears as echogenic interface deep to thyrohyoid membrane, difficult to differentiate from normal laryngeal or hypopharyngeal gas

- **Pyolaryngocele**
  - Thick walled, with echogenic, mobile content
- **Secondary laryngocele**
  - Soft tissue tumor in ipsilateral inferior supraglottic larynx (or larynx may be seen through thyrohyoid membrane or noncalcified thyroid cartilage)

Top Differential Diagnoses

- Thyroglossal duct cyst
- 2nd branchial cleft cyst
- Paratracheal air cyst

Diagnostic Checklist

- Do not forget to look for occult squamous cell carcinoma in low supraglottis or glottic larynx
- Remember that endoscopy is necessary to fully exclude obstructing mass

(Left) Coronal graphic shows a laryngocele ➡ with extralaryngeal extension. There is an isthmus ➡ where the lesion squeezes through the thyrohyoid membrane to the low submandibular space. Note stenosis at the laryngeal ventricle ➡.
(Right) Oblique grayscale US shows a laryngocele ➡ with extralaryngeal extension. US is unable to evaluate the entire extent of a mixed laryngocele as its internal component is obscured by airway gas or thyroid cartilage calcification. (Courtesy A. Momin, MD.)

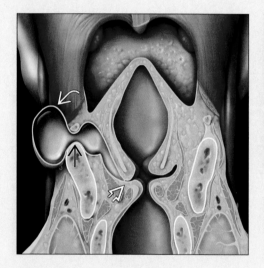
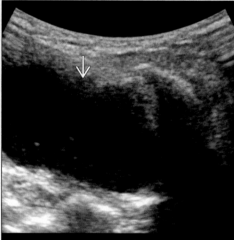

(Left) Corresponding axial grayscale US (same patient) shows a mixed laryngocele ➡ as an anechoic, thin-walled, fluid-filled structure. Note the isthmic waist ➡ at the thyrohyoid membrane and hyoid bone ➡. (Courtesy A. Momin, MD.) (Right) Axial CECT (same patient) shows a mixed laryngocele as well-defined, thin-walled, fluid-filled structure with an isthmus ➡ at the thyrohyoid membrane. Note the intralaryngeal ➡ and extralaryngeal ➡ components lying low in the submandibular space. (Courtesy A. Momin, MD.)

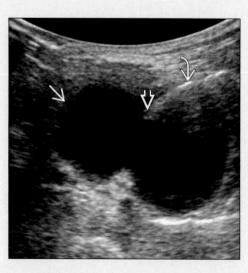
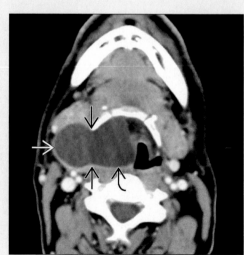

LARYNGOCELE

TERMINOLOGY

Synonyms
- Laryngeal mucocele
- Internal laryngocele = simple laryngocele
- Mixed laryngocele (combined, external) = laryngocele with extralaryngeal extension

Definitions
- Laryngeal saccule
  - Normal mucosal outpouching projecting superiorly from laryngeal ventricle
  - Contains numerous mucous glands
  - Some think function of saccule is to lubricate true cords
- Internal laryngocele
  - Dilated air- or fluid-filled laryngeal saccule
  - Located in paraglottic space of supraglottis
- Mixed laryngocele
  - Extends from paraglottic space through thyrohyoid membrane to low submandibular space (SMS)
  - Contains internal (intralaryngeal) and external (extralaryngeal) components
- Pyolaryngocele
  - Pus-containing superinfected laryngocele
- Secondary laryngocele
  - 15% of all laryngoceles
  - Laryngocele developed secondary to obstructive lesion in glottic or inferior supraglottic larynx
  - Due to tumor, e.g., squamous cell carcinoma (SCCa), post-inflammatory stenosis, trauma, surgery, or amyloid

IMAGING

General Features
- Best diagnostic clue
  - Thin-walled, air- or fluid-filled cystic lesion communicating with laryngeal ventricle
  - ± extralaryngeal extension through thyrohyoid membrane
- Location
  - Internal laryngocele: Supraglottic paraglottic space
  - Mixed laryngocele: Paraglottic space extends through thyrohyoid membrane and SMS
- Size
  - Variable
  - May ↑ with trumpet (forced expiration against closed mouth and nasopharynx) or Valsalva maneuver
- Morphology
  - Circumscribed, thin walled
  - Larger lesions have isthmus when passing outside larynx through thyrohyoid membrane
  - Pyolaryngocele: Thickened walls with adjacent inflammation
  - Secondary laryngocele: Infiltrating mass in low supraglottis or glottis

Ultrasonographic Findings
- External laryngocele
  - Outpouching in lateral or anterior neck with isthmus/waist through thyrohyoid membrane
  - Strong curvilinear echogenic line with mobile posterior shadow if gas filled
  - Anechoic cystic or containing debris if fluid filled
  - Thin walled, representing respiratory mucosa
  - Enlargement with trumpet maneuver
- Internal laryngocele
  - Often inconspicuous on sonography if small or obscured by airway gas or thyroid cartilage calcification
  - Air filled: Echogenic interface deep to thyrohyoid membrane, difficult to differentiate from normal laryngeal or hypopharyngeal gas
  - Fluid filled: May be partially seen as thin-walled, cystic paraglottic lesion at supraglottic level
    - Differentiation from other laryngeal cysts may be difficult due to obscured anatomical origin
      - Use CT for further evaluation
- Pyolaryngocele
  - Thick walled, with echogenic, mobile content
- Secondary laryngocele
  - Soft tissue tumor in ipsilateral inferior supraglottic larynx
    - Larynx may be seen through thyrohyoid membrane or noncalcified thyroid cartilage
  - Vascularity within solid tumor

Radiographic Findings
- Air pocket seen in upper cervical soft tissues
- Soft tissue/fluid density projects against air column in supraglottic region

CT Findings
- CECT
  - Internal laryngocele: Fluid or air density, thin walled, circumscribed, in paraglottic space of supraglottis
    - Absent to minimal peripheral enhancement
    - Paraglottic lesion connects to laryngeal ventricle, best seen on coronal CT
  - Pyolaryngocele: Thick enhancing walls
  - Mixed laryngocele: Paraglottic cyst passes through thyrohyoid membrane into SMS with isthmus/waist at thyrohyoid membrane
  - Secondary laryngocele: Enhancing infiltrative glottic or low supraglottic tumor
    - Laryngocele seen cephalad to tumor

MR Findings
- Low T1W, high T2W, thin walled, with fluid intensity
- Thin walled, with absent to minimal linear peripheral enhancement
- Thick enhancing walls if pyolaryngocele

Nuclear Medicine Findings
- I-131 scan: Rare cause of false-positive uptake mimicking thyroid remnant after thyroidectomy for papillary thyroid carcinoma

Imaging Recommendations
- Best imaging tool: CECT of cervical soft tissues
- Coronal reformatted images best demonstrate relationship to laryngeal ventricle, thyrohyoid membrane, and SMS

DIFFERENTIAL DIAGNOSIS

Thyroglossal Duct Cyst
- Midline cystic mass in vicinity of hyoid bone, embedded in infrahyoid strap muscles
- Variable sonographic appearances

LARYNGOCELE

○ Anechoic, septated, pseudosolid, thick walled if infected, no significant associated vascularity

2nd Branchial Cleft Cyst

- Characteristic location; displaces submandibular gland anteromedially, carotid space medially, and sternocleidomastoid muscle posterolaterally
- Variable sonographic appearances: Anechoic, septated, pseudosolid, thick walled, ± vascularity if infected

Paratracheal Air Cyst

- Often right-sided, thin-walled, air-filled outpouching connected to tracheal wall
- Echogenic mobile pocket of air with posterior shadowing, paratracheal in location
- CT to delineate connection with tracheal lumen

Esophagopharyngeal Diverticulum

- Air- or fluid-filled outpouching off lateral hypopharyngeal wall

Supraglottitis With Abscess

- Thick-walled cystic lesion in anterior neck
- Not connected to laryngeal ventricle or thyrohyoid membrane

PATHOLOGY

General Features

- Etiology
  ○ Commonly acquired, rarely congenital
  ○ Increased intraglottic pressure creates ball-valve phenomenon at communication of laryngeal ventricle with saccule
    ▪ Saccule (appendix of laryngeal ventricle) expands
    ▪ Causes: Glass blowing, playing a wind instrument, excessive coughing
  ○ Secondary laryngoceles from proximal saccular obstruction are less common (15%)
    ▪ Causes: Tumor, post-inflammatory stenosis, trauma, surgery, or amyloid

Gross Pathologic & Surgical Features

- Smooth-surfaced, sac-like specimen

Microscopic Features

- Lined by respiratory epithelium (ciliated, columnar) with fibrous wall

CLINICAL ISSUES

Presentation

- Most common signs/symptoms
  ○ Principal presenting symptom
    ▪ Internal laryngocele: Larger lesions present with hoarseness or stridor
      – When small, often incidental and asymptomatic
    ▪ Mixed laryngocele: Anterior neck mass in low SMS just below angle of mandible
      – May expand with modified Valsalva maneuver
- Other signs/symptoms
  ○ Sore throat, dysphagia, stridor, airway obstruction
- Clinical profile
  ○ Glass blowers, wind instrument players, chronic coughers, weightlifters

Demographics

- Age
  ○ > 50 years old at presentation
- Gender
  ○ More common in males
- Ethnicity
  ○ More common in Caucasians
- Epidemiology
  ○ Bilateral laryngoceles: 30%
  ○ Internal laryngocele is 2x more common than mixed laryngocele

Natural History & Prognosis

- Gradual enlargement over time
- With continued growth, laryngocele penetrates thyrohyoid membrane to enter neck in lower SMS
- Excellent prognosis after removal

Treatment

- Must endoscopically exclude an underlying lesion of true or false cords obstructing laryngeal ventricle
- Isolated internal laryngocele: Endoscopic CO_2 laser resection
- Mixed laryngocele: Requires external surgical procedure

DIAGNOSTIC CHECKLIST

Consider

- If lesion changes size with Valsalva
- If patient is a glass blower, wind instrument player, or chronic cougher

Image Interpretation Pearls

- Best diagnostic clue: Fluid- or air-filled, thin-walled lesion communicating with laryngeal ventricle
- Do not forget to look for occult SCCa in low supraglottic or glottic larynx
  ○ Secondary laryngoceles account for 15% of all laryngoceles
- Coronal plane CECT best shows relationships to laryngeal ventricle and thyrohyoid membrane

SELECTED REFERENCES

1. Conkbayir I et al: Trumpet maneuver in the sonographic diagnosis of an external laryngocele. J Clin Ultrasound. 38(1):56-8, 2010
2. Dursun G et al: Current diagnosis and treatment of laryngocele in adults. Otolaryngol Head Neck Surg. 136(2):211-5, 2007
3. Schmidt M et al: False-positive uptake of I-131 in a laryngocele mimicking thyroid remnant after thyroidectomy for papillary thyroid carcinoma. Clin Nucl Med. 31(11):716-7, 2006
4. Harney M et al: Laryngocele and squamous cell carcinoma of the larynx. J Laryngol Otol. 115(7):590-2, 2001
5. Ahuja AT et al: Lumps and Bumps in the Head and Neck. Cambridge: Cambridge University Press, 2000
6. Nazaroglu H et al: Laryngopyocele: signs on computed tomography. Eur J Radiol. 33(1):63-5, 2000
7. Alvi A et al: Computed tomographic and magnetic resonance imaging characteristics of laryngocele and its variants. Am J Otolaryngol. 19(4):251-6, 1998
8. Arslan A et al: Laryngeal amyloidosis with laryngocele: MRI and CT. Neuroradiology. 40(6):401-3, 1998

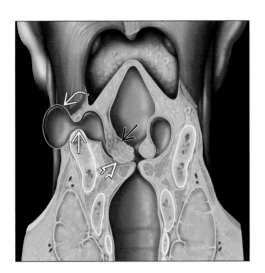

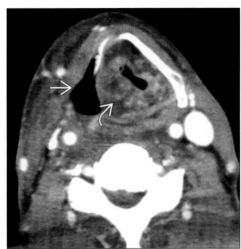

(Left) Coronal graphic shows a laryngocele ➡ with extralaryngeal extension. There is an isthmus ➡ where the lesion squeezes through the thyrohyoid membrane to the low submandibular space. Note stenosis at the laryngeal ventricle ➡ due to an adjacent tumor mass ➡. (Right) Axial CECT shows a well-defined, air-filled laryngocele ➡, paraglottic in location on the right. Note the adjacent tumor mass ➡ identifying it as secondary laryngocele. Secondary laryngoceles account for 15% of all laryngoceles.

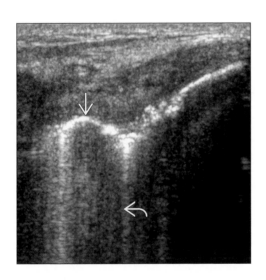

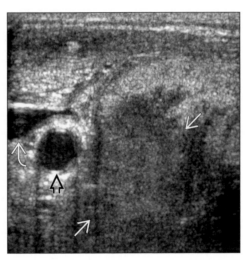

(Left) Axial grayscale US (same patient) shows an external laryngocele as an air-filled echogenic pocket ➡ with marked posterior shadowing ➡. (Right) Axial grayscale US (same patient) shows an ill-defined, hypoechoic heterogeneous laryngeal mass ➡. This is best visualized/evaluated by CECT. Coronal reformatted CT often clearly shows the relationship of a laryngocele to the submandibular space, thyrohyoid membrane or laryngeal ventricle. Note common carotid artery ➡ and internal jugular vein ➡.

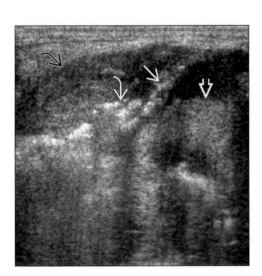

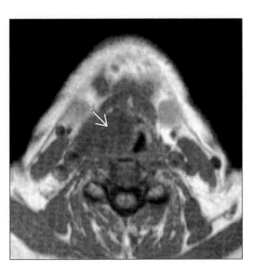

(Left) Axial grayscale US shows a mixed laryngocele. The external component ➡ is filled with fluid, debris, and echogenic gas ➡. The internal component ➡, seen under the laryngeal skeleton, shows homogeneous internal echoes. MR, CECT, or endoscopy is essential to rule out associated tumor. Note the thyroid cartilage ➡. (Right) Axial T1WI MR shows a low-intensity, circumscribed right paraglottic lesion ➡ with mass effect on the laryngeal airway. It abuts but does not extend through the thyrohyoid membrane.

CERVICAL ESOPHAGEAL CARCINOMA

Key Facts

Imaging

- Concentric or eccentric, ill-defined, infiltrative, hypoechoic esophageal mass ± vascularity
- Disrupts layers of esophageal wall
- May contain echogenic foci with "dirty" shadow, which represents air from esophageal lumen
- Frequent extension to hypopharynx or larynx
- Invasion of tracheoesophageal groove, adjacent soft tissue, and thyroid gland is common
- Level VI nodal involvement is most common
- US + FNAC evaluates cervical lymph nodes for metastatic disease
- PET/CT is best imaging tool for staging, monitoring, and surveillance
  - CT: Local disease extent
  - PET: Regional and distant disease
- US evaluates indeterminate lesions (often thyroid nodules) detected on PET

Top Differential Diagnoses

- Hypopharyngeal squamous cell carcinoma
- Thyroid anaplastic carcinoma
- Thyroid non-Hodgkin lymphoma

Pathology

- Strong association with tobacco and alcohol abuse
- > 95% are squamous cell carcinomas

Clinical Issues

- Typically presents with dysphagia, weight loss
- Frequently detected late; poor prognosis
- 15% have synchronous or metachronous tumors
- Distant metastases to liver, lung, pleura, and bones

Diagnostic Checklist

- Cervical node involvement is important for staging and treatment options
- Look for possible 2nd primary malignancy

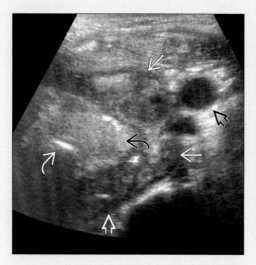
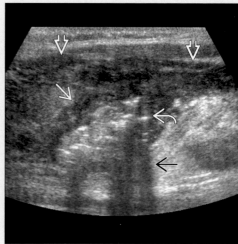

(Left) Transverse grayscale US of the left lower central compartment shows an ill-defined, heterogeneous, hypoechoic mass extending from the cervical esophagus ➡ to the perithyroidal tissue ➡. Normal esophageal layers are lost. Note the trachea ➡, thyroid ➡, and CCA ▷. *(Right)* Corresponding longitudinal US shows an infiltrative, hypoechoic esophageal mass ➡ extending to the anterior visceral space ➡. Note the internal echogenic foci ➡ with "dirty" shadows ➡ representing esophageal intraluminal gas.

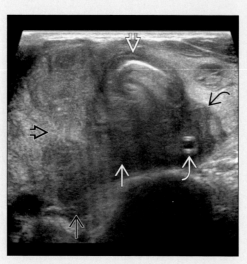
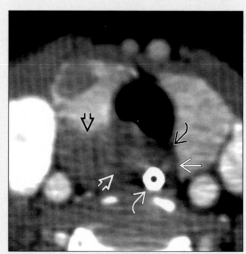

(Left) Transverse grayscale US shows a carcinoma arising from the cervical esophagus ➶ on the left, extending posterior to the trachea ➡ and across the midline ➡ to involve the right thyroid ➹ and adjacent soft tissue ➡. Note the nasogastric tube ➡. *(Right)* Corresponding axial CECT shows a locally invasive hypoenhancing esophageal tumor ➡. Involvement posterior to the trachea ➡ and tracheoesophageal groove ➶ is better delineated than on US. Note the right lobe thyroid invasion ➹ and nasogastric tube ➡.

CERVICAL ESOPHAGEAL CARCINOMA

TERMINOLOGY

Abbreviations
- Cervical esophageal carcinoma (CECa)

Definitions
- Malignancy of lining epithelium of cervical esophagus
  - > 95% are squamous cell carcinomas (SCCa)

IMAGING

General Features
- Primary tumor
  - Location: Lower border of cricoid to thoracic inlet
  - Concentric or eccentric esophageal thickening with ill-defined, infiltrative outer margins
  - Frequent extension to hypopharynx or larynx
  - Local invasion of tracheoesophageal groove, soft tissue of central compartment, and thyroid gland is common
- Metastatic cervical lymph node
  - Upward lymphatic spread is most common in patients with cervical esophageal carcinomas
  - 70% have level VI node involvement at diagnosis

Ultrasonographic Findings
- Primary tumor
  - Concentric or eccentric, ill-defined, infiltrative, hypoechoic esophageal mass ± vascularity
  - Disrupts layers of esophageal wall
  - May contain echogenic foci with "dirty" shadows, which represent air from esophageal lumen (not to be confused with calcification)
    - Movement of gas locules on swallowing in real time
  - Invasion of tracheoesophageal groove and extension posterior to trachea may be obscured by tracheal shadowing
- Metastatic cervical lymph node
  - Similar to metastatic nodes from SCCa of other sites
  - Intranodal necrosis is common
  - Level VI nodal involvement is most common
  - US may not be able to evaluate deep paratracheal lymphadenopathy

Imaging Recommendations
- Best imaging tool
  - PET/CT is best imaging tool for staging, monitoring, and surveillance
    - SCCa is consistently FDG avid
    - Exhibits high sensitivity in detecting regional and distant disease compared with CT, MR, and USG
    - CT is used for evaluation of local disease extent
    - PET is used for regional or distant disease
  - MR is helpful for prevertebral invasion, which is seen as loss of fat planes
  - US is helpful for evaluating indeterminate lesions (often thyroid nodules) detected on PET
    - Also guides FNAC to evaluate cervical lymph nodes for metastatic disease

DIFFERENTIAL DIAGNOSIS

Hypopharyngeal Squamous Cell Carcinoma
- Arises at or above cricoid level
- May extend into esophagus

Thyroid Anaplastic Carcinoma
- Heterogeneous, infiltrative thyroid mass
- In elderly patient with rapidly enlarging neck mass

Thyroid Non-Hodgkin Lymphoma
- Heterogeneous infiltrative thyroid mass ± malignant nodes
- ± features of antecedent Hashimoto thyroiditis

Thyroid Differentiated Carcinoma
- Hypoechoic thyroid mass ± punctate calcification
- Calcification &/or cystic change in adenopathy

PATHOLOGY

General Features
- Etiology
  - Strong association with tobacco and alcohol abuse
  - Increased incidence with caustic stricture, achalasia, prior radiation
  - Association with Plummer-Vinson syndrome
- Associated abnormalities
  - 15% have synchronous or metachronous tumors
    - Especially head and neck SCCa, lung carcinoma

Staging, Grading, & Classification
- AJCC staging as for all esophageal carcinomas
  - T1-T3 are defined by depth of invasion of wall
  - T4a tumor invades resectable structures
  - T4b tumor invades nonresectable structures

CLINICAL ISSUES

Presentation
- Most common signs/symptoms
  - Dysphagia, weight loss

Demographics
- Peak age: 55-65 years
- Gender: M:F = 4:1

Natural History & Prognosis
- Tendency to invade local structures
- Frequently detected late with poor prognosis
- Distant metastases to liver, lung, pleura, and bones
- Overall 5-year survival rate: 10-55%

Treatment
- Preferred
  - Definitive chemoradiotherapy
- Alternative
  - Radical resection of esophagus and hypopharynx with jejunal interposition or gastric pull-up

DIAGNOSTIC CHECKLIST

Image Interpretation Pearls
- Cervical node involvement is important for staging and treatment options
- Look for possible 2nd primary malignancy

SELECTED REFERENCES

1. Ng T et al: Advances in the surgical treatment of esophageal cancer. J Surg Oncol. 101(8):725-9, 2010

VOCAL CORD PARALYSIS

Key Facts

Terminology

- Vocal cord paralysis (VCP), true vocal cord paralysis (TVCP), recurrent laryngeal nerve paralysis (RLNP)
- Immobilization of true vocal cord by ipsilateral vagus (CN10) or recurrent laryngeal nerve dysfunction

Imaging

- Affected cord is flaccid and paramedian in location
- Primary imaging findings are in larynx
- Causative lesions can be anywhere from medulla (CN10 origin) to recurrent laryngeal nerve

Top Differential Diagnoses

- Laryngeal trauma
- Laryngeal and piriform sinus SCCa
- Post-treatment change

Pathology

- Injury to or lesion compressing CN10 anywhere from medulla to recurrent laryngeal nerve
- Most common etiologies: Neoplasm, vascular lesion, trauma, idiopathic, and nonmalignant thoracic pathology

Diagnostic Checklist

- If vocal cord paralysis evident on ultrasound, search for neck neoplasms from larynx, hypopharynx, or thyroid and neck nodal metastases
- CT is useful to look for intrathoracic peripheral lesions causing RLN palsy
- MR is indicated when central-proximal vagal neuropathy is suspected
- Neck neoplasms, arytenoid subluxation/dislocation, and injection laryngoplasty may mimic VCP

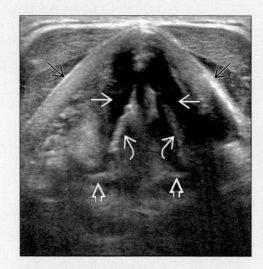
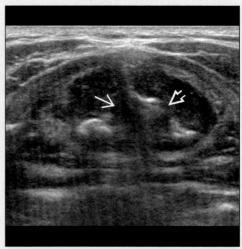

(Left) Axial grayscale ultrasound of true vocal cords at midline transverse plane demonstrates echogenic vocal ligaments ➡, hypoechoic vocalis muscles ➡, arytenoid cartilages ➡, and thyroid laminae ➡. *(Right)* Axial grayscale ultrasound demonstrates complete right cord paralysis with the affected right cord lying in a paramedian position ➡. Note normal abduction of the left cord ➡.

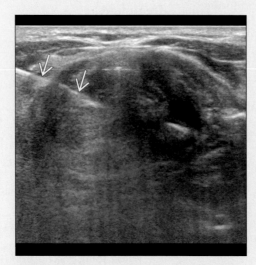
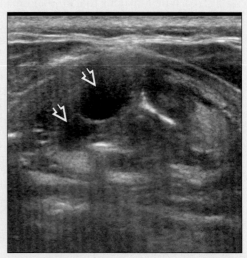

(Left) Ultrasound-guided vocal cord augmentation shows the transcartilaginous insertion of the needle ➡ through the right thyroid lamina into the right paraglottic space. *(Right)* Axial grayscale ultrasound post injection laryngoplasty shows hypoechoic injected material ➡ in right paraglottic space, resulting in "medialization" of the paralyzed right cord in order to regain glottic closure and competence.

VOCAL CORD PARALYSIS

TERMINOLOGY

Abbreviations
- Vocal cord paralysis (VCP), true vocal cord paralysis (TVCP), recurrent laryngeal nerve paralysis (RLNP)

Definitions
- Immobilization of true vocal cord (VC) by ipsilateral vagus (CN10) or recurrent laryngeal nerve dysfunction

IMAGING

General Features
- Best diagnostic clue
  - Affected cord is flaccid and paramedian in location
- Location
  - Primary imaging findings are in larynx
  - Causative lesions can be anywhere from medulla (CN10 origin) to recurrent laryngeal nerve

Ultrasonographic Findings
- Many laryngeal component parts are superficial and have good inherent soft tissue contrast suitable for evaluation by high-resolution ultrasound
- Vocal cords can be visualized by 5 MHz transducers, but scanning frequencies of 7.5 MHz or higher are recommended for better anatomical details
- Midline transverse plane is most useful in assessing movement of the vocal cords, as movement of both sides can be directly compared
  - Despite free edge of true cord having poor reflective angle to sound beam at this angle, image quality will usually suffice for cord mobility evaluation, even in heavily calcified laryngeal cartilage
- Sonographic anatomy: True vocal cords are composed of echogenic vocal ligaments that run along free edge and overlie hypoechoic vocalis muscle
  - False cords overlie echogenic paraglottic fat and sometimes variable hyperechogenicities from laryngeal vestibule
- Visualization of arytenoid cartilages also aids in assessment of symmetry
- Semon law: Partial lesion of recurrent laryngeal nerve affects abduction before adduction; thus, both should be assessed
- Vocal cord movement during quiet breathing: Normal vocal cords abduct on inspiration and relax towards the midline on expiration
- Assessment of voluntary movement during phonation: When patient phonates (such as "eeeee"), normal cord should be seen to adduct and vibrate
  - With cessation of phonation, cords return to their resting position
  - Cord adduction is assessed while patient takes deep inspiration or performs Valsalva maneuver
- Paralysis of posterior cricoarytenoid muscle results in anteromedial subluxation of arytenoid and medialization of posterior aspect of true cord
  - Bilateral paralysis of this muscle causes dyspnea due to inability to abduct vocal cords
- In complete cord paralysis, affected cord lies in paramedian position
- Extracranially, vagus nerve descends posterolateral to internal carotid artery (ICA) in carotid sheath, and is invariably visualized by US

- RLN cannot be consistently or reliably seen on ultrasound
- VCP may result from lesions affecting vagus nerve or RLN
- Identification of VCP on ultrasound should prompt search for neck neoplasms such as carcinoma of larynx or hypopharynx, thyroid, or metastatic lymph nodes
- Best imaging tool
  - Ultrasound may be used to assess vocal cord mobility when laryngoscopy is not readily available or not tolerated by patients
  - Ultrasound also helps guide injections into vocal cord
  - Overall, role of ultrasound in evaluating VC abnormalities is limited

CT Findings
- CECT
  - Paramedian position of affected true vocal cord with ipsilateral ancillary findings
    - Ballooning of laryngeal ventricle = "sail" sign
    - Anteromedial rotation of arytenoid cartilage
    - Medially displaced, thick aryepiglottic fold
    - Enlarged pyriform sinus
    - Cricoarytenoid muscle atrophy
  - If mass along CN10 course from brainstem to jugular foramen
    - CN9, CN11 dysfunction often also evident
      - CN9 injury → loss of ipsilateral pharynx sensation
      - CN11 injury → ipsilateral trapezius and sternocleidomastoid denervation
  - If mass along CN10 in superior carotid space to level of hyoid
    - CN9, CN11, & CN12 dysfunction often evident
      - CN12 injury → ipsilateral tongue denervation

MR Findings
- MR of posterior cranial fossa is indicated when central-proximal vagal neuropathy is suspected

DIFFERENTIAL DIAGNOSIS

Laryngeal Trauma
- Arytenoid dislocation or subluxation may be misdiagnosed as VCP
- May occur after difficult intubation or blunt laryngeal trauma
- True VCP may be caused by endotracheal intubation or arytenoid dislocation when overinflated tube or laterally subluxed arytenoid compresses anterior motor branch of RLN against thyroid cartilage at level of membranous TVC

Laryngeal & Piriform Sinus SCCa
- May mimic VCP by infiltrating aryepiglottic cartilages and causing VC immobilization
- Adjacent fibrosis or malignant infiltration may cause VC fixation while preserving motor innervation
- Soft tissue thickening from tumor may cause apparent medialization of cord that is falsely interpreted as VCP

Post-Treatment Change
- Injection laryngoplasty results in "medialization" of paralyzed cord to regain glottic closure and competence

VOCAL CORD PARALYSIS

PATHOLOGY

General Features

- Etiology
  - Injury to or lesion compressing CN10 anywhere from medulla to recurrent laryngeal nerve
  - Most common etiologies: Neoplasm, vascular lesion, trauma, idiopathic pathology
  - Nonmalignant thoracic causes (cardiovocal [Ortner] syndrome)
    - Atrial septal defect, Eisenmenger complex, patent ductus arteriosus, primary pulmonary hypertension, and aortic aneurysm with stretching of recurrent laryngeal nerve
  - Other causes for RLN palsy in neck include radioactive iodine ablation therapy, external beam radiotherapy, chemotherapy (vinca alkaloids), jugular vein thrombosis, and postsurgical complication
    - In thyroidectomy, carotid endarterectomy, anterior approach to cervical spine; right central venous catheter insertion and median sternotomy for right RLN; left upper lobectomy and cardiac surgery for left RLN
  - ~ 10% of cases are due to central cause, e.g., brain tumors, vascular anomalies, hemorrhage, trauma, or infection
  - Most cases are due to peripheral lesions including intrathoracic neoplasms, vascular lesions, and trauma (including iatrogenic cause)
  - Other causes may include neurological disease, e.g., Guillain-Barré syndrome, multiple sclerosis, poliomyelitis, and other viral neuritis

CLINICAL ISSUES

Presentation

- Most common signs/symptoms
  - Hoarseness, dysphonia, "breathy voice"
- Other signs/symptoms
  - Uncommonly, patients may be asymptomatic with normal voice
  - Aspiration (especially liquids), insufficient cough
  - Foreign body sensation in larynx
  - Shortness of breath sensation, air wasting

Demographics

- Gender
  - No known gender predilection in adults
  - M > F in pediatric age group

Natural History & Prognosis

- VCP due to recurrent nerve or CN10 injury rarely recovers
- Toxic or infectious VCP often self-limited
  - > 80% resolve within 6 months
- Recovery uncommon if no improvement by 9 months

Treatment

- Initially conservative, many "idiopathic" cases will spontaneously improve
- Voice therapy
- Vocal cord augmentation: Material injected to paraglottic space
  - Temporary: Resorbable materials (Gelfoam, hyaluronic acid, collagen)

- Permanent: Fat, calcium hydroxylapatite, Teflon
  - Teflon reserved for terminal patients as > 50% develop granuloma
- Laryngeal framework surgery
  - Medialization thyroplasty with silastic or Gore-Tex implant
  - Arytenoid adduction
  - Laryngeal reinnervation (hypoglossal nerve, ansa cervicalis)

DIAGNOSTIC CHECKLIST

Consider

- If vocal cord paralysis evident on ultrasound, search for neck neoplasms from larynx, hypopharynx, or thyroid and neck nodal metastases
- CT is useful to look for intrathoracic peripheral lesions causing RLN palsy
- MR is indicated when central-proximal vagal neuropathy is suspected

Imaging Pitfalls

- Neck neoplasms, arytenoid subluxation/dislocation, and injection laryngoplasty may mimic VCP

SELECTED REFERENCES

1. Vachha B et al: Losing your voice: etiologies and imaging features of vocal fold paralysis. J Clin Imaging Sci. 3:15, 2013
2. Heikkinen J et al: Cardiovocal Syndrome (Ortner's Syndrome) Associated with Chronic Thromboembolic Pulmonary Hypertension and Giant Pulmonary Artery Aneurysm: Case Report and Review of the Literature. Case Rep Med. 2012:230736, 2012
3. Kwong Y et al: Radiology of vocal cord palsy. Clin Radiol. 67(11):1108-14, 2012
4. Paquette CM et al: Unilateral vocal cord paralysis: a review of CT findings, mediastinal causes, and the course of the recurrent laryngeal nerves. Radiographics. 32(3):721-40, 2012
5. Song SW et al: CT evaluation of vocal cord paralysis due to thoracic diseases: a 10-year retrospective study. Yonsei Med J. 52(5):831-7, 2011
6. Garcia MM et al: Imaging evaluation of vocal cord paralysis. Radiol Bras. 42(5):321-326, 2009
7. Kumar VA et al: CT assessment of vocal cord medialization. AJNR Am J Neuroradiol. 27(8):1643-6, 2006
8. Chin SC et al: Using CT to localize side and level of vocal cord paralysis. AJR Am J Roentgenol. 180(4):1165-70, 2003
9. Aydin K et al: Case report: bilateral vocal cord paralysis caused by cervical spinal osteophytes. Br J Radiol. 75(900):990-33, 2002
10. Miles KA: Ultrasound demonstration of vocal cord movements. Br J Radiol. 62(741):871-2, 1989

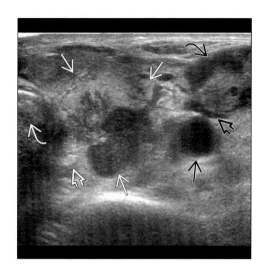
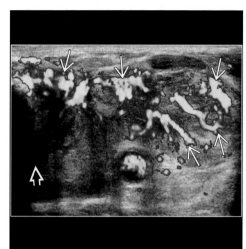

(Left) Axial grayscale ultrasound demonstrates an ill-defined, heterogeneous anaplastic carcinoma in the left lobe of the thyroid ➡ infiltrating the left tracheo-esophageal groove ⬳ and jeopardizing the left RLN. Note the trachea ➡, left CCA ➡, compressed left IJV ⬳, and left cervical metastatic node ➘. *(Right)* Corresponding axial power Doppler shows increased intratumoral vascularity ➡. Again note infiltration of the left tracheo-esophageal groove ⬳, location of RLN.

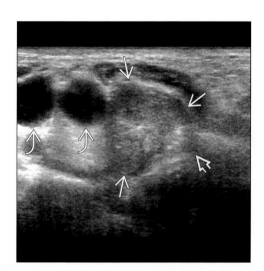
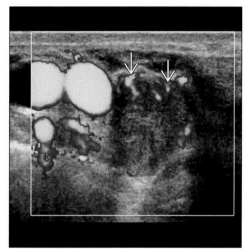

(Left) Transverse grayscale US in a patient with recurrent medullary carcinoma is shown. Paratracheal region is a common site for nodal tumor recurrence ➡, which in this case has invaded right tracheo-esophageal groove ⬳ and right RLN. Note major neck vessels ➡. *(Right)* Corresponding axial power Doppler shows increased vascularity within nodal metastasis ➡. RLN may be affected anywhere along its path. RLN is not reliably seen on US; its location is inferred by identifying tracheo-esophageal groove.

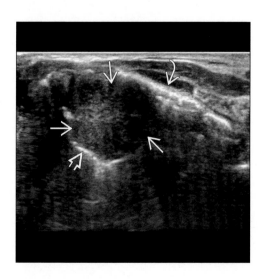
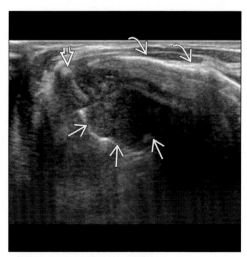

(Left) Axial grayscale ultrasound shows a large left glottic tumor ➡ causing apparent medialization of the left cord ⬳ that may be falsely interpreted as VCP. Note the left thyroid lamina ⬳. Malignant infiltration may cause VC fixation while preserving motor innervation. *(Right)* Grayscale ultrasound shows a laryngeal tumor in the longitudinal plane ➡. Note the hyoid bone ⬳ and thyroid cartilage ➡.

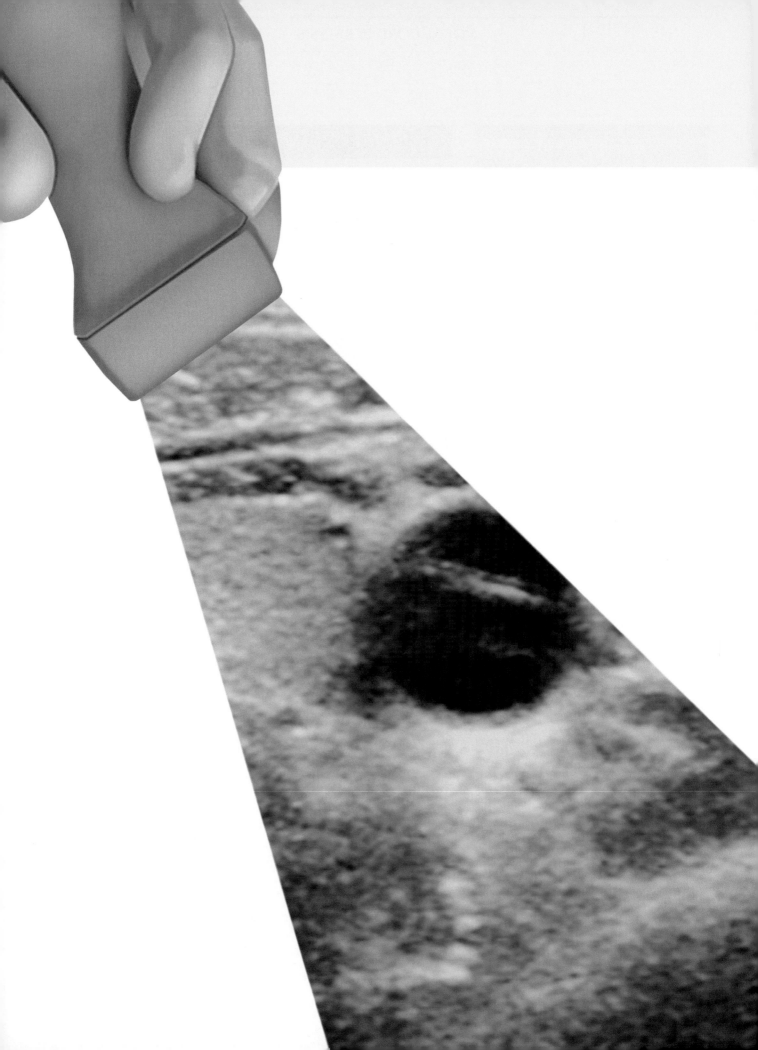

SECTION 6

Vascular

PAROTID VASCULAR LESION

Key Facts

Imaging

- Lesion with cystic or sinusoidal spaces and increased vascular flow on Doppler ultrasound
- Demonstration of dilated vascular channels with high flow allows for accurate diagnosis of AVF
- **Pseudoaneurysm**
  - Round, heterogeneous, hypoechoic mass with well-defined margins
  - Internal calcification (in wall) and cystic spaces within lesion
  - Color flow signal is shown on Doppler ultrasound within cystic spaces; supplying artery may be seen with blood jetting into cystic spaces
- Arteriovenous malformation (AVF)
  - Well-circumscribed cystic lesion with internal septations
  - Enlarged serpiginous vascular channels adjacent to cystic lesion
- Marked intralesional flow on power Doppler with central supplying vessel and enlarged draining vein

Top Differential Diagnoses

- Warthin tumor
- Benign lymphoepithelial lesions
- Venous vascular malformation (in adults)
- Infantile hemangioma (in children)

Diagnostic Checklist

- Pseudoaneurysm and AVF are rare vascular lesions in parotid gland in adults but should be considered in differential diagnosis of parotid mass
- Always evaluate cystic/serpiginous spaces within salivary masses with Doppler as vascular lesions mimic other salivary tumors
- Conventional angiogram is used for planning definitive surgical or endovascular treatment

(Left) Axial grayscale US of a parotid gland shows a pseudoaneurysm as a round, heterogeneous, hypoechoic lesion with well-defined margins ⮕. Note the cystic spaces within ⮕. Initial scan included only grayscale imaging and the lesion was misinterpreted as a salivary tumor. (Right) Subsequent Doppler examination (same patient) shows prominent flow ⮕ within the pseudoaneurysm, revealing its very vascular nature and preventing US-guided biopsy, which could have resulted in torrential bleeding.

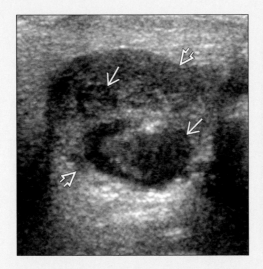
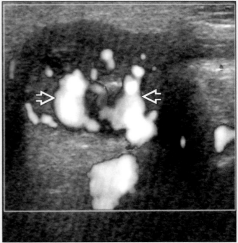

(Left) Coronal T2WI MR (same patient) shows the left parotid pseudoaneurysm as markedly hyperintense ⮕. It was isointense on T1WI (not shown) with signal similar to that of muscles. Glandular neoplasms also tend to be hyperintense on T2WI & isointense on T1WI. (Right) Corresponding coronal T1 C+ FS MR (same patient) shows avid enhancement of the left parotid pseudoaneurysm ⮕. Such intense enhancement is more indicative of a vascular lesion than a glandular neoplasm.

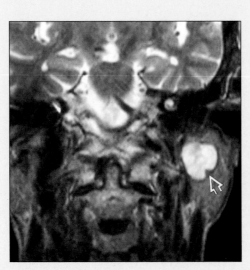
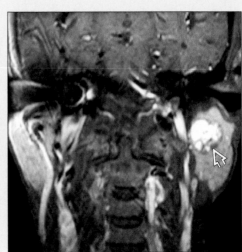

PAROTID VASCULAR LESION

IMAGING

General Features
- Best diagnostic clue
  - Benign lesions with cystic/sinusoidal spaces and ↑ vascular flow on Doppler ultrasound
  - Dilated vascular channels with high flow allows for an accurate diagnosis of arteriovenous fistula (AVF)
- Location
  - May involve both superficial and deep lobes of parotid
- Size
  - Variable, commonly 2-3 cm

Ultrasonographic Findings
- **Pseudoaneurysm**
  - Round, heterogeneous, hypoechoic mass with well-defined margins
  - Internal calcification (in wall) and cystic spaces within lesion
  - Flow/movement of fine echoes may be seen within cystic spaces on grayscale US
  - Color flow signal is seen on Doppler ultrasound within cystic spaces; supplying artery may be seen with blood jetting into cystic spaces
- **AVF**
  - Well-circumscribed cystic lesion with internal septations
  - Multiple enlarged serpiginous vascular channels adjacent to cystic lesion
  - Flow/movement of fine echoes may be seen within cystic spaces on grayscale US
  - Marked intralesional flow on power Doppler with central supplying vessel and enlarged draining vein

MR Findings
- **Pseudoaneurysm**
  - Well-circumscribed, sharp outline/edge
  - Isointense on T1WI, hyperintense on T2WI
  - Avid enhancement after IV gadolinium contrast
- **AVF**
  - Numerous clustered serpiginous signal voids
  - MR angiogram (MRA) shows lesion fed by branches of external carotid artery with venous drainage predominantly via external jugular vein

Angiographic Findings
- **Pseudoaneurysm**
  - Contrast filling, slightly lobulated, saccular outpouching from parent artery
- **AVF**
  - Hypertrophied arterial feeder from external carotid artery and dilated draining veins
  - Smaller new AVF with progressive increase in flow may be seen after embolization of initial AVF

Imaging Recommendations
- Best imaging tool
  - High-resolution ultrasound and MR provide accurate diagnosis
  - Multiplicity, anatomic extent, and involvement of adjacent structures are better demonstrated by MR
- Protocol advice
  - Always evaluate cystic/serpiginous spaces within salivary masses with Doppler as vascular lesions mimic other salivary tumors
  - Conventional angiogram is used for planning definitive surgical or endovascular treatment

DIFFERENTIAL DIAGNOSIS

Warthin Tumor
- Well-defined, hypoechoic, noncalcified mass in apex of superficial lobe of parotid
- Cystic, multiseptated with thick walls, ± posterior enhancement
- Multiplicity of lesions, unilateral or bilateral (20%)
- Color Doppler: Prominent vessels, particularly hilar & septal (may be striking), not within cystic spaces

Benign Lymphoepithelial Lesions
- Cystic lesions not purely cystic but contain internal network of thin septa supplied by vascular pedicles; 40% have mural nodules

Venous Vascular Malformation (VVM)
- Slow-moving debris ("to and fro") on real-time US within dilated channels suggestive of vascular flow
- Phleboliths seen in almost 60% of cases
- Color Doppler: Slow flow within venous, sinusoidal spaces

Infantile Hemangioma
- Should be included in differential diagnosis of pediatric patients
- Prominent hypoechoic vascular channels that "light up" on color Doppler; no phleboliths
- History of rapid enlargement in 1st year of life with subsequent regression

PATHOLOGY

General Features
- Both are rare vascular lesions in parotid gland
- Aneurysms involving external carotid artery and its branches are rare, accounting for 0.4-4% of all aneurysms
- Few cases of aneurysms of external carotid artery and superficial temporal artery presenting as parotid swelling have been reported (traumatic or mycotic in origin)
- Cause of aneurysm in parotid may be idiopathic in absence of preceding history of trauma, surgery, or infection
- Most reported cases of AVF were spontaneous with no preceding history of trauma or surgery

DIAGNOSTIC CHECKLIST

Consider
- Pseudoaneurysm and AVF are rare vascular lesions in parotid gland in adults but should be considered in differential diagnosis of any parotid mass with cystic component

SELECTED REFERENCES

1. Wong KT et al: Vascular lesions of parotid gland in adult patients: diagnosis with high-resolution ultrasound and MRI. Br J Radiol. 77(919):600-6, 2004

PAROTID VASCULAR LESION

(Left) DSA (lateral view) of the left external carotid artery (same patient) shows a pseudoaneurysm ⊳ arising from the distal posterior auricular artery →. (Courtesy S. Yu, MD.) *(Right)* Corresponding oblique view of DSA shows a pseudoaneurysm →. Small, tortuous supplying left posterior auricular artery was then successfully embolized by microcoils proximal to the site of the pseudoaneurysm with no complications. (Courtesy S. Yu, MD.)

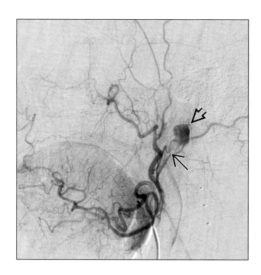
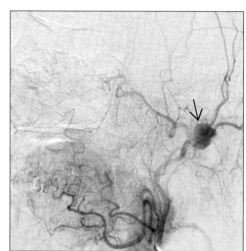

(Left) Axial grayscale US demonstrates the retromandibular vein ⇗, external carotid artery →, and AVF ⊳ in the superficial lobe of the left parotid gland. *(Right)* Corresponding axial power Doppler ultrasound (same patient) shows the retromandibular vein ⇗, external carotid artery →, and AVF ⊳, which is fed by branches from the external carotid artery and drains via the retromandibular vein into the external jugular vein.

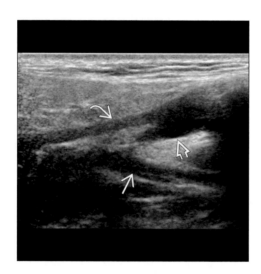
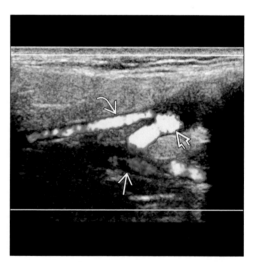

(Left) Axial pulsed Doppler ultrasound (same patient) shows mixed arterial-venous flow signal within AVF. This mixed flow indicates abnormal communication between the arterial & venous systems. *(Right)* Corresponding axial T1WI MR shows a left parotid AVF as signal void ⊳. On high-resolution ultrasound and MR, presence of dilated vascular channels with high flow allows for an accurate diagnosis of an AVF.

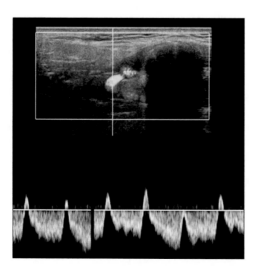
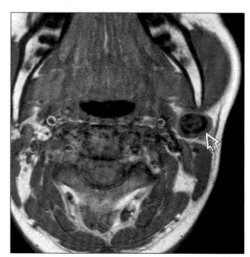

PAROTID VASCULAR LESION

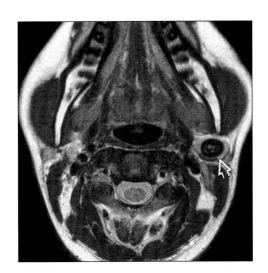

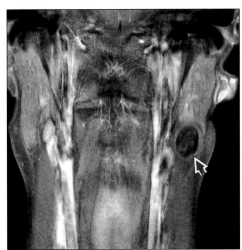

(Left) Axial T2WI MR (same patient) shows a left parotid AVF as signal void ➡. High blood flow results in signal void and should not be mistaken for other hypointense lesions, such as dense calcification. *(Right)* Corresponding coronal T1WI C+ FS MR again shows a left parotid AVF as signal void ➡. MR helps to identify the origin of the feeding artery & venous drainage. DSA is not routinely necessary for diagnosis and is reserved for endovascular treatment planning.

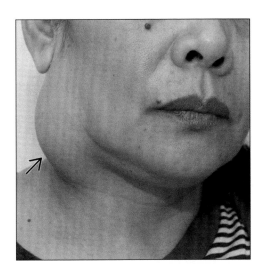

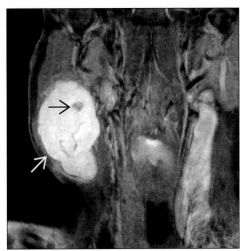

(Left) Clinical photograph shows a large parotid venous vascular malformation (VVM) presenting as a painless right parotid swelling ➡. The overlying skin appears normal with no discoloration, and no pulsation or palpable thrill was demonstrated. *(Right)* Corresponding coronal T1WI C+ FS MR (same patient) shows a right parotid venous vascular malformation ➡ with avid homogeneous enhancement & phlebolith within ➡.

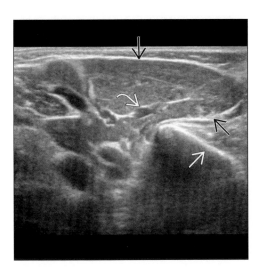

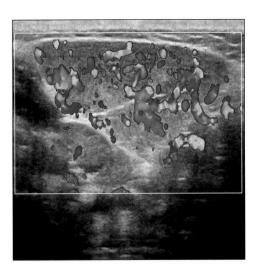

(Left) Axial ultrasound (same patient) shows the right parotid venous vascular malformation ➡ as a heterogeneous hypoechoic lesion with sinusoidal spaces ➡. Slow flow may be seen within sinusoidal spaces on real-time grayscale imaging. The mandibular ramus ➡ is also shown. *(Right)* Corresponding axial color Doppler ultrasound (same patient) shows prominent vascular flow signal within the parotid VVM. Such prominent vascularity may not be seen in VVM with slow flow within.

VENOUS VASCULAR MALFORMATION

Key Facts

Terminology
- Slow-flow, post-capillary lesion composed of endothelial-lined vascular sinusoids

Imaging
- Most common vascular malformation of head and neck
- Soft, compressible mass with multiple serpiginous sinusoidal spaces within
- Mass and sinusoidal spaces ↑ in size on Valsalva, crying, and in dependent position
- Slow-moving debris ("to and fro") on real-time US within dilated channels suggestive of vascular flow
- Hypoechoic with heterogeneous echo pattern
- Phleboliths are seen as focal echogenic foci with dense posterior shadowing (seen in 60% of cases)
- Spectral Doppler: No arterial flow on Doppler, but venous flow may be observed and augmented by compression with transducer

- Color Doppler: Slow flow within venous, sinusoidal spaces
- US cannot evaluate entire extent of large and deep-seated lesions; MR is best for establishing full extent
- Intralesional vascularity is slow and often better seen on grayscale imaging than on Doppler
- On grayscale US, hold transducer gently over lesion and "to and fro" motion of echoes within sinusoidal spaces can be seen
- For color Doppler examination use low wall filter and pulse repetition frequency to increase sensitivity in detecting slow flow

Top Differential Diagnoses
- Lipoma
- Lymphatic malformation
- Ranula (simple or diving)
- Slow-flow arteriovenous malformation

(Left) Clinical photograph shows a patient presenting with painless swelling ➡ just above sternal notch. (Right) Corresponding transverse grayscale US at clinical site shows a well-defined cystic lesion ➔, with large sinusoidal space and uniform fine internal debris ⮕ and septa ➡ within. This debris showed slow "to and fro" motion on real-time grayscale imaging suggesting a diagnosis of venous vascular malformation (VVM). Note the posterior enhancement ➡ indicating the cystic nature of lesion. Normal major neck vessels ➡ are also shown.

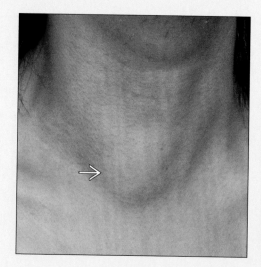
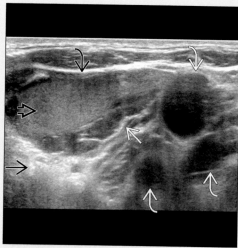

(Left) Transverse grayscale US in the submandibular region (same patient) shows another cystic lesion ➡ with sinusoidal spaces and echogenic phlebolith ➡ confirming VVM at the site. (Right) Corresponding T2WI FS MR shows multiple VVMs ➡, seen as hyperintense lesions throughout the neck. Although US is able to evaluate superficial lesions and confirm their diagnosis, it cannot define the extent of large lesions, identify deep-seated lesions, or confirm multiplicity.

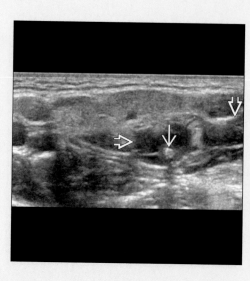
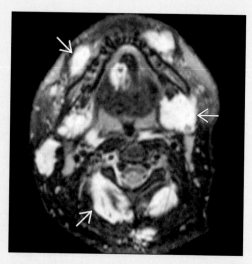

VENOUS VASCULAR MALFORMATION

TERMINOLOGY

Abbreviations
- Venous vascular malformation (VVM)

Definitions
- Slow-flow, post-capillary lesion composed of endothelial-lined vascular sinusoids

IMAGING

General Features
- Best diagnostic clue
  - Lobulated soft tissue mass with phleboliths
- Location
  - Most commonly in buccal region
  - Masticator space, sublingual space, tongue, orbit, and dorsal neck are other common locations
  - May be superficial or deep, diffuse or localized
- Size
  - Variable, may be very large
- Morphology
  - Multilobulated; solitary or multiple
  - May be circumscribed or trans-spatial, infiltrating adjacent soft tissue compartments
  - ± combined lymphatic malformation (LM), i.e., venolymphatic malformation (VLM)

Ultrasonographic Findings
- Soft, compressible mass with multiple serpiginous sinusoidal spaces within
- Mass and sinusoidal spaces increase in size on Valsalva, crying, and in dependent position
- Slow-moving debris ("to and fro") on real-time US within dilated channels suggestive of vascular flow
- Hypoechoic with heterogeneous echo pattern
  - Lesions with small vascular channels are more echogenic and less compressible than lesions with large vascular lumens
    - Small vascular channels have multiple reflecting interfaces making it echogenic
- Phleboliths are seen as focal echogenic foci with dense posterior shadowing (seen in 60% of cases)
- Spectral Doppler: No arterial flow on Doppler, but venous flow may be observed and augmented by compression with transducer
- Color Doppler: Slow flow within venous, sinusoidal spaces

Imaging Recommendations
- Best imaging tool
  - US is ideal initial imaging modality as it clearly identifies VVM, flow within VVM and phleboliths
  - US cannot evaluate entire extent of large and deep seated lesions; MR is best for establishing full extent
- Protocol advice
  - VVMs are compressible and often superficial; US (grayscale & Doppler) must be performed with minimal transducer pressure
  - Intralesional vascularity is slow and often better seen on grayscale imaging than on Doppler
    - On grayscale US, hold transducer gently over lesion and "to and fro" motion of echoes within sinusoidal spaces can be seen

- This is often best clue to nature of lesion, "to and fro" motion is not easily missed
- For color Doppler examination use low wall filter and pulse repetition frequency (PRF) to increase sensitivity in detecting slow flow
  - US ideally follows up patients following treatment and also in patients who may refuse treatment

DIFFERENTIAL DIAGNOSIS

Lipoma
- Encapsulated hypoechoic mass with feathered/striped appearance on US
- No vascularity or phleboliths seen

Lymphatic Malformation (LM)
- Multilocular, trans-spatial mass with cystic spaces, debris, septation, ± fluid levels
- No phleboliths/vascularity within lesion

Ranula (Simple or Diving)
- No phleboliths or vascularity in cystic mass
- Identify extent into submandibular space (SMS), across midline and parapharyngeal space

Slow-Flow Arteriovenous Malformation
- Serpiginous, hypoechoic vascular channels with vascularity on color Doppler
- Arterial and venous signal detected on spectral Doppler

CLINICAL ISSUES

Presentation
- Most common signs/symptoms
  - By definition exist at birth
    - Present clinically in children, adolescents, or young adults
  - Spongy facial soft tissue mass that grows proportionately with patient
  - Mass ↑ in size with Valsalva, bending over, crying
  - Pain, swelling, often on waking due to venous stasis and thrombosis
  - Lesion may enlarge and harden rapidly after trauma or infection

DIAGNOSTIC CHECKLIST

Image Interpretation Pearls
- Presence of phleboliths, sinusoidal vascular spaces, slow flow on grayscale and Doppler US is virtually diagnostic of VVM

SELECTED REFERENCES

1. Harnsberger HR et al: Diagnostic Imaging: Head & Neck. 2nd ed. Salt Lake City: Amirsys, Inc. III-1-10-13, 2011
2. Ahuja AT et al: Accuracy of high-resolution sonography compared with magnetic resonance imaging in the diagnosis of head and neck venous vascular malformations. Clin Radiol. 58(11):869-75, 2003
3. Yang WT et al: Sonographic features of head and neck hemangiomas and vascular malformations: review of 23 patients. J Ultrasound Med. 16(1):39-44, 1997

VENOUS VASCULAR MALFORMATION

(Left) Transverse grayscale US of posterior triangle shows a well-defined, hypoechoic, cystic lesion ⮕ with multiple septi ➡, posterior enhancement ⮔, and sinusoidal spaces within ➡. It showed "to and fro" motion of echoes within on real-time scanning and a slow flow on Doppler (not shown) suggesting a diagnosis of VVM. Differential diagnosis includes lymphatic malformation. *(Right)* Corresponding axial T2WI FS MR confirms location of the lesion and shows fluid level ➡ within.

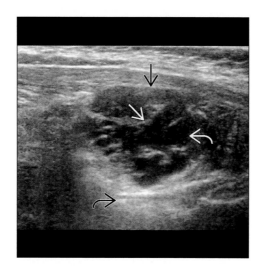
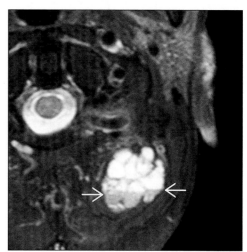

(Left) Transverse grayscale US of the submandibular region shows a well-defined, hypoechoic, cystic lesion ➡ with multiple septi ➡ and sinusoidal spaces within ➡. It showed a "to and fro" motion of echoes within on real-time scanning, suggesting a diagnosis of VVM. *(Right)* Longitudinal power Doppler US shows large vessels ➡ with slow flow within a VVM. In power Doppler US always use low wall filter and PRF to ↑ sensitivity in detecting slow flow. ↑ transducer pressure may obliterate superficial vessels.

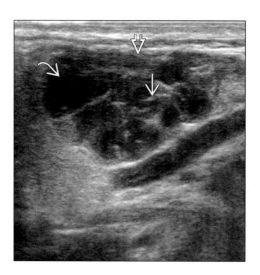
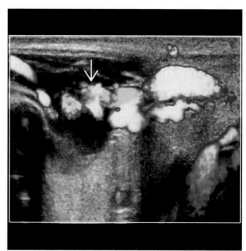

(Left) Transverse grayscale US shows a subtle, hypoechoic, cystic lesion ➡ with multiple septi ➡ and sinusoidal spaces ➡ in the right strap muscles. It showed a "to & fro" motion of echoes within on real-time scanning, suggesting a diagnosis of VVM. Note the right lobe thyroid ⮔ and CCA ➡. *(Right)* Corresponding power Doppler US clearly demonstrates VVM ➡ within the right strap muscles, but no obvious flow is seen within it suggesting very slow flow not picked up by Doppler (not unusual). Note CCA ➡.

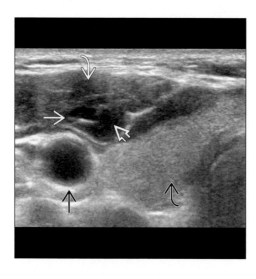
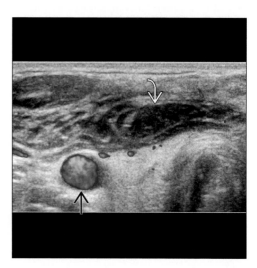

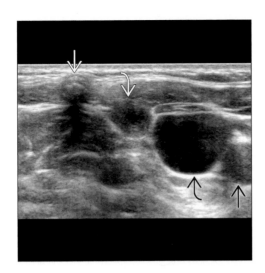

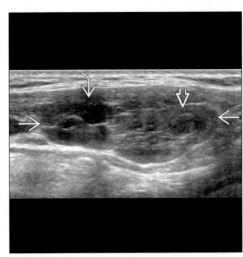

(Left) Transverse grayscale US shows curvilinear, echogenic focus ➡ & a small cystic locule ➡ in right sternomastoid. Note the IJV ➡ and CCA ➡. *(Right)* Corresponding longitudinal grayscale US (same patient) shows a hypoechoic, heterogeneous mass ➡ within the sternomastoid with a focal cystic ➡ area & curvilinear echoes ➡ (calcification). US feature is suggestive of intramuscular VVM. Masseter, digastric, temporalis, and strap muscles are other common sites of intramuscular VVM.

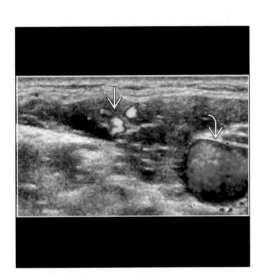

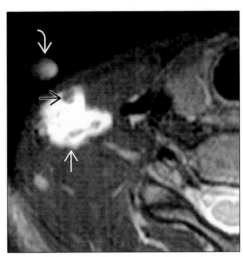

(Left) Transverse power Doppler US (same patient) shows moderately sized vessels ➡ within a sternomastoid VVM. Note the CCA ➡. *(Right)* Corresponding T2WI FS MR shows a VVM ➡ as a hyperintense lesion in the right sternomastoid muscle. Note the phlebolith seen on US is seen on MR as a signal void ➡ area within the VVM. Note the body marker ➡. MR clearly defines the extent of the large VVM, multiplicity, and the presence of deep-seated lesions not visualized by US.

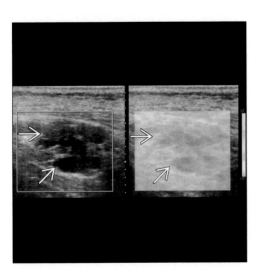

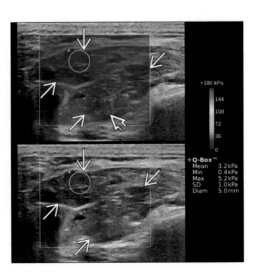

(Left) Transverse grayscale US and strain EI show a cervical VVM ➡. Strain color scale ranges from purple (elastic, soft) to red (inelastic, hard). It is much more elastic than surrounding soft tissues. *(Right)* Transverse grayscale US and SWE of cervical VVM ➡. SWE color scale ranges from blue (0 kPa, soft) to red (180 kPa, stiff). It displays a very low SWE color signal (maximum ~ 5.2 kPa), and some areas lack signal ➡, partly due to the fact that shear waves are not transmitted in nonviscous fluids.

JUGULAR VEIN THROMBOSIS

Key Facts

Terminology

- Chronic internal jugular vein (IJV) thrombosis (> 10 days after acute event) where clot persists within lumen after soft tissue inflammation is gone
- JV thrombophlebitis: Acute-subacute thrombosis of IJV with associated adjacent tissue inflammation

Imaging

- Acute thrombophlebitic phase
  - Loss of fascial planes between IJV & surrounding soft tissues + cellulitis
  - Echogenic intraluminal thrombus, distended, non-compressible IJV
  - Acute thrombus may be anechoic & difficult to distinguish from flowing blood; lack of compressibility & absent color or flow signal on Doppler may be only clues
  - Loss of venous pulsation and respiratory phasicity on spectral Doppler
  - No flow is demonstrated within an echogenic venous thrombus
  - Tumor infiltration of IJV causes tumor thrombus with ↑ vascularity on Doppler US, most commonly from thyroid anaplastic carcinoma or follicular carcinoma
- Chronic phase
  - Collateral veins may be detected
  - Central liquefaction or heterogeneity of thrombus
  - Thrombus tends to be well organized and echogenic
  - May be difficult to separate from echogenic perivascular fatty tissues
  - Absence of phasicity in jugular or subclavian veins may suggest more central nonocclusive thrombus

Top Differential Diagnoses

- Sluggish or turbulent flow in IJV (pseudothrombosis)
- Suppurative lymphadenopathy, neck abscess
- SCCa malignant lymphadenopathy

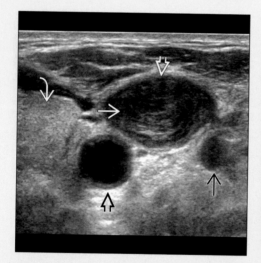 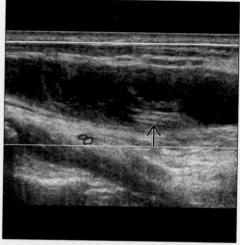

(Left) Transverse grayscale US shows enlarged left internal jugular vein (IJV) ⮑ filled with heterogeneous, laminated intraluminal thrombus ➡. This patient had known H&N squamous cell carcinoma, and thrombosed IJV could well be mistaken for metastatic node. Note the adjacent, round, hypoechoic metastatic node ➡, CCA ⮑, & thyroid gland ➡. *(Right)* Corresponding power Doppler US shows "lesion" to be in fact tubular, consistent with IJV thrombus ➡. Power Doppler US shows absence of flow signal within venous lumen & thrombus.

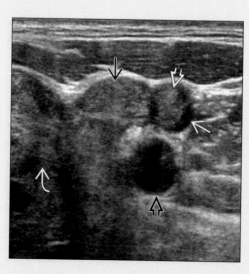 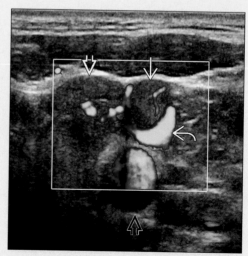

(Left) Transverse grayscale US shows a tumor thrombus in the left IJV ➡, arising from a malignant thyroid mass ➡ and extending into the IJV via the middle thyroid vein ➡ (also filled with thrombus & distended). Note remnant lumen of the vein ➡ and CCA ⮑. *(Right)* Corresponding transverse power Doppler US shows vascularity within the IJV thrombus ➡ & in the middle thyroid vein thrombus ➡, suggesting these to be tumor thrombi. Note flow signal within remnant lumen of the IJV ➡ and CCA ⮑.

JUGULAR VEIN THROMBOSIS

TERMINOLOGY

Abbreviations
- Jugular vein thrombosis (JVT)

Definitions
- JVT: Chronic internal jugular vein (IJV) thrombosis (> 10 days after acute event) where clot persists within lumen after soft tissue inflammation is gone
- Jugular vein thrombophlebitis: Acute to subacute thrombosis of IJV with associated adjacent tissue inflammation (myositis and fasciitis)

IMAGING

General Features
- Best diagnostic clue
  - Luminal clot in IJV with (thrombophlebitis) or without (thrombosis) associated soft tissue inflammatory changes
- Size
  - IJV may be smaller than normal in chronic phase or enlarged in acute-subacute phase
- Morphology
  - Ovoid to round IJV luminal filling defect

Ultrasonographic Findings
- Technique
  - Patient in supine position with neck slightly extended and turned to opposite side
  - Axial and longitudinal images should be obtained
  - Transducer pressure should be kept to a minimum to avoid IJV collapse
  - Lower IJV, medial subclavian vein, and their confluence to form brachiocephalic vein is accessible by US by scanning in coronal plane at supraclavicular fossa
- Right IJV is normally larger than left IJV, due to right side dominance of cerebral venous drainage
- A valve may normally be identified at distal IJV
- Acute thrombophlebitic phase
  - Loss of fascial planes between IJV and surrounding soft tissues + cellulitis
  - Echogenic intraluminal thrombus causing distension of IJV, which becomes incompressible
  - Acute thrombus may be anechoic and difficult to distinguish from flowing blood, in which case lack of compressibility and absent color or flow signal on Doppler may be only clues
  - Valsalva maneuver may also render thrombus more conspicuous
  - Loss of venous pulsation and respiratory phasicity on spectral Doppler
  - No flow is demonstrated within an echogenic venous thrombus
  - Tumor infiltration of IJV causes tumor thrombus that shows ↑ vascularity on Doppler ultrasound, most commonly from thyroid carcinoma (anaplastic carcinoma or follicular carcinoma)
- Chronic phase
  - Collateral veins may be detected
  - Central liquefaction or heterogeneity of thrombus are also signs of chronicity
  - Thrombus tends to be well organized and echogenic

- May be difficult to separate from echogenic perivascular fatty tissues
- Absence of phasicity in jugular or subclavian veins may suggest more central nonocclusive thrombus
- Advantage of ultrasound: Noninvasive imaging for rapid diagnosis and serial follow-up during treatment
  - Tumor thrombus in IJV is highly associated with pulmonary metastases due to direct exposure of circulation to malignant cells; surveillance for pulmonary deposits is thus warranted
- Limitations of ultrasound: Nonvisualization of IJV cephalad to mandible; fresh clot lacks inherent echogenicity
- Common cause of false-positive finding is sluggish venous flow resulting in internal echoes within IJV being mistaken for thrombus; as such, it is important to evaluate in orthogonal planes and to elicit compressibility and Doppler flow for confirmation

Radiographic Findings
- Radiography
  - Central venous catheters in neck region increases risk of JVT

CT Findings
- NECT
  - Acute thrombus is hyperdense
- CECT
  - Acute-subacute IJV thrombophlebitis (< 10 days)
    - Nonenhancing central filling defect (central low attenuation) within enlarged IJV
    - Acute thrombus is hyperdense and may not be seen on CECT
    - Inflammation-induced loss of soft tissue planes surrounding thrombus-filled IJV
    - Peripheral enhancement of vessel wall (vasa vasorum)
    - Edema fluid in retropharyngeal space (RPS) as secondary sign
  - Chronic IJV thrombosis (> 10 days)
    - Well-marginated, tubular thrombus fills IJV without adjacent inflammation
    - Tubular/linear enhancement of prominent collateral veins bypassing thrombosed IJV
- CTA
  - Filling defect in jugular vein
  - In chronic phase, large venous collaterals may be seen

MR Findings
- T1WI
  - IJV thrombus signal intensity depends on composition of clot (age)
  - Fat-suppressed sequences show acute thrombus as isointense
    - Subacute clot often high signal (methemoglobin)
- T2WI
  - Acute thrombus (early hours of acute event) in IJV lumen bright
  - Subacute IJV thrombus low signal
- T2* GRE
  - Luminal thrombus may display susceptibility artifact ("blooms") with low signal appearing larger than IJV
- T1WI C+
  - Acute-subacute IJV thrombophlebitis
    - Low signal clot fills enlarged IJV

JUGULAR VEIN THROMBOSIS

- IJV wall enhancement ± enhancement of adjacent soft tissues
  - ○ Chronic jugular vein thrombosis
    - Filling defect in normal-sized IJV
    - Partial recanalization may allow contrast to outline clot in IJV
    - Venous collaterals around clotted IJV will be low signal or enhance depending on flow rate
- MRV
  - ○ Acute-subacute jugular vein thrombophlebitis: Clotted IJV is absent
  - ○ Chronic jugular vein thrombosis
    - IJV on thrombosed side absent or small and irregular (partially recanalized)
    - Mature venous collaterals may be prominent

DIFFERENTIAL DIAGNOSIS

Sluggish or Turbulent IJV Flow (Pseudothrombosis)

- Fully compressible with flow signal on Doppler ultrasound; slow flow is visible on grayscale imaging as mobile echoes with layering in dependent portion

Suppurative Lymphadenopathy

- Multiple focal cystic masses along IJV ± clinical signs of infection

Squamous Cell Carcinoma (SCCa) Metastatic Nodes

- Multiple focal, necrotic, and nonnecrotic masses along IJV, known head and neck SCCa

Neck Abscess

- Focal fluid collection with thick walls, debris ± adjacent soft tissue inflammatory change

PATHOLOGY

General Features

- Etiology
  - ○ Jugular vein thrombosis pathogenesis: 3 mechanisms for thrombosis
    - Endothelial damage from indwelling line or infection, altered blood flow, and hypercoagulable state
    - Venous stasis from compression of IJV in neck (nodes) or mediastinum (SVC syndrome) can incite JVT
    - Migratory IJV thrombophlebitis (Trousseau syndrome) associated with malignancy (pancreas, lung, and ovary)
      - Elevated factor VIII and accelerated generation of thromboplastin cause hypercoagulable state

Microscopic Features

- Jugular vein thrombosis different from intraparenchymal hematoma
  - ○ JVT: Lamination of thrombus occurs
    - No hemosiderin deposition
    - Delay in evolution of blood products (especially methemoglobin)

CLINICAL ISSUES

Presentation

- Most common signs/symptoms
  - ○ Acute-subacute thrombophlebitis phase (< 10 days)
    - Swollen, hot, tender neck mass with fever
    - Often mistaken for neck abscess clinically
  - ○ Chronic jugular vein thrombosis phase
    - Palpable tender cord in peripheral neck
    - Often mistaken for metastatic lymph nodes
  - ○ Possible patient histories
    - May be spontaneous clinical event
    - Previous neck surgery, trauma, central venous catheterization, drug abuse, hypercoagulable state, or malignancy

Demographics

- Age
  - ○ Older, sicker patient population

Natural History & Prognosis

- IJV thrombophlebitis gives way to thrombosis over 7-14 day period with decreased soft tissue swelling
- Prognosis related to cause of IJV thrombosis
- IJV thrombosis itself is self-limited
  - ○ Venous collaterals forming to circumvent occluded internal jugular vein

Treatment

- Aggressive intravenous antibiotics given to treat any underlying infection
- Anticoagulant therapy only used in severe cases
  - ○ Significant thromboembolism to lungs is rare

DIAGNOSTIC CHECKLIST

Consider

- Do not mistake acute-subacute IJV thrombophlebitis for infection or chronic IJVT for tumor or lymphadenopathy

SELECTED REFERENCES

1. Felstead AM et al: Thrombosis of the internal jugular vein: A rare but important operative finding. Br J Oral Maxillofac Surg. 48(3):195-6, 2010
2. Binnebösel M et al: Internal jugular vein thrombosis presenting as a painful neck mass due to a spontaneous dislocated subclavian port catheter as long-term complication: a case report. Cases J. 2:7991, 2009
3. Chen MH et al: Prolonged facial edema is an indicator of poor prognosis in patients with head and neck squamous cell carcinoma. Support Care Cancer. Epub ahead of print, 2009
4. Chlumský J et al: Spontaneous jugular vein thrombosis. Acta Cardiol. 64(5):689-91, 2009
5. Deganello A et al: Necrotizing fasciitis of the neck associated with Lemierre syndrome. Acta Otorhinolaryngol Ital. 29(3):160-3, 2009
6. Ball E et al: Internal jugular vein thrombosis in a warfarinised patient: a case report. J Med Case Reports. 1:184, 2007
7. Ascher E et al: Morbidity and mortality associated with internal jugular vein thromboses. Vasc Endovascular Surg. 39(4):335-9, 2005

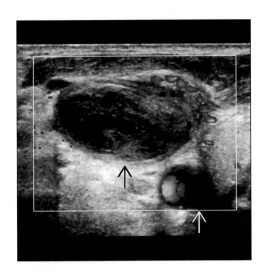

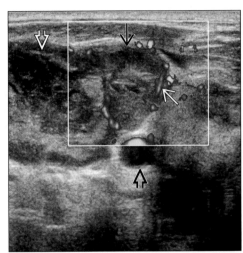

(Left) Transverse color Doppler US shows large, laminated thrombus in distended IJV ➡. Note absence of any flow signal within lumen & in thrombus, suggesting a bland venous thrombus rather than a tumor within IJV. Note the CCA ➡. *(Right)* Transverse power Doppler US shows tumor thrombus with increased vascularity ➡ within the IJV ➡. Note adjacent, necrotic metastatic node ➡ and CCA ➡. Modern transducers are sensitive in identifying such small vessels within tumor thrombi.

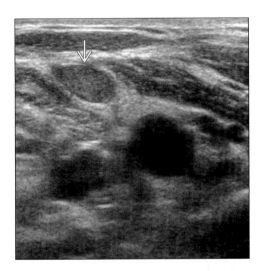

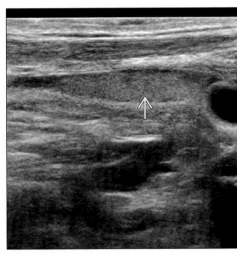

(Left) Transverse grayscale US shows homogeneous echoes within IJV ➡ mimicking a solid node. Sluggish IJV flow may be seen in cardiac failure, and, on real-time US, "to and fro" motion is detected within debris of this "pseudothrombus." *(Right)* Corresponding longitudinal US shows layering of debris in dependent portion of IJV ➡. Patency is further evaluated by demonstrating compressibility, flow signal on Doppler, or by changing the patients's position. This "thrombus" disappears when the patient sits up.

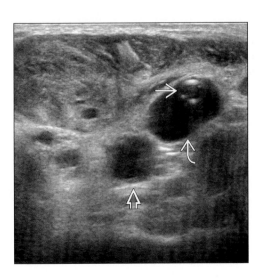

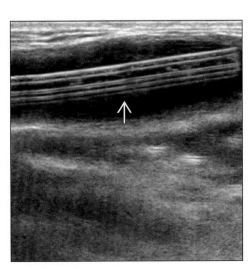

(Left) Transverse grayscale US shows a circular echogenic focus ➡ in the right IJV ➡. Note the CCA ➡. Initial impression may suggest this to be an IJV thrombus. *(Right)* Corresponding longitudinal grayscale US shows the round structure to be tubular ➡ and consistent with indwelling line within the IJV. It should not be mistaken for an intraluminal thrombus or intimal flap in carotid artery dissection.

CAROTID ARTERY DISSECTION IN NECK

Key Facts

Terminology

- Carotid artery dissection (CAD): Tear in carotid artery wall allows blood to enter & delaminate wall layers

Imaging

- Extracranial internal carotid artery dissection (ICAD) > > intracranial ICAD or common carotid artery dissection
- 20% of ICADs are bilateral or involve vertebral arteries
- Pathognomonic findings of dissection: Intimal flap or double lumen
- Turbulent flow caused by fluttering movement of intimal flap
- Smooth tapering stenosis is typical sonographic appearance of ICAD, often occurs in young patients with no visible atherosclerotic plaque
- High ICAD beyond reach of ultrasound may only manifest as ↑ flow resistance in Doppler waveform and ↓ flow velocity due to distal obstruction

- Flap may be obscured by color blooming artifact on color Doppler and better seen on grayscale imaging
- False lumen commonly demonstrates low peak flow velocity and reversed diastolic flow direction
- "Slosh" phenomenon of systolic forward-and-backward flow proximal to dissection is highly typical but not pathognomonic

Top Differential Diagnoses

- Fibromuscular dysplasia
- Traumatic internal carotid artery pseudoaneurysm

Clinical Issues

- Ipsilateral pain in face, jaw, head, or neck
- Oculosympathetic palsy (miosis & ptosis, partial Horner syndrome), bruit (40%), pulsatile tinnitus
- Ischemic symptoms (cerebral or retinal TIA or stroke)
- Lower cranial nerve palsies (especially CN10)

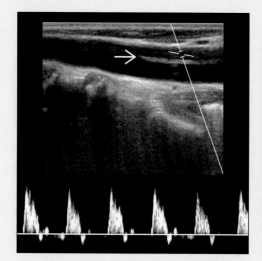
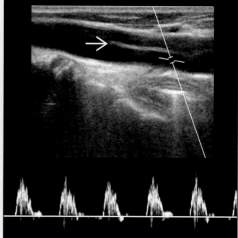

(Left) Longitudinal pulsed Doppler US shows a common carotid artery dissection (CCAD) with 2 lumina separated by a thick dissection membrane ➡. *(Right)* Longitudinal pulsed Doppler US shows a CCAD with 2 lumens separated by a thick dissection membrane ➡. Doppler waveforms of these 2 lumens both show high-resistance flow with rapid systolic upstroke and low forward flow during diastole.

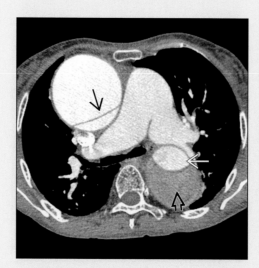
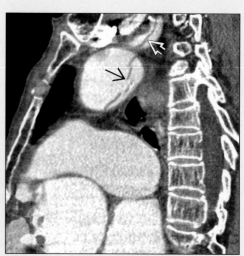

(Left) Dissection commonly originates from the thoracic aorta and extends into the carotid arteries, as shown on this axial CECT study. Note the dissection membrane ➡ and thrombosed false lumen ➡. The larger thrombosed false lumen causes narrowing of the true lumen ➡. *(Right)* Corresponding sagittal CECT reconstructed image (same patient) again demonstrates the intimal flap ➡. Note the extension of the dissection into the left CCA ➡.

CAROTID ARTERY DISSECTION IN NECK

TERMINOLOGY

Abbreviations
- Carotid artery dissection (CAD)
- Common carotid artery dissection (CCAD)
- Internal carotid artery dissection (ICAD)

Definitions
- CAD: Tear in carotid artery wall allows blood to enter and delaminate wall layers and create a false lumen

IMAGING

General Features
- Best diagnostic clue
  - Pathognomonic findings of dissection: Intimal flap or double lumen (seen in < 10%)
  - Aneurysmal dilatation is seen in 30%, commonly in distal subcranial segment of ICA
  - Flame-shaped ICA occlusion (acute phase)
  - Smooth tapering ICA stenosis
- Location
  - ICADs most commonly originate in ICA 2-3 cm distal to carotid bulb and variably involve distal ICA
  - CAD commonly starts in aortic arch and usually extends only to carotid bifurcation but may also extend into ICA

Ultrasonographic Findings
- Technique
  - Patient in supine position with neck slightly extended and head turned away from side being examined
  - High-frequency linear transducer should be used: 5-12 MHz transducer for imaging and 3-7 Mhz transducer for Doppler
  - Cervical carotid arteries are examined by grayscale, color Doppler imaging in both axial and longitudinal planes, and spectral Doppler waveform analysis in longitudinal plane
  - Regions of interest include both CCA from origins to bifurcations and both ICAs and ECAs as cephalad as feasible
  - Differentiation of extracranial ICA and ECA
    - Extracranial ICA has no branch while 1st branch of ECA, superior thyroid artery, is readily identifiable on ultrasound
    - ICA runs lateral or posterolateral to ECA in 90% of cases
    - ICA has larger caliber than ECA
    - Doppler waveform of ICA is of low resistance with high diastolic component while that of ECA is of high resistance with low or no diastolic component
    - "Tapping" maneuver of superficial temporal artery will trigger prominent disturbance in ECA Doppler waveform
- Double lumen of carotid artery with thin to thick intervening dissection membrane ± thrombus formation; may show localized increase in arterial diameter
- Thin dissection membranes (when intima dissected from vessel wall) may be seen moving freely within arterial lumen
- False lumen in CCAD may be blind-ended and thrombosed or patent while false lumen in ICAD is almost always thrombosed
- Smooth tapering stenosis is typical sonographic appearance of ICAD, often occurs in young patients with no visible atherosclerotic plaque
- Turbulent flow caused by fluttering movement of intimal flap
- Flap may be obscured by color blooming artifact on color Doppler and better seen on grayscale imaging
- False lumen commonly demonstrates low peak flow velocity and reversed diastolic flow direction
- High ICAD beyond reach of ultrasound may only manifest as increased flow resistance in Doppler waveform and reduced flow velocity due to distal obstruction
  - High-resistance spectral waveforms show rapid systolic upstroke, possible flow reversal in early diastole and low or no forward flow during diastole
  - Normal CCA and ICA show low-resistance spectral waveform with slower increase in flow velocity in systole, gradual decrease in flow velocity in diastole, and continued forward flow during entire cardiac cycle
  - It should be noted that widening of carotid bulb with disturbance of laminar flow in CCA will cause flow reversal in normal carotid bulb
- "Slosh" phenomenon of systolic forward-and-backward flow proximal to dissection is highly typical but not pathognomonic
- Ultrasound should be used for serial follow-up of patients with carotid dissection to assess therapeutic response to anticoagulant therapy
  - US follow-up of patients with ICAD on after anticoagulation demonstrates recanalization in up to 70% of cases

CT Findings
- CECT
  - Narrowing of dissected artery ± aneurysmal dilatation
  - May show dissection flap ± double lumen
- CTA
  - Shows narrowing of arterial lumen ± aneurysmal dilatation
  - May show intramural thrombus as low-attenuation crescent
  - May show dissection flap ± double lumen

MR Findings
- T1WI
  - T1 MR with fat saturation: Intramural hematoma (hyperintense crescent adjacent to arterial lumen)
- T2WI
  - Aneurysmal form: Laminated stages of thrombosis (with intervening layers of methemoglobin and hemosiderin)
- MRA
  - Vessel tapering ± aneurysmal dilatation of dissected carotid artery

Angiographic Findings
- Pathognomonic: Intimal flap + double lumen (true and false)
- Carotid artery lumen stenosis with slow flow
- Abrupt reconstitution of lumen
- Dissecting aneurysm or pseudoaneurysm
- Flame-shaped, tapered occlusion is usually acute

CAROTID ARTERY DISSECTION IN NECK

Imaging Recommendations

- Best imaging tool
  - Angiography remains gold standard for CAD
  - CTA and MRA emerging as superior technologies to image intramural and extraluminal dissection components
  - Ultrasound serves as quick and noninvasive initial imaging evaluation
- Protocol advice
  - Aim of ultrasound assessment in CAD
    - Delineate extent of dissection as far as possible
    - Assess patency, direction, and characteristics of flow within true and false lumens
    - Document patency of ECA and ICA
    - Evaluate degree of any stenosis

DIFFERENTIAL DIAGNOSIS

Carotid Fibromuscular Dysplasia

- Clinical: Young female with transient ischemic attack (TIA)
- Imaging: "String of beads" and long segment stenosis
  - May have associated ICAD

Traumatic ICA Pseudoaneurysm

- Clinical: History of recent or remote trauma
- Imaging: Dissecting aneurysm may be indistinguishable from traumatic pseudoaneurysm

PATHOLOGY

General Features

- Etiology
  - Dissections usually arise from intimal tear, blood enters artery wall → intramural hematoma (false lumen)
  - Secondary to severe trauma, iatrogenic injury, or underlying vessel wall weakness (arteriopathy such as fibromuscular dysplasia, genetic syndromes)
  - False lumen may be blind ended or recommunicate with true lumen distally
  - ICAD may be spontaneous
- ICA most common cervical artery to dissect
  - Extracranial ICA more likely to dissect than intracranial

CLINICAL ISSUES

Presentation

- Most common signs/symptoms
  - Ipsilateral pain in face, jaw, head, or neck
  - Oculosympathetic palsy (miosis and ptosis, partial Horner syndrome)
  - Ischemic symptoms (cerebral or retinal TIA or stroke)
  - Bruit (40%)
- Other signs/symptoms
  - Lower cranial nerve palsies (especially CN10)
  - Pulsatile tinnitus
  - Hyperextension or neck rotation (yoga, vigorous exercise, cough, vomiting, sneezing, resuscitation, neck manipulation)
  - Congenital Horner syndrome with traumatic delivery
- Clinical profile
  - Head and neck pain, partial Horner syndrome, TIA-stroke triad (~ 33%)

Demographics

- Age
  - 30-55 years
  - Average: 40 years
- Epidemiology
  - Annual incidence 2.5-3 per 100,000
  - Extracranial ICAD > > intracranial ICAD or CCAD
  - 20% of ICADs are bilateral or involve vertebral arteries

Natural History & Prognosis

- 90% of stenoses resolve
- 70% of occlusions are recanalized
- 33% of aneurysms decrease in size
- Risk of recurrent dissection = 2% (1st month), then 1% per year (usually in another vessel)
- Risk of stroke due to thromboembolic disease ↑; related to severity of initial ischemic insult
- Death from ICAD < 5%
- Serious neurological complications are more common in traumatic carotid dissection than in atraumatic dissection

Treatment

- Antithrombotic and antihypertensive drug therapy
- Intravenous heparin + oral warfarin (Coumadin) (unless contraindicated by hemorrhagic stroke)
- Antiplatelet therapy in asymptomatic patients and stable imaging findings for 6 months
- Endovascular stent placement rarely used
- Surgical treatment now rare option
  - Used when refractory to maximal medical and endovascular therapy
  - Interposition graft
  - Relatively high morbidity and mortality

DIAGNOSTIC CHECKLIST

Image Interpretation Pearls

- CAD may present as luminal occlusion, stenosis, or aneurysmal dilatation (pseudoaneurysm)

SELECTED REFERENCES

1. Ansari SA et al: Endovascular treatment of distal cervical and intracranial dissections with the neuroform stent. Neurosurgery. 62(3):636-46; discussion 636-46, 2008
2. Chandra A et al: Spontaneous dissection of the carotid and vertebral arteries: the 10-year UCSD experience. Ann Vasc Surg. 21(2):178-85, 2007
3. Wu HC et al: Spontaneous bilateral internal carotid artery dissection with acute stroke in young patients. Eur Neurol. 56(4):230-4, 2006
4. Biondi A et al: Progressive symptomatic carotid dissection treated with multiple stents. Stroke. 36(9):e80-2, 2005
5. Edgell RC et al: Endovascular management of spontaneous carotid artery dissection. J Vasc Surg. 42(5):854-60; discussion 860, 2005
6. Sturzenegger M et al: Ultrasound findings in carotid artery dissection: analysis of 43 patients. Neurology. 45(4):691-8, 1995

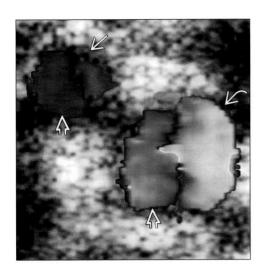

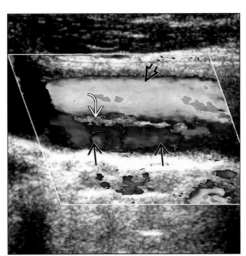

(Left) Axial color Doppler ultrasound shows dissection extending into the internal ➡ and external ➡ carotid arteries, with retrograde diastolic flow within the false lumen ➡. *(Right)* Longitudinal color Doppler ultrasound shows a CCAD with turbulent flow within the false lumen ➡. Note the thick echogenic dissection membrane ➡ and true lumen ➡.

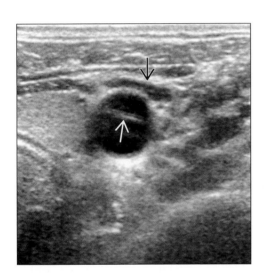

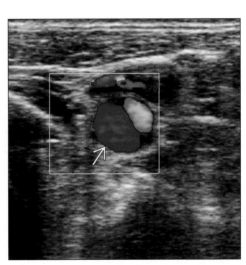

(Left) Axial grayscale ultrasound demonstrates a CCAD. Note the echogenic intimal flap ➡ and internal jugular vein ➡. *(Right)* Corresponding axial color Doppler ultrasound shows retrograde diastolic flow within the patent false lumen ➡.

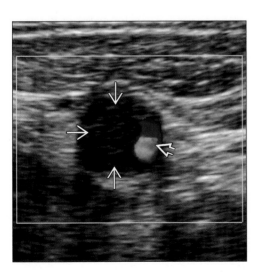

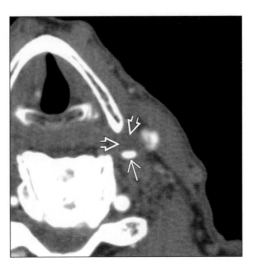

(Left) Axial color Doppler ultrasound shows the thrombosed false lumen ➡ of dissection of the CCA causing narrowing of the true lumen, which is still patent with flow signal ➡. *(Right)* Corresponding axial CECT shows the thrombosed nonenhancing false lumen ➡ of dissection of the left CCA causing narrowing of the patent enhancing true lumen ➡.

CAROTID STENOSIS/OCCLUSION

Key Facts

Imaging

- Characterization of plaques
  - Uniformly echolucent or predominantly echolucent; fatty or fibrofatty; ↑ risk of embolization
  - Uniformly/mildly echogenic and predominantly echogenic; fibrous; ↓ risk of embolization
  - Highly echogenic with distal shadowing, focal/diffuse; calcified; ↓ risk of embolization
  - Ulcerated: Focal crypt in plaque with sharp or overhanging edges; ↑ risk of embolization
- Grading of internal carotid artery (ICA) stenosis
  - < 50% stenosis: Peak systolic velocity (PSV) < 125 cm/s (end diastolic velocity [EDV] < 40 cm/s; PSV ratio [PSVR] < 2.0)
  - 50-69% stenosis: PSV 125-229 cm/s (EDV 40-99 cm/s; PSVR 2-3.9)
  - ≥ 70% stenosis: PSV ≥ 230 cm/s (EDV ≥ 100 cm/s; PSVR ≥ 4.0)

- Near occlusion: High-/low-velocity (trickle) flow
- Occlusion: Absent flow
- Common carotid artery (CCA) and ECA stenosis
  - No well-established Doppler criteria for grading stenosis
  - Measuring stenosis on color-coded images may underestimate degree of stenosis
- Diagnostic pitfalls
  - Trickle flow at near occlusion may be undetected
  - ICA stenosis may be underestimated due to poor cardiac function or tandem stenoses
  - Contralateral ICA stenosis may be overestimated due to crossover collateral flow
  - Moderate carotid stenosis may be underestimated due to normalization of flow at bulb

Diagnostic Checklist

- Correlate grayscale, color Doppler, and spectral Doppler findings when evaluating carotid stenosis

(Left) Longitudinal spectral Doppler US shows a tight stenosis at the proximal internal carotid artery (ICA) causing significant focal increase in flow velocity (> 700 cm/s). Aliasing artifacts are depicted within the stenotic lumen. Findings are predictive of a > 70% stenosis. (Right) Longitudinal spectral Doppler US shows total ICA occlusion. The proximal ICA segment is devoid of any Doppler signals ➦, whereas high-resistance monophasic waveforms are detected in the preocclusive segment.

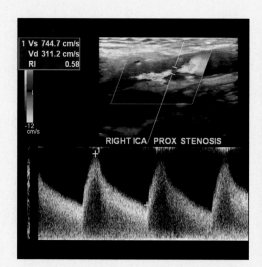
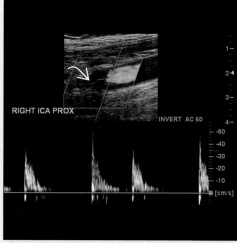

(Left) Longitudinal power Doppler ultrasound shows near occlusion at the proximal ICA with a slender residual lumen ➦. Compared with color Doppler, power Doppler is more sensitive to delineating the residual lumen with low-velocity flow. (Right) Corresponding spectral Doppler ultrasound shows "to and fro" flow within the severely stenotic segment due to high-flow resistance. The findings are suggestive of near occlusion.

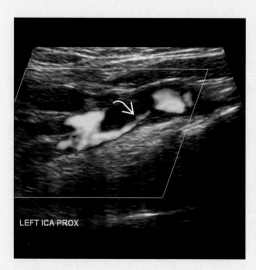
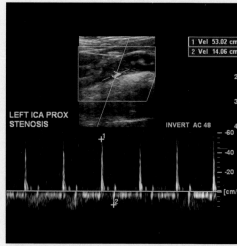

CAROTID STENOSIS/OCCLUSION

TERMINOLOGY

Definitions
- Stenosis: Narrowing of luminal diameter or area
- Occlusion: Complete blockage

IMAGING

General Features
- Best diagnostic clue
  - Stenosis: ↑ focal flow velocity on spectral Doppler
  - Occlusion: Absent flow on color or spectral Doppler
- Location
  - Predominantly at proximal internal carotid artery (ICA) near its origin
  - Less frequent: Common carotid artery (CCA) except as post-radiotherapy complication for H&N cancers
- Size
  - Stratification of ICA stenosis
    - < 50%, ≥ 50-69%, or ≥ 70-99% stenosis
    - Occlusion or near occlusion
- Morphology
  - Residual lumen: Concentric, eccentric, or irregular
  - Pattern of echogenicity: Uniformly echolucent, predominantly echolucent (> 50% of plaque), predominantly echogenic (> 50% of plaque), uniformly echogenic
  - Plaque ulceration

Ultrasonographic Findings
- Grayscale ultrasound
  - Atherosclerotic plaque
    - Increased risk of embolization
      - Heterogeneous: Focal or scattered areas of hypoechogenicity
      - Ulcerated: Focal crypt in plaque with sharp or overhanging edges
      - Uniformly echolucent or predominantly echolucent; fatty or fibrofatty
    - Decreased risk of embolization
      - Homogeneous: Uniform mid-level echotexture
      - Calcified: Highly echogenic with distal shadowing; focal/diffuse; dystrophic
      - Uniformly or mildly echogenic and predominantly echogenic; fibrous
  - Stenosis: Plaque formation + luminal narrowing
  - Occlusion: Echogenic material filling lumen
- Color Doppler: Useful for guiding site of interrogation and angle correction during velocity measurement
  - May depict blood flow in crypt of ulcerated plaque
  - Stenosis < 50%: Relatively uniform intraluminal color hues at and distal to stenosis
  - Stenosis ≥ 50-69%: Mildly disturbed intraluminal color hues at and distal to stenosis
  - Stenosis ≥ 70-99%: Color scale shift or aliasing due to elevated velocity at stenosis with significant poststenotic turbulence
  - Near occlusion: High-/low-velocity (trickle) flow
  - Occlusion: Absent color flow
  - Moderate stenosis: May normalize disturbed flow at carotid bulb
- Power Doppler: Useful for detecting low-velocity flow at and distal to near occlusion
  - Differentiates between near occlusion and occlusion

- Spectral Doppler: Useful for estimating degree of stenosis with velocity parameters
  - Peak systolic velocity (PSV) is most popular and recommended; primary parameter for grading ICA stenosis
  - PSVR ratio (PSVR) = PSV (ICA stenosis/normal CCA)
  - PSVR and end diastolic velocity (EDV): 2° parameter when ICA PSV may not reflect extent of stenosis
  - Grading of ICA stenosis
    - < 50% stenosis: PSV < 125 cm/s (EDV < 40 cm/s; PSVR < 2.0)
    - ≥ 50-69% stenosis: PSV 125-229 cm/s (EDV 40-99 cm/s; PSVR 2-3.9)
    - ≥ 70-99% stenosis: PSV ≥ 230 cm/s (EDV ≥ 100 cm/s; PSVR ≥ 4.0)
    - Near occlusion: Variable velocity
      - May be much lower than expected due to high flow resistance
      - Diagnosis based on color Doppler appearance and damped Doppler waveforms at or distal to stenosis
    - Occlusion: Absent flow on color or spectral Doppler
      - Artery filled with intraluminal echogenic material
    - Ancillary Doppler findings secondary to ICA occlusion or high-grade stenosis
      - Ipsilateral CCA: ↑ resistance flow
      - Ipsilateral CCA: ↓ resistance flow if external carotid artery (ECA) is a collateral
      - Ipsilateral ECA: ↓ resistance flow if it is a collateral
      - Ipsilateral ICA: Dampened/irregular waveforms distal to high-grade stenosis
      - Contralateral CCA & ICA: ↑ velocity ↓ resistance flow if crossover collateralization present
    - Moderate stenosis may be underestimated at carotid bulb due to normalization of flow
- CCA stenosis: No defined Doppler criteria but ICA criteria seem to work
  - Direct measurement on cross-sectional US images is usually feasible
  - Direct measurement on color-coded images may underestimate degree of stenosis due to color bleed
  - Ancillary Doppler waveform findings secondary to CCA occlusion/high-grade stenosis
    - Ipsilateral ICA: Low-resistance low-velocity waveforms; antegrade flow
    - Ipsilateral ECA: Low-resistance low-velocity waveforms; retrograde flow
    - Hemodynamic change across stenosis is helpful to detect a significant stenosis
- ECA stenosis: Limited studies available for grading
  - Hemodynamic change across stenosis is helpful to detect a significant stenosis

MR Findings
- MRA
  - Combination of MRA and US may replace DSA
  - MRA may over- or underestimate degree of carotid stenosis due to flow turbulence

Angiographic Findings
- DSA: Gold standard for documentation of carotid stenosis/occlusion
  - Accepted ICA stenosis measurement protocol
    - (1- maximal ICA diameter stenosis/diameter of post-bulbar ICA) x 100%

CAROTID STENOSIS/OCCLUSION

○ May underestimate degree of stenosis due to underestimation of outer luminal diameter at stenosis with post-bulbar diameter
○ ≥ 70% diameter stenosis on angiogram warrants carotid endarterectomy (CEA)

Imaging Recommendations

- Best imaging tool
  ○ Color Doppler US ± MRA
- Protocol advice
  ○ Always use PSV as primary parameter for grading of ICA stenosis; use power Doppler to detect trickle flow for excluding occlusion
  ○ Always apply PSVR and EDV in doubtful cases when PSV alone cannot reflect severity of stenosis
    ▪ Underestimation of stenosis % due to poor cardiac function or tandem stenoses
    ▪ Overestimation of stenosis % due to crossover collateralization in contralateral arteries

DIFFERENTIAL DIAGNOSIS

Bulb Flow Artifacts

- Areas of static flow may mimic plaque formation
- Complex flow pattern in carotid bulb (normal finding)
- Undisturbed flow in carotid bulb sign of plaque filling

Carotid Dissection

- CCA: Extends from arch and ends at bifurcation
  ○ 2 CCA lumina with blood flow in 1 or both
  ○ Possible oscillating membrane
- ICA: Begins near skull base and extends inferiorly; may not reach bifurcation
  ○ Long stenosis or occlusion on color/power Doppler
  ○ High-resistance flow proximal to dissection

Neointimal Hyperplasia Post-CEA or Stenting

- Smooth, tapered narrowing in treated area
- Uniform medium echogenic wall thickening

PATHOLOGY

General Features

- Etiology
  ○ Complex, multifactorial
    ▪ Genetic: Lipid metabolism dyscrasia
    ▪ Underlying disease, esp. diabetes and hypertension
    ▪ Lifestyle: Smoking, diet
    ▪ Anatomic or mechanical factors: Most severe at ICA origin
    ▪ Inflammation: ↑ recognized pathogenic factor
    ▪ Infection: Possible *Chlamydia* or *Helicobacter* association
- Genetics
  ○ Probably multigenetic

Gross Pathologic & Surgical Features

- Fatty or inflammatory material narrowing lumen

Microscopic Features

- Subendothelial deposition of lipid (fatty streak)
- Lipid deposits incite inflammatory response
- Macrophages ingest lipid → foam cells
- Inflammation → migration or transformation of smooth muscle cells

○ Subendothelial fibrous cap is formed
- Continued plaque growth and inflammation damage fibrous plaque
  ○ Inflammation or damage to cap → platelet or thrombus aggregation → embolization

CLINICAL ISSUES

Presentation

- Most common signs/symptoms
  ○ Transient ischemic attack (TIA), stroke, amaurosis fugax

Demographics

- Age
  ○ Elderly > 60 years old; clinically significant stenosis uncommon < 50 y/o
- Gender
  ○ Male predominance, possibly due to lifestyle &/or genetics
- Epidemiology
  ○ Carotid atherosclerosis is a major cause of morbidity/ mortality
    ▪ Up to 40% of deaths in elderly
    ▪ 90% of large cerebral infarcts caused by embolization (not all carotid)
    ▪ High-grade carotid stenosis in 30% of carotid territory strokes

Natural History & Prognosis

- TIA, by definition, has no permanent sequelae
- Stroke: Silent, neurological defect, permanent or with partial recovery

Treatment

- Current clinical practice (based on major carotid endarterectomy trials)
  ○ ≥ 70% or preocclusive ICA stenosis: CEA or carotid stenting, symptomatic or asymptomatic
  ○ ≥ 50% but < 70% of ICA stenosis: Intervention if symptomatic
  ○ < 50% stenosis: Treatment with antiplatelet agents
  ○ Occlusion: No ipsilateral therapy; possible intervention for contralateral disease
- Supportive for stroke

DIAGNOSTIC CHECKLIST

Consider

- Stenosis when disturbed flow is absent at carotid bulb
- Stenosis ≥ 70% when abnormally high/low carotid flow velocity detected in presence of plaque
- Occlusion when carotid flow is absent

Image Interpretation Pearls

- Presence of aliasing artifacts at stenosis with poststenotic turbulence or trickle flow within a stenotic segment is indicative of critical stenosis

SELECTED REFERENCES

1. von Reutern GM et al: Grading carotid stenosis using ultrasonic methods. Stroke. 43(3):916-21, 2012

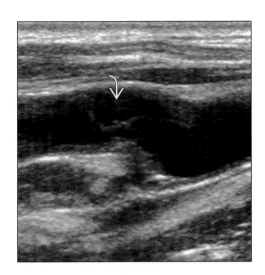

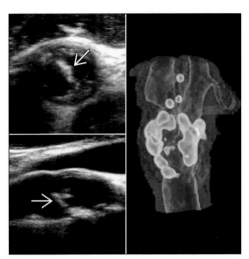

(Left) Longitudinal ultrasound shows a predominantly hypoechoic plaque ⇗ at the proximal ICA. Its low echogenicity is due to a large amount of lipid content within it. Such a plaque is known to be associated with an increased risk of embolic event. *(Right)* Transverse (left upper) and longitudinal (left lower) ultrasound shows an irregular plaque mimicking an ICA dissection with a flap ⇒ separating the lumen. Corresponding 3D CT reconstruction shows it is an irregular calcified plaque.

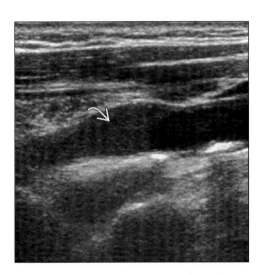

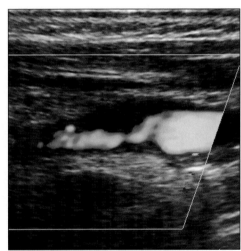

(Left) Longitudinal ultrasound shows a subtle hypoechoic fibrofatty plaque ⇗ at the proximal ICA. *(Right)* Corresponding power Doppler ultrasound shows the plaque causing a high-grade stenosis at the proximal ICA. Note the plaque is so echo-poor that it is difficult to see it on ultrasound and may be easily missed without the aid of color Doppler.

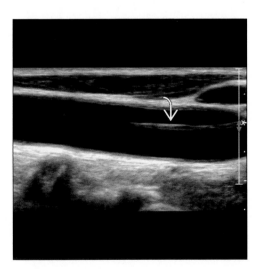

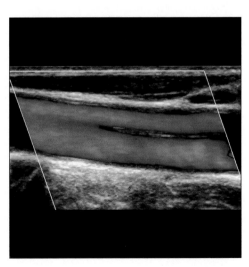

(Left) Longitudinal ultrasound shows CCA dissection with a thin intraluminal flap ⇗ dividing the mid CCA into 2 arterial lumina. *(Right)* Corresponding longitudinal color Doppler ultrasound shows color flow in both arterial lumina, confirming a dissection.

(Left) Longitudinal ultrasound shows an ulcerative plaque in the CCA. Note that there is a focal crypt ➦ within the plaque with sharp overhanging edges ➡, which is characteristic of an ulcer. *(Right)* Corresponding color Doppler ultrasound shows blood flow within the cavity ➤ of the ulcerative plaque.

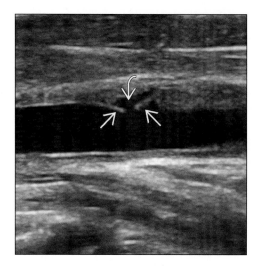
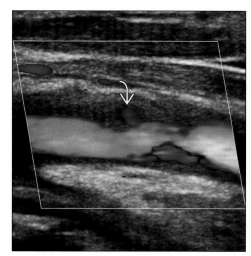

(Left) Longitudinal color Doppler ultrasound shows trickle flow ➡ within a stenotic plaque at the proximal ICA. Features are suggestive of a near occlusion. *(Right)* Corresponding spectral Doppler shows low-velocity monophasic flow within the residual lumen. Findings are consistent with near occlusion.

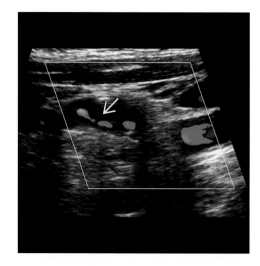
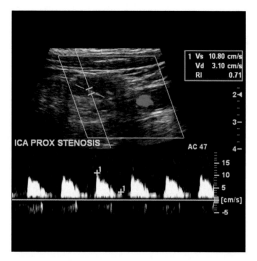

(Left) Longitudinal spectral Doppler shows normal flow velocities within a stenotic ICA segment (~ 60 cm/ s), which is predictive of a stenosis of < 50%. *(Right)* Corresponding ultrasound shows the luminal diameter reduction of the stenosis is 70%. The discrepancy in degree of stenosis as estimated by PSV and direct measurement may be due to poor patient cardiac output, tandem stenosis, and drop of PSV at a stenosis approaching near occlusion.

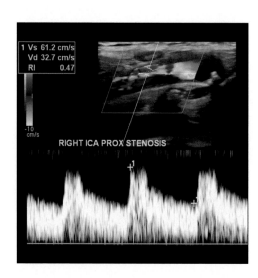
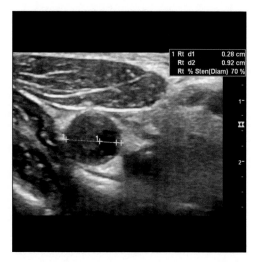

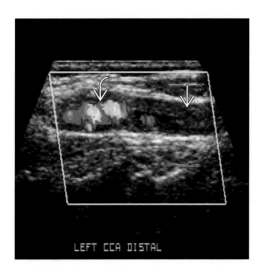

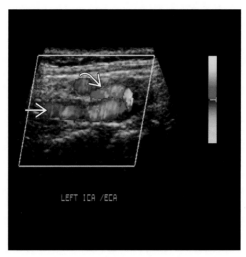

(Left) Longitudinal color Doppler ultrasound shows CCA occlusion with revascularization near the bifurcation. Note the distal CCA segment is absent of color signals ➡ whereas color signals are present at the bifurcation ➡. *(Right)* Color Doppler ultrasound of the same CCA occlusion shows retrograde flow in respective external carotid artery (ECA) ➡ supplying ipsilateral ICA where the flow is antegrade ➡. Note that the ECA is a common collateral pathway secondary to CCA occlusion.

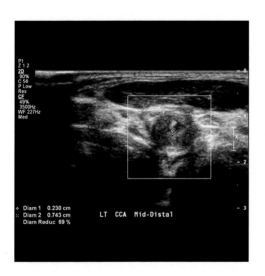

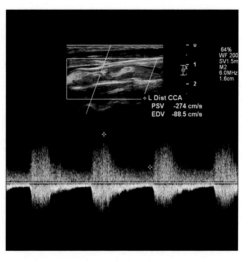

(Left) Transverse color Doppler US shows severe CCA stenosis estimated on cross section of the stenotic segment with the use of color Doppler. Caution must be taken to optimize color settings so as to avoid color bleed over the vessel wall, resulting in underestimation of degree of stenosis. *(Right)* Corresponding spectral Doppler shows significant increase in flow velocities within the stenotic segment with turbulence. Findings are consistent with a hemodynamically significant stenosis.

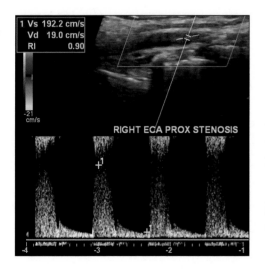

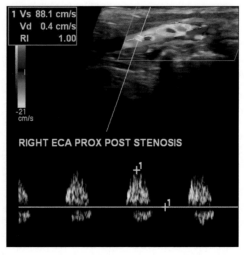

(Left) Spectral Doppler ultrasound shows severe ECA stenosis with significant increase in focal flow velocities with turbulence. *(Right)* Corresponding spectral Doppler ultrasound shows significant drop in flow velocities at the poststenotic segment. Although there is limited data for grading ECA stenosis, hemodynamic change across a stenosis provides a clue to the diagnosis of a significant stenosis.

VERTEBRAL STENOSIS/OCCLUSION

Key Facts

Imaging

- Plaque formation: Proximal vertebral artery (VA) > distal VA
- Grayscale imaging
  - Chronic occlusion: Contracted vessel caliber; VA may be hard to demonstrate
- Spectral Doppler
  - Stenosis: Significant focal ↑ in peak systolic velocity (PSV) + poststenotic turbulence or dampened flow
  - Occlusion: Absent Doppler signals; vertebral venous (VV) signals may be prominent
  - Asymmetrical VA velocities may be due to difference in vessel caliber or unilateral occlusive disease
  - Mild subclavian steal (SS): Systolic deceleration
  - Moderate SS: Alternating flow
  - Complete SS: Flow reversal
  - Dynamic test with affected arm exercise is recommended to test severity of subclavian steal

- Color Doppler
  - Stenosis: Aliasing or trickle flow at stenosis
  - Occlusion: Absent Doppler signals ± surrounding neck collaterals
  - Mild SS: Antegrade or minimal retrograde flow
  - Moderate SS: Bidirectional flow
  - Severe SS: Predominantly retrograde flow

Top Differential Diagnoses

- VA hypoplasia, subclavian steal, collateral artery, arteriovenous fistula

Diagnostic Checklist

- Check for presence of intraluminal plaque with abnormal ↑ or ↓ of PSV and neck arterial collaterals
- Consider alteration of VA flow velocity, flow asymmetry, and flow resistance as causes for stenosis/occlusion if it cannot be accounted for by VA size

---

(Left) Spectral Doppler ultrasound shows dampened waveforms of the V2 segment with delayed upstroke and reduced flow velocities. Findings are indicative of significant proximal arterial stenosis or occlusion *(Right)* Spectral Doppler ultrasound shows high-resistance waveforms with sharp upstroke and low end-diastolic velocity of the normal-sized V2 segment. Findings may be due to significant distal stenosis. Note that flow resistance is usually higher than normal in hypoplastic vertebral artery (VA).

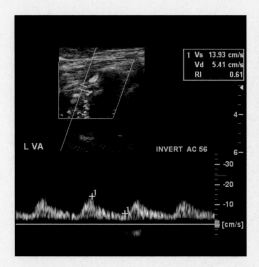 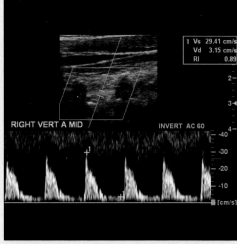

(Left) Spectral Doppler ultrasound shows abnormal biphasic flow in a small VA. The finding is suspicious of near or total arterial occlusion in the distal segment. *(Right)* Spectral Doppler ultrasound shows monophasic waveforms with sharp upstroke and absent diastolic components of the V2 segment. The finding is typical in preocclusive arterial segment.

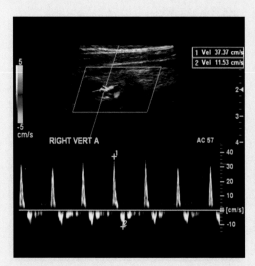 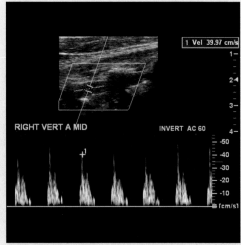

VERTEBRAL STENOSIS/OCCLUSION

TERMINOLOGY

Abbreviations

- Vertebral artery (VA) is divided into 4 segments
  - V1: Preinterforaminal segment (origin to point before entering transverse foramen of 6th cervical vertebra (C6)
  - V2: Interforaminal segment between C6 and C2
  - V3: Atlas loop segment (C2 to dura)
  - V4: Intracranial segment (dura to basilar artery [BA])

Definitions

- Luminal narrowing or blockage due to plaque formation, thrombosis, or dissection

IMAGING

General Features

- Best diagnostic clue
  - Stenosis: Focal ↑ in peak systolic velocity (PSV) at stenosis with poststenotic turbulent/dampened flow
  - Occlusion: Absent Doppler flow signals ± surrounding arterial collaterals
- Location
  - Plaque formation: Proximal VA > distal VA
    - Origin (most common)
    - High-grade stenosis in V2 and V3 is uncommon
    - Stenosis in V4 usually involves origin of BA
  - Dissection: Distal V1 (most common)
  - Thrombosis: Variable
- Size
  - Normal VA diameter: 2-4 mm
  - Hypoplasia: No consensus on definition but < 2 mm is widely accepted

Ultrasonographic Findings

- Grayscale imaging
  - Limited in depiction and characterization of plaque and detection of ostial stenosis
  - Stenosis: Luminal narrowing by hypoechoic plaque
  - Occlusion: Hypoechoic material filling arterial lumen
  - Chronic occlusion: Contracted vessel caliber; VA may be hard to demonstrate
- Spectral Doppler
  - Normal VA Doppler waveform resembles a scaled-down waveform of internal carotid artery
  - Normal VA PSV range: 20-60 cm/s
  - Stenosis: Significant focal ↑ in PSV + poststenotic turbulence or dampened flow
    - No standardized flow velocity criteria available to document degree of stenosis
    - US is insensitive for detection of mild stenosis
    - Moderate: Focal flow velocity ↑
    - High grade: Focal flow velocity markedly ↑ + aliasing + poststenotic disturbance/dampened flow ± prestenotic high-resistance flow
  - Occlusion: Absent Doppler signals; vertebral venous (VV) signals may be prominent
  - Proximal or distal stenosis/occlusion: Altered spectral Doppler waveform or flow resistance
  - Elevated VA flow velocity may indicate collateral pathway or compensatory increased flow due to contralateral VA hypoplasia or stenosis/occlusion
  - Asymmetrical VA flow velocities may be due to difference in vessel caliber or unilateral occlusive disease
  - Subclavian steal (SS) due to ipsilateral proximal subclavian artery stenosis/occlusion is best demonstrated by abnormal VA flow direction
    - Mild steal: Systolic deceleration
    - Moderate steal: Alternating flow
    - Complete steal: Flow reversal
    - Dynamic test with affected arm exercise is recommended to test severity of subclavian steal
      - May enhance steal after arm exercise
    - Bilateral steal is rare; caused by bilateral proximal subclavian or left subclavian + innominate artery stenosis or occlusion
- Color Doppler
  - Valuable for detection of VA stenosis/occlusion, secondary collateralization, and subclavian steal
  - Stenosis: Aliasing or trickle flow at stenosis
  - Occlusion: Absent Doppler signals ± surrounding neck collaterals
  - Subclavian steal
    - Mild: Antegrade or minimal retrograde flow
    - Moderate: Bidirectional flow
    - Severe: Predominantly retrograde flow
- Transcranial color Doppler (TCCD)
  - Useful in assessing patency of V4 segment and BA
  - Acoustic window: Transoccipital approach through foramen magnum
  - Severe subclavian steal: Reversed flow in BA + VA

MR Findings

- MRA
  - Similar to ultrasound, both are limited in demonstrating ostial stenosis
  - Tends to overestimate ostial stenosis at VA

Angiographic Findings

- DSA
  - Selective angiography remains gold standard
  - More sensitive than MRA and ultrasound for VA ostial stenosis
  - Delayed imaging performed to demonstrate reconstitution of VA through cervical collaterals

Imaging Recommendations

- Best imaging tool
  - Color Doppler is ideal for screening VA occlusive disease and evaluation of subclavian steal
  - DSA is best to evaluate VA stenosis/occlusion
- Protocol advice
  - Ultrasound is first-line investigation for VA disease
  - Selective vertebral angiography as preoperative investigation
- Technique
  - V1: Technically difficult to assess due to
    - Obscuration by clavicle especially on left
    - Vessel tortuosity
    - Confusion with other arterial branches
      - Mastoid tapping helps to differentiate VA from adjacent arteries
      - Flow disturbance appears on VA Doppler waveforms with mastoid tapping
    - Difficult to obtain accurate angle correction

VERTEBRAL STENOSIS/OCCLUSION

○ V2: Easily accessible; partially obscured by bony structures
  ▪ Provide indirect assessment of proximal and distal segments
  ▪ Examination of VA usually starts at V2 segment
○ V3: Not routinely examined unless V2 findings are abnormal
○ V4: Examined transcranially

DIFFERENTIAL DIAGNOSIS

Collateral Artery
- Occluded VA is usually reconstituted via cervical collaterals with flow direction towards VA

VA Hypoplasia
- ↑ risk of ischemic posterior circulation stroke
- Flow resistance is higher than normal because
  ○ Flow friction ↑ in small artery
  ○ Hypoplastic VA often supplies only ipsilateral posterior inferior cerebellar artery

Subclavian Steal
- Moderate steal with alternating flow may mimic "to and fro" flow in preocclusive segment

Arteriovenous Fistula (AVF)
- Abnormal communication between VA and VV
- High-velocity turbulent flow at AVF on color Doppler may be confused with high-grade stenosis

Extrinsic Bony Compression
- Caused by osteophytes, edge of transverse foramina, or intervertebral joints

PATHOLOGY

General Features
- Etiology
  ○ Atherosclerosis (primary)
  ○ Fibrous band in neck
  ○ Fibromuscular dysplasia
  ○ VA dissection
  ○ Vasculitis, giant-cell arteritis (most common)
  ○ Extrinsic compression by osteophytes, edge of transverse foramina, or intervertebral joints
    ▪ V2 segment most commonly affected during rotation and extension of neck
- VA stenosis accounts for 20% of posterior circulation ischemic stroke, mostly due to microembolization
- VA stenosis rarely causes hemodynamic stroke
- V4 stenosis is strongly associated with brainstem infarction

Gross Pathologic & Surgical Features
- Very few pathological in-vivo specimens available, as endarterectomy for vertebral stenosis is rare

CLINICAL ISSUES

Presentation
- Most common signs/symptoms
  ○ Vertebrobasilar insufficiency (VBI)
    ▪ Dizziness, vertigo, drop attack
    ▪ Diplopia, perioral numbness

▪ Alternating paresthesias, dysarthria, imbalance
▪ Tinnitus, dysphasia
○ Stroke (cerebellar, brainstem, posterior hemispheric)

Demographics
- Age
  ○ Mean: 62.5 years
- Gender
  ○ M > F
- Epidemiology
  ○ No population-based prevalence data for extracranial VA stenosis
  ○ More prevalent in Japanese, Chinese, and African Americans than Caucasians

Natural History & Prognosis
- Atherosclerosis
  ○ Atheroma formation with small lipid deposition in intima
  ○ Atheroma progression with ↑ lipid pool → narrowing of arterial lumen
  ○ Rupture of plaque → thrombus formation
    ▪ Healing and fibrosis of rupture plaque → further luminal narrowing
    ▪ Total arterial occlusion
    ▪ Thromboembolic stroke
- Prognosis is good after VA reconstruction
  ○ Combined stroke and death rate < 4%
- Fair prognosis for acute vertebrobasilar occlusion
  ○ Mortality rate ↓ from 90% to 60%

Treatment
- Symptomatic VBI but not fit for surgery: Long-term anticoagulation
- Acute VB occlusion
  ○ Atherothrombotic: Combined therapy of intravenous abciximab and intraarterial fibrinolysis + percutaneous transluminal angioplasty/stenting
  ○ Embolic occlusions: Mechanical catheter devices, such as basket or snare devices or rheolytic systems
- Chronic VB occlusion
  ○ Surgical intervention only in symptomatic patients
  ○ V1: Reconstruction with transposition of proximal VA onto common carotid artery (most common)
  ○ V1: Endarterectomy and bypass (less common)
  ○ V2: Elective surgical reconstruction rarely undertaken
  ○ V3 & V4: Surgical reconstruction, bypass, or transposition

DIAGNOSTIC CHECKLIST

Consider
- Alteration of VA flow velocity, flow asymmetry, and flow resistance as cause for stenosis/occlusion if it cannot be accounted for by VA size

Image Interpretation Pearls
- Presence of intraluminal plaque with abnormal ↑ or ↓ of PSV or flow resistance and neck arterial collaterals

SELECTED REFERENCES

1. Katsanos AH et al: Is vertebral artery hypoplasia a predisposing factor for posterior circulation cerebral ischemic events? A comprehensive review. Eur Neurol. 70(1-2):78-83, 2013

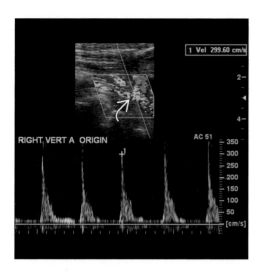

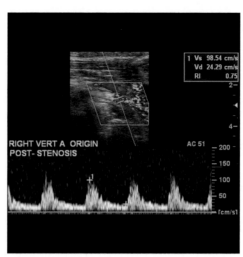

(Left) Spectral Doppler ultrasound shows an aliasing artifact ⬈ and abnormal increase in focal PSV (~ 300 cm/s) at the origin of the VA. Findings are indicative of significant stenosis. The most common site of VA stenosis is at its origin. *(Right)* Spectral Doppler ultrasound at the corresponding post-stenotic segment shows significant drop in PSV of the flow. This finding is characteristic of hemodynamically significant stenosis.

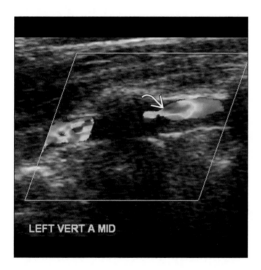

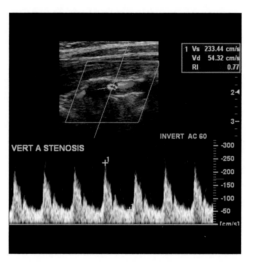

(Left) Color Doppler ultrasound shows stenotic V2 segment with aliasing artifact ⬈, which is the signature of significant stenosis and guides sonographers toward the site of maximal stenosis on color Doppler. *(Right)* Corresponding spectral Doppler ultrasound at the site of aliasing gives a PSV of 233.4 cm/s, which is well beyond the normal range of VA flow velocities (20-60 cm/s). This is suggestive of hemodynamically significant stenosis.

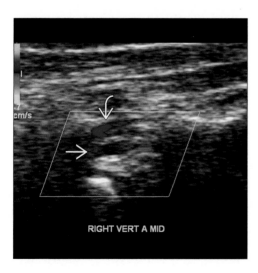

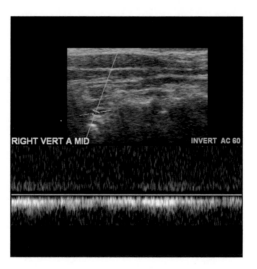

(Left) Longitudinal color Doppler ultrasound shows a VA occlusion. The occluded VA segment is devoid of any color flow signals ⮕, while flow signals are depicted in the adjacent VV ⬈. *(Right)* Corresponding spectral Doppler ultrasound shows no arterial signals on Doppler waveform, while venous signals appear below baseline.

(Left) Color Doppler ultrasound shows an occluded V1 segment ➡. Note that no color flow signals are apparent. *(Right)* Corresponding color Doppler ultrasound shows reconstitution of flow in the V2 segment ➡ by multiple cervical arterial collaterals ➡ secondary to proximal VA occlusion.

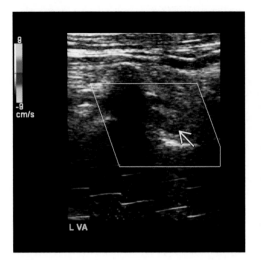

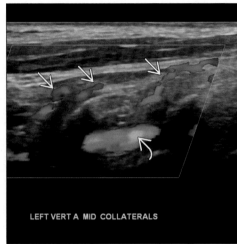

(Left) Spectral Doppler ultrasound of VA shows systolic deceleration in mild subclavian steal where a "notch" ➡ appears in waveforms during systole. Mild steal occurs with significant but not severe stenosis at the origin of the ipsilateral subclavian artery. *(Right)* Spectral Doppler ultrasound of VA shows moderate subclavian steal with transient reversed flow ➡ during systole. This bidirectional flow is caused by more severe stenosis at the origin of the ipsilateral subclavian artery.

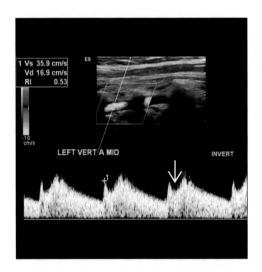

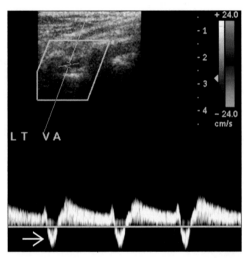

(Left) Spectral Doppler ultrasound of VA shows severe subclavian steal with complete flow reversal. This finding is due to subtotal stenosis or occlusion at the origin of the ipsilateral subclavian artery *(Right)* Spectral Doppler ultrasound of the corresponding ipsilateral subclavian artery at its origin shows dampened waveforms with delayed upstroke and reduced PSV. Findings are consistent with subtotal stenosis.

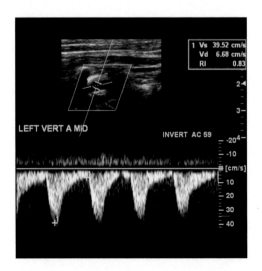

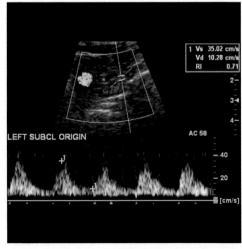

VERTEBRAL STENOSIS/OCCLUSION

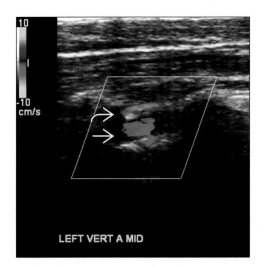

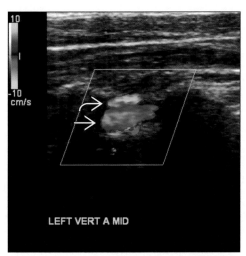

(Left) Color Doppler ultrasound shows normal antegrade flow in VA ➦ as depicted in red, and normal venous flow ➥ as denoted in blue in a patient with vertigo. Doppler ultrasound was requested to rule out vertebrobasilar insufficiency. *(Right)* Corresponding color Doppler ultrasound of VA shows transient retrograde flow indicative of moderate subclavian steal. Note both VA ➦ and VV ➥ flow direction is the same, denoted in blue.

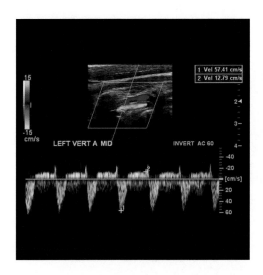

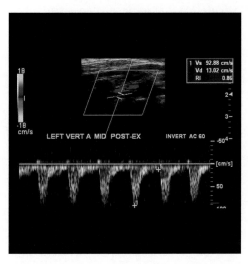

(Left) Spectral Doppler ultrasound shows bidirectional VA flow suggestive of moderate subclavian steal with the patient's affected arm at rest. *(Right)* Spectral Doppler ultrasound of corresponding VA shows enhanced retrograde flow with complete flow reversal after exercise of the affected arm. Dynamic functional test of the affected arm is important to test severity of subclavian steal.

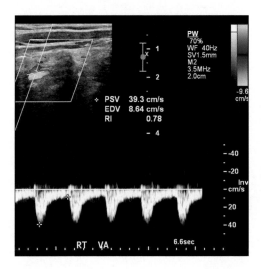

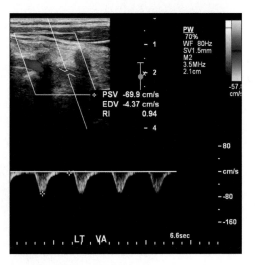

(Left) Spectral Doppler ultrasound shows a rare case of bilateral subclavian steal in which right VA flow shows complete flow reversal in both systole and diastole. *(Right)* Corresponding spectral Doppler of contralateral VA shows less steal with flow reversal only in systole, and stagnant flow in diastole. Bilateral steal is usually caused by bilateral proximal subclavian or innominate artery + left subclavian artery stenosis or occlusion.

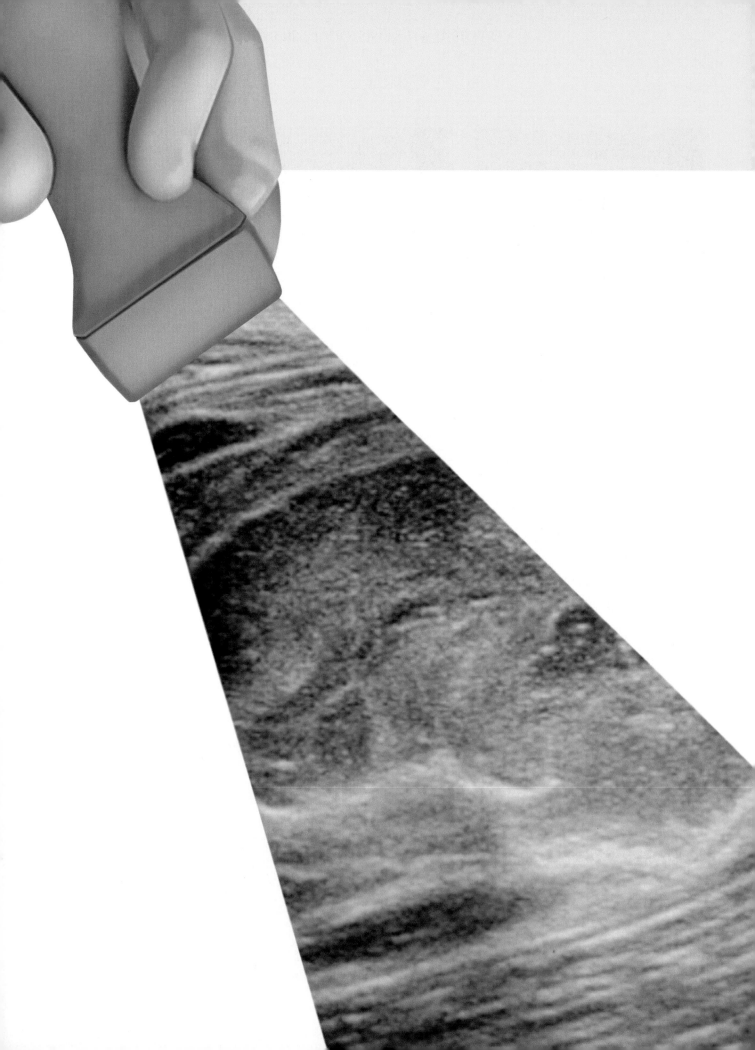

SECTION 7
Post-Treatment Change

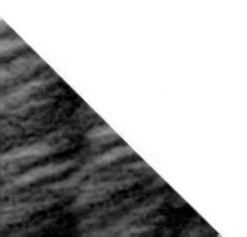

EXPECTED CHANGES IN THE NECK AFTER RADIATION THERAPY

Key Facts

Terminology

- Early radiation complications occur during course of XRT or within 90 days after treatment; mostly reversible
- Late radiation complications become apparent > 90 days after completion of treatment, take months to years to develop, and are often irreversible

Imaging

- Early: Diffuse edema of all soft tissues of superficial and deep face and neck
- Late: Atrophy of all radiated soft tissues and glands
- Examine both sides of neck and evaluate
- XRT-induced sialadenitis, thyroiditis, lymph node changes, and vasculopathy
- XRT-induced lymph node changes and vasculopathy
- XRT-induced secondary malignancies and osteoradionecrosis

Clinical Issues

- Oral pain from mucosal inflammation
- Myositis of masticator space → trismus
- Glandular atrophy

Diagnostic Checklist

- Severe XRT changes make evaluating scan difficult
- Residual or recurrent tumor may be easily missed, and meticulous examination technique is essential
- Imaging changes are dependent on XRT dose and rate, irradiated tissue volume, and time interval from completion of treatment
- Edema/inflammation most severe in 1st few months; many of these changes diminish/resolve (tissue atrophy does not resolve)
- Focal thickening or solid mass may suggest persistent/recurrent tumor/nodes
- Focal inflammatory changes suggest secondary infection or other complication

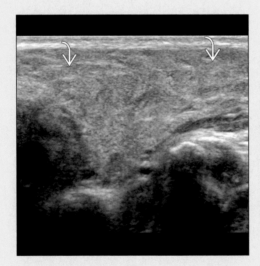
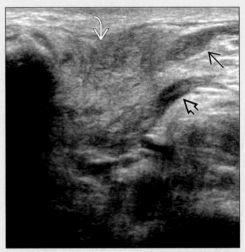

(Left) Transverse grayscale US shows XRT-induced acute parotitis. The parotid gland is diffusely enlarged with a hypoechoic, heterogeneous, parenchymal echo pattern ⤵ and no duct dilatation. These glands are often tender and transducer pressure is kept to minimum. *(Right)* Transverse grayscale US shows XRT-induced parotid atrophy. Gland is atrophic and hypoechoic with a heterogeneous, parenchymal echo pattern ⤵ and no duct dilatation. Note atrophic sternomastoid ➔ & posterior belly of digastric ⟱ muscles.

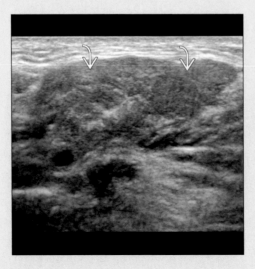
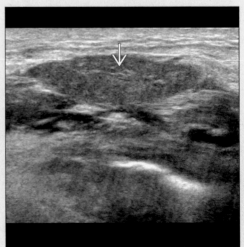

(Left) Transverse grayscale US shows XRT-induced acute submandibular sialadenitis. Note that the gland is diffusely enlarged with a hypoechoic, heterogeneous, parenchymal echo pattern ⤵ and no duct dilatation. *(Right)* Transverse grayscale US shows chronic sialadenitis of the submandibular gland, which appears atrophic with a heterogeneous, hypoechoic echo pattern ➔. At this stage there are usually clinical symptoms of xerostomia. Often such changes are bilateral, and the glands are firm on palpation.

EXPECTED CHANGES IN THE NECK AFTER RADIATION THERAPY

TERMINOLOGY

Abbreviations
- Radiation therapy (XRT)

Definitions
- Early radiation complications occur during course of XRT or within 90 days after treatment and are mostly reversible
- Late radiation complications become apparent > 90 days after completion of treatment, take months to years to develop, and are often irreversible

IMAGING

General Features
- Best diagnostic clue
  - Early: Diffuse edema of all soft tissues of superficial and deep face and neck
  - Late: Generalized atrophy of all radiated soft tissues and glands

Ultrasonographic Findings
- Early changes due to XRT
  - Skin and superficial muscle thickening, subcutaneous edema ("cobblestone/pavement" appearance)
  - Major salivary glands are often included in radiation field during XRT of head and neck neoplasms
  - Acute sialadenitis
    - Salivary glands are enlarged and hypoechoic
    - Heterogeneous echo pattern, no duct dilatation
    - ± increased vascularity on color Doppler
    - Tender on transducer pressure
    - ± adjacent inflammatory nodes
- Late changes due to XRT
  - Soft tissue fibrosis of neck
  - Chronic sialadenitis
    - Functional impairment and structural distortion results in xerostomia
    - Atrophic, small salivary glands, heterogeneous hypoechoic parenchyma, no duct dilatation
    - Usually no increased vascularity in Doppler
  - Radiation-induced vasculopathy
    - Accelerated atherosclerosis of carotid artery and thrombosis of IJV are well-known vascular complications of XRT
    - Latency period from 4 months to 20 years
    - Sonographic appearances of XRT-induced vasculopathy are indistinguishable from other atherosclerotic diseases
    - Often bilateral and conform to radiation field
    - Pseudoaneurysm of ICA is rare complication
  - Osteoradionecrosis
    - Ultrasound may detect osteoradionecrosis of mandible by demonstrating focal cortical disruption and possibly sequestra formation
    - Any associated soft tissue mass raises suspicion of tumor
  - Radiation-induced secondary malignancies
    - Rare; incidence of 0.037% for postradiation osteosarcoma in nasopharyngeal carcinoma patients
    - Latency from 4-27 years (mean: 13.3)
    - Various types of radiation-induced malignancies, including sarcomas, SCCa, and lymphoma
    - Diagnostic criteria
      - Lesion located in radiation field
      - No previous primary malignancy at site
      - Latency period of at least 3 years after completion of XRT
    - Variable appearances, commonly aggressive, and rapidly enlarging, ill-defined hypoechoic mass, ± ↑ vascularity on Doppler
    - Ossification may be seen in osteogenic tumors
  - Thyroiditis induced by XRT
    - Thyroid abnormalities induced by XRT include primary hypothyroidism, Graves disease (± ophthalmopathy), silent thyroiditis, Hashimoto thyroiditis, benign adenoma, and thyroid cancer
    - Thyroid storm after IMRT also reported
    - Radiation-induced thyrotoxicosis is usually transient while hypothyroidism is usually permanent
    - Thyroid damage starts to be seen within first 6 months, though peak incidence of hypothyroidism is at 2-3 years after treatment (50% within first 5 years after XRT)
    - Shorter latency associated with higher radiation dose
    - Early: Enlarged, hypoechoic, heterogeneous parenchyma, ↑ vascularity
    - Late: Atrophic, hypoechoic, heterogeneous parenchyma, ↓ vascularity
  - Changes in lymph nodes after XRT
    - Early: ↓ size, hypoechoic, heterogeneous, ↓ vascularity, and adjacent soft tissue edema
    - Late: ↓ size, hypoechoic, ± normal shape, bright fibrotic streaks in cortex, ± reappearance of hilum
    - Persistent/recurrent disease: Presence of nodes at previously uninvolved sites, ↑ size, vascularity, persistence of cystic necrosis, adjacent soft tissue edema
    - Post XRT hypertrophy: Nodes in known nonradiated sites, ↑ size, cortical hypertrophy, well defined, solid, ± round/elliptical, hilar vascularity

CT Findings
- CECT
  - Early (1-4 months): Diffuse edema of all tissues of neck
    - Thickened skin and platysma
    - Reticulation of subcutaneous and deep fat planes
    - Diffuse thickening and enhancement of mucosa, prominent submucosal edema
    - Swollen, ill-defined contours of parotid and submandibular gland (SMG)
  - Late (≥ 12 months): Diffuse fibrosis of all neck tissues
    - Thinning of subcutaneous and deep fat planes
    - Aryepiglottic (AE) fold and paralaryngeal fat edema remains in ~ 2/3 of patients
    - Glandular tissues (submandibular, parotid, thyroid) atrophy; often maintain increased enhancement
    - Radiated lymph nodes and lymphoid tissues atrophy

MR Findings
- T2 and T1 C+ accentuate changes seen on CECT
  - MR has greater sensitivity to soft tissue inflammation and to contrast enhancement
- Early: Extensive T2 hyperintensity and enhancement of most tissues

EXPECTED CHANGES IN THE NECK AFTER RADIATION THERAPY

- ○ Neck appears "watery" and diffusely inflamed
- ○ Muscles may show T2 hyperintensity
- ○ Symmetric diffuse enhancement of mucosa
- ○ Increased enhancement of salivary glands
- Late: Most soft tissues return to near-normal signal but appear atrophic
- ○ Timeline for tissue normalization not defined but likely takes longer than CECT
- ○ Decrease in enhancement of mucosal and glandular tissues

Nuclear Medicine Findings

- PET/CT
- ○ Carbon 11-methionine PET may allow assessment of individual response of major salivary glands to XRT
- ○ PET done within 10-12 weeks after completion of radiation therapy is associated with high false-positive results due to postradiation edema and inflammation
- Scintigraphy, in particular with SPECT, is useful for assessment of salivary excretory function

DIFFERENTIAL DIAGNOSIS

Oral Cavity Abscess

- Ludwig angina: Infection spreads through floor of mouth, forming multiple loculations

Acute Parotitis

- Inflammation of gland, often with extensive facial cellulitis
- Typically unilateral; hypoechoic, heterogeneous gland, ± calculus, duct dilatation, ↑ vascularity

SMG Sialadenitis

- Inflammation of SMG often associated with calculi
- Typically unilateral, hypervascular, hypoechoic, dilated duct, ± impacted calculus

PATHOLOGY

General Features

- Etiology
- ○ XRT destroys endothelial cells lining and small blood vessels
  - Early: Results in ischemia, edema, inflammation
  - Late: Results in tissue fibrosis
  - Tissues ill equipped to deal with extreme stressors → XRT complications
- Associated abnormalities
- ○ Chemotherapy may be given concurrently to sensitize tissues to XRT
  - Increases severity of acute side effects
  - Probably increases frequency of late effects
  - Improves overall results

CLINICAL ISSUES

Presentation

- Most common signs/symptoms
- ○ Oral pain from mucosal inflammation
  - Reduced saliva flow compounds
- ○ Myositis of masticator space → trismus
  - May occur early with myositis or late with fibrosis
- ○ Glandular atrophy

- Parotid atrophy → xerostomia
- Thyroid atrophy → hypothyroidism; may be subclinical
  - Seen in 26-48% of head and neck SCCa patients

Demographics

- Age
- ○ Any age, although SCCa, for which most XRT is given, is primarily a disease of adults > 45 years

Natural History & Prognosis

- Severity and duration of radiation reactions are correlated with treatment technique, cumulative dose, and volume of irradiated tissues, and may be aggravated by lifestyle factors such as smoking and alcohol, as well as individual radiosensitivity

DIAGNOSTIC CHECKLIST

Consider

- Imaging changes are dependent on XRT dose and rate, irradiated tissue volume, and time interval from completion of treatment
- ○ Edema and inflammation most pronounced in 1st few months
- ○ Many of these changes diminish/resolve
- ○ Tissue atrophy does not resolve

Image Interpretation Pearls

- Radiation changes are generally readily identifiable as such
- ○ Symmetric diffuse edema → symmetric diffuse fibrosis
- Be aware of asymmetric changes from unilateral XRT
- Severe XRT changes make evaluating scan difficult
- ○ Residual or recurrent tumor may be easily missed

Reporting Tips

- Look for focal thickening or solid mass to suggest residual or recurrent tumor/nodes
- ○ Evaluate specifically along jugular chains, submandibular space, and posterior triangle
- ○ More focal inflammatory changes suggest secondary infection or other complication

SELECTED REFERENCES

1. Glastonbury CM et al: The postradiation neck: evaluating response to treatment and recognizing complications. AJR Am J Roentgenol. 195(2):W164-71, 2010
2. Murphy BA et al: Mucositis-related morbidity and resource utilization in head and neck cancer patients receiving radiation therapy with or without chemotherapy. J Pain Symptom Manage. 38(4):522-32, 2009
3. Popovtzer A et al: Anatomical changes in the pharyngeal constrictors after chemo-irradiation of head and neck cancer and their dose-effect relationships: MRI-based study. Radiother Oncol. 93(3):510-5, 2009
4. Hermans R: Posttreatment imaging in head and neck cancer. Eur J Radiol. 66(3):501-11, 2008
5. Ahuja A et al: Echography of metastatic nodes treated by radiotherapy. J Laryngol Otol. 113(11):993-8, 1999
6. Ahuja A et al: The sonographic appearance and significance of cervical metastatic nodes following radiotherapy for nasopharyngaeal carcinoma. Clin Radiol. 51(10):698-701, 1996

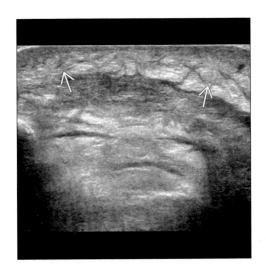

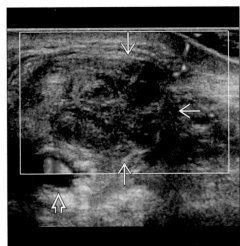

(Left) Transverse US shows typical post-radiation change in superficial soft tissues with generalized soft tissue thickening & prominent subcutaneous edema ➡, giving it a "cobblestone" appearance. *(Right)* Transverse power Doppler US shows focal, ill-defined, hypoechoic, heterogeneous lesion ➡ with cystic necrosis anterior to carotid ➡ in patient receiving XRT for nasopharyngeal carcinoma. Differentials include abscess formation & persistent metastatic node. Guided FNAC confirmed abscess.

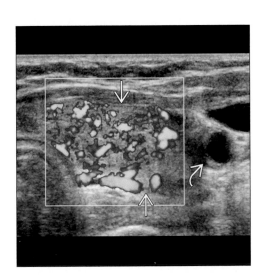

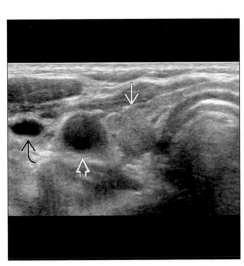

(Left) Transverse power Doppler US shows XRT-induced thyroiditis. Thyroid gland ➡ is diffusely enlarged with a rounded contour, heterogeneous echo pattern, and increased vascularity. Note the associated carotid wall thickening ➡. *(Right)* Transverse grayscale US shows chronic sequela of thyroiditis from XRT. Thyroid ➡ is atrophic, heterogeneously hypoechoic, and was hypovascular on color Doppler (not shown). Such patients are often hypothyroid. Note the carotid ➡ & IJV ➡.

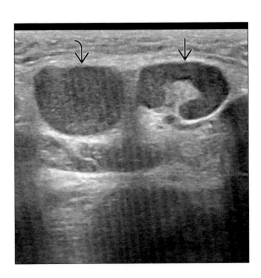

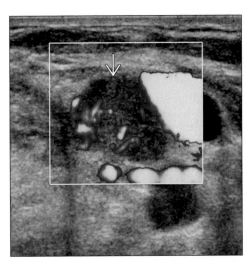

(Left) Axial grayscale US in a patient with XRT for NPC a few years ago shows enlarged, solid, well-defined, hypoechoic nodes with hypertrophied cortex. One node shows echogenic hilum ➡ and another none ➡, mimicking a metastatic node (FNAC benign). Submental and paratracheal regions are common sites for such hypertrophic nodes (post RT for NPC), possibly due to midline shunting of lymphatic flow. *(Right)* Axial power Doppler shows hypertrophic paratracheal node ➡ with malignant vascularity.

EXPECTED CHANGES IN THE NECK AFTER RADIATION THERAPY

(Left) Transverse grayscale US shows atherosclerotic plaque ⮞ causing narrowing of the right CCA ⮞ lumen by 50%. Atherosclerosis is known to be accelerated by XRT. (Right) Transverse power Doppler US shows complete occlusion of the left CCA by calcified thrombus ⮞. It is not uncommon to identify accelerated atherosclerosis in relatively young patients after XRT to the neck, severe enough to cause almost complete occlusion of carotid arteries despite being relatively asymptomatic.

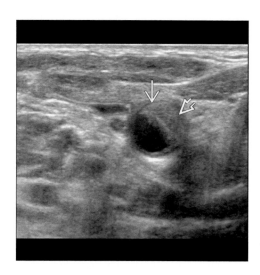
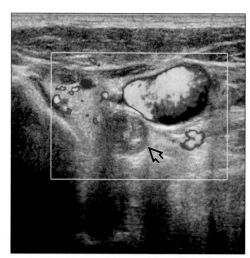

(Left) Transverse grayscale US in a patient after XRT for NPC presents with a palpable left upper neck mass. On US, the palpable mass ⮞ has extensive thickening and atherosclerotic change involving the carotid artery. Note CCA lumen ⮞. (Right) Longitudinal grayscale US (same patient) clearly demonstrates the true nature of the lesion, seen as dense atherosclerotic plaques ⮞ within CCA lumen ⮞. Note the posterior acoustic shadows from densely calcified plaques ⮞.

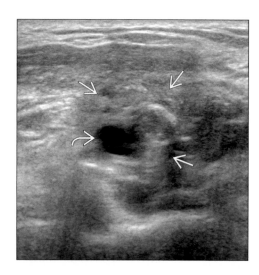
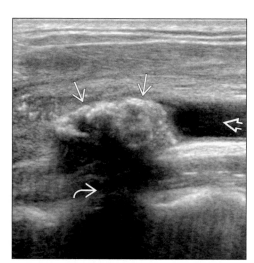

(Left) Longitudinal grayscale US shows the normal, smooth mandibular contour is replaced by cortical irregularity, disruption with stepping, and echogenic foci suspicious of sequestra ⮞. Features are suggestive of mandibular osteoradionecrosis. (Right) Transverse power Doppler US shows a metastatic deposit in sternocleidomastoid muscle ⮞. Metastatic deposits may be present at sites other than surgical bed & nodal groups, and meticulous technique & attention to detail is essential to evaluate post-XRT neck.

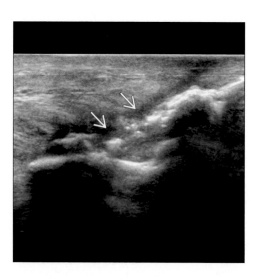
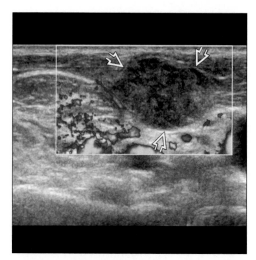

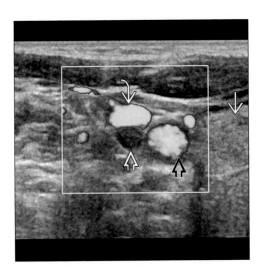

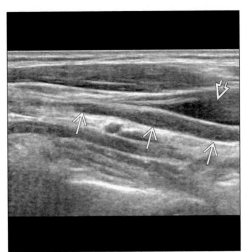

(Left) Transverse power Doppler US in a patient with previous XRT for NPC shows thickened right vagus nerve ⊳. Post-radiotherapy thickening of vagus nerve is commonly observed and may be mistaken for abnormal lymph node and lead to unnecessary FNAC. Note IJV ⊳, CCA ⊳, and thyroid ➔. Similarly, post-XRT thickened brachial plexus may be mistaken for metastatic nodes in supraclavicular fossa. (Right) Corresponding longitudinal grayscale US shows entire thickened vagus nerve ➔. Note the IJV ⊳.

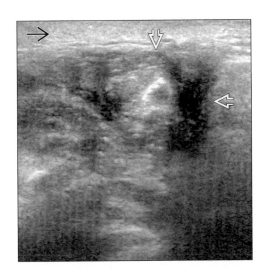

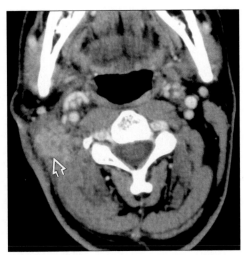

(Left) Transverse grayscale US in a patient with XRT for head and neck carcinoma shows an ill-defined recurrent tumor ⊳ embedded within fibrotic neck tissues. Note subcutaneous edema ➔. Due to its high resolution, US identifies these recurrences and readily guides FNAC for confirmation. (Right) Corresponding axial CECT shows the recurrent tumor as an ill-defined area of mild enhancement ➔. Recurrent tumors may be quite subtle in post-radiotherapy neck due to distorted anatomy and extensive fibrosis.

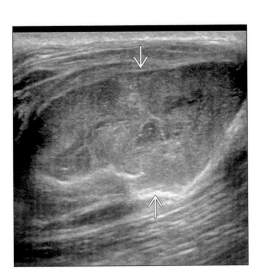

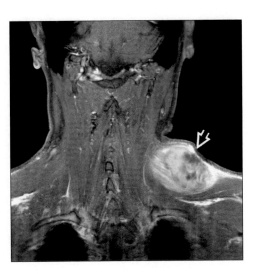

(Left) Oblique grayscale US shows a well-defined, heterogeneous, solid mass ➔ in the left trapezius muscle. This site was included in the radiation field although not involved by the tumor. XRT was completed 5 years ago. This finding is suspicious of radiation-induced tumor. (Right) Corresponding coronal T1WI C+ FS MR shows avid, heterogeneous enhancement of a smoothly marginated tumor ➔ in the trapezius muscle. Biopsy confirmed malignant fibrous histiocytoma.

POSTSURGICAL CHANGES IN THE NECK

Key Facts

Terminology

- Postsurgical imaging findings include altered anatomy from surgical resection/reconstruction, residual/recurrent tumor, and postoperative complications

Imaging

- Postoperative US requires sound technique, meticulous attention to detail, knowledge of appearance of expected changes; often used in conjunction with CT/MR & guided FNAC
- Aim of postoperative US surveillance is to identify expected postop changes, potential postop complications, and to differentiate these from tumor recurrence
- Postoperative complications detected by US may include seroma, hematoma, abscess, fistula
- Most surgery-related complications occur in early postop period

Clinical Issues

- Tumor recurrence, especially those deep to flap reconstructions, are not readily accessible by visual examination or physical palpation; imaging surveillance is therefore required for early detection, and US serves as quick and noninvasive first-line modality for such purpose
- Perineural tumor spread/recurrence in head and neck is most commonly observed in squamous cell carcinoma (SCCa), and less frequently in adenoid cystic carcinoma, malignant lymphoma, and malignant schwannoma; best demonstrated on MR due to its superior soft tissue contrast
- Risk factors for surgical complications include preoperative radiotherapy or chemoradiation, previous tracheostomy, advanced age, medical complications, malnutrition, anemia, smoking, and alcoholism

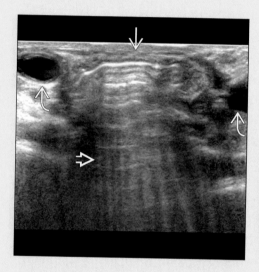
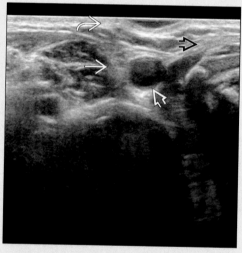

(Left) Transverse grayscale US shows free jejunal flap ➡ with a hypoechoic bowel wall, hyperechoic mucosal folds, and reverberation artifacts ⇶ from intraluminal bowel gas. Note common carotid artery ➡. *(Right)* Transverse grayscale US in a patient with RND shows right internal carotid artery (ICA) ➡. Expected positions of right submandibular gland ⊟, IJV ➡, and SCM muscle ➡ are empty from previous resection. RND involves removal en bloc of all ipsilateral nodes levels I-V, these 3 structures, and the spinal accessory nerve.

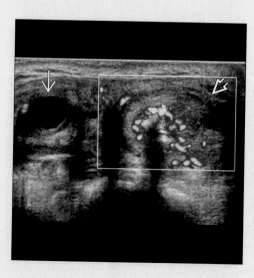
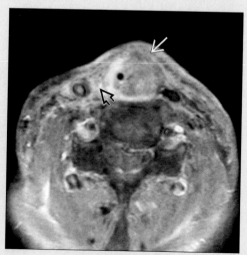

(Left) Transverse power Doppler US shows tumor recurrence at anastomosis of bowel interposition appearing as eccentric, irregular wall thickening with increased vascularity ➡. Note adjacent right ICA ➡ with surrounding soft tissue thickening due to scar/fibrosis and obliteration of fat planes. *(Right)* Corresponding axial T1WI C+ MR shows anastomotic recurrent tumor as ill-defined, poorly enhancing, eccentric thickening ➡. Fibrotic thickening around the right carotid sheath is again seen ⊟.

POSTSURGICAL CHANGES IN THE NECK

TERMINOLOGY

Definitions

- Postsurgical imaging findings include altered anatomy from surgical resection and reconstruction, residual or recurrent tumor, and postoperative complications

IMAGING

Ultrasonographic Findings

- Aim of postop US surveillance is to identify expected postop changes, potential postop complications, and to differentiate these from tumor recurrence
- Postop complications detected by US may include seroma, hematoma, abscess, and fistula
- Altered anatomy
  - Tissue transfer
    - Most commonly used for pharyngoesophageal reconstruction after pharyngolaryngoesophagectomy (PLO)
    - May involve gastric pull-up, colonic transposition, free jejunal interposition, or free radial forearm flap
    - Free jejunal autotransplantation may be most common
    - Interposed bowel shows alternating hypoechoic/hyperechoic wall/mucosal folds standing out against heterogeneous hypoechoic contents in bowel lumen
    - Bowel peristalsis and reverberation artifacts from intraluminal bowel gas are often seen
    - Mesentery with vascular arcades and lymph nodes are also readily identifiable
    - Mesenteric nodes may be prominent but usually reactive due to postop environmental change (malignant change is known to occur, often associated with tumor recurrence)
    - Jejunal free flap based on jejunal artery from SMA is susceptible to ischemia
    - Differential diagnosis may include Zenker diverticulum
    - Reconstructed myocutaneous flap for replacement of part of trachea and cricoid cartilage may be seen after surgery for aggressive thyroid cancer
  - Neck dissection
    - Absence of tissues resected together with neck nodes
    - Radical neck dissection includes removal en bloc of all ipsilateral nodes levels I-V, including
      - (1) sternocleidomastoid muscle, (2) IJV, (3) submandibular gland, and (4) spinal accessory nerve
    - Modified radical neck dissection involves en bloc removal of all ipsilateral nodes with sparing of 1 or more of the other 4 structures
    - Extended radical neck dissection includes removal of additional nodes (levels VI & VII) &/or nonlymphatic structures (e.g., ICA, CN10, & CN12)
    - Soft tissue thickening from fibrosis or scar is seen around carotid sheath obliterating fat planes
- Residual or recurrent tumor
  - Residual nodal metastases may be seen in immediate postop period due to incomplete preop work-up
  - Tumor recurrence typically occurs within first 2 years post treatment

- May also be seen within weeks after surgery before adjuvant RT due to accelerated repopulation
- Most common sites for recurrence are at surgical bed and its margins
- Sonographic appearances of metastatic nodes
  - Metastatic nodes tend to be round, except for focal intranodal tumor deposition in which node may show eccentric cortical hypertrophy
  - Tumor deposition results in ↑ heterogeneity in acoustic impedance between node and its adjacent tissues and gives rise to sharp, nodal borders
  - Ill-defined, unsharp borders of metastatic nodes imply extracapsular spread, which indicates poor prognosis
  - Loss of normal hyperechoic hilar architecture may be seen in 69-95% of metastatic nodes
  - Head and neck (H&N) squamous cell carcinoma (SCCa) metastatic nodes are hypoechoic, whereas papillary thyroid carcinoma metastatic nodes are hyperechoic when compared to muscles
  - Calcifications are commonly seen in metastatic nodes from papillary and medullary thyroid cancers but are rare in SCCa metastatic nodes
  - Intranodal necrosis is a common finding in SCCa metastatic nodes
  - Presence of peripheral vascularity is highly suggestive of metastatic nodes, which may show both peripheral or mixed (hilar and peripheral) vascularity on color or power Doppler
  - Spectral Doppler usually shows high intranodal vascular resistance (RI > 0.8, PI > 1.6) in metastatic nodes
  - Location
    - Carcinomas in oral cavity: Level I, II, & III nodes
    - Carcinomas in oropharynx (OP) and supraglottic larynx: Level II, III, & IV nodes
    - Carcinomas in nasopharynx (NP), hypopharynx, and tongue base: Level II, III, IV, & V nodes
    - Thyroid cancer: Level III, IV, & VI nodes
    - Carcinomas in NP, OP, tongue base, and supraglottic larynx often show bilateral nodal metastases
    - Level IIA (jugulodigastric group) is most frequently involved nodal group
  - Nodal size alone is not very useful criteria, although in patients with known H&N cancer enlarging node on serial studies is highly suspicious of metastasis
  - Differential diagnosis of nodal metastases
    - Non-Hodgkin lymphoma nodes: Multiple, round, hypoechoic, well-defined nodes with pseudocystic or reticulated pattern, marked hilar and peripheral vascularity
    - Tuberculous nodes: Multiple, hypoechoic, heterogeneous nodes with intranodular necrosis, nodal matting, adjacent soft tissue edema, avascular or displaced hilar vascularity
    - Reactive nodes: Elliptical, solid, hypoechoic nodes with normal echogenic hila and low-resistance hilar vascularity
  - Sonographic appearances of recurrent tumors
    - Low-grade tumors may appear well defined and solid with predominantly homogeneous echo pattern

POSTSURGICAL CHANGES IN THE NECK

- High-grade tumors tend to be more ill defined and hypoechoic with heterogeneous architecture due to necrosis or hemorrhage
- Extracapsular spread with invasion of adjacent tissues may be seen
- ± recurrent metastatic nodes may also be present
- Profuse chaotic intratumoral vascularity often shown on color or power Doppler
- Potential postoperative complications
  - Most surgery-related complications occur in early postoperative period
  - Seroma
    - After surgery, focal collections due to serous retention may be seen, often adjacent to flaps
    - Such serous retentions tend to resolve spontaneously and require no further treatment
    - Sonographically these seromas appear as well-defined, homogeneous, anechoic collections with posterior acoustic enhancement
    - No eccentric wall thickening, internal septation, or solid component if simple
    - Echogenic debris, if present, suggests hemorrhagic component
    - ± increased wall vascularity if secondarily infected
  - Hematoma
    - Acute hematoma may appear echogenic
    - Subacute hematoma may show fluid-fluid level
    - Complicated cystic collection with internal septations due to fibrinous strands or heterogeneous solid lesion
    - Posterior acoustic enhancement
    - No internal blood flow on color or power Doppler; healing stage may show peripheral vascularity
  - Abscess
    - Appears as ill-defined, irregular, uni-/multilocular collection with thick walls, septa, internal debris, surrounding soft tissue edema, and loss of normal fascial planes
    - Increased vascularity on color Doppler is usually present at abscess wall and adjacent soft tissues
    - Prominent inflammatory nodes may be seen in vicinity
    - Potential complication may include venous thrombophlebitis and carotid involvement
    - Abscess with extension beyond accessibility of US should be evaluated by CT/MR before aspiration or surgical drainage
    - Differential diagnosis includes necrotic metastatic nodal mass with superimposed infection
    - FNAC helps to establish diagnosis and provides specimens for laboratory analysis
  - Fistula
    - Seen as hypoechoic tracts connecting 2 or more epithelial-lined cavities
    - ± ↑ vascularity on color Doppler if infected
    - Deep extent of fistula may not be visualized by US
    - Chylous fistula is seen in 1-2% of post-neck dissection patients, especially those with level IV node dissection, usually in left lower neck

CT Findings

- Myocutaneous flaps gradually show denervation atrophy, volume loss, and fatty change with variable enhancement pattern, which do not predict failure of flap reconstruction

- Recurrent tumors appear as infiltrating lesions with attenuation similar to muscles and enhancement; lesions with lower attenuation than that of muscles are less likely to be malignant and are often due to edema

MR Findings

- Diffusion-weighted imaging (DWI) may be useful in differentiating tumor recurrence from early, normal post-treatment changes
- High signal on DWI with ↓ value for ADC is suspicious of tumor recurrence due to restricted proton movement in extracellular space from tumor hypercellularity
- ↑ ADC is seen in inflammation, necrosis, or submucosal fibrosis from ↑ interstitial space and low cellularity

Imaging Recommendations

- Protocol advice
  - Postoperative US requires sound technique, meticulous attention to detail, knowledge, and appearance of expected changes
    - Often used in conjunction with CT/MR, which globally evaluate postsurgical change better
    - Distorted anatomy makes scanning difficult and may restrict transducer contact particularly in early postoperative phase
      - Operative scars, wounds, tubes, etc. may also restrict US access
    - US-guided aspiration is immensely useful in confirming nature of abnormalities and draining collections/abscesses

CLINICAL ISSUES

Natural History & Prognosis

- Tumor recurrence, especially those deep to flap reconstructions, are not readily accessible by visual examination or physical palpation
  - Imaging surveillance is therefore required for early detection, and US serves as quick and noninvasive first-line modality for such purpose
- Perineural tumor spread/recurrence in H&N is most commonly observed in SCCa, and less frequently in adenoid cystic carcinoma, malignant lymphoma, and malignant schwannoma
  - Best demonstrated on MR due to its superior soft tissue contrast
- Risk factors for surgical complications include preoperative radiotherapy or chemoradiation, previous tracheostomy, advanced age, medical complications, malnutrition, anemia, smoking, and alcoholism
- Reported surgical complication rates in H&N after radiotherapy is 37-74% and after chemoradiation is 46-100%
- Reported incidence of pharyngocutaneous fistula is 3-65% after total laryngectomy

SELECTED REFERENCES

1. Saito N et al: Posttreatment CT and MR imaging in head and neck cancer: what the radiologist needs to know. Radiographics. 32(5):1261-82; discussion 1282-4, 2012

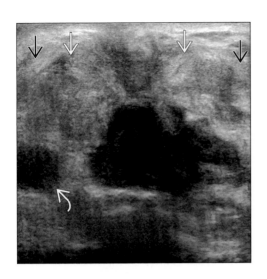

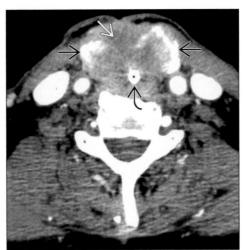

(Left) Transverse grayscale US shows another example of recurrent tumor at gastric pull-up anastomosis appearing as an infiltrative hypoechoic mass ➡ invading both lobes of the thyroid ➡. There is loss of normal bowel signature. US-guided FNAC confirmed diagnosis. Note the CCA ➡. *(Right)* Corresponding axial CECT shows recurrent tumor is ill defined and poorly enhancing ➡ on CT, with invasion of thyroid ➡. Endogastric tube ➡ is completely encased by the tumor. CECT better shows tumor extent.

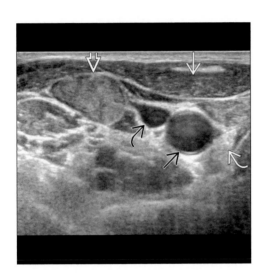

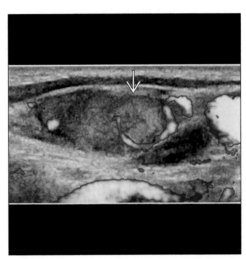

(Left) Axial grayscale US following total thyroidectomy shows a residual cervical chain metastatic node ➡, hyperechoic to muscle ➡. The right thyroid bed is clear ➡. Incomplete preoperative work-up may lead to understaging and incomplete surgery. Note the CCA ➡ & IJV ➡. *(Right)* Corresponding longitudinal Doppler US shows ↑ intranodal vascularity. Papillary thyroid cancer metastatic nodes ➡ are hyperechoic to muscle and may contain punctate microcalcification, similar to primary tumor.

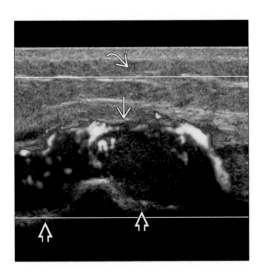

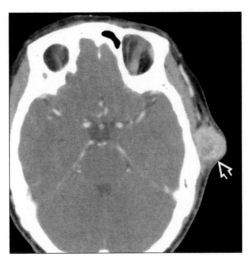

(Left) Longitudinal power Doppler US shows an irregular, hypoechoic mass ➡ with profuse vascularity over the skull vault ➡ and under the surgical flap ➡. Appearances are highly suspicious for tumor recurrence at the margin of the surgical bed. *(Right)* Corresponding CECT (same patient) shows a suspicious tumor recurrence as an avidly enhancing mass overlying the skull vault under the surgical flap ➡. US-guided biopsy confirmed local tumor recurrence.

POSTSURGICAL CHANGES IN THE NECK

(Left) Longitudinal grayscale US in a patient with recent head and neck surgery shows an ill-defined, irregular, hypoechoic, heterogeneous lesion with thick walls and internal debris ➡ anterior to the sternomastoid muscle ➡. Note edematous soft tissues and loss of normal fascial planes. *(Right)* Corresponding power Doppler US shows profuse vascularity within the lesion ➡. Sonographic appearances are suggestive of early abscess formation/phlegmon.

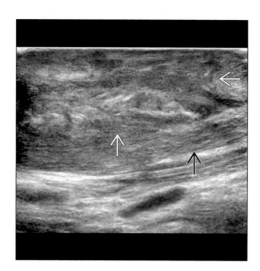 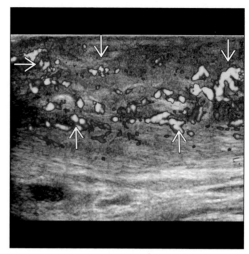

(Left) Axial CECT (same patient) shows the abscess as an ill-defined, heterogeneous mass ➡ with poorly enhancing necrotic component, adjacent inflammatory change, and loss of fascial planes. *(Right)* Corresponding PET/CT fusion images show the abscess to be intensely and homogeneously hypermetabolic ➡. Both inflammatory/infectious lesions and malignant lesions may show ↑ metabolism and be indistinguishable on FDG-PET alone. Biopsy revealed actinomycotic abscess.

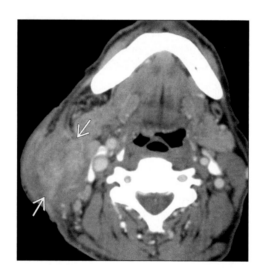 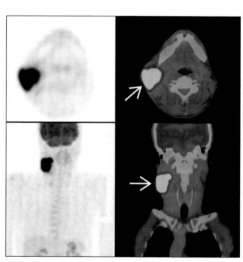

(Left) Transverse grayscale US shows another neck abscess as an ill-defined, irregular, hypoechoic mass ➡ with internal debris and necrosis. Note the left lobe of the thyroid ➡, left CCA ➡, and IJV ➡. *(Right)* Corresponding longitudinal grayscale US shows the abscess ➡ with internal necrosis ➡ inseparable from the sternomastoid anteriorly ➡. US can be used to target liquefied component for aspiration to reduce size and obtain a specimen for confirmatory laboratory tests.

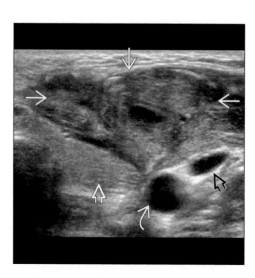 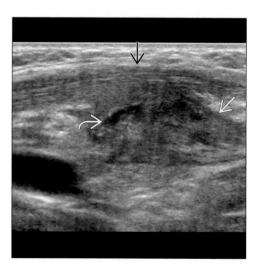

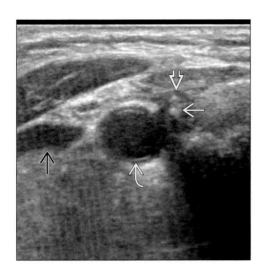

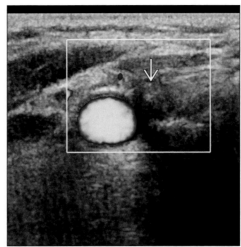

(Left) Transverse grayscale US in a patient with previous total thyroidectomy for papillary carcinoma shows presence of hypoechoic soft tissue ➡ with small echogenic foci ➡ in the right thyroid bed. Note the CCA ➡ & IJV ➡. *(Right)* Corresponding transverse power Doppler US shows no abnormal vascularity in the focal, soft tissue lesion ➡. Differential diagnosis includes suture granuloma, recurrent papillary thyroid cancer. Guided biopsy confirmed suture granuloma.

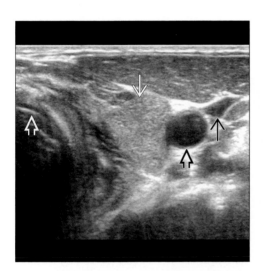

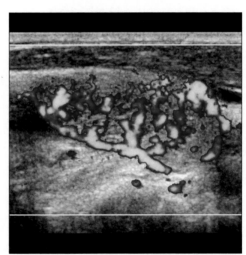

(Left) Post-thyroidectomy remnant thyroid may become hypertrophic, as in this patient with subtotal thyroidectomy for refractory thyrotoxicosis, with remaining thyroid becoming roundish in contour and slightly enlarged ➡. Note the CCA ➡, IJV ➡, and trachea ➡ on transverse grayscale US. *(Right)* Corresponding power Doppler US shows marked vascularity in thyroid remnant, a common feature in the thyroid hypertrophy following surgery for thyrotoxicosis.

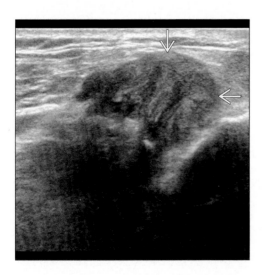

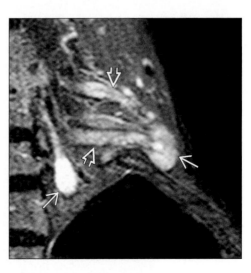

(Left) Axial grayscale US in a postoperative neck demonstrates a focal, nodular lesion ➡ at the lower posterior triangle, paraspinal in location. In another plane, thickened brachial plexus elements were seen in continuity with this lesion (not shown in this image). Findings suggested stump neuroma. *(Right)* Corresponding coronal T2WI FS MR confirms stump neuromas ➡ and thickened brachial plexus ➡, all with high T2 signal. No confirmatory FNAC was necessary.

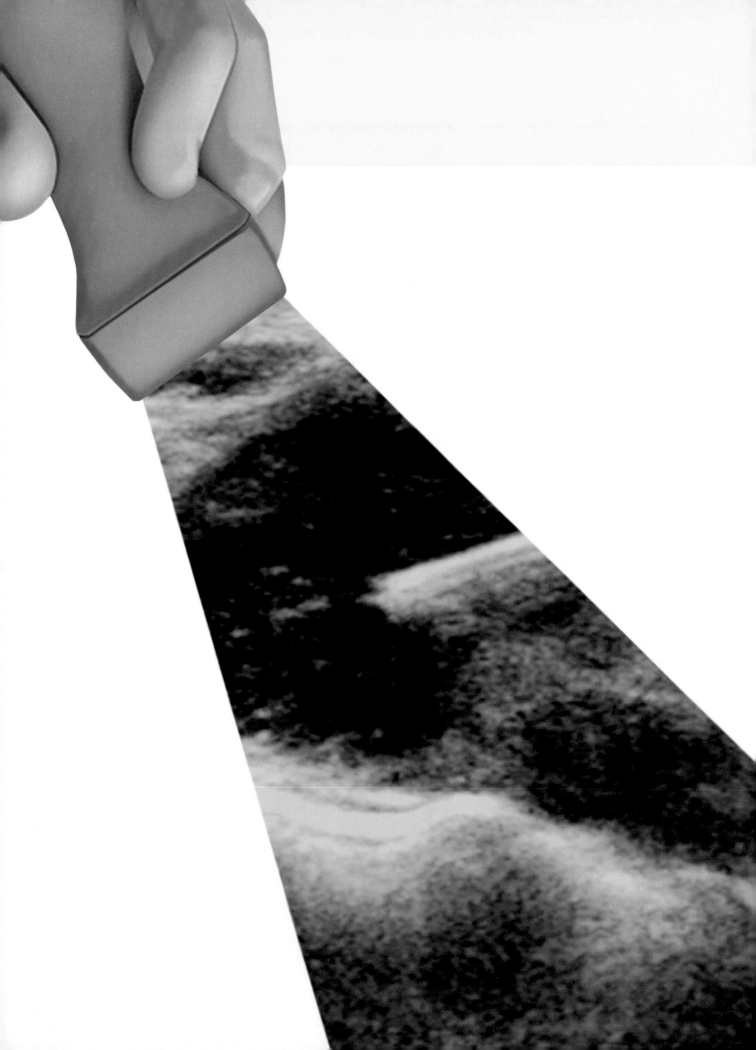

SECTION 8
Intervention

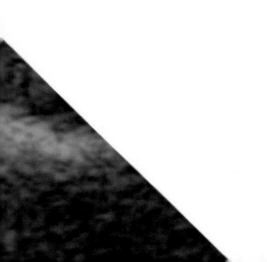

ULTRASOUND-GUIDED INTERVENTION

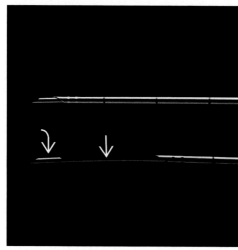

Photo shows inner stylet of side-cutting needle with specimen notch ➡. Part of stylet ➡ beyond may protrude outside target for optimal positioning, potentially raising risk of iatrogenic injury to adjacent structures.

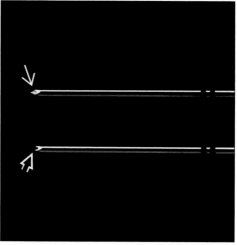

The tip ➡ of an end-cutting needle is shown with inner stylet in situ inside outer trocar. Note the serrated tip ➡ of the outer trocar after removal of the inner stylet. This configuration safely obtains better specimens.

TERMINOLOGY

Definitions
- Besides its diagnostic purpose, ultrasound is frequently used to guide interventions in neck
  - Some ultrasound-guided procedures can be safely performed in a general radiology department for management of head and neck (H&N) neoplasms

PROCEDURE

Ultrasound-Guided Core Biopsy
- Treatment planning of neoplastic disease requires pathological confirmation, classification, and grading of disease, and percutaneous ultrasound biopsy is usually preferred approach for suspected malignant tumors in neck
  - FNAC of H&N lesions
    - May be nondiagnostic in 10-30% of cases and gives incomplete classification, particularly in lymphomas
  - Repeating the FNAC may aggravate patient anxiety and frustration and still be inadequate
    - Thus, ultrasound-guided core needle biopsy is often preferred alternative
  - Some institutes actually adopt core needle biopsy as first-line approach in obtaining tissue samples in neck
- Core biopsy needles can be divided into 2 main types, according to design of cutting mechanism: **Side-cutting** and **end-cutting** needles
  - **Side-cutting needles** are composed of outer cutting shaft and inner stylet with a specimen notch
    - Needle tip is positioned at edge of target tissue
    - Inner stylet is then introduced into target tissue, part of which will thus prolapse into specimen notch
    - Outer cutting shaft is then advanced, usually by spring-loaded mechanism, to resheath inner stylet to cut out specimen core

- Part of outer shaft as well as stylet distal to specimen notch may protrude beyond target for optimal positioning of specimen notch
  - This is a major drawback of side-cutting needles because there is increased risk of iatrogenic injury to adjacent tissues
- Extra care should be exercised when performing biopsy of neck lesions using this type of needle, as major neurovascular structures are often in very close proximity to lesions
- In addition, volume of tissue sample obtained in each pass is limited by size of specimen notch, and multiple passes are often required in order to obtain adequate samples
  - **End-cutting needles** consist of inner stylet and outer trocar
    - Needle tip is positioned within sampling tissue at target area
    - After removal of inner stylet, trocar is connected via tube to syringe
    - Trocar is then rotated and moved "to and fro," while applying suction to syringe, to obtain tissue samples
    - Reintroduction of stylet or saline flush is used to dispose specimen from needle
    - Technique of using end-cutting needles is very similar to that of using fine needles for aspiration cytology
    - Safe for biopsy of even small lesions adjacent to vital structures, given that needle tract is well delineated and needle tip is kept within target area under real-time ultrasound monitoring
    - Adequate tissue samples can often be obtained in 1 pass using end-cutting needles, with long cores of tissues being retrieved by cutting-suction mechanism
    - Different designs of end-cutting needle tip configurations are available
      - Serrated or slotted type and more acute bevel angle appear to give better yields

Key Facts

Procedure

- Technique of using end-cutting needles is very similar to that of using fine needles for aspiration cytology
  - Safe for biopsy of even small lesions adjacent to vital structures, given that needle tract is well delineated and needle tip is kept within target area under real-time ultrasound monitoring
  - End-cutting needles may also be used under ultrasound guidance for biopsy of deep-seated lesions via intraoral approach
- Ultrasound-guided percutaneous ethanol injection ablation of neck nodal metastases from papillary thyroid carcinoma is one of the most frequently performed treatments in neck
  - Inexpensive outpatient procedure, much less invasive than surgical exploration
  - Can be repeated without increased technical difficulty and with minimal or no morbidity
  - Considered to be effective and basically risk-free alternative for this patient group
- Aim of symptomatic relief for unilateral vocal cord palsy is to attain medialization of paralyzed vocal cord by bringing it to midline or near-midline position so as to restore glottis competence on phonation and swallowing by functional contralateral vocal cord
  - Ultrasound can be used to guide accurate needle positioning in this transcartilaginous approach
- Ultrasound-guided radiofrequency ablation is used mainly for local control of recurrent well-differentiated thyroid carcinoma and is considered safe and effective alternative for treatment of nodal recurrence not suitable for surgery

---

- Large tissue samples with preserved architecture obtained by core needle biopsies almost always provide accurate histopathological diagnosis
  - Published data suggest excellent results with use of side-cutting needles, widely regarded as safe and effective technique for biopsy of H&N lesions, such as
    - Lymphadenopathy
    - Salivary gland and thyroid tumors
- End-cutting needles may also be used under ultrasound guidance for biopsy of deep-seated lesions via intraoral approach
  - 18-g or 20-g needles are usually ideal for biopsy of lymphadenopathy or salivary gland lesions, whereas smaller (22-g) needles are usually employed for thyroid lesions, smaller lesions, or deep-seated lesions via intraoral approach

Percutaneous Ethanol Injection Ablation of Neck Nodal Metastases From Papillary Thyroid Carcinoma

- Ultrasound-guided interventions also include therapeutic procedures
  - Ultrasound-guided percutaneous ethanol injection ablation of neck nodal metastases from papillary thyroid carcinoma is one of the most frequently performed treatments in neck
- Total thyroidectomy with regional neck nodal excision is primary treatment of choice for papillary carcinoma of thyroid and is often followed by radioactive iodine-131 ablation of remnant tumors
  - Nevertheless, it is not uncommon for new or previously unknown neck nodal metastases to be identified on follow-up of patients
  - Further radioiodine therapy is usually of limited efficacy in treatment of recurrent papillary thyroid carcinoma
  - Moreover, repeated surgical explorations become difficult due to fibrotic scars
  - In this context, percutaneous ultrasound-guided ethanol injection serves as a useful, less invasive treatment for patients with limited neck nodal metastases
- Patient selection criteria
  - < 5 nodal metastases amenable to percutaneous ethanol injection
  - Poor surgical candidates
  - Patients preferring no further surgery
  - Patients unresponsive to previous radioiodine therapy
- Each metastatic node is punctured and injected at multiple sites under real-time ultrasound guidance to attain complete treatment
  - Absolute alcohol is used
    - Total volume injected varies with size of nodes
  - Deepest part of node is injected first, then needle tip is repositioned
  - Injection is repeated until whole node is sufficiently filled or until ethanol begins to back-diffuse along needle tract into surrounding tissues
  - Excessive diffusion of ethanol may cause collateral damage to adjacent tissues and should be avoided
    - Especially when there are adjacent neurovascular structures
  - At least 2 sessions are scheduled for each patient
  - Nodes are mostly solid before 1st injection
    - Thus, injected ethanol tends to back-diffuse early before complete treatment can be attained
  - Nodes become more necrotic a few weeks later, and subsequent injections will then be able to fill up nodes completely
- Post-treatment patients should be followed up by ultrasound every 6-8 weeks
  - End-point is reached when node size has decreased/ become static in size and when there is no residual flow on power Doppler
    - Some recommend that post-treatment evaluation must include contrast-enhanced ultrasound to establish absence of intranodal vascularity
  - Transient hoarseness and mild pain may be seen in some patients, but major complication (e.g., nerve damage) is very rare
- Percutaneous ethanol injection is outpatient procedure of low cost, much less invasive than surgical exploration, and can be repeated many times without increased technical difficulty and with minimal or no morbidity

- Considered to be effective and basically risk-free alternative for this patient group
- Surgical reexploration and radioiodine treatment may then be reserved for those patients with more disseminated or aggressive form of papillary thyroid carcinoma

Ultrasound-Guided Vocal Cord Injection for Unilateral Vocal Cord Paralysis

- Ultrasound is also useful in guiding treatment of complication of malignant disease
  - As exemplified by ultrasound-guided vocal cord injection for unilateral vocal cord paralysis
- Vocal cord palsy caused by tumor involvement of recurrent laryngeal nerve is a common debilitating problem seen in patients suffering from neck and mediastinal neoplasms
  - Aim of symptomatic relief for unilateral vocal cord palsy is to attain medialization of paralyzed vocal cord by bringing it to midline or near-midline position
    - Goal is to restore glottis competence on phonation and swallowing by functional contralateral vocal cord, thereby alleviating symptoms of hoarseness and aspiration
- Due to its relative simplicity, transcutaneous vocal cord injection is usually preferred over traditional laryngeal framework surgery
  - Needle may be introduced through cricothyroid membrane toward undersurface of vocal cord or via thyrohyoid notch to reach endolaryngeal space and then vocal cord under endoscopic guidance
  - With direct visualization, it is possible to guide site for optimal injection, but in some patients angulation of anatomy may prevent needle entry
- Alternative approach is to insert needle directly through thyroid cartilage to access vocal fold
  - Theoretically, such transcartilaginous entry eliminates any anatomical constraint to reach vocal fold
    - With exception of heavily calcified/ossified thyroid cartilage
  - However, this is a submucosal approach and therefore essentially a blind procedure that often makes accurate needle positioning difficult
    - Especially in patients with thick neck soft tissues, in whom external judgment of level of vocal cords is almost impossible
- Ultrasound can be used to guide accurate needle positioning in this transcartilaginous approach
  - False vocal cords and vocal ligament (free edge of true cord) are hyperechoic due to high fibrous contents, whereas true vocal cords are hypoechoic due to high muscle content
  - Level of vocal cords is approximately at midpoint between thyroid notch and lower border of thyroid cartilage at midline
- Localization of vocal fold can be further confirmed by referring to phasic vocal cord movement of normal side during respiration
  - Ultrasound can therefore provide real-time guidance for entry and direction of advancement of needle to ensure optimal placement for vocal cord injection

- Entry site is paramedian with angulation toward center of vocalis muscle
- Ultrasound can also assess location and adequacy of vocal cord medialization during and after injection
- Different biocompatible materials may be used for injection
- Radiesse contains synthetic calcium hydroxyapatite (CaHA) microspheres (25-45 µm) suspended in aqueous gel carrier
- Restylane (small particle-size hyaluronic acid [SPHA]) contains animal- or bacterial-derived variations of naturally occurring extracellular glycosaminoglycan in various human tissues like vocal cord lamina propria

Ultrasound-Guided Radiofrequency Ablation (RFA)

- Percutaneous RFA is an established treatment modality for various H&N lesions
  - e.g., locoregional control of recurrent well-differentiated thyroid carcinoma and benign thyroid nodules
- Mechanism of RFA: Oscillating current is sent to target lesion via active tip, and current returns by large area dispersive electrode attached to another part of body
  - Because of relative small size of needle tip, high field density is created around it with induction of micromovement of tissue ions by oscillating current
    - This generates frictional heat that will cause thermal ablation when cytotoxic threshold is reached
      - Threshold temperature is usually > 60°C
  - Dissipation of thermal energy to adjacent tissues by conduction may induce further coagulation necrosis or reversible hyperthermia depending on temperature reached
  - Time it takes to induce irreversible cellular damage varies inversely with temperature
    - At 60-100°C, there is almost instant cellular damage
  - Multipronged expandable electrode or single, straight electrode may be used
    - Straight electrode is usually preferred because of its smaller needle bore and ease of manipulation for complete lesion ablation
    - Most current straight electrodes are equipped with internal cooling system to improve RF energy dissipation and prevent tissue charring
    - Radius of thermocoagulation is reported to increase from 8 mm to 10-12 mm by incorporation of internal cooling system
  - It should be noted that fibrosis and calcification are intrinsic hindrances to thermal ablation
  - Also, for predominantly cystic lesions, ethanol is usually better alternative
- Local anesthesia is usually adequate for pain control
  - Premedication is purposely avoided since continuous verbal communication with patient during procedure helps to identify thermal injury to recurrent laryngeal nerve by detection of hoarseness of voice
- Transisthmic approach is proposed for RFA treatment of thyroid lesions
- Electrode should be advanced with whole needle tract, including needle tip, being visualized by ultrasound

- Care must be taken to avoid iatrogenic injury of structures in "danger triangle" deep to medial aspect of thyroid gland, where recurrent laryngeal nerve, trachea, and esophagus reside
- Infusion of dextrose or normal saline between target lesion and the nerve may help prevent of nerve injury
- Any voice change detected during RFA procedure indicates that ablation should be stopped immediately
- Coughing resulting from heat irritation of trachea also signifies that procedure should be halted
- Transient echogenicity generated during RFA treatment likely represents coagulation necrosis and tissue vaporization, and indicates successful thermocoagulation
  - Needle tip should be positioned to ablate lesions from deep to superficial and from remote to close, with multiple repositions to achieve complete treatment of larger lesions, as indicated by complete echogenic change of lesions after RFA
  - Ablation should begin with lower voltages (such as 30 W for 1 cm active tip or 50 W for 1.5 cm active tip), with stepwise increment of power by 5-10 W up to a maximum of 100-110 W if there is no transient formation of echogenic change
  - Transient pain and heat sensation is commonly experienced by patients during RFA
    - It is usually well tolerated and can be reduced by lowering or shutting down power temporarily
  - Patient should be observed for 1-3 hours after procedure, with light compression applied by ice pack to treatment site
  - Complications from ultrasound-guided RFA are uncommon, with hoarseness of voice being most significant
  - Recovery usually occurs within 3 months, but residual dysphonia tends to be permanent
  - Local neck swelling and discomfort are common but usually self-limiting and tend to resolve in 1-2 weeks
  - Hematoma may result from mechanical injury and, if large, may necessitate postponement of RFA
  - A few cases of skin burn were reported, all at puncture site of superficial lesions with protruded active tips, and were minor
- Post-RFA patients should be followed up with biochemical and ultrasound assessment
  - Ultrasound criteria for treatment response include shrinkage in lesion size and reduction/absence of internal vascularity if present before treatment
  - Progressive involution may be observed in 1st few months and up to a year
  - Enlargement of lesion after initial shrinkage is highly suspicious of recurrence and warrants tissue sampling for evaluation
- Ultrasound-guided RFA is used mainly for local control of recurrent well-differentiated thyroid carcinoma and is considered to be a safe and effective alternative for treatment of nodal recurrence not suitable for surgery
- It has been suggested that RFA is superior to ethanol for treating well-differentiated thyroid carcinoma recurrence as it results in better disease control with fewer treatment sessions

SELECTED REFERENCES

1. Yuen HY et al: A short review of basic head and neck interventional procedures in a general radiology department. Cancer Imaging. 13(4):502-11, 2013
2. Ng SK et al: Combined ultrasound/endoscopy-assisted vocal fold injection for unilateral vocal cord paralysis: a case series. Eur Radiol. 22(5):1110-3, 2012
3. Yuen HY et al: Use of end-cutting needles in ultrasound-guided biopsy of neck lesions. Eur Radiol. 22(4):832-6, 2012
4. Hay ID et al: The coming of age of ultrasound-guided percutaneous ethanol ablation of selected neck nodal metastases in well-differentiated thyroid carcinoma. J Clin Endocrinol Metab. 96(9):2717-20, 2011
5. Udelsman R: Treatment of persistent or recurrent papillary carcinoma of the thyroid--the good, the bad, and the unknown. J Clin Endocrinol Metab. 95(5):2061-3, 2010
6. Wong KT et al: Biopsy of deep-seated head and neck lesions under intraoral ultrasound guidance. AJNR Am J Neuroradiol. 27(8):1654-7, 2006
7. Lewis BD et al: Percutaneous ethanol injection for treatment of cervical lymph node metastases in patients with papillary thyroid carcinoma. AJR Am J Roentgenol. 178(3):699-704, 2002

ULTRASOUND-GUIDED INTERVENTION

(Left) Under ultrasound guidance, the tip of the end-cutting needle ➡ is positioned within the target sampling tissue. The needle is rotated and moved "to and fro" while applying suction to obtain tissue samples. The technique is very similar to that of using fine needles for aspiration cytology. **(Right)** Adequate tissue samples can often be obtained in 1 pass by using end-cutting needle, with long cores of tissue ➨ being retrieved by the cutting-suction mechanism.

Ultrasound-Guided Biopsy Using End-Cutting Needle

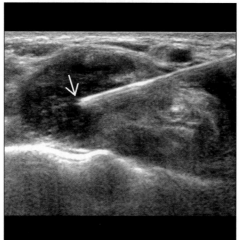

Biopsy Specimens Obtained Using End-Cutting Needles

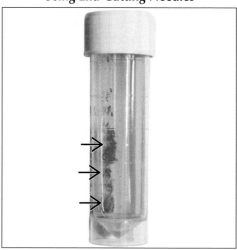

(Left) Transverse power Doppler US of supraclavicular fossa in a patient with previous surgery for thyroid papillary carcinoma shows a recurrent metastatic node ➡ from papillary thyroid carcinoma with prominent increased vascularity. Note its proximity to major vessels ➨. **(Right)** Corresponding grayscale US shows needle insertion under US guidance into a recurrent metastatic node for ethanol injection. Note the needle track ➡ and increased echogenicity ➨ from injected ethanol.

Ultrasound-Guided Alcohol Ablation of Nodal Recurrence of Papillary Thyroid Carcinoma

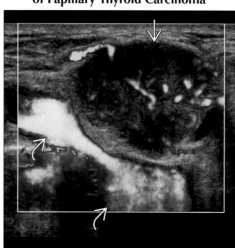

Ultrasound-Guided Alcohol Ablation of Nodal Recurrence of Papillary Thyroid Carcinoma

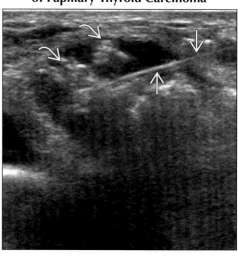

(Left) Pre-alcohol ablation appearance of nodal metastasis from papillary thyroid carcinoma shows a heterogeneous hypoechoic mass with chaotic increased vascularity ➨. **(Right)** Post-treatment end-point is reached (same patient) when the node ➡ size has decreased/become static and when there is no residual flow detected on power Doppler or contrast-enhanced ultrasound.

Assessment of Response to Alcohol Ablation

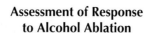

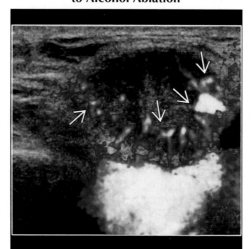

Assessment of Response to Alcohol Ablation

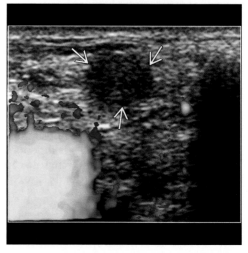

ULTRASOUND-GUIDED INTERVENTION

Ultrasound-Guided Vocal Cord Injection

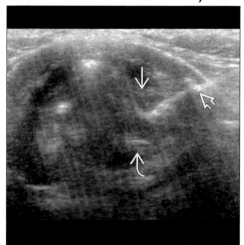

Ultrasound-Guided Vocal Cord Injection

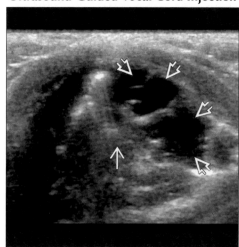

(Left) Transverse grayscale ultrasound shows transcartilaginous puncture of the left vocal cord ➡. Note the needle ⇉ and arytenoid cartilage ➡. Ultrasound guides the needle into the vocal cord, making the procedure safe. *(Right)* Transverse grayscale ultrasound after injection (same patient) shows medialization of the left vocal cord ➡ post injection. Left vocal cord is now filled with anechoic material ⇉. In addition to needle guidance, ultrasound also readily aids in follow-up of such patients.

Principles of RFA

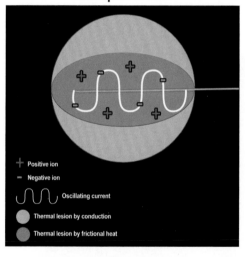

+ Positive ion
− Negative ion
〜 Oscillating current
● Thermal lesion by conduction
● Thermal lesion by frictional heat

Transisthmic Approach for RFA of Thyroid Lesions

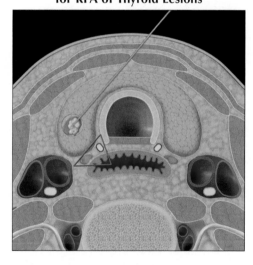

(Left) Oscillating current is sent to a target lesion via an active needle tip. A high field density is created in this small area where micromovements of tissue ions are induced to create frictional heat for thermal ablation. *(Right)* The electrode is inserted along a path that allows visualization of the whole needle tract on ultrasound. The active tip is positioned to avoid injury to structures in the danger triangle (red line) deep to the medial aspect of the thyroid.

Radiofrequency Ablation of Thyroid Nodule

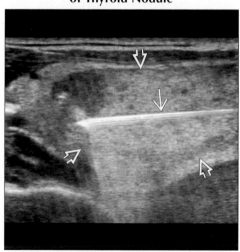

Thyroid Nodule Post Radiofrequency Ablation

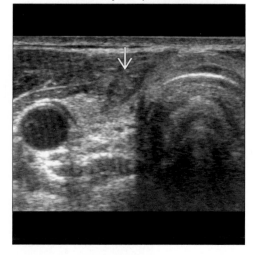

(Left) Oblique grayscale ultrasound shows an electrode ➡ positioned within a target thyroid nodule ➡ under ultrasound guidance and ready for radiofrequency ablation. (Courtesy W. Cho, MD.) *(Right)* Transverse grayscale follow-up ultrasound demonstrates marked shrinkage in the size of thyroid nodule ➡ after radiofrequency ablation. (Courtesy W. Cho, MD.)

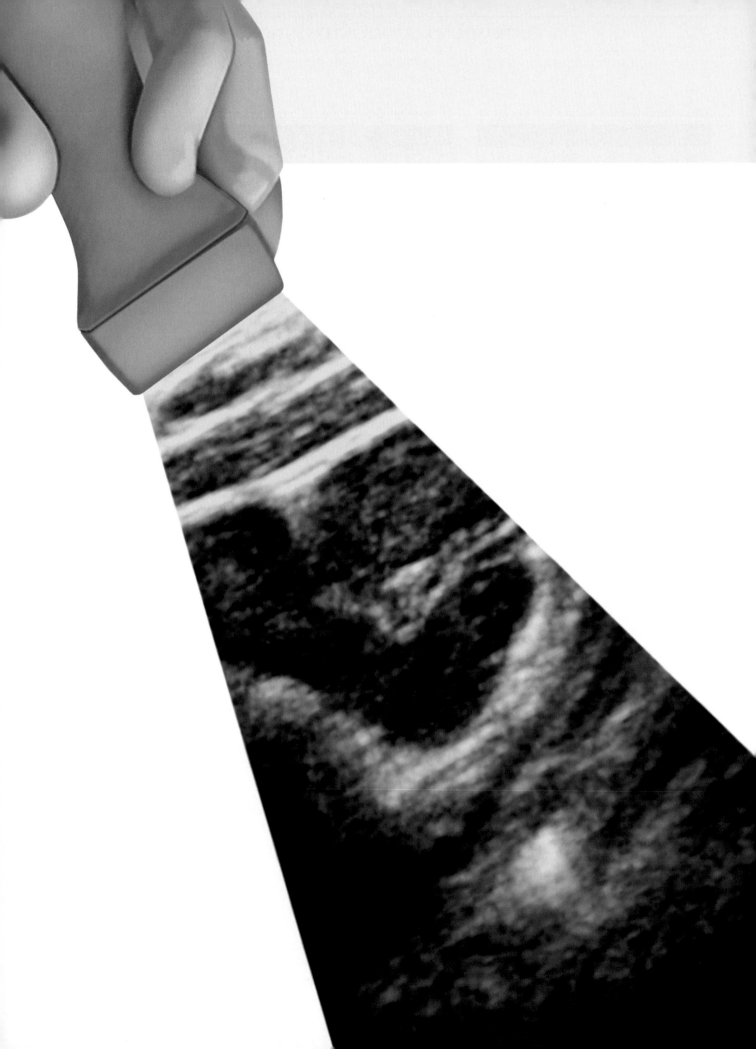

SECTION 1
Head and Neck

MIDLINE NECK MASS

DIFFERENTIAL DIAGNOSIS

Common
- Lymph Nodes
- Thyroid Mass
- Pyramidal Lobe (Mimic)
- Thyroglossal Duct Cyst
- Ranula

Less Common
- Dermoid/Epidermoid
- Laryngocele
- Lateral Pharyngeal Diverticulum
- Hypopharyngeal Tumor
- Postoperative
  - Parastomal Recurrence
  - Colonic Interposition, Jejunal Pull-Up

Rare but Important
- Ectopic Thyroid

ESSENTIAL INFORMATION

Key Differential Diagnosis Issues
- During routine US of head and neck, central compartment is often overlooked
  - To avoid mistakes, establish scanning protocol that routinely includes central compartment
  - Shadowing from hyoid, laryngeal cartilage, and tracheal ring may obscure visualization of lesions in midline
    - Pay meticulous attention to detail and technique at this site to avoid mistakes
- Most abnormalities at this location are site specific and have typical US features
- Patient's demographic information (e.g., age, sex) and clinical history are important for diagnosis
  - Thyroglossal duct cyst (TDC), dermoid/epidermoid more common in young age group
  - History of relevant surgical procedures provides clue toward colonic interposition/jejunal pull-up/ parastomal recurrence

Helpful Clues for Common Diagnoses
- **Lymph Nodes**
  - Normal lymph nodes (LNs) in central compartment generally small and obscured by tracheal ring shadowing
  - Malignant nodes in this compartment receive drainage from specific sites and give clue to origin of primary tumor (thyroid, larynx)
    - Large, round, hyper- to hypoechoic, loss of normal echogenic hilum, peripheral vascularity
    - Intranodal punctate calcification ± cystic necrosis from primary papillary thyroid carcinoma
  - Hypertrophied/reactive nodes in postradiation patients (particularly with nasopharyngeal carcinoma) or those with autoimmune thyroid disease
    - Lymph nodes are benign looking with elliptical shape, hypertrophied cortex, normal hilar architecture, and vascularity
    - Submental and paratracheal LNs in patients who have received radiotherapy in lateral neck
    - Para-/pretracheal LNs in patient with autoimmune thyroid disease
- **Thyroid Mass**
  - Thyroid is major organ in central neck
  - Thyroid nodules in isthmus are common, usually benign in nature
    - Hyperplastic nodules/adenomatous nodules as part of multinodular change are most common
    - Usually there is evidence of multinodular change in both lobes of thyroid
  - Solitary thyroid neoplasm is less common
    - Clues suspicious of malignancy include ill-defined/ infiltrative margin, hypoechoic, solid mass, presence of tracheal invasion ± regional metastatic lymph nodes
- **Pyramidal Lobe (Mimic)**
  - 10-30% of patients have "3rd" lobe: Pyramidal lobe
    - Should be recognized as anatomic variant
  - Isolated island of tissue with fine bright echo pattern of thyroid gland, superior to thyroid lobes/isthmus
  - Secondary to ascent from isthmus or adjacent part of either lobe (more often left lobe)
- **Thyroglossal Duct Cyst**
  - Occurs anywhere along thyroglossal duct: Infrahyoid (75%) > hyoid (20%) > suprahyoid (15%)
    - Suprahyoid TDC at base of tongue or posterior floor of mouth
    - At hyoid level: Anterior/ventral to hyoid
    - Infrahyoid: Embedded in strap muscles; often paramedian
  - Noninfected, nonhemorrhagic
    - Anechoic, thin-walled cyst, fine internal debris ± fluid level
    - Posterior enhancement or pseudosolid appearance
    - No vascular solid component on Doppler
  - Infected, hemorrhagic
    - Thick, irregular walls
    - Hypoechoic and heterogeneous in echo pattern
    - Presence of debris ± fluid-fluid level
    - Vascularity in walls and septa
  - Thick wall or soft tissue may represent functioning thyroid tissue, infection, or malignant change (thyroid carcinoma in 1-4%)
    - Guided fine-needle aspiration and cytology (FNAC) for any TDC with solid component confirms diagnosis
  - Evaluate thyroid bed for presence or absence of normal thyroid tissue
- **Ranula**
  - Retention cyst in sublingual space (SLS), epithelial lining
  - Simple ranula
    - Confined within SLS, above mylohyoid muscle
  - Diving ranula
    - When simple ranula ruptures from SLS into submandibular space (SMS)
  - Uninfected ranula
    - Thin walled, anechoic, posterior enhancement
  - Ranula with previous hemorrhage/infection
    - Thick and irregular wall
    - Internal debris/fluid level
  - Color Doppler: Avascular; vascularity in thick wall/ adjacent soft tissue if infected

Helpful Clues for Less Common Diagnoses
- **Dermoid/Epidermoid**
  - Dermoid: Round, well-defined, with internal echoes ± posterior enhancement
    - Heterogeneous ± fluid-fluid level; pseudosolid with fat content and osseo-dental structures

- Look for any soft tissue growth as 5% develop squamous cell carcinoma
  - ○ Epidermoid: Well defined and homogeneously echogenic due to fat content, posterior enhancement
    - Pseudosolid appearance with uniform internal echoes due to cellular material within
    - With intermittent transducer pressure, swirling motion of debris is seen on real-time scanning
  - ○ Color Doppler: Both dermoid and epidermoid show no significant vascularity within lesion or its wall
  - ○ In absence of osseo-dental structures, one cannot sonographically definitively distinguish dermoid from epidermoid
  - ○ Define location for both: Supramylohyoid (sublingual) vs. inframylohyoid (submandibular) on ultrasound
    - Determines intraoral vs. external operative approach
- **Laryngocele**
  - ○ 26% external, 40% mixed: Completely or partially protruded through thyrohyoid membrane
  - ○ Seen as mobile echogenic lines (air) in characteristic location, exacerbated on blowing
    - Contain fluid ± debris, thickened walls
  - ○ Rule out laryngeal ventricle obstruction by tumor in patients with no relevant clinical history (trumpet players, glass blowers)
- **Lateral Pharyngeal Diverticulum**
  - ○ Mobile echogenic lines (gas) or fluid-filled space
  - ○ Empties on compression
  - ○ Better demonstrated by barium/water soluble contrast examination/CT
- **Hypopharyngeal Tumor**
  - ○ Pyriform fossae are inferolateral to hyoid
    - Visualization depends on size of tumor and presence/absence of sound attenuation by adjacent laryngeal structures
  - ○ Ill-defined, solid, hypoechoic tumor filling fossa
  - ○ Look for metastatic regional lymph nodes on either side of neck
- **Postoperative**
  - ○ **Parastomal Recurrence**

- Hypoechoic, soft tissue mass ± vascularity at surgical site
- May be difficult to differentiate from postoperative granulation tissue
- Evaluate regional nodal status, confirm recurrent tumor by FNAC
  - ○ **Colonic Interposition, Jejunal Pull-Up**
    - Need to know patient history to avoid misdiagnosis
    - Look for "gut signature": Concentric echogenic/hypoechoic rings
    - Evaluate presence of any abnormal nodes in accompanying mesentery

Helpful Clues for Rare Diagnoses
- **Ectopic Thyroid**
  - ○ Anywhere along course of thyroglossal duct
  - ○ Only functioning thyroid tissue in 70-80% of cases
    - Check thyroid bed for any thyroid tissue
  - ○ Multinodular goiter changes may occur; 3% malignant change to papillary carcinoma
  - ○ Scintigraphy to confirm diagnosis and detect functioning tissue at any other location in neck

Alternative Differential Approaches
- Evaluate lesions by specific/common location in neck, from cranial to caudal
- Lymph nodes occur at any level in midline/paramidline (often obscured by shadowing from bone, cartilage)
- Floor of mouth/suprahyoid neck
  - ○ Ranula, TDC, dermoid, epidermoid, ectopic thyroid
- Infrahyoid neck
  - ○ TDC, ectopic thyroid, thyroid masses, hypopharyngeal diverticula/tumor, laryngocele, parastomal recurrence, postoperative change

SELECTED REFERENCES
1. Ahuja AT et al: Diagnostic Imaging: Ultrasound. 1st ed. Salt Lake City: Amirsys.11-2-5, 2007

Lymph Nodes

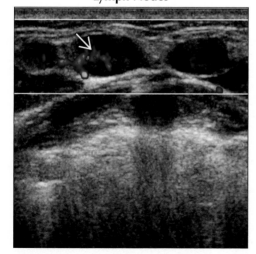

Transverse power Doppler ultrasound shows hypertrophied midline submental neck lymph nodes in a patient with previous radiation therapy. Note central vascularity ➡ and absence of peripheral vascularity.

Lymph Nodes

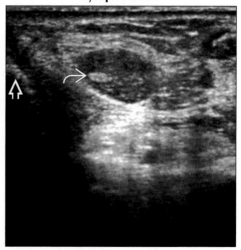

Transverse ultrasound shows a hypertrophied node in the suprasternal region with preserved hilar architecture ➡. Note the trachea ➡.

Lymph Nodes

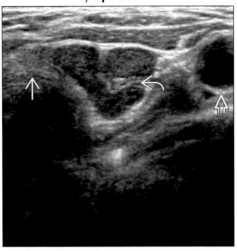

Lymph Nodes

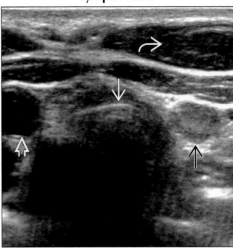

(Left) Transverse ultrasound shows a well-defined, hypoechoic, hypertrophic node in the left paratracheal location in a patient with previous radiation therapy. Note normal hilar architecture ➽ (trachea ➡, left common carotid artery [CCA] ➔).
(Right) Transverse ultrasound shows an enlarged node ➔ in the left paratracheal region. Note this node is hyperechoic compared to the adjacent muscle ➽, suggesting a metastatic node from papillary thyroid carcinoma (trachea ➡, right CCA ➔).

Pyramidal Lobe (Mimic)

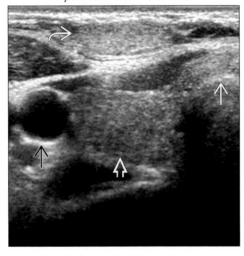

Pyramidal Lobe (Mimic)

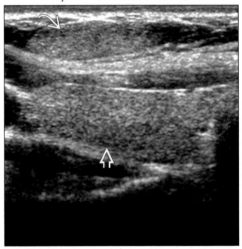

(Left) Transverse ultrasound shows an island of soft tissue ➽ with similar echogenicity to the normal thyroid gland ➔. Note its anterior location, just off midline (CCA ➔, trachea ➡). The appearance is consistent with a pyramidal lobe. (Right) Longitudinal ultrasound in the same patient shows the island of thyroid tissue ➽ and its relation to the thyroid gland ➔. Although pyramidal lobes are more typical on the left, in this patient, the lobe was on the right.

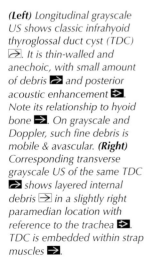

(Left) Longitudinal grayscale US shows classic infrahyoid thyroglossal duct cyst (TDC) ➔. It is thin-walled and anechoic, with small amount of debris ➽ and posterior acoustic enhancement ➔. Note its relationship to hyoid bone ➡. On grayscale and Doppler, such fine debris is mobile & avascular. (Right) Corresponding transverse grayscale US of the same TDC ➽ shows layered internal debris ➔ in a slightly right paramedian location with reference to the trachea ➔. TDC is embedded within strap muscles ➔.

Thyroglossal Duct Cyst

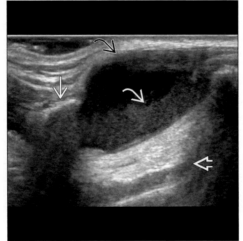

Thyroglossal Duct Cyst

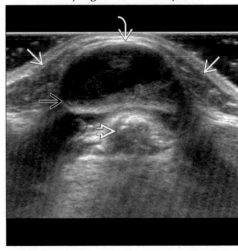

Thyroglossal Duct Cyst

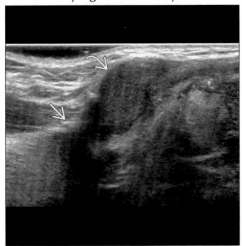

Thyroglossal Duct Cyst

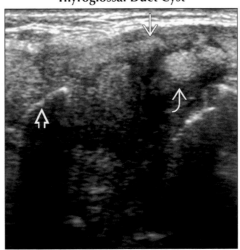

(Left) Longitudinal grayscale US shows an infrahyoid TDC ➡ with a pseudosolid appearance, the typical and common appearance of all congenital neck cysts. Note the hyoid ➡. *(Right)* Longitudinal grayscale US shows an infrahyoid TDC ➡ with irregular solid soft tissue ➡, suspicious of malignant change (confirmed on FNAC). In patients with solid tissue in TDC, Doppler for vascularity and guided FNAC is indicated to rule out any malignant change. Note the hyoid ➡.

Thyroglossal Duct Cyst

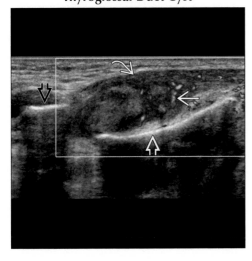

Thyroglossal Duct Cyst

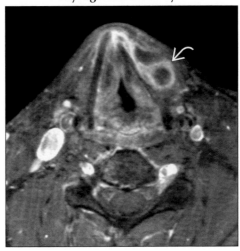

(Left) Longitudinal grayscale US shows infrahyoid, paramedian TDC ➡ with heterogeneous pseudosolid appearance and internal vascularity ➡. Patient presented with pain & swelling after recent FNAC of this lesion. US appearance is consistent with superimposed infection. Note thyroid cartilage ➡ and hyoid bone ➡. *(Right)* Corresponding axial T1WI C+ FS MR of TDC ➡ shows a thick, enhancing wall, consistent with US finding of infected TDC. Note its left paramedian location.

Dermoid/Epidermoid

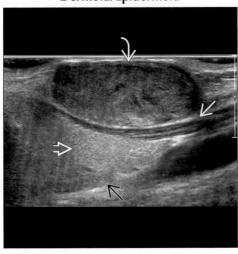

Dermoid/Epidermoid

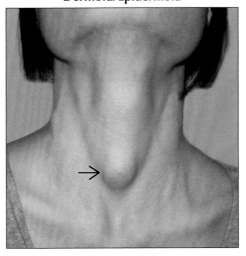

(Left) Longitudinal oblique grayscale US of neck shows dermoid cyst ➡ with heterogeneous pseudosolid appearance and mild posterior acoustic enhancement ➡. Note its location is superficial to strap muscles ➡ and thyroid gland ➡, well away from the hyoid bone. *(Right)* Clinical photograph of the same patient shows midline location of the dermoid cyst ➡. Clinical examination revealed no relation with swallowing.

MIDLINE NECK MASS

Dermoid/Epidermoid

(Left) Transverse ultrasound shows an epidermoid ➡ at the floor of the mouth. Note the uniform, echogenic, homogeneous echo pattern of the epidermoid cyst. Also present are the sublingual glands ➡. (Right) Axial T2WI MR with fat suppression in the same patient shows the homogeneous fluid signal ➘ typically seen in an epidermoid. On this MR, TDC is included in the differential, but the US appearance is more suggestive of an epidermoid.

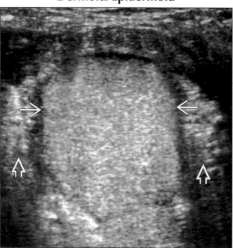

Dermoid/Epidermoid

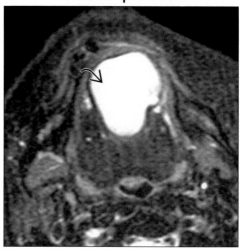

Laryngocele

(Left) Transverse ultrasound of the right paramedian region of the neck shows a curvilinear echogenic interface ➡ and "dirty" posterior acoustic shadowing ➘, consistent with a laryngocele. Note the thyroid cartilage ➡. (Right) Transverse ultrasound through the thyrohyoid membrane shows an irregular soft tissue laryngeal mass ➡ and an associated laryngocele ➡, seen as echogenic foci representing air. Note the left thyroid cartilage ➡.

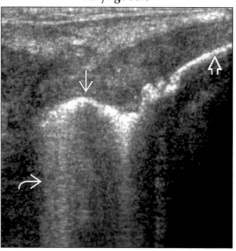

Laryngocele

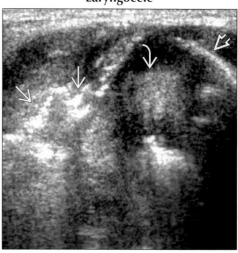

Laryngocele

(Left) Axial CECT in the same patient shows the air-filled laryngocele ➡ and soft tissue mass in the right vocal cord ➘. Note arytenoid ➘ and left thyroid cartilage ➡. CT better evaluates laryngocele and any associated abnormality. (Right) Transverse grayscale US shows jejunal interposition ➘ in a patient with previous carcinoma of larynx. Note carotid arteries ➡ lateral to the graft and vertebral body ➘ posteriorly. Small mesenteric nodes may be seen along with bowel.

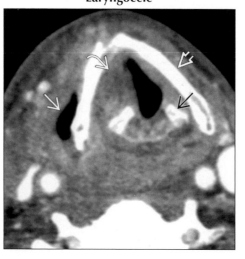

Thyroglossal Duct Cyst

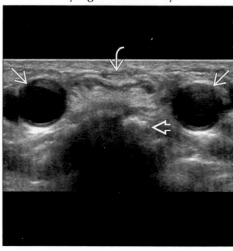

Colonic Interposition

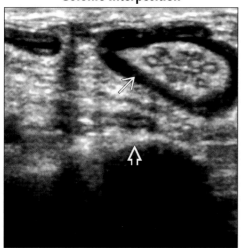

Colonic Interposition, Jejunal Pull-Up

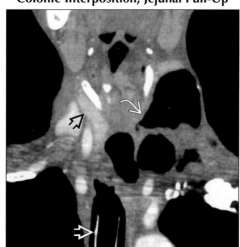

(Left) Transverse ultrasound at the midline of the neck shows a mass ➡ with a "bowel" signature, a colonic pull-up in this patient. Note the vertebral body ➡. It is helpful to be familiar with a patient's surgical history to avoid mistaking this for an abnormality. (Right) Coronal reformat CECT of the same patient shows the loops of the colon ➡ (gas-filled) in the left paramedian region. Note the tracheostomy tube ➡ and right lobe of the thyroid gland ➡.

Parastomal Recurrence

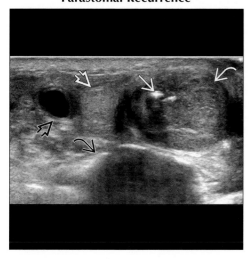

Parastomal Recurrence

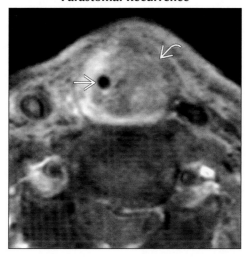

(Left) Transverse grayscale US shows parastomal recurrence ➡, seen as eccentric wall thickening relative to the location of a feeding tube ➡. Some thyroid tissue is seen adjacent to the parastomal recurrence ➡. Note CCA ➡ and vertebral body ➡. (Right) Corresponding transverse T1WI C+ FS MR of parastomal recurrence ➡ shows heterogeneous, eccentric wall enhancement and a displaced feeding tube ➡.

Ectopic Thyroid

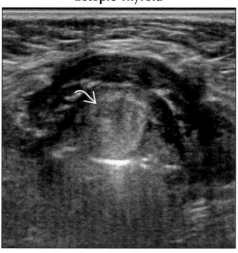

Ectopic Thyroid

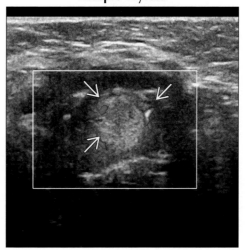

(Left) Transverse grayscale US shows a sublingual thyroid ➡ in an infant presenting with congenital hypothyroidism. Note fine, homogeneous, echogenic pattern similar to normal thyroid tissue. Thyroid bed was empty (not shown). The findings were confirmed by thyroid scintigraphy. (Right) Corresponding transverse power Doppler ultrasound of the same lesion shows internal vascularity ➡, as opposed to a dermoid/epidermoid cyst.

CYSTIC NECK MASS

DIFFERENTIAL DIAGNOSIS

Common
- Neck Abscess
- Metastatic Lymph Node
  - Squamous Cell Carcinoma (SCCa)
  - Papillary Carcinoma of Thyroid

Less Common
- Venous Vascular Malformation (VVM)
- Lymphatic Malformation
- Acute Suppurative Thyroiditis
- Thyroglossal Duct Cyst
- Simple Ranula (SR)
- Diving Ranula (DR)

Rare but Important
- Dermoid
- Epidermoid
- 2nd Branchial Cleft Cyst (2nd BCC)
- 1st Branchial Cleft Cyst (1st BCC)
- Thymic Cyst

ESSENTIAL INFORMATION

Key Differential Diagnosis Issues
- Cystic masses in head & neck are site specific; therefore, location of mass is a clue to its diagnosis
- Asymptomatic adult male
  - Solitary metastatic node from H&N SCCa is much more common than 2nd BCC, even at known site of 2nd BCC
- Asymptomatic adult woman
  - Consider possibility of metastatic node from papillary thyroid cancer
- Guided fine-needle aspiration and cytology (FNAC) is crucial to diagnosis
- If abscess is detected on ultrasound, CT & MR may be indicated to evaluate
  - Exact anatomical location, extent, and mediastinal involvement if any
  - Relation of abscess to carotid artery and risk of carotid blow-out

Helpful Clues for Common Diagnoses
- **Neck Abscess**
  - Clinical features of acute infection in majority of cases (fever, tenderness, ↑ white cell count)
  - Grayscale ultrasound features
    - Thick-walled, irregular outlines with hypoechoic/necrotic center
    - Floating low-level echoes representing pus/inflammatory debris
    - ± echogenic foci with "comet tail" artifacts representing gas
    - ± enlarged inflammatory lymph nodes
    - Thickening or edema of overlying skin, subcutaneous tissue, and soft tissue
    - Marked local tenderness on probe pressure
  - Doppler ultrasound features
    - Hypervascular walls with avascular center
    - Hypervascularity in adjacent inflammatory tissues
  - US-guided aspiration of liquefied contents helps to identify infective organism

- CT may be required if suspicion of extension to deep neck spaces (e.g., parapharyngeal or retropharyngeal spaces) or mediastinum
- **Metastatic Lymph Node**
  - Known history of primary malignancy provides a clue for diagnosis
  - **Squamous Cell Carcinoma (SCCa)**
    - Location of nodes is site specific and depends on site of primary tumor in head and neck
    - Solid, round with heterogeneously hypoechoic echo pattern
    - Loss of hilar architecture (69-95%)
    - ± intranodal cystic or coagulation necrosis
    - ± extracapsular spread: Indistinct border, infiltration of adjacent soft tissue
    - Calcification in metastatic SCCa nodes is uncommon
    - Doppler: Abnormal, chaotic, peripheral vascularity
  - **Papillary Carcinoma of Thyroid**
    - Round or ovoid with large cystic areas
    - Solid components contain punctate calcification and internal vascularity
    - Primary carcinoma is often in ipsilateral thyroid lobe; appearance similar to metastatic node

Helpful Clues for Less Common Diagnoses
- **Venous Vascular Malformation (VVM)**
  - Often multiple with multicompartment involvement
  - Thin walled, multiseptated with serpiginous cystic spaces
  - Presence of phleboliths is characteristic
  - Variable hypoechoic stromal component
    - May mimic muscle or intermuscular fat on ultrasound
  - Slow venous flow
    - May be seen only on grayscale; too slow to be seen on color Doppler
  - ↑ transducer pressure may compress and obscure abnormality
  - MR is indicated to detect multiplicity, extent of abnormality
    - May extend into mediastinum
- **Lymphatic Malformation**
  - Children > > adult, present with soft neck mass
  - Cystic hygroma > cavernous or capillary lymphatic malformation
  - Commonly in posterior triangle; septate with multicompartment and trans-spatial involvement
  - Thin-walled, multiloculated, anechoic, cystic mass
  - Thick walled and debris if complicated by infection or hemorrhage
  - No grayscale flow movement (as in VVM)
  - Doppler: If uninfected, no vascularity within wall or septa
  - MR may be indicated to evaluate anatomical extent in neck and mediastinal/axillary involvement
  - US helps to guide sclerotherapy and follow-up after treatment
- **Acute Suppurative Thyroiditis**
  - Seen in children with history of recurrent infection/abscess at same site; left > right
  - Clinical symptoms and signs of acute infection
  - Left lobe (95%) > > right lobe (5%)
  - Perithyroidal ± intrathyroidal abscess, typically around upper pole of left lobe
    - Thick-walled, heterogeneous, liquefied pus
    - Tiny echogenic foci representing gas within

- ▪ Perithyroidal soft tissue thickening and edematous changes
  - ○ Barium study after acute episode to identify underlying pyriform fossa fistula
- **Thyroglossal Duct Cyst**
  - ○ Occurs anywhere along thyroglossal duct, midline in location; may be paramedian in location
  - ○ Infrahyoid (75%) > hyoid > suprahyoid level
  - ○ Noninfected: Well-defined, anechoic cyst with posterior enhancement; homogeneous pseudosolid appearance
  - ○ Infected/hemorrhagic: Thick-walled, heterogeneous, presence of debris ± fluid level
- **Simple Ranula (SR)**
  - ○ Retention cyst confined to sublingual space
  - ○ Uninfected: Thin-walled, unilocular, anechoic
  - ○ May appear thick-walled with internal echoes if infected
- **Diving Ranula (DR)**
  - ○ Simple ranula (+ epithelial lining) ruptures into submandibular space forming pseudocyst (no epithelial lining)
  - ○ Uninfected: Thin-walled, unilocular, anechoic lesion involving sublingual and submandibular spaces
  - ○ Uni-/multilocular internal debris and thick walls if infected

Helpful Clues for Rare Diagnoses

- **Dermoid**
  - ○ Commonly midline in position
  - ○ Mixed internal echoes from echogenic fat content and calcifications with dense posterior acoustic shadowing
  - ○ May appear pseudosolid or heterogeneous with fat content and osteodental structures
- **Epidermoid**
  - ○ Less common than dermoid cyst
  - ○ Often well defined, homogeneous, cystic with posterior enhancement
  - ○ May appear as pseudosolid in appearance due to cellular material within

- ○ With intermittent transducer pressure, swirling motion of debris may be seen on real-time scanning
- **2nd Branchial Cleft Cyst (2nd BCC)**
  - ○ 95% of all branchial anomalies
  - ○ Typically posterior to submandibular gland, along anteromedial border of sternocleidomastoid muscle
    - ▪ Superficial to common carotid artery (CCA) and internal jugular vein
  - ○ US may demonstrate associated track or fistula and characteristic extension of cyst between internal carotid artery (ICA) and external carotid artery (ECA)
  - ○ Typically well defined, anechoic, thin walls, posterior acoustic enhancement, or pseudosolid (avascular)
  - ○ May be become infected or hemorrhagic
    - ▪ Complex cyst with thick irregular walls, septa, debris, ± vascularity
  - ○ Mimic metastatic nodes with large cystic component
    - ▪ FNAC or excisional biopsy essential to differentiate from metastatic node
- **1st Branchial Cleft Cyst (1st BCC)**
  - ○ 8% of all branchial anomalies
  - ○ In/around parotid gland, external auditory canal (EAC), and angle of mandible
  - ○ Typically seen in middle-aged woman with recurrent parotid abscesses
  - ○ Anechoic, thin walls, posterior acoustic enhancement, or pseudosolid
  - ○ MR to exclude deep sinus tract through EAC to temporal bone
- **Thymic Cyst**
  - ○ Uncommon; occurs anywhere from angle of mandible to superior mediastinum along carotid sheath
  - ○ Well-defined anechoic cyst, commonly below level of thyroid, left > > right
  - ○ Aspiration yields clear watery fluid

SELECTED REFERENCES

1. Ibrahim M et al: Congenital cystic lesions of the head and neck. Neuroimaging Clin N Am. 21(3):621-39, viii, 2011
2. Wong KT et al: Imaging of cystic or cyst-like neck masses. Clin Radiol. 63(6):613-22, 2008

Neck Abscess

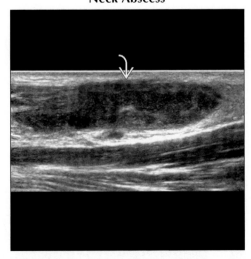

Longitudinal grayscale US shows a subcutaneous abscess ⤴ with thick-walled, cystic appearance and internal debris. Multiple matted, necrotic nodes were seen in ipsilateral posterior triangle.

Neck Abscess

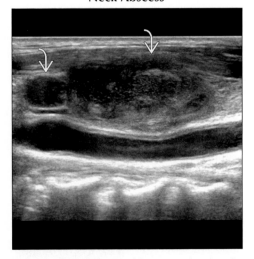

US (same patient) shows 2 of the necrotic lymph nodes ⇗ in the adjacent posterior triangle as a cause of the subcutaneous abscess. Sonographic feature indicates TB lymphadenitis, confirmed by FNAC.

Neck Abscess

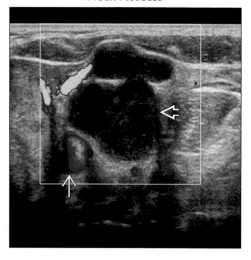

Neck Abscess

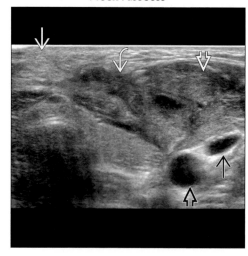

(Left) Transverse power Doppler US shows a classic "collar stud" abscess arising from TB lymphadenitis ➡. It is thick walled with internal debris and avascular on Doppler. US clearly defines its location and relation to common carotid artery (CCA) ➡. *(Right)* Transverse grayscale US shows postoperative abscess ➡ in a patient presenting with fever 5 days after surgery. Note its relation to CCA ➡, internal jugular vein (IJV) ➡, and sternomastoid muscle ➡ and postoperative soft tissue change ➡.

Metastatic Lymph Node

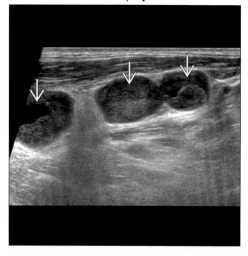

Squamous Cell Carcinoma (SCCa)

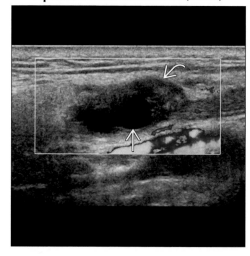

(Left) Longitudinal grayscale US shows multiple metastatic nodes from undifferentiated carcinoma of the nasopharynx. Note intranodal necrosis ➡ and absence of nodal matting or adjacent soft tissue edema and abscess formation (features of TB adenitis). *(Right)* Longitudinal power Doppler US shows metastatic node ➡ from head & neck primary SCCa. Intranodal necrosis, coagulation, and cystic necrosis ➡ is common in metastatic SCCa lymphadenopathy.

Papillary Carcinoma of Thyroid

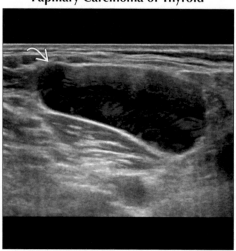

Papillary Carcinoma of Thyroid

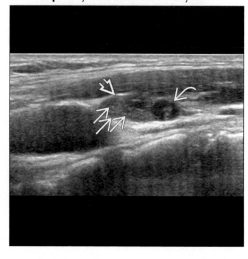

(Left) Transverse grayscale US shows a large cystic node ➡ with no obvious solid component in a patient with history of thyroidectomy for papillary carcinoma. FNAC confirmed metastasis from papillary carcinoma. *(Right)* Longitudinal grayscale US of the same patient shows another metastatic node ➡ inferior to the cystic neck mass. Note cystic change ➡ and fine punctate calcification ➡ in the solid component. Appearances are typical of metastasis from papillary thyroid carcinoma.

Venous Vascular Malformation (VVM)

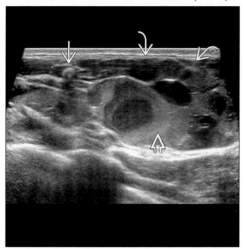

Venous Vascular Malformation (VVM)

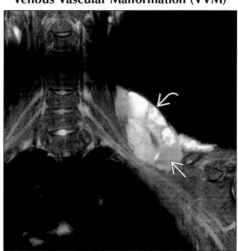

(Left) Transverse grayscale US of the left supraclavicular fossa shows a cystic, septate, trans-spatial lesion ➡. Note phlebolith ➡ and fine echogenic debris ➡ within, which showed slow "to and fro" motion on real-time grayscale US, features typical of slow-flow VVM. (Right) Corresponding coronal T2WI FS MR confirms location, extent, and multiseptated cystic appearance ➡ of VVM. Heterogeneous signal represents sedimentation of blood cells ➡ due to slow flow.

Lymphatic Malformation

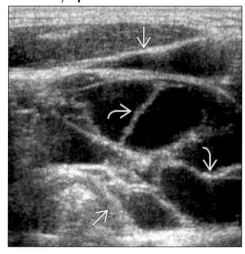

Lymphatic Malformation

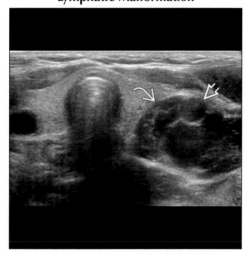

(Left) Transverse grayscale US of posterior triangle shows a thin-walled, septate ➡, multiloculated cystic mass ➡. Note cystic spaces are compartmentalized rather than serpiginous, and no phleboliths are present (vs. VVM). US features indicate lymphatic malformation (LM). (Right) Transverse grayscale US shows LM ➡ extending from prevertebral space to carotid space. Trans-spatial extension is typical for LM, and its extent is better defined by CT/MR. Note CCA ➡.

Acute Suppurative Thyroiditis

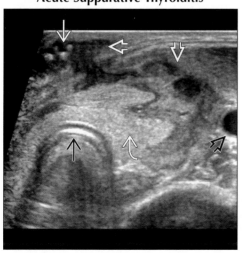

Acute Suppurative Thyroiditis

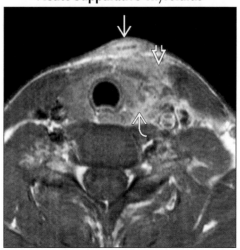

(Left) Transverse grayscale US shows a neck abscess ➡ in perithyroidal soft tissue, suggesting acute suppurative thyroiditis. Echogenic foci ➡ represent gas, which may be due to communication with pyriform sinus or infection by gas-forming organism. Note thyroid ➡, trachea ➡, and CCA ➡. (Right) Corresponding axial T1WI C+ MR shows superficial abscess ➡ and enhancing thyroid ➡ and perithyroid tissue ➡, consistent with acute suppurative thyroiditis.

CYSTIC NECK MASS

Diving Ranula (DR)

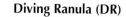

(Left) Transverse grayscale US of left floor of the mouth shows a cystic lesion extending from sublingual space ➡, across mylohyoid muscle ➡, to submandibular space ➡. The lesion is unilocular and thin walled with mobile, echogenic debris, features of diving ranula. Simple ranula is confined to sublingual space. Note submandibular gland ➡. *(Right)* Corresponding transverse T2WI MR clearly demonstrates sublingual ➡ and submandibular ➡ space involvement, typical of diving ranula.

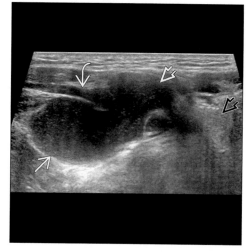

Diving Ranula (DR)

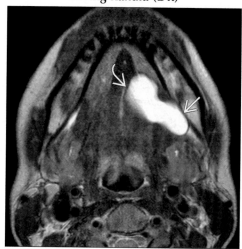

Dermoid

(Left) Transverse ultrasound of the lower neck shows a cystic, midline epidermoid cyst ➡. It is thin walled with faint internal debris ➡ and posterior acoustic enhancement ➡. *(Right)* Transverse grayscale US of the midline lower neck shows a well-defined, unilocular, thin-walled, heterogeneous cystic lesion ➡ with posterior enhancement. It is superficial to strap muscles ➡ and not related to hyoid bone (not shown), as opposed to thyroglossal duct cyst. Note thyroid gland ➡ and trachea ➡.

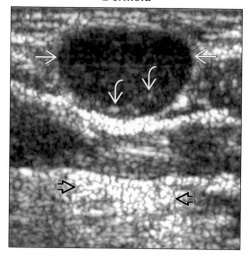

Dermoid

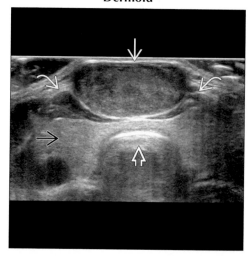

2nd Branchial Cleft Cyst (2nd BCC)

(Left) Transverse grayscale US shows typical 2nd BCC ➡ as a thin-walled, unilocular cystic lesion with low-level internal debris posterior to submandibular gland ➡ (SMG), under medial edge of sternomastoid muscle ➡, and superficial to carotid bifurcation ➡ (classic location). *(Right)* Corresponding transverse power Doppler US of 2nd BCC ➡ shows no vascularity in its walls or adjacent soft tissues. Its location anterior to carotid bifurcation ➡ is confirmed.

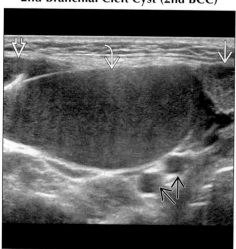

2nd Branchial Cleft Cyst (2nd BCC)

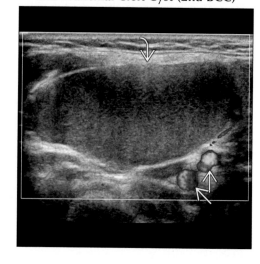

2nd Branchial Cleft Cyst (2nd BCC)

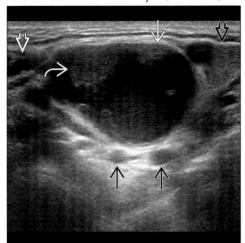

2nd Branchial Cleft Cyst (2nd BCC)

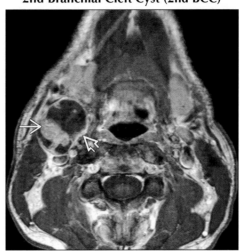

(Left) Transverse grayscale US shows a cystic mass ➡️ *with a solid mural nodule* ➡️ *in the typical location of 2nd BCC. Differential diagnosis includes metastatic node (from H&N SCCa, thyroid papillary carcinoma) and infected 2nd BCC. FNAC confirmed metastatic node from H&N SCCa. Note sternomastoid* ➡️, *submandibular gland* ➡️, *and carotid bifurcation* ➡️. *(Right) Corresponding transverse T1WI C+ MR confirms irregular wall thickening* ➡️ *and enhancing mural nodule* ➡️, *consistent with necrotic metastatic node.*

1st Branchial Cleft Cyst (1st BCC)

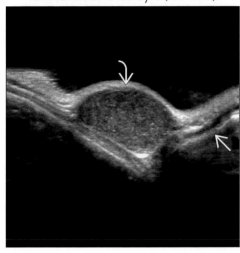

1st Branchial Cleft Cyst (1st BCC)

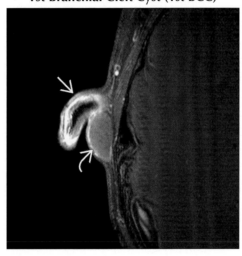

(Left) Longitudinal grayscale US of right retroauricular region shows typical pseudosolid appearance of congenital neck cyst ➡️ *located adjacent to pinna* ➡️. *It was avascular on Doppler ultrasound (not shown). Location and US features are typical for simple 1st BCC. (Right) Corresponding transverse T1WI C+ MR shows thin, enhancing wall, consistent with an uncomplicated BCC* ➡️ *and its relation to pinna* ➡️. *A "beak" pointing to the external auditory canal may be seen on MR.*

Thymic Cyst

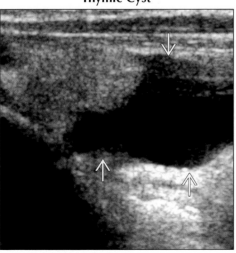

Thymic Cyst

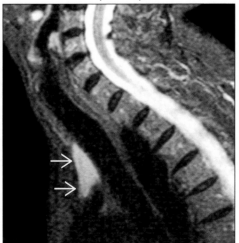

(Left) Longitudinal ultrasound of the suprasternal region shows an irregular midline unilocular cyst ➡️, *representing a thymic cyst, which is more common on the left. Aspiration of such a cyst yields clear watery fluid. These are usually discovered incidentally. (Right) Sagittal T2WI MR with fat suppression of the midline suprasternal region in the same patient shows homogeneous fluid signal within the thymic cyst* ➡️.

NON-NODAL SOLID NECK MASS

DIFFERENTIAL DIAGNOSIS

Common
- Nerve Sheath Tumor
- Lipoma
  - Madelung Disease

Less Common
- Carotid Body Paraganglioma

Rare but Important
- Ectopic Thyroid

ESSENTIAL INFORMATION

Key Differential Diagnosis Issues
- Most common solid masses in neck are normal/abnormal lymph nodes
  - Look for clues that mass represents lymph nodes
    - Along lymph node chains, with hilar architecture, vascularity, multiplicity, bilaterality
  - Clinical history helpful
    - Known head and neck or infraclavicular tumor
    - Symptoms and signs of infection/inflammation
    - ↑ white cell count, fever
  - Typical features of abnormal lymph nodes
    - Papillary thyroid carcinoma nodes: Hyperechoic, intranodal punctate calcifications, peripheral and chaotic intranodal vascularity, cystic necrosis
    - Lymphomatous nodes: Solid, "reticulated" internal architecture, hilar > peripheral vascularity
    - Tuberculous nodes: Matting, soft tissue edema, cystic necrosis, displaced hilar vascularity
- Once non-nodal nature of mass is established, evaluate mass based on its location and specific characteristics
  - Nerve sheath tumors (NST) occur at known location of nerve: Vagus, brachial plexus, sympathetic chain
  - Soft and compressible nature with feathered or striped appearances are highly suggestive of lipoma
  - Location of carotid body paraganglioma (CBP) is a specific and very good clue to diagnosis
- MR/CT may be indicated for further evaluation
  - In patients with CBP, rule out glomus jugulare and vagale as US cannot evaluate these
  - For better anatomical delineation of large lesions which cannot be completely assessed by US
  - Aids lesion characterization (e.g., typical "salt and pepper" appearance of CBP; fat signal intensity and uniform signal loss on fat-suppression sequence suggest lipoma)

Helpful Clues for Common Diagnoses
- Nerve Sheath Tumor
  - Benign tumor of Schwann cells that wraps around nerve
  - Commonly arises from vagus nerve, brachial plexus, or small cutaneous nerve
  - Transverse scan to identify tumor
    - Supplemented by longitudinal scan to evaluate continuity/nerve thickening and vascularity
  - Identification of tapering end/continuation with nerve is often tedious and requires meticulous technique
    - Use light pressure on long-axis scan to prevent slipping of tumor off scan plane
  - Grayscale US features
    - Well circumscribed, fusiform/oval-shaped ± tapering end(s), hypoechoic
    - Often shows posterior enhancement (despite being solid), "pseudocystic"
    - May or may not show sharply defined focal intratumoral cystic areas
    - May or may not show mass effect on adjacent vessels (common carotid artery [CCA] and internal jugular vein [IJV] may be draped over anterior surface of tumor with sympathetic NST, separation of CCA and IJV with vagal NST)
    - Continuity with nerve/thickening of adjacent nerve is diagnostic
  - Color Doppler US
    - Prominent intratumoral vascularity; better evaluated on longitudinal scan
    - Use light transducer pressure to avoid compression of intratumoral vessels
  - FNAC is usually not necessary if continuation with thickened nerve is seen
  - CT/MR is indicated for
    - Equivocal US findings
    - Better anatomical delineation and relationship of the nerve in large tumor
  - CT features
    - NECT: Well-circumscribed soft tissue density mass in carotid space adjacent to CCAs/ICAs and IJV
    - CECT: Uniform enhancement; focal areas of absent enhancement if intratumoral cystic change present
  - MR features
    - T2WI: Signal higher than muscle; sometimes with intratumoral cysts with areas of high signal
    - T1 C+: Dense uniform enhancement is typical
    - Intratumoral/nonenhancing cysts often present in larger lesions
  - If US, CT, or MR findings are equivocal, FNAC may be considered
- Lipoma
  - Clinical diagnosis usually made, US mainly to confirm clinical diagnosis
  - Occurs at any neck site
    - Posterior cervical space and submandibular space are most common
  - Intermuscular > intramuscular
  - May involve multiple contiguous spaces (trans-spatial)
  - Grayscale US features
    - Well-defined, soft, compressible mass
    - Typically hypoechoic in neck (isoechoic to muscles); echogenic type of lipoma/angiolipoma is more commonly seen in trunk and limbs
    - Multiple, thin, echogenic lines oriented parallel to transducer/skin in both transverse and longitudinal planes; feathered or striped appearance (compared with striation of muscles seen only in longitudinal plane)
    - No evidence of calcification, nodularity, necrosis, posterior acoustic enhancement/attenuation
    - Displacement but no infiltration/stranding of adjacent structures
  - Color Doppler US
    - Absence/paucity of vascularity
  - Liposarcoma should be suspected if soft tissue stranding present ± vascularity ± necrosis ± calcification
    - Presence of adjacent soft tissue stranding

- Presence of nodular mass, septation, and vascularity within lesion
- Cystic/necrotic areas and calcifications within
- MR indicated to evaluate full extent; subsequent US-guided FNAC or excision for pathological diagnosis
  - **Madelung Disease**
    - Benign symmetrical lipomatosis
    - Diffuse lobulated lipomas in cervical and shoulder regions bilaterally
    - As fat is unencapsulated, US not able to define degree of involvement
    - May mask underlying neck malignancy; CT and MR better define distribution of fat, compression of vital structures, and examination of deeper structures

Helpful Clues for Less Common Diagnoses

- **Carotid Body Paraganglioma**
  - Solid vascular tumor at carotid bifurcation is 1st clue to diagnosis
  - Always evaluate contralateral side as tumor may be bilateral
  - Grayscale features
    - Round/oval hypoechoic mass straddling carotid bifurcation
    - Typically blurred outlines despite its superficial location (probably due to dispersion of sound by multidirectional high-velocity flow within tumor)
    - Homogeneous parenchymal echo pattern ± serpiginous vessels within
    - Heterogeneous parenchymal echo pattern in larger tumors due to necrosis or hemorrhage within
    - No evidence of calcification or internal necrosis
    - Large tumors may completely encase bifurcation
  - Color/power Doppler
    - Profuse intratumoral vascularity
    - Deeper components may appear avascular as they are not well interrogated with Doppler
    - External and internal carotid arteries are splayed (by large enough tumors) and often encased without any narrowing

- Use gentle transducer pressure to avoid compressing intratumoral vessels
  - Characteristic signal pattern on MR
    - T1WI : "Salt and pepper" appearances; "salt" = high signal area due to subacute blood; "pepper" = hypointense punctate foci due to high flow within intratumoral vessels
    - T1 C+: Intense enhancement

Helpful Clues for Rare Diagnoses

- **Ectopic Thyroid**
  - May occur anywhere along tract of thyroglossal duct
    - Related to embryogenesis and inferior migration of the primordial thyroid gland
    - May be associated with thyroglossal duct cyst/fistula
  - Represents functioning thyroid tissue in only 70-80%
  - US features
    - Midline dorsum of tongue near foramen cecum (majority) > thyroglossal duct > trachea
    - Well-defined solid mass with fine echogenic parenchymal pattern and vascularity (resembling thyroid tissue)
    - May or may not show empty thyroid bed
    - May or may not show changes of multinodular goiter
  - Malignancy in 3%, typically papillary carcinoma
    - Papillary carcinoma: Solid, hypoechoic, ill-defined, vascular tumor ± punctate calcification, cystic necrosis, associated lymph nodes
    - FNAC required if there is any suspicious solid nodule or mass
  - Scintigraphy to confirm diagnosis and detect functioning tissue at any other location in neck

SELECTED REFERENCES

1. Yasumatsu R et al: Diagnosis and management of extracranial head and neck schwannomas: a review of 27 cases. Int J Otolaryngol. 2013:973045, 2013
2. Demattè S et al: Role of ultrasound and color Doppler imaging in the detection of carotid paragangliomas. J Ultrasound. 15(3):158-63, 2012

Nerve Sheath Tumor

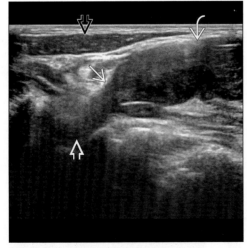

Longitudinal oblique US shows a solid, hypoechoic mass ➡ with the tapering end ➡ deep to the sternomastoid muscle ➡ and connected to the exiting thickened nerve ➡, suggestive of nerve sheath tumor (NST).

Nerve Sheath Tumor

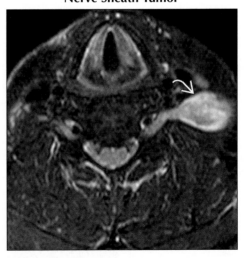

Corresponding axial T1WI C+ FS MR confirms an avidly enhancing schwannoma ➡. US readily identifies nature of lesion; however, CT/MR better assess multiplicity and anatomic extent.

Nerve Sheath Tumor

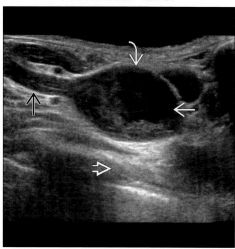

Nerve Sheath Tumor

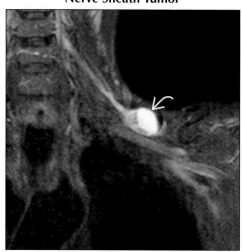

(Left) Longitudinal oblique US of left supraclavicular fossa shows a spindle-shaped hypoechoic nodule ➔ with cystic area ➔ and posterior enhancement ➔ continuous with exiting nerve root (C6) ➔, which are classic features of nerve sheath tumors (NST). A cystic area of variable size is a common finding in NST. *(Right)* Corresponding coronal T2WI FS MR confirms C6 NST ➔. US is an ideal imaging tool to evaluate NSTs in the neck as it identifies continuation with the involved nerve, which has a fibrillary pattern on US.

Nerve Sheath Tumor

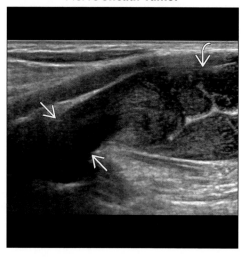

Nerve Sheath Tumor

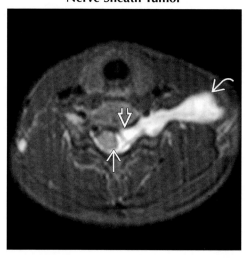

(Left) Longitudinal oblique grayscale US of the left supraclavicular fossa shows a large NST ➔. Note the heterogeneous, hypoechoic, noncalcified appearance and continuity with markedly thickened nerve root ➔. *(Right)* Corresponding axial T2WI FS MR shows extension of the NST ➔ into the spinal canal ➔, causing spinal cord compression ➔. Although US identifies the lesion, CT/MR better delineate intraspinal extension and any other associated small NSTs.

Lipoma

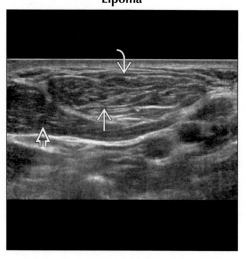

Lipoma

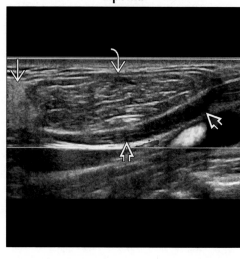

(Left) Transverse grayscale US shows a well-defined mass ➔ superficial to the sternomastoid muscle ➔. It has a striated/feathered echo pattern with echogenic lines ➔ parallel to the transducer. *(Right)* Corresponding longitudinal power Doppler US ➔ shows no internal vascularity, and intralesional echogenic lines remain parallel to transducer. Grayscale and Doppler features are typical of lipoma. Note tail of parotid gland ➔ and sternomastoid muscle ➔.

Lipoma

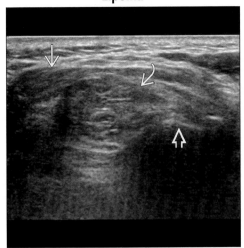

Lipoma

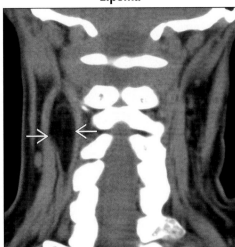

(Left) Transverse grayscale US of the posterior neck shows a well-defined hypoechoic mass ⮕ with a striated/feathered appearance. It is deep to the levator scapulae muscle ⮕, consistent with an intermuscular lipoma. Note the transverse process ⮕. There is no evidence of heterogeneous solid component or abnormal vascularity (not shown) to suggest sarcomatous change. (Right) Corresponding coronal NECT clearly identifies an intermuscular lipoma ⮕ composed entirely of fat density.

Madelung Disease

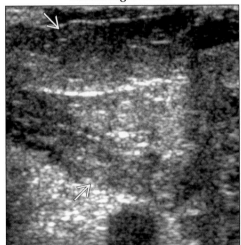

Madelung Disease

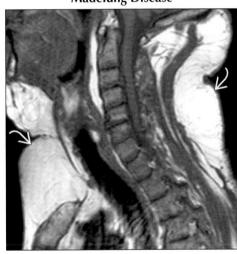

(Left) Transverse US shows a large, soft, compressible, hypoechoic mass ⮕ in the subcutaneous layer of the neck with extensive involvement, consistent with Madelung disease. (Right) Sagittal T1WI MR in the same patient shows extensive lipomatosis ⮕ in the neck. Although US readily establishes the diagnosis, CT or MR better evaluates the extent of involvement and presence of any associated tumor, which may be masked by lipomatosis.

Carotid Body Paraganglioma

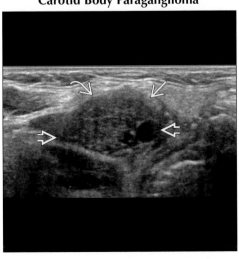

Carotid Body Paraganglioma

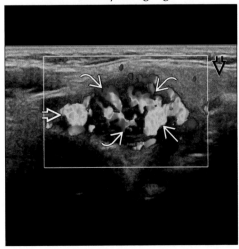

(Left) Transverse grayscale US shows the typical appearance of a right carotid body paraganglioma (CBP) ⮕ with fine, heterogeneous parenchymal pattern splaying and encasing carotid arteries ⮕. The border is typically indistinct ⮕ on US despite the sharply marginated nature of the tumor. (Right) Corresponding transverse color Doppler US shows typically profuse intratumoral vascularity ⮕ with arteriovenous shunts. Note internal carotid artery ⮕, external carotid artery ⮕, and submandibular gland ⮕.

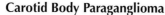

Carotid Body Paraganglioma

(Left) Transverse grayscale US shows a carotid body paraganglioma (CBP) ➡ splaying and displacing the carotid arteries ⮕ medially. Although the carotid arteries are not significantly encased in this patient, other features of carotid body tumor (including a fine, heterogeneous hypoechoic pattern and indistinct border ⮕) are present. *(Right)* Corresponding transverse power Doppler US shows profuse intratumoral vascularity ➡. Location, grayscale & Doppler features help to identify CBP. Note the carotid arteries ⮕.

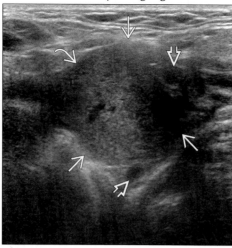

Carotid Body Paraganglioma

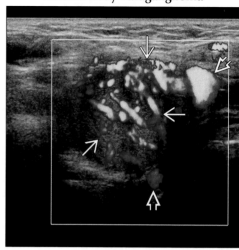

Carotid Body Paraganglioma

(Left) Axial T1WI C+ FS MR (same patient) shows typical avid contrast enhancement in the CBP ➡ and small flow voids ➡ consistent with a highly vascular lesion. MR also evaluates presence of any other glomus tumors in the head & neck (i.e., glomus jugulare, vagale, and tympanicum). *(Right)* Corresponding axial FDG-18 PET/CT shows high uptake within a CBP ➡. Most paragangliomas are shown to be FDG avid and therefore mimic a malignant lesion on PET.

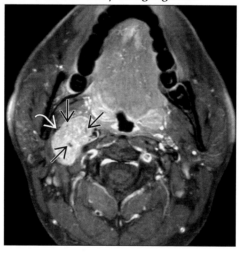

Carotid Body Paraganglioma

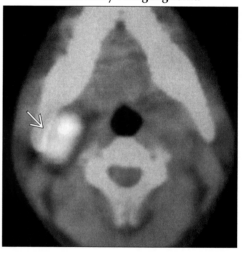

Carotid Body Paraganglioma

(Left) Axial NECT shows a well-defined, homogeneously hypodense mass ➡ in the left upper cervical region. *(Right)* Axial CECT shows avid contrast enhancement ⮕ of the mass, close to that of the adjacent vessels. The carotid arteries ⮕ are splayed and partially encased. The features are typical of a CBP. The coverage on CT/MR should extend from temporal bones to the lower neck.

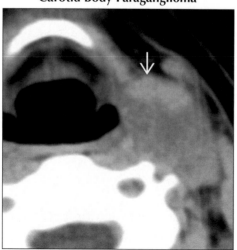

Carotid Body Paraganglioma

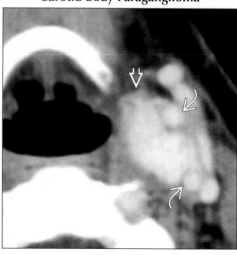

Carotid Body Paraganglioma

NON-NODAL SOLID NECK MASS

Ectopic Thyroid

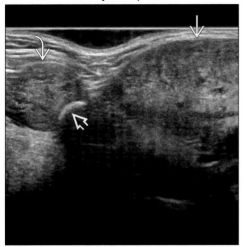

Ectopic Thyroid

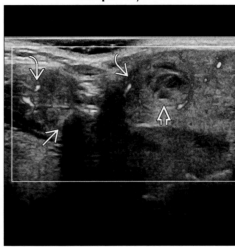

(Left) Longitudinal grayscale US shows hypoechoic midline nodules above ⇗ and below ⇒ the hyoid bone ⇒. *(Right)* Corresponding longitudinal power Doppler US shows scattered internal vascularity ⇒ within the nodules. Note the presence of a cystic, heterogeneous nodule ⇒ below the hyoid bone ⇒. Sonographic appearances of the nodules are reminiscent of nodular change in thyroid parenchyma, multinodular goiter (MNG).

Ectopic Thyroid

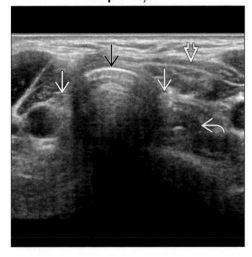

Ectopic Thyroid

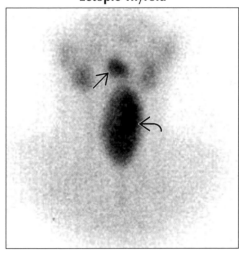

(Left) Transverse grayscale US *(same patient)* confirms an empty thyroid bed ⇒. Note the cervical esophagus ⇒ immediately deep to the strap muscles ⇒. Trachea ⇒ is shown. *(Right)* Corresponding anteroposterior Tc-99m pertechnetate thyroid scan shows a large area of uptake in the left paramedian region of the mid-upper neck ⇒ and further "hot" nodule in the suprahyoid neck ⇒, consistent with ectopic thyroid tissue corresponding to US.

Ectopic Thyroid

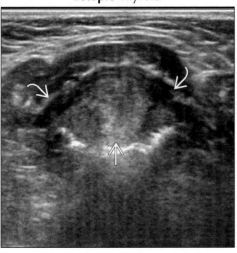

Ectopic Thyroid

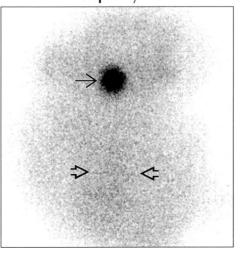

(Left) Transverse grayscale US in an infant presenting with congenital hypothyroidism shows a well-defined, round nodule ⇒ with a fine echogenic pattern (reminiscent of thyroid parenchymal echo pattern) in the midline floor of the mouth. Note mylohyoid muscle ⇒. The thyroid bed was empty (not shown). *(Right)* Corresponding anteroposterior Tc-99M pertechnetate thyroid scan shows tracer accumulation in the midline floor of the mouth, consistent with sublingual thyroid ⇒. Note the empty thyroid bed ⇒.

SOLID NECK LYMPH NODE

DIFFERENTIAL DIAGNOSIS

Common
- Reactive Lymph Node
- Metastatic Lymph Node
- Lymphoma

Less Common
- Calcified Lymph Node
- Tuberculous Infection
- Autoimmune Disease
  - Systemic Lupus Erythematosus (SLE)
  - Rheumatoid Arthritis (RA)

Rare but Important
- Kikuchi Disease
- Kimura Disease
- Rosai-Dorfman Syndrome

ESSENTIAL INFORMATION

Key Differential Diagnosis Issues
- No single sonographic criterion is absolute for malignancy or benignity of lymph nodes; US features to be assessed include
  - Shape: Elliptical/round
  - Border: Well-/ill-defined
  - Echogenicity: Hypoechoic/isoechoic/hyperechoic
  - Internal architecture: Presence/absence of echogenic hilus, intranodal necrosis, calcification
  - Vascularity on power Doppler: Presence/absence and distribution of vascularity, peripheral/hilar/mixed vascularity
  - Other associated features: ± invasion of adjacent structures, matting, soft tissue edema
- Size is not reliable predictor of malignancy
  - Serial change in size on follow-up examination is more relevant
  - US is able to identify small nodes, which ↑ sensitivity but ↓ specificity
    - Addition of guided fine-needle aspiration and cytology (FNAC) ↑ specificity
- Findings suggestive of nodal abnormality
  - Round shape, absent hilus, intranodal necrosis, intranodal punctate calcification, reticulation, and disorganized intranodal vascularity
- Distribution of lymph nodes provides useful information
  - Tuberculous node: Often unilateral, predominance in posterior triangle and supraclavicular fossa
  - Lymphomatous node: Frequently bilateral involvement ± other sites (e.g., groin, axillae)
  - Metastatic nodes: In neck are site specific, their distribution is related to location of primary tumor

Helpful Clues for Common Diagnoses
- **Reactive Lymph Node**
  - Commonly seen in children, smokers, and patients with allergic rhinitis and recent upper respiratory tract infection
  - Common sites: Submandibular, posterior triangle > internal jugular chain > supraclavicular fossa and intraparotid region
  - Distribution often bilateral and symmetrical
  - Elliptical, homogeneously hypoechoic with normal echogenic hilar architecture

- Vascularity is central, i.e., from hilus, branching to cortex with tapering ends
  - Dual hila sometimes seen
  - No peripheral vascularity
- No intranodal necrosis or calcification
- Static or shows serial reduction in nodal size on follow-up
- **Metastatic Lymph Node**
  - Location is commonly ipsilateral to primary tumor and in known draining sites of primary tumor
    - Always evaluate for contralateral lymphadenopathy as this may alter staging and management
  - Round, ± focal cortical eccentric enlargement (eccentric cortical hypertrophy)
    - Most are hypoechoic (except metastatic nodes from papillary carcinoma, iso-/hyperechoic to muscle)
    - Intranodal necrosis: Cystic (hypoechoic) or coagulation necrosis (echogenic, mimicking hilus but not continuous with surrounding fat)
    - Necrotic nodes common in metastases from head and neck SCCa, papillary thyroid carcinoma
  - Calcification: Punctate in papillary carcinoma; coarse, dense shadowing in metastatic medullary carcinoma, and post-treatment nodes
  - Margins are well defined in malignant nodes, ill defined in inflammatory nodes due to periadenitis (also in postradiation nodes)
    - If node shows all features of malignancy but ill-defined margins, suggests extracapsular spread (poorer prognosis)
  - Nodal matting and soft tissue edema may be seen in post-treatment nodes
  - Disorganized intranodal vascularity
    - Absent hilar flow to peripheral vascularity (not originating from hilum), displaced vessels, focal avascular areas
- **Lymphoma**
  - Multiple and bilateral involvement
  - Enlarged round node, ± multiple, hilar architecture often preserved
  - Diffuse cortical hypertrophy with reticulated pattern (seen with newer high-frequency transducers)
  - Acoustic enhancement behind solid nodes ("pseudocystic" pattern)
    - Due to uniform cellular infiltration within nodes, produces fewer interfaces and facilitates passage of sound
  - ± surrounding tissue edema
  - Intranodal necrosis is uncommon
  - Lack of intranodal calcification
  - Marked intranodal vascularity: Exaggerated hilar and peripheral vessels (hilar > peripheral)
    - Peripheral vascularity alone is rare (vs. metastatic node)
  - Biopsy confirms diagnosis

Helpful Clues for Less Common Diagnoses
- **Calcified Lymph Node**
  - Small foci of calcification: TB, papillary carcinoma
  - Coarse calcification: Old TB infection, post-treatment nodes, metastasis from medullary thyroid carcinoma
- **Tuberculous Infection**
  - Sonographic features very similar to malignant lymph nodes except
    - More oval than round

- Necrosis and matting are seen earlier, i.e., in smaller nodes, and are common features
- Surrounding edema more prominent
- Coarse shadowing from calcification may be present (different from punctate calcification seen in metastatic papillary carcinoma)
- Necrotic content may discharge to form cold abscess with characteristic "collar stud" appearance
○ Necrosis may be focal, ill defined, and difficult to see
- Absent or displaced vascularity (at site of necrosis) is supportive evidence
○ Appearances closely mimic metastatic nodes ± superimposed infection or pyogenic nodes
- FNA establishes definitive diagnosis
- **Autoimmune Disease**
○ Prominent lymph nodes common in patients with autoimmune disease
- RA and connective tissue diseases such as Sjögren syndrome, SLE, dermatomyositis
○ Variable sonographic appearance of nodes
- Reactive in majority of cases
- Cortical hypertrophy, profuse hilar vascularity seen with more active disease
○ Prominent lymph nodes in other sites (e.g., axillae, groin) as well
○ ↑ risk of lymphoma in RA, Sjögren syndrome, ± SLE and dermatomyositis

Helpful Clues for Rare Diagnoses

- **Kikuchi Disease**
○ Typically young Asian female (20-30 years old)
○ Nodes commonly in posterior triangle
○ Oval, hypoechoic, normal hilar architecture ± cortical necrosis, no matting or soft tissue edema
○ May or may not be surrounded by echogenic rim
○ Profuse hilar vascularity + displaced/absent vascularity in necrotic areas
- **Kimura Disease**
○ Typically in young Asian male (20-30 years old)
○ Nodes (± multiple) within parotid and in vicinity of salivary glands
○ Round, well defined, homogeneous, hypoechoic, ± normal echogenic hilus, ± intranodal necrosis

○ Associated soft tissue masses, salivary and subcutaneous in head and neck (in proximity of salivary glands)
- **Rosai-Dorfman Syndrome**
○ Typically 10- to 20-year-old blacks with massive lymphadenopathy
○ Grayscale and power Doppler features mimic malignant/lymphomatous nodes
- Round, solid, absent hilus, peripheral/mixed vascularity
○ Diagnosis relies on histology

SELECTED REFERENCES

1. Giacomini CP et al: Ultrasonographic evaluation of malignant and normal cervical lymph nodes. Semin Ultrasound CT MR. 34(3):236-47, 2013
2. Herd MK et al: Lymphoma presenting in the neck: current concepts in diagnosis. Br J Oral Maxillofac Surg. 50(4):309-13, 2012
3. Lo WC et al: Ultrasonographic differentiation between Kikuchi's disease and lymphoma in patients with cervical lymphadenopathy. Eur J Radiol. 81(8):1817-20, 2012
4. Sofferman RA et al: Ultrasound of the Thyroid and Parathyroid Glands. New York: Springer. 211-228, 2012
5. Khanna R et al: Usefulness of ultrasonography for the evaluation of cervical lymphadenopathy. World J Surg Oncol. 9:29, 2011
6. Furukawa MK et al: Diagnosis of lymph node metastases of head and neck cancer and evaluation of effects of chemoradiotherapy using ultrasonography. Int J Clin Oncol. 15(1):23-32, 2010
7. Ahuja AT et al: Ultrasound of malignant cervical lymph nodes. Cancer Imaging. 8:48-56, 2008
8. Ahuja AT et al: Diagnostic Imaging: Ultrasound. 1st ed. Salt Lake City: Amirsys.11-40-53, 2007
9. Chan JM et al: Ultrasonography of abnormal neck lymph nodes. Ultrasound Q. 23(1):47-54, 2007
10. Ahuja AT et al: Sonographic evaluation of cervical lymph nodes. AJR Am J Roentgenol. 184(5):1691-9, 2005
11. King AD et al: Necrosis in metastatic neck nodes: diagnostic accuracy of CT, MR imaging, and US. Radiology. 230(3):720-6, 2004
12. Ying M et al: Accuracy of sonographic vascular features in differentiating different causes of cervical lymphadenopathy. Ultrasound Med Biol. 30(4):441-7, 2004

Reactive Lymph Node

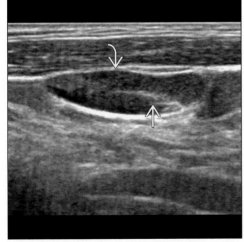

Longitudinal grayscale US shows typical reactive node ➤ in posterior triangle. It is elliptical (short-/long-axis ratio < 1/2), solid, and noncalcified with hypoechoic cortex and normal echogenic hilus ➡.

Reactive Lymph Node

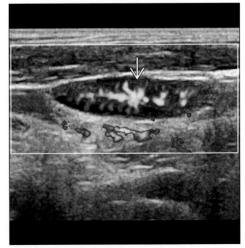

Corresponding longitudinal power Doppler US shows typical hilar vascular pattern ➡: Vessels branching out from the nodal hilum and absent peripheral vessels.

SOLID NECK LYMPH NODE

Reactive Lymph Node

Reactive Lymph Node

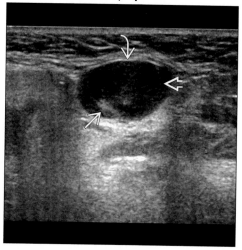

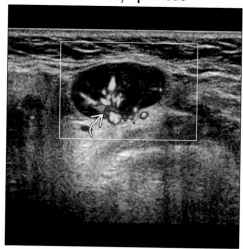

(Left) Transverse grayscale US shows hypertrophied submandibular node ➔ in a post-RT patient. Note cortical hypertrophy ➔ & rounded appearance. Echogenic hilum ➔ is visible & the border remains well defined. *(Right)* Corresponding transverse power Doppler US shows prominent hilar vascular pattern ➔. After radiation therapy, midline cervical nodes (submental, pre-/paratracheal) often undergo hypertrophy because of lymphatic redirection. Guided FNAC helps to exclude metastasis.

Metastatic Lymph Node

Metastatic Lymph Node

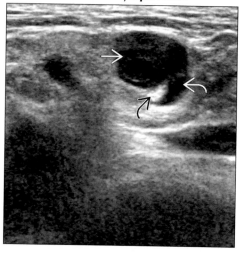

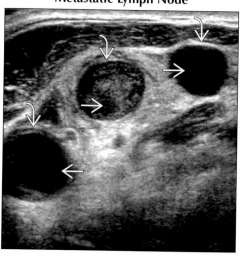

(Left) Transverse grayscale US shows eccentric cortical hypertrophy ➔ in metastatic lymph node (LN). The echogenic hilus ➔ is displaced by hypertrophied cortex. Note nonhypertrophied part of node ➔. FNA should be directed toward the hypertrophied area. *(Right)* Transverse grayscale US shows multiple metastatic LNs ➔ from head and neck squamous cell carcinoma (SCCa). They are round, well defined, and heterogeneously hypoechoic with areas of intranodal necrosis ➔ and absent echogenic hilus.

Metastatic Lymph Node

Metastatic Lymph Node

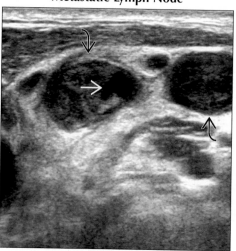

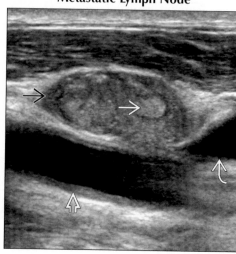

(Left) Transverse grayscale US shows multiple metastatic nodes ➔. Note that they are round, hypoechoic, and heterogeneous with loss of hilar architecture and intranodal eccentric cystic necrosis ➔. *(Right)* Longitudinal grayscale US shows metastatic LN ➔ with heterogeneous echo pattern. Note presence of focal echogenic area representing coagulative necrosis ➔, which is not continuous with perinodal soft tissues (vs. echogenic hilus). Note CCA ➔ and compressed internal jugular vein ➔.

SOLID NECK LYMPH NODE

Metastatic Lymph Node

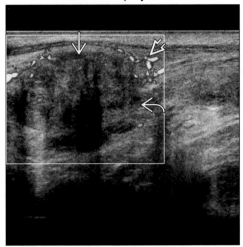

Metastatic Lymph Node

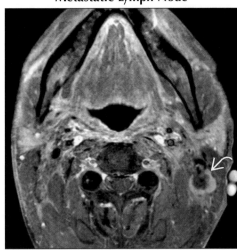

(Left) Longitudinal power Doppler US shows metastatic node ➡ from nasopharyngeal carcinoma with ill-defined margins and peripheral vascularity ➡. Its ill-defined border ➡ indicates extracapsular spread. Metastatic nodes are usually sharply defined compared to blurred margins in inflammatory nodes (due to periadenitis). *(Right)* Corresponding axial T1WI C+ FS MR confirms necrotic node ➡ in apex of left posterior triangle, a known common location of metastatic node from nasopharyngeal carcinoma.

Lymphoma

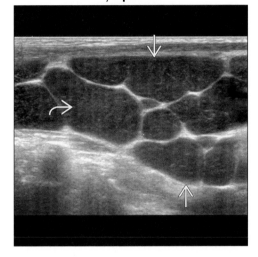

Lymphoma

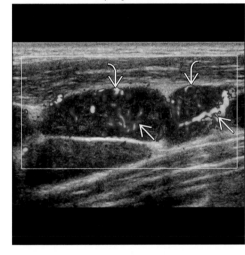

(Left) Longitudinal grayscale US shows multiple, solid, noncalcified, hypoechoic nodes ➡ with absent echogenic hilus. Note faint granular/reticulated echo pattern ➡ of these nodes in a patient with non-Hodgkin lymphoma. Extracapsular spread, cystic necrosis, and matting are relatively uncommon. *(Right)* Longitudinal power Doppler US shows multiple hilar ➡ and peripheral ➡ vessels. Hilar vascularity is > peripheral vascularity and is typically seen in lymphomatous nodes.

Lymphoma

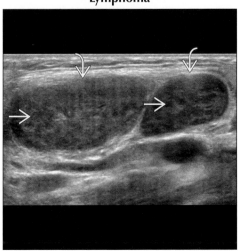

Lymphoma

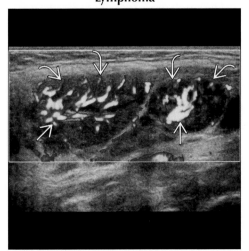

(Left) Longitudinal grayscale US shows multiple enlarged, solid, rounded, well-defined, noncalcified, hypoechoic nodes ➡ in the posterior triangle of a young adult patient. Note typically reticulated intranodal echo pattern ➡ typical of lymphomatous nodes. *(Right)* Corresponding longitudinal power Doppler ultrasound shows prominent hilar ➡ and peripheral vessels ➡ (hilar > peripheral vascularity), commonly seen in lymphomatous nodes.

SOLID NECK LYMPH NODE

(Left) Oblique US of midcervical chain shows echogenic focus ➥ with posterior shadow ➥ in small cervical node, consistent with calcification. Note Doppler box is used with power signal turned down to use fundamental grayscale US. Patient has history of treated TB, and US features are consistent with post-treatment, calcified node. **(Right)** Transverse grayscale US shows postradiation therapy node ➥ with calcification ➥. No abnormal vascularity was seen on Doppler FNA confirmed benign nature.

Calcified Lymph Node

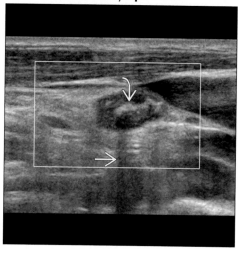

Calcified Lymph Node

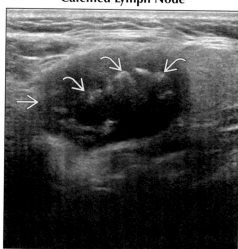

(Left) Transverse grayscale US shows a solitary, hypoechoic, heterogeneous, predominantly solid node in TB lymphadenitis ➥ (± tiny focus of necrosis ➥). TB lymphadenitis usually involves multiple posterior triangle nodes, and necrosis and abscess occur early. **(Right)** Corresponding transverse power Doppler US shows hilar ➥ and peripheral vessels ➥. Hilar vascularity in TB lymphadenitis is often displaced by focal avascular areas of caseous necrosis.

Tuberculous Infection

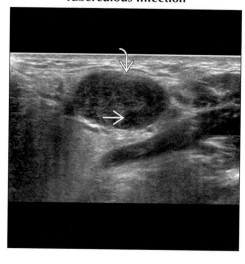

Tuberculous Infection

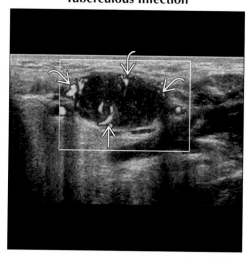

(Left) Longitudinal grayscale US shows multiple enlarged nodes ➥ with normal hilar architecture ➥ in the posterior triangle of a young Asian woman. Note the absence of necrosis, matting, and soft tissue edema. Location and grayscale features suggest Kikuchi disease. **(Right)** Corresponding longitudinal power Doppler US shows prominent vascularity radiating from the hilum ➥ in a benign vascular pattern. No vascularity is seen in adjacent soft tissues. Guided FNAC confirmed Kikuchi disease.

Kikuchi Disease

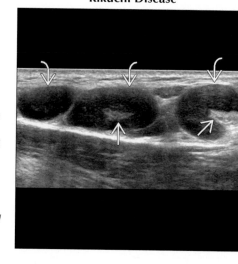

Kikuchi Disease

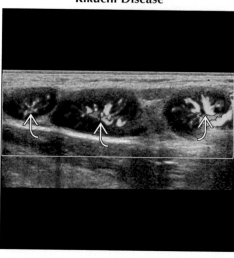

SOLID NECK LYMPH NODE

Kimura Disease

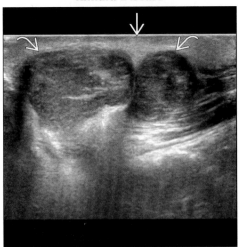

Kimura Disease

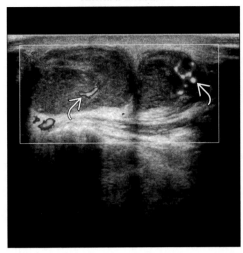

(Left) Transverse grayscale US shows enlarged nodes ➡ in the apex of the posterior triangle in an adult Asian male patient. Associated subcutaneous thickening in the upper neck ➡ and earlobe was present as well as multiple intraparotid nodes. (Right) Longitudinal power Doppler US shows sparse intranodal vascularity ➡. In the clinical context, US features and distribution in the neck/ perisalivary region are suspicious for Kimura disease, subsequently confirmed by FNA.

Kimura Disease

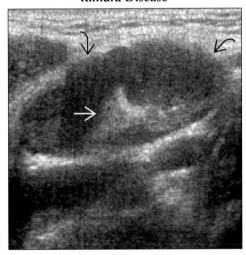

Kimura Disease

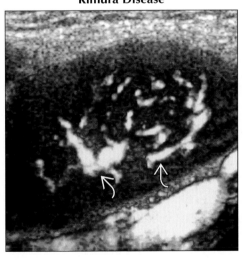

(Left) Longitudinal ultrasound in the same patient shows an enlarged, solid, hypoechoic node ➡ in the posterior triangle. The cortex is diffusely hypertrophied, but the echogenic hilar architecture ➡ is preserved. (Right) Longitudinal power Doppler ultrasound in the same patient shows profuse hilar vascularity ➡. Together with the intraparotid soft tissue mass, the features are suggestive of Kimura disease.

Rosai-Dorfman Syndrome

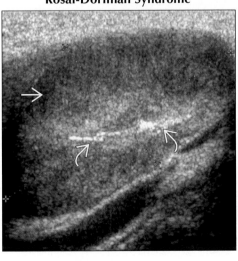

Rosai-Dorfman Syndrome

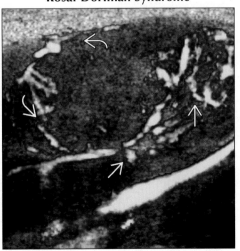

(Left) Longitudinal US shows a markedly enlarged lymph node in an African adolescent. Note the node's solid, hypoechoic echo pattern ➡. The echogenic hilum ➡ is preserved. (Right) Longitudinal power Doppler ultrasound in the same patient shows both central ➡ and peripheral ➡ vascularity. The ultrasound findings and clinical setting suggest Rosai-Dorfman syndrome, but metastatic lymphadenopathy must be excluded. The biopsy confirmed the diagnosis.

NECROTIC NECK LYMPH NODE

DIFFERENTIAL DIAGNOSIS

Common
- Metastatic Lymph Node, Squamous Cell Carcinoma (SCCa)
- Tuberculous Lymphadenitis

Less Common
- Metastatic Lymph Node, Papillary Thyroid Carcinoma

ESSENTIAL INFORMATION

Key Differential Diagnosis Issues
- Punctate calcification within solid component of necrotic lymph node is characteristic of metastasis from papillary carcinoma of thyroid

Helpful Clues for Common Diagnoses
- **Metastatic Lymph Node, Squamous Cell Carcinoma (SCCa)**
  - Primary: Head and neck SCCa, esophagus, lung, distant or unknown primary
    - Primary head and neck SCCa follows expected nodal drainage of tumor
  - Round, single or multiple, heterogeneous, hypoechoic, loss of normal hilar architecture
    - Reported in 69-95% of involved nodes
  - Cystic necrosis is common; can be small to entirely cystic (discrete or coalescent)
  - Coagulative necrosis seen as echogenic foci/areas
  - Calcification is rare (punctate or coarse)
  - Doppler: Peripheral and mixed (hilar and peripheral) vascularity, absent vascularity in necrotic areas
- **Tuberculous Lymphadenitis**
  - Common in young adults and new immigrants to endemic area
  - Posterior triangle ± discharging sinus ± low-grade fever ± constitutional symptoms
  - Multiple heterogeneous hypoechoic lymph nodes, ovoid > rounded
  - Early necrosis seen as small cortical hypoechoic area with displaced vascularity
  - Larger necrotic nodes tend to mat together and have associated soft tissue edema/periadenitis (scrofula)
  - Nodal calcification is not seen in acute disease (except in recurrent disease in previously affected/treated/incompletely treated node)
  - Color Doppler: Displaced hilar vascularity in 50%, avascular in 19%, capsular vascularity (supply from perinodal inflammatory tissue)
  - Discharge of contents of necrotic node into soft tissues forms large subcutaneous abscess
    - "Collar stud" abscess
  - Following FNAC, send specimen for culture, PCR to establish diagnosis

Helpful Clues for Less Common Diagnoses
- **Metastatic Lymph Node, Papillary Thyroid Carcinoma**
  - Round or ovoid with cystic areas
  - Solid component contains punctate calcification and internal vascularity
  - Color Doppler: Increased chaotic vascularity in solid component
  - Primary tumor with suspicious features (ill-defined margin, solid, hypoechoic, punctate calcification, chaotic intranodular vascularity, invasion of adjacent structures) in ipsilateral thyroid lobe
    - Sometimes primary tumor may be occult
  - Lymph nodes in expected drainage areas
    - Anterior compartment and along internal jugular vein, single or multiple
  - Exclude contralateral neck node metastasis in tumors close to midline
  - FNAC should be directed toward solid area with punctate calcification
  - Cystic fluid may be sent for thyroglobulin estimation

SELECTED REFERENCES

1. Ahuja AT et al: Diagnostic Imaging: Ultrasound. 1st ed. Salt Lake City: Amirsys. 11-42-47, 2007

Metastatic Lymph Node, Squamous Cell Carcinoma (SCCa)

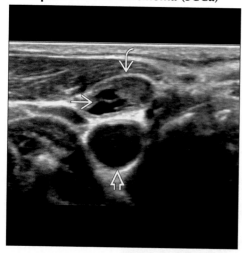

Transverse US shows metastatic node ➡ from H&N SCCa with intranodal necrosis ➡. Modern transducers accurately identify small nodes and evaluate internal architecture & relation to major vessels such as CCA ➡.

Metastatic Lymph Node, Squamous Cell Carcinoma (SCCa)

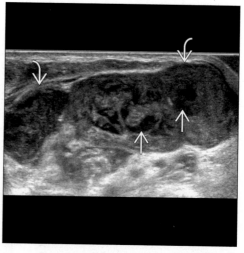

Longitudinal grayscale US shows multiple metastatic nodes from SCCa ➡. Note absent hilar architecture and presence of areas of intranodal cystic necrosis ➡.

Tuberculous Lymphadenitis

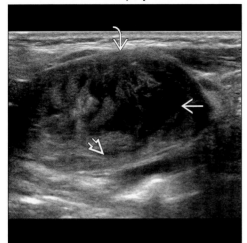

Tuberculous Lymphadenitis

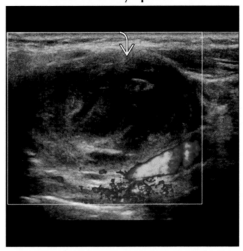

(Left) Longitudinal grayscale US of a tuberculous node ➡ shows large areas of intranodal necrosis ➡ within the node and irregular walls ➡, common features of TB. Necrosis occurs early in TB lymphadenitis. (Right) Corresponding longitudinal power Doppler US shows no vascularity within the necrotic node ➡ due to caseous necrosis & endarteritis (causing occlusion of vessels), features of tuberculous lymphadenitis.

Tuberculous Lymphadenitis

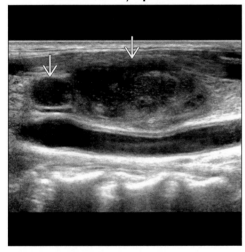

Metastatic Lymph Node, Papillary Thyroid Carcinoma

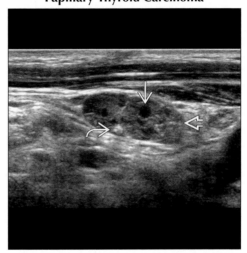

(Left) Longitudinal grayscale US shows multiple necrotic nodes ➡ with no normal intervening soft tissues (nodal matting). Soft tissue edema and nodal matting due to periadenitis are common features of TB nodes. (Right) Longitudinal grayscale US shows a small, hyperechoic node ➡ with well-defined borders, foci of internal necrosis ➡, and punctate calcification ➡. US features are typical for a metastatic node from a thyroid papillary carcinoma.

Metastatic Lymph Node, Papillary Thyroid Carcinoma

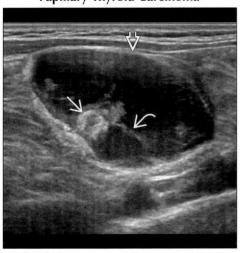

Metastatic Lymph Node, Papillary Thyroid Carcinoma

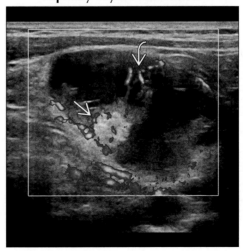

(Left) Transverse grayscale US shows a large, predominantly cystic node ➡ with intranodal septa ➡ and solid component within. Note the fine echogenic foci ➡ within the solid component of the node. US features are strongly suspicious for a metastatic node from a thyroid papillary carcinoma. (Right) Corresponding power Doppler US shows the presence of abnormal vascularity within septa ➡ and solid component ➡. US-guided FNAC confirmed a metastatic node from a thyroid papillary carcinoma.

DIFFUSE SALIVARY GLAND ENLARGEMENT

DIFFERENTIAL DIAGNOSIS

Common
- Acute Sialadenitis
  - Calculus Sialadenitis
  - Infective Sialadenitis
- Chronic Sialadenitis

Less Common
- Sjögren Syndrome (SJS)
- Sarcoidosis
- Benign Lymphoepithelial Lesion (BLEL)
- Lymphatic Malformation
- Hemangioma/Venous Vascular Malformation (VVM)
- Kuttner Tumor
- Kimura Disease

Rare but Important
- Metastasis
- Lymphoma

ESSENTIAL INFORMATION

Key Differential Diagnosis Issues
- Submandibular glands scanned in transverse, longitudinal, and oblique planes to demonstrate abnormality and anatomy
- For parotid glands, transverse scans define location of abnormality in relation to external carotid artery and retromandibular vein
  - Longitudinal scans help to evaluate parenchyma and parotid tail
- US does not evaluate pathology in deep lobe of parotid gland as gland is obscured by mandible
  - CT or MR best evaluate deep parotid lobe

Helpful Clues for Common Diagnoses
- **Acute Sialadenitis**
  - Acute inflammation of salivary glands (4 types)
    - Bacterial: Localized infection, unilateral involvement, may become suppurative
    - Viral: Usually from systemic viral infection, 75% bilateral parotid gland involvement
    - Calculus-induced: Unilateral with obstructing stone
    - Autoimmune: Acute episode of chronic disease
  - Clinical signs and symptoms of sepsis (fever, pain, and swelling), ↑ white cell count
  - Diffusely heterogeneous hypoechoic echo pattern, enlarged gland with hypervascularity ± abscess
  - ± ductal dilatation, ± echogenic ductal stone, ± posterior shadowing
    - Parotid calculi may be difficult to detect on US; NECT much more sensitive
  - Tender on probe pressure
  - Uncontrolled disease may progress to abscess formation
    - Ill-defined, thick-walled hypoechoic mass with liquefied component ± gas
  - Presence of reactive lymph nodes (LNs)
    - Mildly enlarged, elliptical, preserved echogenic hilum and hilar vascularity
  - Calculus-induced disease: Submandibular > parotid
    - Submandibular saliva is thicker, more mucinous, and alkaline than parotid
- **Chronic Sialadenitis**

- Atrophic gland with heterogeneous, hypoechoic echo pattern
- Enlarged gland with cystic dilatation of ducts and subsequent parenchymal atrophy
  - Indistinguishable from SJS and BLEL
  - Sialadenitis often involves 1 gland rather than multiple (vs. SJS and BLEL)

Helpful Clues for Less Common Diagnoses
- **Sjögren Syndrome (SJS)**
  - Parotid > submandibular > sublingual ± lacrimal gland; bilateral involvement
  - Early phase
    - Normal-sized or diffusely enlarged glands, normal parenchymal pattern
  - Intermediate phase
    - Diffusely enlarged glands + multiple cysts of similar size and solid masses (representing parenchymal destruction and lymphoid aggregates)
    - Microcystic (cysts < 1 mm, may be missed) or macrocystic pattern
  - May be indistinguishable from BLEL on US, but tonsillar hyperplasia and reactive cervical LNs not features of SJS
  - Diagnosis is clinical and serological and confirmed with biopsy
  - Imaging to confirm/exclude salivary gland involvement and surveillance for lymphomatous change
- **Sarcoidosis**
  - Clinical evidence of uveitis and facial paralysis (Heerfordt disease)
  - Nonspecific US appearances
    - Affects submandibular > parotid glands
  - May be seen as diffuse hypoechogenicity with normal-sized or enlarged gland
  - Associated with neck node enlargement
- **Benign Lymphoepithelial Lesion (BLEL)**
  - Mainly involves parotid glands, associated with tonsillar hyperplasia and reactive lymphadenopathy
  - 5% of HIV-positive patients develop BLEL of parotids
  - Diffuse enlargement of gland with multiple cysts, mixed cystic and solid lesions, &/or solid nodules
    - Cysts are thin walled ranging from a few mm up to 3.5 cm
    - Solid lesions: Ill-defined masses representing lymphoid aggregates
- **Lymphatic Malformation**
  - Congenital lymphatic malformation
  - More commonly presented in childhood
  - May involve adjacent spaces (i.e., trans-spatial)
    - MR may be needed to map extent of involvement prior to treatment
  - Uninfected: Thin-walled, multiseptated anechoic cystic lesion
  - Infected/hemorrhagic: Thick-walled, heterogeneous internal echoes, ± debris, ± fluid level
- **Hemangioma/Venous Vascular Malformation (VVM)**
  - US appearance reflects histology
    - Hemangioma: Small vessels with ↑ stromal component
    - VVM: Sinusoidal spaces with ↓ stroma
  - Phleboliths may be seen; more in slow-flow lesions such as VVM

- Doppler shows internal vascularity in medium to high-flow vessels
  - Slow flow often better seen on grayscale as "to and fro" motion of debris/contents within VVM
- **Kuttner Tumor**
  - Chronic sclerosing sialadenitis
  - Submandibular > > > parotid gland
    - Bilateral involvement is common
  - Diffuse "cirrhotic" gland
    - Diffusely heterogeneous, hypoechoic parenchymal echo pattern with lobulated contours
  - Focal "geographic" pattern
    - Focal, ill-defined, hypoechoic areas (simulating malignancy) in gland
  - Doppler US: Preserved architecture with hypervascularity in involved areas
    - No mass effect by hypoechoic "mass"
- **Kimura Disease**
  - Subcutaneous masses ± salivary gland (parotid > submandibular) masses ± lymphadenopathy in young Asian males
  - Masses may be ill/well defined and hypoechoic with variable vascularity on Doppler
  - Background glandular parenchyma may be heterogeneous

Helpful Clues for Rare Diagnoses

- **Metastasis**
  - Note: Parotid gland contains nodes and is, therefore, site of nodal metastases
  - Common 1° tumor: Malignant melanoma, squamous cell carcinoma in face, lateral scalp, external auditory meatus, and nasopharyngeal carcinoma
  - US: Solitary/multiple hypoechoic nodules, solid, ± ill-defined, ± skin/subcutaneous/extraparotid extension
  - Multiplicity and history of known head and neck malignant 1° should raise suspicion
- **Lymphoma**
  - Primary: More common in Sjögren syndrome, rheumatoid arthritis, and patients on immunosuppressants

- Secondary: In 1-8% of patients with systemic lymphoma
- 80% involve parotid glands (both 1° and 2°)
- Nodal involvement: Enlarged lymph node + reticulated pattern or microcystic appearance + posterior enhancement + central > peripheral vascularity
- Parenchymal involvement: Diffuse, heterogeneous, hypoechoic pattern (mimicking sialadenitis) or as ill-defined, irregular, hypoechoic, hypervascular mass

Alternative Differential Approaches

- Approach by differentiation of echo pattern/nature of enlarged salivary gland
  - Cystic: Chronic sialadenitis, SJS, BLEL, lymphatic malformation ± hemangioma/VVM
  - Diffuse hypoechoic infiltration: Acute calculus or infective sialadenitis ± metastasis
  - Tumor-like: Hemangioma, Kimura disease, Kuttner tumor, metastasis, lymphoma

SELECTED REFERENCES

1. Abdullah A et al: Imaging of the salivary glands. Semin Roentgenol. 48(1):65-74, 2013
2. Burke CJ et al: Imaging the major salivary glands. Br J Oral Maxillofac Surg. 49(4):261-9, 2011
3. Sodhi KS et al: Role of high resolution ultrasound in parotid lesions in children. Int J Pediatr Otorhinolaryngol. 75(11):1353-8, 2011
4. Katz P et al: Clinical ultrasound of the salivary glands. Otolaryngol Clin North Am. 42(6):973-1000, Table of Contents, 2009
5. Zenk J et al: Diagnostic imaging in sialadenitis. Oral Maxillofac Surg Clin North Am. 21(3):275-92, 2009
6. Lee YY et al: Imaging of salivary gland tumours. Eur J Radiol. 66(3):419-36, 2008
7. Ahuja AT et al. Diagnostic Imaging: Ultrasound. 1st ed. Salt lake City: Amirsys. 11-54-71, 2007
8. Madani G et al: Inflammatory conditions of the salivary glands. Semin Ultrasound CT MR. 27(6):440-51, 2006

Calculus Sialadenitis

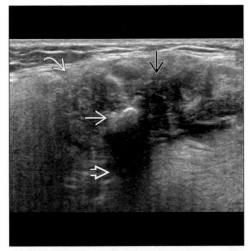

Transverse US shows curvilinear echogenic interface ➡ with strong posterior acoustic shadow ⮞ at glandular hilum, consistent with calculus. Note associated SMG ➡ sialadenitis + swollen, heterogeneous parenchyma ➡.

Calculus Sialadenitis

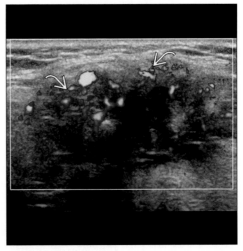

Corresponding power Doppler US shows hypervascularity ➡, consistent with acute calculus sialadenitis. 85% of calculi occur in the submandibular gland.

DIFFUSE SALIVARY GLAND ENLARGEMENT

Infective Sialadenitis

Infective Sialadenitis

(Left) Longitudinal US in a patient with sepsis and unilateral parotid swelling shows the gland ➡ is diffusely enlarged and heterogeneously hypoechoic with branching tubular structures representing dilated salivary ducts ➡.
(Right) Corresponding power Doppler US confirms dilated parotid ducts ➡ and diffuse hypervascularity ➡. Culture of parotid discharge confirmed methicillin-resistant Staphylococcus aureus (MRSA) parotiditis.

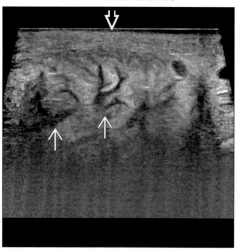

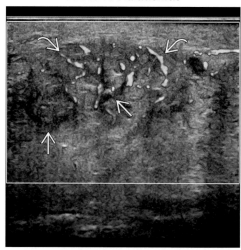

Chronic Sialadenitis

Chronic Sialadenitis

(Left) Transverse ultrasound shows an enlarged parotid gland with a multicystic ➡ appearance. The cystic spaces are interconnecting ➡, which would not be seen in Sjögren syndrome (SJS) or benign lymphoepithelial lesion (BLEL). Note the parenchymal atrophy (mandible ➡).
(Right) Coronal T2WI MR with fat suppression (sialogram) in the same patient shows cystic spaces ➡ along the branches of the parotid ducts ➡, representing cystic dilatation of intraglandular ducts due to chronic sialadenitis.

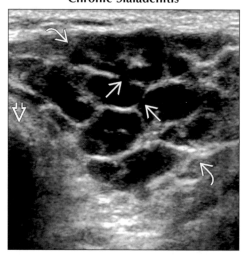

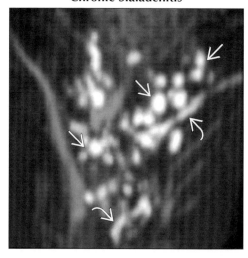

Sjögren Syndrome (SJS)

Sjögren Syndrome (SJS)

(Left) Longitudinal grayscale US of a woman with Sicca syndrome shows diffusely enlarged parotid with multiple hypoechoic foci ➡ of similar size seen throughout the gland. *(Right)* Transverse grayscale US of the same patient shows similar changes in the submandibular gland (SMG) ➡. Both parotid and SMG were involved bilaterally. US appearances are consistent with SJS, confirmed by labial biopsy. Hypoechoic foci may represent combination of sialectasia and lymphoid hyperplasia.

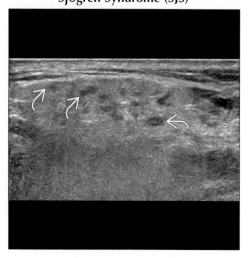

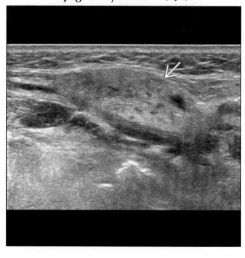

DIFFUSE SALIVARY GLAND ENLARGEMENT

Benign Lymphoepithelial Lesion (BLEL)

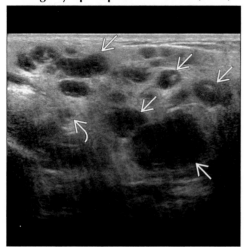

Benign Lymphoepithelial Lesion (BLEL)

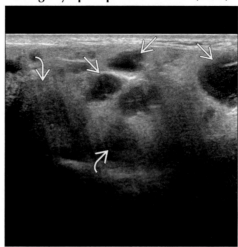

(Left) Transverse grayscale US shows BLEL. Diffusely enlarged parotid with multiple thin-walled cysts ➡ and ill-defined solid nodules ➡ of variable size are seen scattered throughout the gland. Cysts = ductal obstruction; ill-defined nodules = lymphoid aggregate. *(Right)* Longitudinal grayscale US of contralateral parotid shows symmetrical involvement with cysts ➡ and ill-defined nodules ➡. BLEL may be bilateral in up to 50% patients. (Courtesy R. Kadasne, MD.)

Benign Lymphoepithelial Lesion (BLEL)

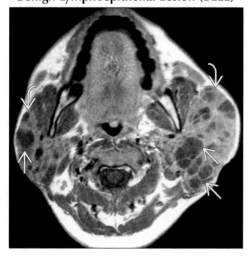

Benign Lymphoepithelial Lesion (BLEL)

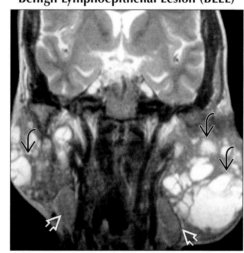

(Left) Axial T1WI C+ MR shows BLEL involvement of both parotid glands ➡. Cystic areas ➡ of variable sizes that do not enhance. *(Right)* Coronal T2WI MR in the same patient shows hyperintense cystic spaces ➡ in both parotid glands. Note that the submandibular glands ➡ are not involved despite severe parotid disease as compared with Sjögren syndrome. MR evaluates the deep lobe of parotid better than US.

Lymphatic Malformation

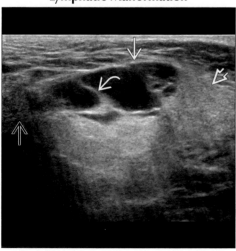

Lymphatic Malformation

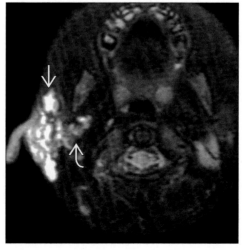

(Left) Transverse grayscale US of the right parotid gland ➡ shows lymphatic malformation (LM) ➡ in superficial lobe. It is thin walled and multiseptated ➡ with anechoic content and posterior enhancement. There was no phlebolith or internal flow on grayscale/Doppler (vs. venous vascular malformation). Note mastoid process ➡. *(Right)* Corresponding axial T2WI MR of the same LM shows involvement of both superficial ➡ and deep ➡ lobe of parotid. MR is indicated to evaluate LM due to its propensity for trans-spatial involvement.

DIFFUSE SALIVARY GLAND ENLARGEMENT

Hemangioma/Venous Vascular Malformation (VVM)

Hemangioma/Venous Vascular Malformation (VVM)

(Left) Transverse grayscale US of the right parotid shows an irregular, hypoechoic mass ⮑ with multiple sinusoidal spaces ➡. Phlebolith ⮑ and apparent debris, which shows slow "to and fro" flow on real-time scanning, are typical for slow-flow VVM. (Right) Corresponding T2WI MR reveals involvement of entire parotid ➡ with extension to posterior triangle ⮑ and another component ➡ in tonsillar fossa. MR/CT evaluate multifocal and trans-spatial extent better than US.

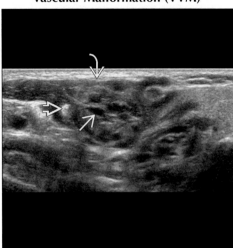
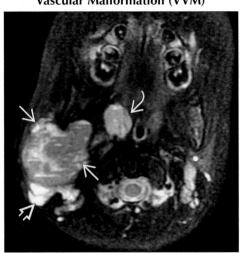

Kuttner Tumor

Kuttner Tumor

(Left) Longitudinal grayscale US of submandibular gland ➡ shows diffuse enlargement, rounded contour, and heterogeneous, "cirrhotic" parenchyma. Note mandible ➡ and submandibular lymph node ⮑. (Right) Corresponding power Doppler US shows diffuse, nondisplaced hypervascularity ➡. Both submandibular glands were involved symmetrically on both sides while parotid glands were spared in this patient. Sonographic pattern is consistent with Kuttner tumor, confirmed by FNA.

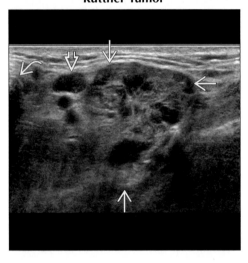
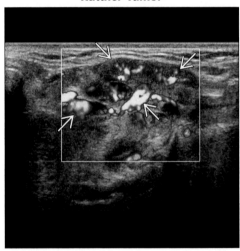

Kimura Disease

Kimura Disease

(Left) Transverse ultrasound shows a large, solid, fairly well-defined, hypoechoic mass ➡ in the parotid gland. Note the presence of a similar smaller mass ⮑. Shadowing from the mandible ➡ is also visible. (Right) Axial T1WI C+ MR in the same patient shows the parotid mass ➡ and multiple subcutaneous soft tissue masses ➡ in the periparotid region. Biopsy confirmed Kimura disease in this young Chinese man.

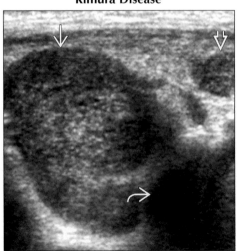
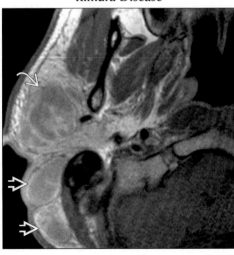

DIFFUSE SALIVARY GLAND ENLARGEMENT

Kimura Disease

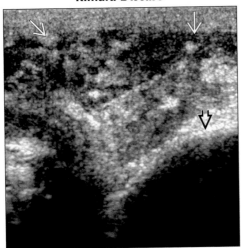

Kimura Disease

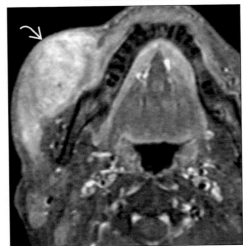

(Left) Transverse ultrasound shows a hypoechoic, heterogeneous, subcutaneous mass ⊡ in the soft tissues anterior to the mandible ⊡. *(Right)* Axial T1WI C+ MR with fat suppression in the same patient shows avid enhancement of the subcutaneous mass ➡. Kimura disease may manifest as salivary masses (parenchymal mass or lymph nodes) or subcutaneous nodules and nodes in the vicinity of salivary glands in Asian males.

Metastasis

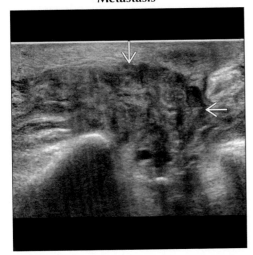

Metastasis

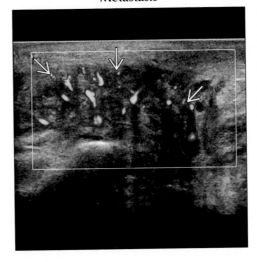

(Left) Transverse grayscale US of the left parotid gland shows a diffusely enlarged, heterogeneously hypoechoic parotid gland ➡. *(Right)* Corresponding Doppler US shows diffuse hypervascularity ➡. There is no ductal dilatation, and multiple malignant nodes were present in ipsilateral cervical chain. Sonographic features are suspicious for malignant infiltration, and guided FNAC confirmed parotid metastasis from undifferentiated nasopharyngeal carcinoma.

Lymphoma

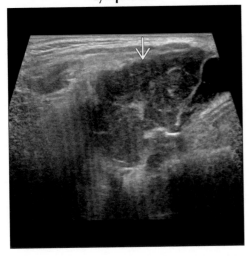

Lymphoma

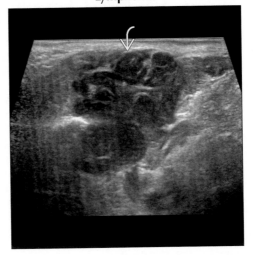

(Left) Transverse grayscale US in a patient with tender left parotid gland swelling shows a large, hypoechoic, heterogeneous parotid mass ➡ in the superficial lobe. *(Right)* Corresponding longitudinal grayscale US ➡ shows lobulated contour and heterogeneous, reticulated architecture. This was associated with multiple cervical lymphadenopathy with reticulated appearance (not shown). Sonographic features are suspicious for lymphoma. FNAC confirmed low-grade B cell lymphoma of the parotid gland.

FOCAL SALIVARY GLAND MASS

DIFFERENTIAL DIAGNOSIS

Common
- Benign Mixed Tumor (BMT)
- Warthin Tumor
- Intraparotid Lymph Node

Less Common
- Sialocele
- Lipoma
- Venous Vascular Malformation (VVM)
- Lymphatic Malformation
- Abscess
- Tuberculous Infection
- Kuttner Tumor
- Salivary Gland Malignancy
  - Mucoepidermoid Carcinoma (MECa)
  - Adenoid Cystic Carcinoma
  - Adenocarcinoma
- Metastasis

Rare but Important
- Lymphoma
- Acinic Cell Carcinoma
- Pseudoaneurysm
- 1st Branchial Cleft Cyst

ESSENTIAL INFORMATION

Key Differential Diagnosis Issues
- US ideal to evaluate submandibular lesions due to their superficial location
  - Unable to evaluate parotid deep lobe lesions or deep lobe extension of superficial lobe abnormality
- Use high-frequency (> 7.5 MHz) transducer
  - Benign tumors have well-defined edges, and malignant tumors have ill-defined edges
  - Internal architecture: Benign tumors are homogeneous, and malignant tumors are heterogeneous (hemorrhage and necrosis)
    - Low-grade MECa may mimic benign tumor (homogeneous, well defined)
    - Warthin tumor often cystic with septa and heterogeneous architecture
  - Malignant tumors more likely to have adjacent soft tissue & nodal involvement
    - ± prominent intratumoral vessels and high resistance (RI > 0.8, PI > 2.0)
- US useful in identifying tumor, predicting malignancy, and guiding biopsy
  - CECT/MR best delineate tumor extent, perineural extension, and nodal disease

Helpful Clues for Common Diagnoses
- **Benign Mixed Tumor (BMT)**
  - US features: Well defined, hypoechoic, lobulated, or bosselated surface, and intratumoral vascularity (mainly venous)
    - Cystic change and hemorrhage often seen in larger tumors (> 3 cm)
    - Dystrophic calcification seen occasionally in longstanding tumor
    - Posterior acoustic enhancement: Tumor offers few interfaces and allows sound to penetrate easily

- If left untreated, may undergo malignant transformation (9.5% for BMTs present more than 15 years)
  - Treatment by elective excision
- **Warthin Tumor**
  - Arise from intraparotid nodes
    - Typically seen in tail of parotid; rarely involves other salivary glands
    - Multiplicity of lesions, unilateral or bilateral (20%)
  - US features: Well-defined, heterogeneous hypoechoic mass, posterior acoustic enhancement, ± septa, and intratumoral vascularity ("hilar")
    - Cystic change more common than BMT
    - May look solid and mimic BMT
    - Malignant change (carcinoma or lymphoma) reported in < 1%
  - May be treated expectantly
- **Intraparotid Lymph Node**
  - Reactive intraparotid lymph nodes are common finding (particularly in children)
    - Echogenic hilar architecture and vascularity are preserved
  - Small lymph node with undetectable vascularity may be difficult to differentiate from small salivary tumor
  - Metastatic nodes (from scalp cancers, nasopharyngeal carcinoma [NPC]): Round, solid, hypoechoic, ± intranodal necrosis, peripheral vascularity

Helpful Clues for Less Common Diagnoses
- **Sialocele**
  - Focal collection of saliva in glands
    - Leak from ductal system due to previous obstruction or inflammation
  - Unilocular, thin walled, with internal echogenic debris (± mobile) and no vascularity
  - Indistinguishable from 1st branchial cleft cyst (BCC)
    - Aspirated fluid sent for amylase (↑ in saliva vs. 1st BCC)
- **Lipoma**
  - 10% of all parotid tumors
  - Hypoechoic relative to surrounding parotid parenchyma
    - Linear, hyperechoic "feathery" striation, parallel to transducer in both transverse and longitudinal planes
    - Soft and compressible by pressure with transducer
    - No significant vascularity on Doppler
- **Venous Vascular Malformation (VVM)**
  - Soft and compressible mass
  - Sinusoidal thin-walled spaces with grayscale flow/motion ± phleboliths, ± slow flow on Doppler
  - MR to map extent of lesion prior to treatment
- **Lymphatic Malformation**
  - Congenital malformation of lymphatics
  - Often found in multiple contiguous spaces, i.e., trans-spatial involvement
  - Noninfected lymphangioma: Multiseptate, anechoic, cystic mass with thin, avascular wall, ± debris, ± fluid level, and no intratumoral vascularity
  - Infected/hemorrhagic lymphangioma: Heterogeneous echo pattern with internal debris, thick walls with vascularity, ± fluid-fluid level
- **Abscess, Tuberculous Infection**
  - Clinical signs of infection (fever, pain and tenderness), ↑ white cell count
  - Nodal &/or parenchymal involvement

- ○ Ill-defined mass (inflammatory phlegmon) ± abscess, ± involvement of other neck nodes
- ○ US provides guidance for aspiration
- **Kuttner Tumor**
  - ○ Chronic sclerosing sialadenitis
  - ○ Commonly affect salivary glands on both sides
  - ○ Cirrhotic/geographic pattern, hypoechoic areas with nondisplaced hypervascularity
    - ▪ Submandibular > > > parotid involvement
- **Salivary Gland Malignancy**
  - ○ Several histologic types: Adenoid cystic, mucoepidermoid, adenocarcinoma
  - ○ Low-grade malignancy indistinguishable from benign tumors, so search carefully for features of malignancy
    - ▪ Ill-defined border, hypoechoic, necrosis
    - ▪ Abnormal vascularity
    - ▪ Invasion of adjacent structures (e.g., skin, subcutaneous tissue, masseter, etc.)
    - ▪ Adjacent malignant nodes
  - ○ Diagnosis made with US-guided FNAC
- **Metastasis**
  - ○ Hypoechoic mass(es) with malignant sonographic features at known sites of intraparotid nodes
  - ○ Multiplicity and history of known primary tumor raises suspicion

Helpful Clues for Rare Diagnoses

- **Lymphoma**
  - ○ Nodal or parenchymal involvement
    - ▪ Parenchymal involvement may be seen as focal mass or diffuse enlargement
    - ▪ May have reticulated appearances, lack of intranodal necrosis
    - ▪ ↑ vascularity within lymphomatous nodes, hilar > peripheral
  - ○ Note association with systemic lymphoma, Sjögren syndrome, rheumatoid arthritis, and immunosuppression
- **Acinic Cell Carcinoma**

- ○ Represents only 2–4% of all major salivary gland tumors; however, it is 2nd most common malignant parotid tumor
    - ▪ 80–90% occur in parotid gland
  - ○ Middle-aged patients predominant, but it is also 2nd most frequent pediatric malignant salivary gland tumor
  - ○ US appearance is similar to other salivary gland malignancies but tends to be multifocal
- **Pseudoaneurysm**
  - ○ Related to previous injury or infection
  - ○ Round, hypoechoic lesion with anechoic center and eccentric soft tissue density hematoma
    - ▪ Presence of arterial flow into anechoic center
    - ▪ Supplying artery can be identified on US
  - ○ Exclude this diagnosis before biopsy; evaluate all salivary masses with Doppler
- **1st Branchial Cleft Cyst**
  - ○ Seen in children; appearance similar to sialocele, but sinus tract may be seen
  - ○ Evaluate temporal bone to exclude associated abnormality/tract

SELECTED REFERENCES

1. Abdullah A et al: Imaging of the salivary glands. Semin Roentgenol. 48(1):65-74, 2013
2. Rong X et al: Differentiation of pleomorphic adenoma and Warthin's tumor of the parotid gland: ultrasonographic features. Acta Radiol. Epub ahead of print, 2013
3. Burke CJ et al: Imaging the major salivary glands. Br J Oral Maxillofac Surg. 49(4):261-9, 2011
4. Lee YY et al: Imaging of salivary gland tumours. Eur J Radiol. 66(3):419-36, 2008
5. Ahuja AT et al: Diagnostic Imaging: Ultrasound. 1st ed. Salt Lake City: Amirsys. 11-58-85, 2007
6. Thoeny HC: Imaging of salivary gland tumours. Cancer Imaging. 7:52-62, 2007
7. Madani G et al: Inflammatory conditions of the salivary glands. Semin Ultrasound CT MR. 27(6):440-51, 2006
8. Madani G et al: Tumors of the salivary glands. Semin Ultrasound CT MR. 27(6):452-64, 2006

Benign Mixed Tumor (BMT)

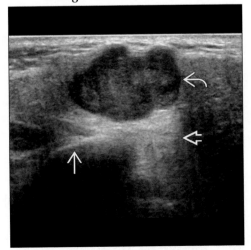

Transverse grayscale US of parotid gland shows typical appearance of BMT ➡: Well defined, hypoechoic, and bosselated with posterior acoustic enhancement ➡. Note the mandible ➡.

Benign Mixed Tumor (BMT)

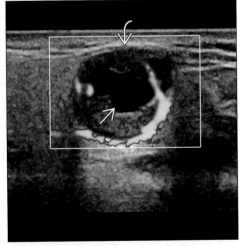

Power Doppler US shows parotid BMT ➡ with cystic change ➡ and intratumoral vascularity (usually of low resistance; RI < 0.8, PI < 2.0). US features mimic low-grade salivary gland malignancy and FNAC is required.

FOCAL SALIVARY GLAND MASS

Warthin Tumor

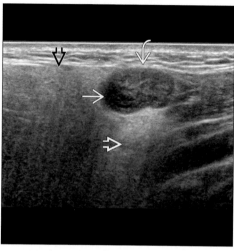

Warthin Tumor

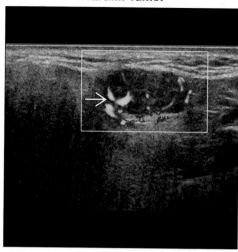

(Left) Longitudinal grayscale US shows biopsy-proven Warthin tumor ➡ in tail of the parotid gland ⇥, a common site of intraparotid node. The tumor is well defined and hypoechoic with cystic change ➡ and posterior acoustic enhancement ⇥. *(Right)* Corresponding power Doppler US shows intratumoral vascularity reminiscent of nodal hilar vessels ➡. US appearance and location are typical for Warthin tumor. High-resolution US better characterizes such small lesions compared to CT/MR.

Warthin Tumor

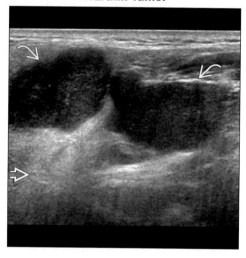

Warthin Tumor

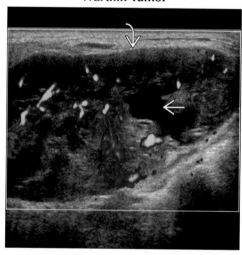

(Left) Longitudinal grayscale US of parotid gland in a smoker shows 2 well-defined, hypoechoic, heterogeneous nodules ➡ with posterior enhancement in tail of the parotid gland ⇥. Features suggest multiple Warthin tumors, confirmed by FNAC. *(Right)* Longitudinal power Doppler US of a large Warthin tumor ➡ in parotid apex shows a heterogeneous nodule with cystic change ➡ and vascularity within (usually low-resistance type, not routinely done in clinical practice).

Sialocele

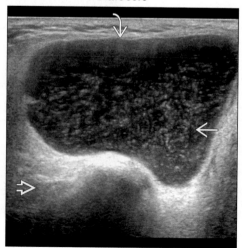

Sialocele

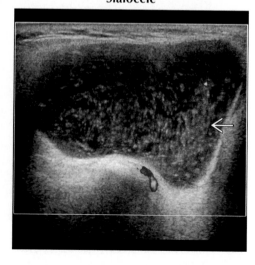

(Left) Transverse grayscale US shows parotid sialocele ➡. Note the thin-walled, unilocular cystic appearance with mobile internal debris on real-time scanning ➡ and posterior acoustic enhancement ⇥. *(Right)* Corresponding transverse power Doppler US shows no internal vascularity to suggest solid component. Movement of internal debris ➡ is exaggerated due to stronger ultrasound pulses. The sonographic appearance could be confused with 1st branchial cleft cyst (BCC).

Lipoma

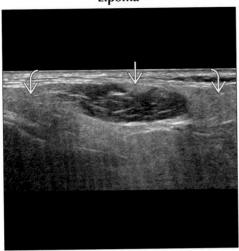

Venous Vascular Malformation (VVM)

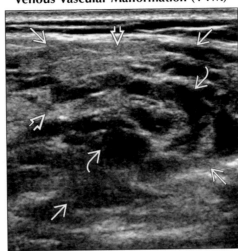

(Left) Transverse grayscale US of parotid gland ➜ shows elliptical, solid, hypoechoic nodule ➜ with linear echogenic lines parallel to the transducer surface and a striped/feathered appearance, typical of lipoma. These echogenic lines remain parallel to the transducer in all scanning planes. (Right) Longitudinal ultrasound shows a parotid VVM. The border ➜ is well defined and lobulated, and a soft tissue stromal component ➜ and sinusoidal vascular spaces ➜ are seen.

Venous Vascular Malformation (VVM)

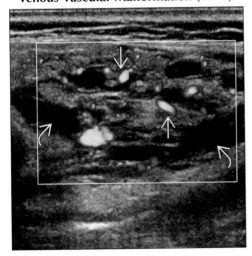

Abscess

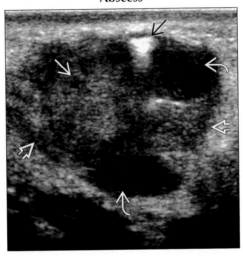

(Left) Longitudinal power Doppler ultrasound in the same patient shows vascularity in smaller vessels ➜, though it is absent in the larger vascular spaces ➜ due to slow flow. Grayscale US better evaluates slow flow as motion/movement within the VVM. (Right) Transverse ultrasound shows an echogenic focus with a "comet tail" artifact ➜ representing gas within a parotid gland abscess ➜. Also note the presence of internal debris ➜ and necrosis ➜.

Tuberculous Infection

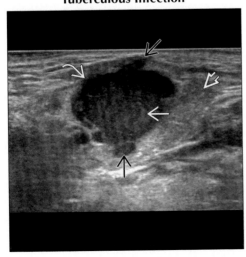

Tuberculous Infection

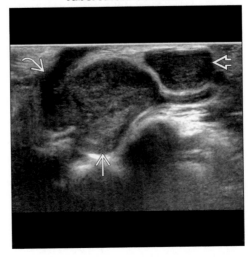

(Left) Transverse grayscale US in a patient presenting with fever and painful submandibular gland (SMG) ➜ mass shows an irregular, thick-walled abscess ➜ with internal debris ➜ and discharging sinus ➜ into adjacent soft tissues. FNA confirmed tuberculous abscess. (Right) Longitudinal grayscale US of parotid gland shows a well-defined, heterogeneous tuberculous abscess ➜ with internal debris and discharging sinus ➜ into soft tissues/skin surface. Note adjacent periparotid tuberculous node ➜.

FOCAL SALIVARY GLAND MASS

Kuttner Tumor

Kuttner Tumor

(Left) Transverse grayscale US shows an enlarged, rounded, hypoechoic, heterogeneous, "cirrhotic" looking SMG ➡ mimicking a mass lesion. *(Right)* Corresponding power Doppler US shows profuse, nondisplaced internal vascularity ➡. Grayscale and Doppler features are typical for Kuttner tumor (confirmed by FNA). Mucosal-associated lymphoid tumor (MALToma) of salivary gland is the main differential, and a biopsy may be helpful to distinguish between them.

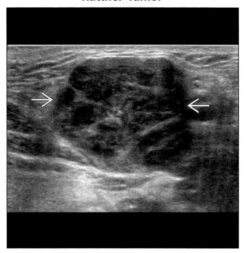

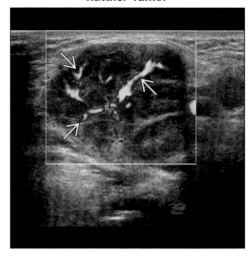

Salivary Gland Malignancy

Salivary Gland Malignancy

(Left) Transverse grayscale US in a patient with previous partial parotidectomy shows a heterogeneous, hypoechoic nodule ➡ with an irregular border ➡ abutting a surgical scar ➡, features suspicious for malignancy. Guided FNA confirmed carcinoma ex-pleomorphic adenoma. *(Right)* Transverse grayscale US shows a hypoechoic mass ➡ in the parotid gland ➡. Ill-defined border ➡, heterogeneous appearance, and breaching of parotid capsule ➡ are features suspicious for malignancy. FNA confirmed high-grade salivary duct carcinoma.

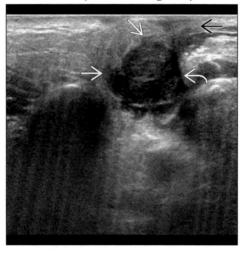

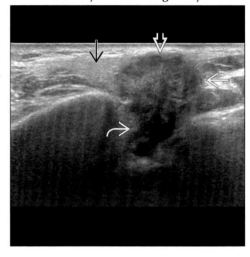

Mucoepidermoid Carcinoma (MECa)

Metastasis

(Left) Longitudinal grayscale US shows low-grade MECa ➡ in the parotid gland. US appearance is similar to a benign salivary gland tumor, except for the soft sign of a partly ill-defined edge ➡ and intratumoral cystic necrosis ➡. *(Right)* Longitudinal grayscale US shows metastatic intraparotid node from carcinoma of tongue. Note cystic necrosis ➡, ill-defined border ➡, and adjacent abnormal node ➡, clues to diagnosis.

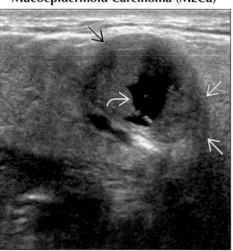

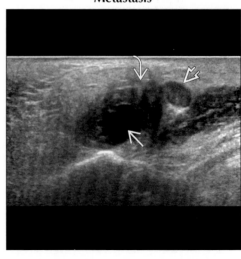

FOCAL SALIVARY GLAND MASS

Lymphoma

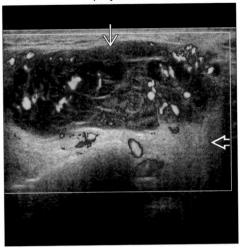

Lymphoma

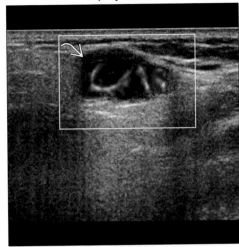

(Left) Transverse power Doppler US shows parotid MALToma ➡ seen as a discrete, ill-defined, hypoechoic, heterogeneous noncalcified mass with posterior enhancement ⮞ and marked intratumoral vascularity. Ill-defined borders and hypervascularity are suspicious for malignant mass. (Right) Longitudinal power Doppler US shows small parotid MALToma ➡. Sonographic features are similar to small Warthin tumor/ intraparotid lymphadenopathy. In this case, diagnosis was made after FNA.

Pseudoaneurysm

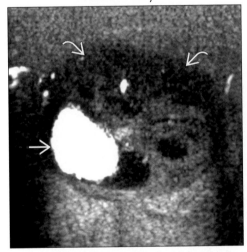

Pseudoaneurysm

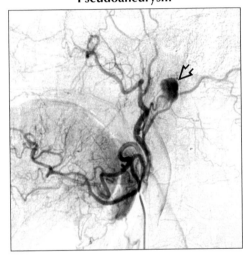

(Left) Transverse power Doppler ultrasound (shown in black and white) shows an intraparotid pseudoaneurysm ➡ arising from the external carotid artery. The majority of the lumen is thrombosed ⮞. Color/power Doppler of a parotid mass should always be performed to avoid inadvertent biopsy of a pseudoaneurysm. (Right) Angiography of the external carotid artery in the same patient confirms the pseudoaneurysm ⮞ with residual lumen. The lesion was subsequently successfully embolized.

1st Branchial Cleft Cyst

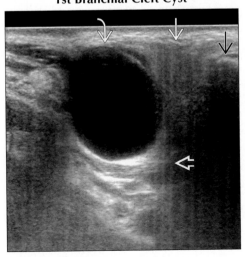

1st Branchial Cleft Cyst

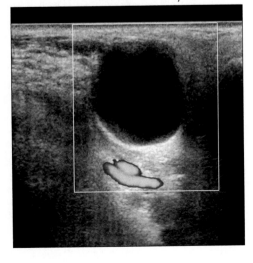

(Left) Transverse grayscale US shows 1st branchial cleft cyst ➡, seen as a thin-walled, unilocular, anechoic cyst with posterior acoustic enhancement ⮞. US appearance is indistinguishable from sialocele. Clinical features and FNAC may help to differentiate between the two. Note the mandible ➡ and normal parotid tissue ⮞. (Right) Corresponding transverse power Doppler US shows absent vascularity within walls of the cyst, consistent with its simple cystic nature.

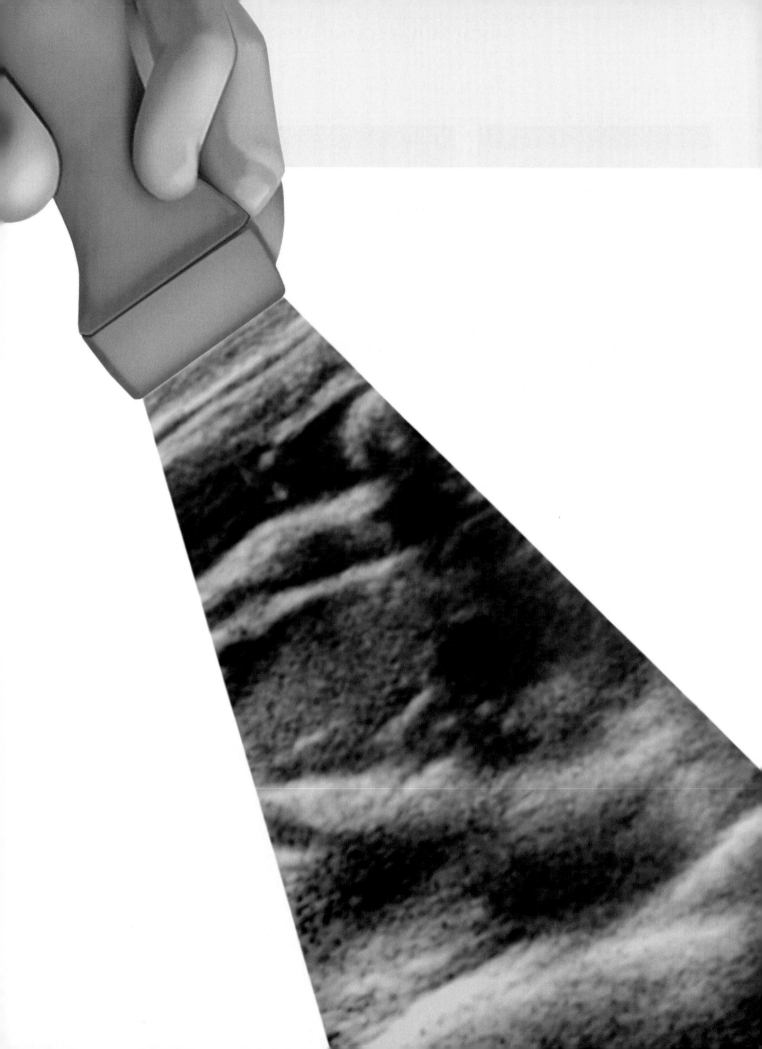

SECTION 2
Thyroid and Parathyroid

DIFFUSE THYROID ENLARGEMENT

DIFFERENTIAL DIAGNOSIS

Common
- Multinodular Goiter
- Graves Disease
- Hashimoto Thyroiditis

Less Common
- de Quervain Thyroiditis
- Acute Suppurative Thyroiditis
- Anaplastic Thyroid Carcinoma

Rare but Important
- Thyroid Metastasis
- Lymphoma
- Leukemia

ESSENTIAL INFORMATION

Key Differential Diagnosis Issues
- Most diagnoses are made clinically, so US should be targeted to answer specific questions
  - Is US done to confirm diagnosis &/or guide biopsy?
    - Will additional CT or MR help?
  - Is US done to evaluate associated abnormalities &/or complications?
    - In multinodular goiter (MNG), US is done to identify presence of thyroid cancer; look for features of malignant nodule, ± lymph node
    - In Hashimoto thyroiditis, US done to look for any developing non-Hodgkin lymphoma (NHL) in gland or lymph nodes

Helpful Clues for Common Diagnoses
- **Multinodular Goiter**
  - Most common cause of diffuse thyroid enlargement (symmetric/asymmetric)
  - Typical MNG: Multiple heterogeneous nodules
    - Multiplicity of nodules, bilateral diffuse involvement
    - Solid nodules are often isoechoic, small proportion being hypoechoic
    - Thin, sharply defined hypoechoic halo
    - Heterogeneous internal echo pattern with cystic change, septation, internal debris; avascular solid component due to organized blood clot; "spongiform" appearance
    - Dense shadowing calcification (curvilinear, dysmorphic, coarse)
    - Nodules with "comet tail" artifacts: Highly suggestive of colloid nodule
  - Color Doppler
    - Peripheral vascularity > intranodular vascularity
    - Septa and intranodular solid portions may be avascular: Represents organizing blood clot
  - Look carefully for presence of malignant nodule against background of multinodularity
  - Features of suspicious malignant nodule
    - Ill-defined margin
    - Solid, hypoechoic, taller than wide in configuration
    - Presence of punctate calcification
    - Hypervascular and predominantly intranodular in distribution on color Doppler
    - ± extracapsular, vascular infiltration
    - ± associated malignant regional lymph nodes
- **Graves Disease**

- Most common type of autoimmune thyroiditis
- Diagnosis based on laboratory findings of hyperthyroidism and raised circulating thyroglobulin and thyroperoxidase antibodies
- Mild/moderate diffuse, symmetric enlargement of thyroid gland, including isthmus with rounded contour
- Hypoechoic, heterogeneous, "spotty" parenchymal echo pattern
- Heterogeneity may appear nodular, mimicking MNG
- Color Doppler: Marked, diffuse parenchymal hypervascularity, "thyroid inferno"
- Spectral Doppler: Increase in peak flow velocity (up to 120 cm/s) as measured in inferior thyroid artery
- **Hashimoto Thyroiditis**
  - Chronic lymphocytic thyroiditis
  - Diagnosis based on clinical (diffuse goiter and euthyroid/hypothyroid) and serology tests (antimicrosomal antibodies, antithyroglobulin, thyroid peroxidase)
  - Gradual painless enlargement of thyroid with euthyroid (majority), hypothyroid (20%), or hyperthyroid (5%) status
    - Hypothyroid with atrophic gland at end stage
  - Diffuse, hypoechoic, heterogeneous, micronodular echo pattern
  - Characteristic echogenic fibrous septa in chronic cases, seen as multiple echogenic horizontal lines
  - Avascular in acute phase and hypervascular in chronic, hypothyroid phase (due to stimulation by TSH)
    - Flow velocities within normal limits (as opposed to ↑ in Graves disease)
  - Always evaluate thyroid and lymph nodes (± FNAC) for known risk of developing NHL in chronic cases

Helpful Clues for Less Common Diagnoses
- **de Quervain Thyroiditis**
  - Typical history: Acute onset painful thyroid swelling preceded by upper respiratory tract infection 2-3 weeks prior
  - Transient hyperthyroidism (50%), but paradoxical low radioiodine uptake due to severe glandular destruction
  - Acute phase
    - Mildly enlarged thyroid gland, with focal ill-defined hypoechoic heterogeneous area
    - Transducer pressure elicits pain
    - Inflammatory nodes in its vicinity
    - Hypovascularity of nodule on power Doppler
  - Subacute phase
    - Evolves to affect rest of gland, which becomes diffusely hypoechoic and heterogeneous
    - Residual localized tenderness on transducer pressure
    - Mild to moderate hypervascularity; hypoechoic areas may be avascular due to severe glandular destruction
  - Clinical recovery correlates well with sonographic recovery
- **Acute Suppurative Thyroiditis**
  - Clinical history of repeated neck/thyroid abscesses on left (95%)
  - Predominantly affects children and young adults
  - Clinical symptoms of fever, anterior neck pain and tenderness; raised white cell count

- ○ Starts as perithyroidal abscess, subsequently involving thyroid gland, upper pole > lower pole
- ○ Ill-defined, hypoechoic, inflammatory thyroid "mass" ± liquefied center representing abscess
- ○ Must identify underlying fistula tract from pyriform fossa sinus after acute episode (barium, CECT)
- **Anaplastic Thyroid Carcinoma**
  - ○ Clinical diagnosis: Rapidly enlarging mass with obstructive symptoms in patient with known MNG
  - ○ Role of US is to confirm diagnosis, guide needle biopsy, evaluate extrathyroid spread, and identify malignant nodes
  - ○ Invasive, hypoechoic, heterogeneous thyroid mass, ± focal calcification (50%), ± necrosis against background of MNG
  - ○ ± extracapsular spread, malignant cervical lymph nodes, ± tumor thrombus in internal jugular vein
  - ○ Color Doppler
    - Prominent chaotic intranodular vascularity
    - Necrotic tumor may be avascular/hypovascular (vascular infiltration/occlusion)

Helpful Clues for Rare Diagnoses

- **Thyroid Metastasis**
  - ○ Rapid onset goiter/hoarseness/dysphagia in patient with known malignancy
    - Breast, kidney, lung, colon most common
  - ○ Invariably associated with widely disseminated disease
  - ○ Nonspecific appearance
    - In absence of relevant history, cannot be differentiated from anaplastic carcinoma, other thyroid primary, lymphoma, or leukemia without biopsy
  - ○ Solitary/multiple, solid, hypoechoic nodules with intranodular vascularity or diffuse infiltration (mild goiter with heterogeneous hypoechoic parenchyma)
  - ○ Infiltrative type may be subtle and easily missed; disseminated disease and neck nodes provide useful clues
- **Lymphoma**
  - ○ Primary thyroid lymphoma is rare

- Typically seen in patients with longstanding Hashimoto thyroiditis
- ○ Rapidly enlarging thyroid mass
- ○ Solid, ill-defined, hypoechoic, noncalcified mass
  - 80% solitary, often large (5-10 cm)
- ○ Diffuse involvement: Goiter with heterogeneous echo pattern or minimal change in echo pattern (often missed)
- ○ ± local infiltration, lymphomatous cervical nodes (hypoechoic with reticulated pattern/"pseudocystic" appearance)
- ○ Color Doppler: Nonspecific, hypovascular, or chaotic intranodular vessels
- **Leukemia**
  - ○ Thyroid lesion similar to lymphoma or metastatic involvement
    - Diffuse infiltrative pattern; multifocal nodular pattern
  - ○ Lymphadenopathy does not show "reticulated" or "pseudocystic" appearance

SELECTED REFERENCES

1. Alzahrani AS et al: Role of ultrasonography in the differential diagnosis of thyrotoxicosis: a noninvasive, cost-effective, and widely available but underutilized diagnostic tool. Endocr Pract. 18(4):567-78, 2012
2. Chung AY et al: Metastases to the thyroid: a review of the literature from the last decade. Thyroid. 22(3):258-68, 2012
3. Sofferman RA et al: Ultrasound of the Thyroid and Parathyroid Glands. New York: Springer. 61-150, 2012
4. Anderson L et al: Hashimoto thyroiditis: Part 1, sonographic analysis of the nodular form of Hashimoto thyroiditis. AJR Am J Roentgenol. 195(1):208-15, 2010
5. Anderson L et al: Hashimoto thyroiditis: Part 2, sonographic analysis of benign and malignant nodules in patients with diffuse Hashimoto thyroiditis. AJR Am J Roentgenol. 195(1):216-22, 2010
6. Ito Y et al: Thyroid ultrasonography. World J Surg. 34(6):1171-80, 2010
7. Ahuja AT et al. Diagnostic Imaging: Ultrasound. 1st ed. Salt Lake City: Amirsys Publishing, Inc. 11-16-35, 2007
8. Doi Y et al: Primary thyroid lymphoma associated with Graves' disease. Thyroid. 14(9):772-6, 2004

Multinodular Goiter

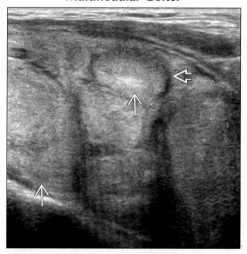

Longitudinal US shows diffuse thyroid enlargement with multiple solid, homogeneous, noncalcified, isoechoic nodules ⇨ of varying size. Most nodules are surrounded by a complete hypoechoic halo ⇨.

Multinodular Goiter

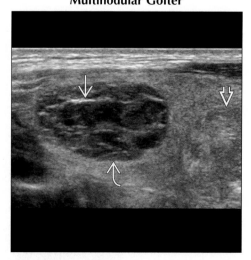

Transverse US shows an isoechoic nodule ⇨ and cystic nodule ⇨ with internal septations ⇨ (spongiform appearance). Cystic change and septation are often seen in benign hyperplastic nodules due to degeneration.

DIFFUSE THYROID ENLARGEMENT

Graves Disease

Graves Disease

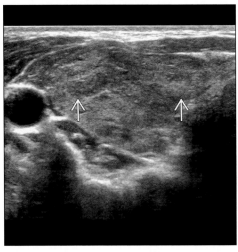
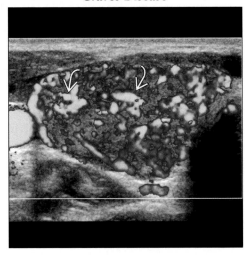

(Left) Transverse grayscale US shows diffuse enlargement of thyroid gland with heterogeneous, "nodular," hypoechoic parenchymal echo pattern ➡, consistent with Graves disease. (Right) Transverse power Doppler US shows diffuse hypervascularity ➡ within the gland, the commonly described "thyroid inferno" of Graves disease. These vessels show high velocity on spectral Doppler (not shown), unlike the normal velocity seen in Hashimoto thyroiditis.

Graves Disease

Graves Disease

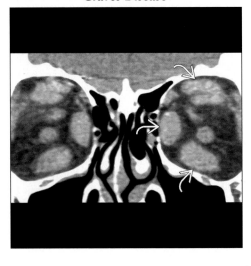
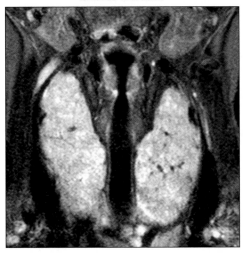

(Left) Coronal reformatted CT of the orbits shows hypertrophy of multiple extraocular muscles ➡, consistent with Graves ophthalmopathy. (Right) Coronal T2WI MR with fat suppression shows diffuse enlargement of the thyroid gland in a patient with Graves disease. The extent of the enlargement and absence of associated tracheal compression are clearly demonstrated. CT/MR are useful in evaluating a massively enlarged thyroid.

Graves Disease

Graves Disease

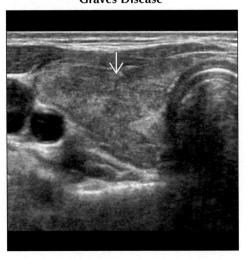
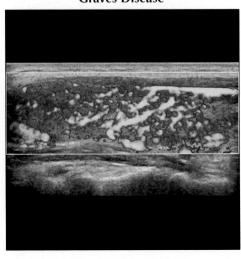

(Left) Transverse grayscale US shows mild thyroid enlargement ➡. The parenchymal echoes are non-nodular, relatively homogeneous, hypoechoic, and faintly "spotty." This is a common grayscale appearance of the thyroid in Graves disease. (Right) Longitudinal power Doppler US shows "thyroid inferno." If the gland is extremely vascular, one may have to use high pulse repetition frequency and filters to evaluate vascularity and eliminate artifacts.

Hashimoto Thyroiditis

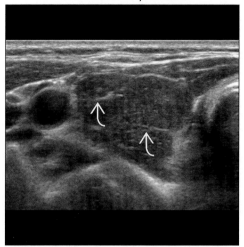

Hashimoto Thyroiditis

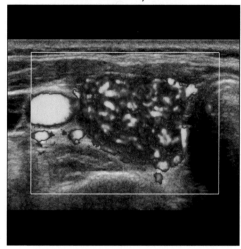

(Left) Transverse grayscale US of the thyroid gland shows multiple horizontal echogenic lines ➡ representing fibrous septa in Hashimoto thyroiditis. Rule out any suspicion of developing non-Hodgkin lymphoma in the thyroid & neck nodes in patients with chronic disease. (Right) Transverse power Doppler US shows marked hypervascularity (TSH effect) throughout the gland. Vessels show normal flow velocities compared to vessels with high velocities in Graves disease.

de Quervain Thyroiditis

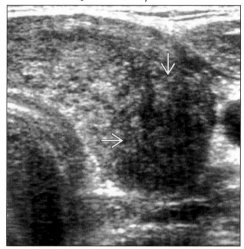

de Quervain Thyroiditis

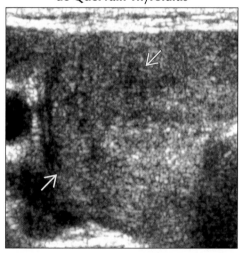

(Left) Transverse US shows diffuse thyroid enlargement with a focal, heterogeneous, hypoechoic area ➡ in this young patient with acute painful thyroid swelling preceded by an upper respiratory tract infection. This appearance and history is consistent with de Quervain thyroiditis. (Right) Transverse US in the same patient a few days later shows ill-defined, hypoechoic heterogeneity ➡ in the contralateral lobe.

Acute Suppurative Thyroiditis

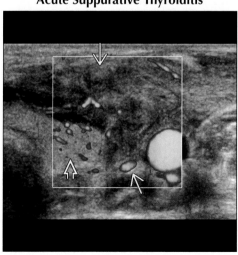

Acute Suppurative Thyroiditis

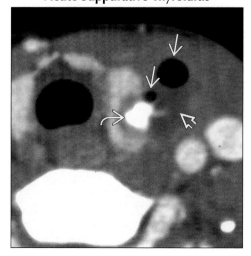

(Left) Transverse power Doppler US shows a perithyroidal abscess ➡ around the left lobe of the thyroid ➡. Acute suppurative thyroiditis is more common on the left side. (Right) Corresponding axial CECT in the same patient shows a left perithyroidal abscess with nonenhancing necrotic component ➡. Note gas ➡ and barium ➡ (from prior barium swallow) reaching the abscess via the left pyriform sinus fistula.

DIFFUSE THYROID ENLARGEMENT

(Left) Double contrast barium image of the hypopharynx shows the left pyriform sinus fistula ➡ in a patient with acute suppurative thyroiditis. The examination was performed after the acute episode subsided. *(Right)* Transverse US shows an anaplastic carcinoma in the left lobe of the thyroid. The tumor ➡ is poorly defined, solid, hypoechoic, and infiltrating most of the left lobe. It appears to have an extrathyroid extension posteriorly ➡.

Acute Suppurative Thyroiditis

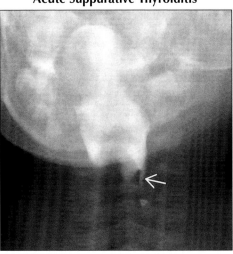

Anaplastic Thyroid Carcinoma

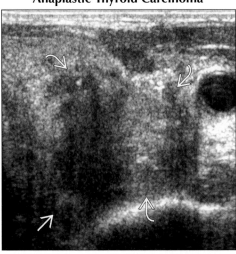

(Left) Transverse US in the same patient shows the tumor extending to the right thyroid bed ➡ via the prevertebral space and the tumor's association with multiple metastatic nodes ➡ in the contralateral neck. *(Right)* Axial CECT of the thyroid in the same patient clearly shows diffuse infiltration of the left lobe of the thyroid ➡ by the anaplastic carcinoma, with extrathyroid spread crossing the midline ➡ and encasing the left common carotid artery ➡.

Anaplastic Thyroid Carcinoma

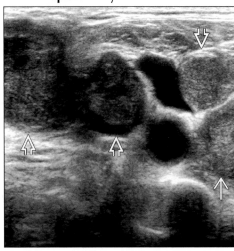

Anaplastic Thyroid Carcinoma

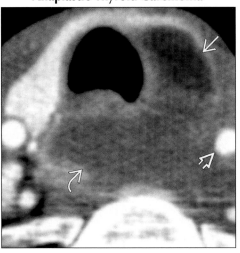

(Left) Transverse grayscale US shows an ill-defined, heterogeneous, hypoechoic, anaplastic carcinoma ➡ encasing the left CCA ➡. Extrathyroid extension is better evaluated with CT or MR (not shown). FNAC is best done using US to guide the needle. *(Right)* Transverse power Doppler US of the right lobe of thyroid shows mild diffuse enlargement with a focal ill-defined, vascular, hypoechoic area ➡ in this patient with known disseminated carcinoma. US-guided FNAC showed metastasis.

Anaplastic Thyroid Carcinoma

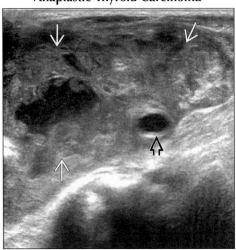

Thyroid Metastasis

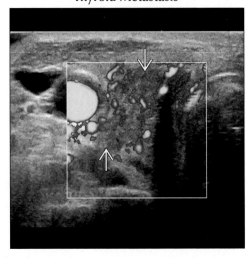

DIFFUSE THYROID ENLARGEMENT

Thyroid Metastasis

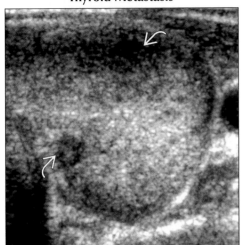

Thyroid Metastasis

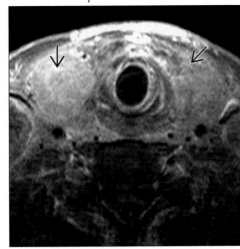

(Left) Transverse US shows multiple hypoechoic nodules ⊅ of the left lobe. Thyroid metastases are invariably associated with disseminated disease from lung, bone, liver, and lymph nodes. (Right) Axial T1WI C+ MR in the same patient shows a goiter with mild heterogeneous thyroid parenchymal intensity ⊅. Note that the metastatic lesions are subtle on MR though clearly seen on the US.

Lymphoma

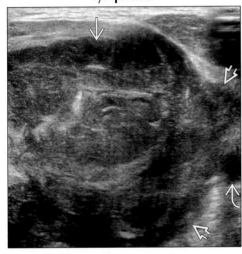

Lymphoma

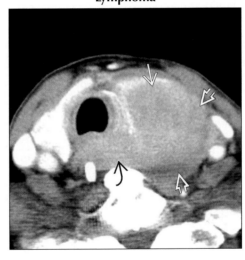

(Left) Transverse grayscale US shows a diffusely enlarged, heterogeneous, hypoechoic thyroid gland ⊅. The thyroid capsule is interrupted with extrathyroid extension of the tumor ⊅. Note the CCA ⊅. (Right) Corresponding axial CECT shows a hypoenhancing left lobe thyroid tumor ⊅ with diffuse infiltration of left neck soft tissues ⊅ and esophagus ⊅ (with nasogastric tube). These findings are typical of lymphomatous involvement of the neck soft tissues & thyroid.

Leukemia

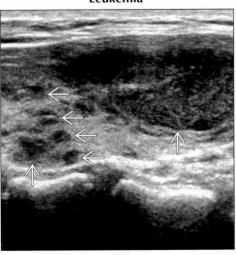

Leukemia

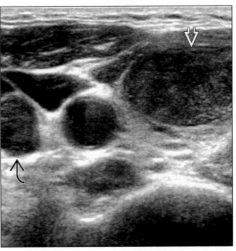

(Left) Longitudinal US shows thyroid involvement by chronic lymphocytic leukemia, seen as multiple ill-defined hypoechoic areas ⊅ scattered in the gland. The appearance is nonspecific and mimics other thyroid malignancies. (Right) Transverse US in the same patient shows the mass ⊅ in the right lobe of the thyroid and associated malignant lymph node ⊅. Clinical correlation is crucial as US appearance is nonspecific.

ISO-/HYPERECHOIC THYROID NODULE

DIFFERENTIAL DIAGNOSIS

Common
- Multinodular Goiter
- Postoperative Hypertrophy

Less Common
- Follicular Lesion
  - Follicular Adenoma
  - Follicular Carcinoma
  - Hürthle Cell Neoplasm

ESSENTIAL INFORMATION

Key Differential Diagnosis Issues
- Likelihood of malignancy ↑ as echogenicity ↓
  - Review of malignant nodules shows 4% are hyperechoic, 26% isoechoic, and 63% hypoechoic
- Benign thyroid nodules very common; therefore, solitary hypoechoic nodule is statistically more likely to be benign

Helpful Clues for Common Diagnoses
- **Multinodular Goiter**
  - May show predominantly hyperplastic nodules, colloid nodules, or a combination
  - Hypoechoic halo and perinodular vascularity help to delineate hyperplastic nodules
  - Usually, there are multiple benign nodules (well-defined margin, cystic nodules with "spongiform" appearance, peripheral/perinodular vascularity) in the rest of thyroid gland
- **Postoperative Hypertrophy**
  - Postoperative recurrence/residual multinodular goiter is common
  - Sonographic appearance is otherwise similar to preoperative multinodular goiter
  - History of previous thyroid surgery/surgical scar should reveal diagnosis

Helpful Clues for Less Common Diagnoses
- **Follicular Lesion**

- Imaging or fine-needle aspiration and cytology (FNAC) unable to differentiate benign follicular adenoma from follicular carcinoma
  - Differentiation made after surgery based on vascular & capsular invasion; therefore, they are commonly considered together as follicular lesion
- Ultrasound features of follicular adenoma
  - Well-defined oval, solid nodule, iso-/hyperechoic, ± small area of cystic change
  - Calcification is rare
  - Perinodular > intranodular vascularity
- Features more indicative of carcinoma
  - Ill-defined border, hypoechoic or hypoechoic portion of otherwise iso-/hyperechoic nodule, ± heterogeneous (necrotic, cystic) areas
  - Marked chaotic intranodular vascularity
  - Frank extrathyroid, vascular invasion
- **Hürthle Cell Neoplasm**
  - Adenoma or carcinoma, like follicular lesions, cannot be distinguished with imaging or FNAC
  - Association seen with Hashimoto thyroiditis, nodular goiter
  - Metastasize more often than follicular carcinoma
  - Sonographic appearance is similar to that of follicular lesion (grayscale & Doppler)

SELECTED REFERENCES

1. Sofferman RA et al: Ultrasound of the Thyroid and Parathyroid Glands. New York: Springer. 61-150, 2012
2. Bonavita JA et al: Pattern recognition of benign nodules at ultrasound of the thyroid: which nodules can be left alone? AJR Am J Roentgenol. 193(1):207-13, 2009
3. Moon WJ et al: Are there any specific ultrasound findings of nodular hyperplasia ("leave me alone" lesion) to differentiate it from follicular adenoma? Acta Radiol. 50(4):383-8, 2009
4. Moon WJ et al: Benign and malignant thyroid nodules: US differentiation--multicenter retrospective study. Radiology. 247(3):762-70, 2008
5. Ahuja AT et al: Diagnostic Imaging: Ultrasound. 1st ed. Salt Lake City: Amirsys. 11-28-31, 2007
6. Marqusee E et al: Usefulness of ultrasonography in the management of nodular thyroid disease. Ann Intern Med. 133(9):696-700, 2000

Multinodular Goiter

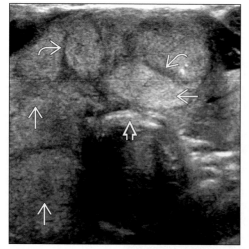

Transverse ultrasound shows diffuse thyroid enlargement. Multiple isoechoic nodules ➡ are delineated by the presence of a hypoechoic halo ➡. Note the trachea ➡.

Postoperative Hypertrophy

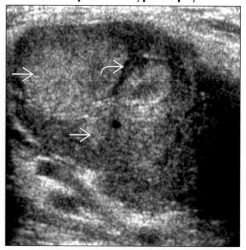

Longitudinal ultrasound shows a thyroid mass with lobulated contour. Note multiple isoechoic thyroid nodules ➡ and a hypoechoic halo ➡. The patient had history of hemithyroidectomy for multinodular goiter.

ISO-/HYPERECHOIC THYROID NODULE

Follicular Adenoma

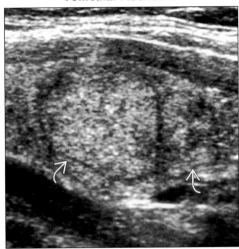

Follicular Adenoma

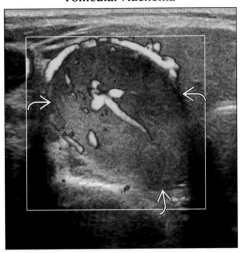

(Left) Longitudinal ultrasound shows well-defined, completely haloed, isoechoic nodules ➦ in the thyroid. They are solid, homogeneous, and without cystic change, colloid or punctate calcifications. The findings suggest a follicular lesion. (Right) Transverse power Doppler ultrasound shows a nodule ➦ with similar grayscale characteristics and perinodular/ halo vascularity. Surgical pathology confirmed follicular adenomas in both cases.

Follicular Carcinoma

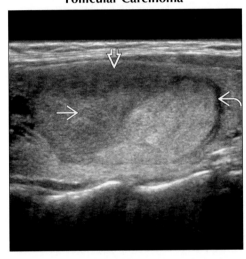

Follicular Carcinoma

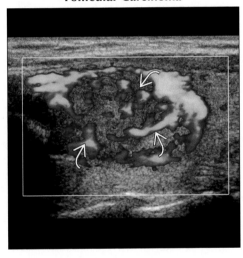

(Left) Longitudinal grayscale ultrasound shows a solid, heterogeneous thyroid nodule ➦ with indistinct borders ➥. There is a hypoechoic component ➦ within the nodule, suspicious of follicular carcinoma. (Right) Corresponding longitudinal power Doppler ultrasound in the same patient shows profuse chaotic intratumoral vascularity ➦. Thyroidectomy showed follicular carcinoma. Imaging and FNAC are unable to differentiate benign from malignant follicular lesions.

Hürthle Cell Neoplasm

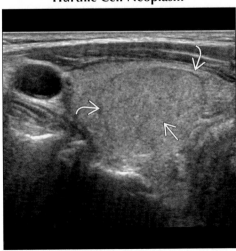

Hürthle Cell Neoplasm

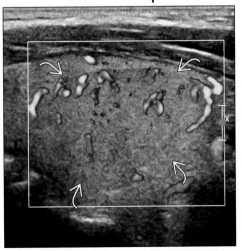

(Left) Transverse grayscale ultrasound shows a well-defined, solid, homogeneous, isoechoic nodule ➦ with a complete hypoechoic halo ➦. The appearance suggests a follicular lesion, and surgery showed Hürthle cell adenoma. (Right) Transverse power Doppler ultrasound shows another isoechoic Hürthle cell adenoma ➦. Moderate intratumoral vascularity is seen. Occasionally, Hürthle cell adenoma may be avascular (unlike follicular).

HYPOECHOIC THYROID NODULE

DIFFERENTIAL DIAGNOSIS

Common
- Multinodular Goiter (MNG)

Less Common
- Papillary Carcinoma
- Follicular Carcinoma
- Medullary Carcinoma
- de Quervain Thyroiditis
- Acute Suppurative Thyroiditis

Rare but Important
- Anaplastic Carcinoma
- Lymphoma
- Metastasis

ESSENTIAL INFORMATION

Key Differential Diagnosis Issues
- In routine clinical practice, most common hypoechoic thyroid nodules are part of multinodular goiter (MNG)
  - Adenomatous, hyperplastic, colloid nodules
  - However, many malignant nodules are also seen against background of MNG
    - Main reason for US in MNG is to identify presence of malignancy in thyroid
    - Anaplastic carcinomas, though rare, invariably occur against background of MNG
- Essential to be familiar with US appearance of thyroid cancers; papillary carcinoma is most common
- Crucial to identify malignant features in hypoechoic nodule and combine US with FNAC for definitive diagnosis
- US features to be assessed for thyroid nodule include
  - Margin: Well-/ill-defined; haloed (thin/thick)
  - Echogenicity: Hypo-/iso-/hyperechoic
  - Internal architecture: Solid/cystic/mixed; septation; presence of calcification (coarse/punctate); presence of colloid
  - Shape: Taller than wide shape suggests malignancy
  - Vascularity: Avascular/perinodular/intranodular vascularity
  - Associated features: Regional lymphadenopathy, jugular venous thrombus, tumor invasion of adjacent structures
- Overlap of features between benign and malignant thyroid nodules
  - Combination of sonographic features (grayscale and Doppler) will help identify malignant hypoechoic thyroid nodule
- Benign features
  - Well defined, completely haloed, cystic change, septation, presence of colloid, dense/dysmorphic calcification, predominant perinodular vascularity
- Malignant features
  - Ill defined, irregular, punctate calcification, necrosis, marked intranodular vascularity, local invasion, lymphadenopathy, internal jugular vein (IJV) thrombus

Helpful Clues for Common Diagnoses
- **Multinodular Goiter (MNG)**
  - Most common cause of hypoechoic nodule
  - Degenerative nodules
    - Degenerative change in hyperplastic nodules

- Cystic change → septation → entirely cystic ± colloid deposits
- Well defined ± being completely haloed
- Colloid nodules
  - Thin walled, well defined, cystic
  - Echogenic foci with "comet tail" artifacts are characteristic
  - Thick septations ± aggregates of debris
- Background parenchymal heterogeneity (± intranodular hemorrhage) may occur in both degenerative and colloid types
- Other nodules/areas with dense/dysmorphic shadowing calcification may be present in both types
- Colloid nodules/septa are relatively avascular on Doppler
  - Degenerative nodules with cystic change show predominant perinodular vascularity
  - Solid portions in hyperplastic nodules may be quite vascular

Helpful Clues for Less Common Diagnoses
- **Papillary Carcinoma**
  - Painless, enlarging thyroid/neck mass (lymphadenopathy) or incidental finding on thyroid US
  - Hypoechoic, ill defined, ± cystic change
  - Characteristic punctate calcification (psammoma bodies)
  - Large and locally advanced tumor shows invasion of adjacent structures (e.g., strap muscles, trachea)
  - Color Doppler: Hypervascular with disorganized intranodular vascularity
  - Metastatic nodes show features of primary: Punctate calcification, cystic change, and disorganized vascularity
    - Large completely cystic node mimics benign lesion (e.g., 2nd branchial cleft cyst), FNAC indicated
  - ± jugular venous invasion/thrombosis
- **Follicular Carcinoma**
  - Cannot be definitively differentiated from adenoma on either imaging or cytology
  - In most cases, develops from preexisting adenoma
  - Excision is required for definitive diagnosis (to detect any vascular or capsular invasion)
  - Most follicular lesions are iso-/hyperechoic on US
  - US features suggestive of carcinoma
    - Ill-defined border, hypoechoic areas in otherwise iso-/hyperechoic nodule, irregular thick walls, disorganized vascularity, extrathyroid soft tissue, and vascular involvement
    - Metastatic disease in bones, lungs; less commonly in nodes
- **Medullary Carcinoma**
  - Multifocal and bilateral > solitary > diffusely infiltrative
  - Hypoechoic solid tumor, often well defined, frequently located in lateral upper 2/3 of gland in sporadic form
  - Echogenic foci (80-90%) = amyloid + calcification
  - Hypoechoic lymph nodes with coarse shadowing calcification along mid and low IJV chain and superior mediastinum
  - Indistinguishable from papillary carcinoma (more common) on US; diagnosis made by FNAC
    - Differentiating clue: Central coarse calcification and denser shadowing compared with punctate calcification in papillary carcinoma

HYPOECHOIC THYROID NODULE

- **de Quervain Thyroiditis**
  - Typical history + ill-defined hypoechoic noncalcified mass ± internal necrosis
  - Progressive involvement of thyroid parenchyma
  - Vascularity due to inflammatory hyperemia, avascular in necrotic region
  - Localized tenderness with transducer pressure
- **Acute Suppurative Thyroiditis**
  - Acute onset painful thyroid swelling ± recurrent episodes, left (95%) > > right (5%)
  - Starts as perithyroidal inflammation/abscess
  - Late involvement of thyroid gland
  - Ill-defined, hypoechoic internal debris ± gas, soft tissue edema/abscess
  - To exclude underlying pyriform sinus fistula by barium swallow or endoscopy after acute infection has resolved

Helpful Clues for Rare Diagnoses

- **Anaplastic Carcinoma**
  - Rapidly enlarging lower neck mass (± obstructive symptoms) in elderly female with long history of goiter
  - Usually locally advanced disease at clinical presentation
  - US features: Large, ill-defined hypoechoic mass with background MNG
    - Necrosis (78%), dense amorphous/ring calcification (58%), abnormal intratumoral vascularity
    - Extracapsular spread with extensive local invasion with nodal (80%) and distant metastasis
  - US-guided FNAC to confirm diagnosis; CT for extent and extrathyroid involvement
- **Lymphoma**
  - Rapidly enlarging lower neck mass in longstanding Hashimoto thyroiditis
  - Ill-defined mass; often large or diffuse infiltration ± local invasion
  - Necrosis, calcification, and hemorrhage are rare
  - Associated lymphomatous nodes, reticulated/pseudosolid

- **Metastasis**
  - Most patients have known primary and disseminated disease
  - Ill-defined hypoechoic mass; solitary > multifocal > diffuse infiltrative
  - In absence of known primary, lacks specific sonographic features

SELECTED REFERENCES

1. Frates MC et al: Subacute granulomatous (de Quervain) thyroiditis: grayscale and color Doppler sonographic characteristics. J Ultrasound Med. 32(3):505-11, 2013
2. Sofferman RA et al: Ultrasound of the Thyroid and Parathyroid Glands. New York: Springer. 61-150, 2012
3. Anil G et al: Thyroid nodules: risk stratification for malignancy with ultrasound and guided biopsy. Cancer Imaging. 11:209-23, 2011
4. Moon HJ et al: A taller-than-wide shape in thyroid nodules in transverse and longitudinal ultrasonographic planes and the prediction of malignancy. Thyroid. 21(11):1249-53, 2011
5. Kwak JY et al: Value of US correlation of a thyroid nodule with initially benign cytologic results. Radiology. 254(1):292-300, 2010
6. Moon HJ et al: Can vascularity at power Doppler US help predict thyroid malignancy? Radiology. 255(1):260-9, 2010
7. Bonavita JA et al: Pattern recognition of benign nodules at ultrasound of the thyroid: which nodules can be left alone? AJR Am J Roentgenol. 193(1):207-13, 2009
8. Moon WJ et al: Are there any specific ultrasound findings of nodular hyperplasia ("leave me alone" lesion) to differentiate it from follicular adenoma? Acta Radiol. 50(4):383-8, 2009
9. Moon WJ et al: Benign and malignant thyroid nodules: US differentiation--multicenter retrospective study. Radiology. 247(3):762-70, 2008
10. Ahuja AT et al: Diagnostic Imaging: Ultrasound. 1st ed. Salt Lake City: Amirsys Publishing, Inc. 11-6-35, 2007
11. Hoang JK et al: US Features of thyroid malignancy: pearls and pitfalls. Radiographics. 27(3):847-60; discussion 861-5, 2007
12. Frates MC et al: Management of thyroid nodules detected at US: Society of Radiologists in Ultrasound consensus conference statement. Radiology. 237(3):794-800, 2005

Multinodular Goiter (MNG)

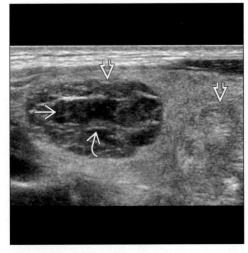

Longitudinal grayscale US shows multiple nodules ➡. Such cystic change ➡ and septation ➡ are characteristic of hyperplastic nodules (spongiform appearance). Overall findings are consistent with MNG.

Multinodular Goiter (MNG)

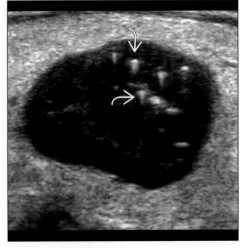

Transverse grayscale US shows a typical thin-walled colloid cyst/nodule with multiple suspended echogenic foci and "comet tail" artifacts ➡.

HYPOECHOIC THYROID NODULE

Papillary Carcinoma

Papillary Carcinoma

(Left) Longitudinal grayscale US shows an ill-defined, solid, hypoechoic thyroid nodule ➡. Note the spiculated border ➡ and conglomeration of fine calcifications ➡, suggesting papillary carcinoma. *(Right)* Corresponding transverse US in the same patient shows solid, hypoechoic, metastatic nodes ➡ from papillary carcinoma with punctate calcifications ➡. The appearance is very similar to the primary tumor ➡ in the thyroid. Note common carotid artery (CCA) ➡ and internal jugular vein (IJV) ➡.

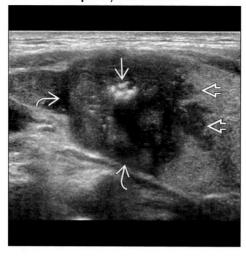

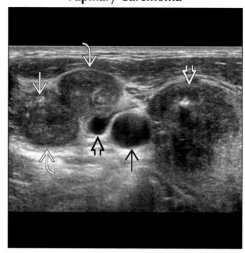

Papillary Carcinoma

Papillary Carcinoma

(Left) Transverse grayscale US shows a large, hypoechoic, infiltrative papillary carcinoma with punctate calcification ➡ and ipsilateral metastatic lymphadenopathy ➡. Note the irregular ill-defined border ➡ and probable extracapsular spread ➡. Note CCA ➡. *(Right)* Corresponding transverse power Doppler US shows marked disorganized internal vascularity in in the primary tumor ➡ and metastatic lymphadenopathy ➡. Note CCA ➡.

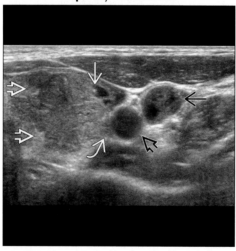

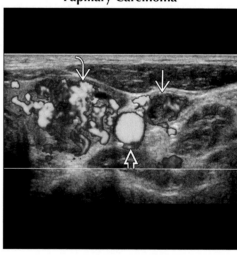

Follicular Carcinoma

Follicular Carcinoma

(Left) Longitudinal US shows an ovoid, solid, hypoechoic thyroid nodule. The homogeneous echo pattern is suggestive of a follicular lesion. The partially indistinct border ➡ and hypoechogenicity are suspicious of malignant change. Excision showed follicular carcinoma. *(Right)* Axial NECT in the same patient shows multiple lung metastases ➡ from follicular carcinoma. Some patients with follicular carcinoma may 1st present with metastases.

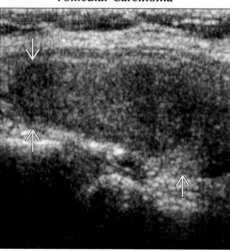

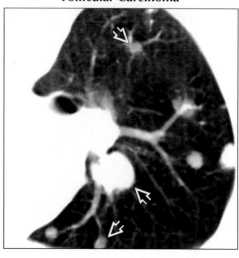

HYPOECHOIC THYROID NODULE

Follicular Carcinoma

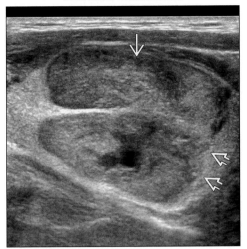

Follicular Carcinoma

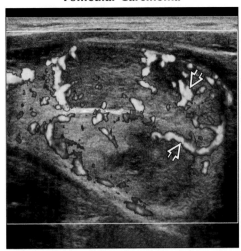

(Left) Longitudinal grayscale US shows a solid, hypoechoic, noncalcified thyroid nodule ➡️. The partially ill-defined border ➤ and heterogeneity are suspicious of malignant change in a follicular lesion. (Right) Corresponding longitudinal power Doppler US in the same patient shows profuse intratumoral vascularity ➤. The ill-defined border and abnormal intranodular vascularity are clues to the malignant nature of the nodule.

Medullary Carcinoma

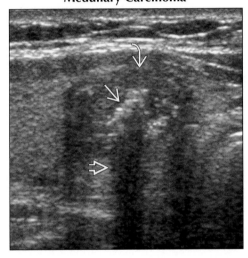

Medullary Carcinoma

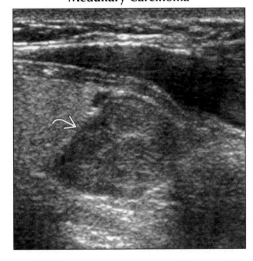

(Left) Longitudinal grayscale US shows an ill-defined, solid hypoechoic nodule ➡️. Note internal foci of dense calcifications ➡️ with posterior shadowing ➤. Note its similarity to papillary carcinoma. Central, dense calcification is the clue to medullary thyroid carcinoma. (Right) Longitudinal grayscale US in the same patient shows a solid, hypoechoic, well-defined parathyroid adenoma ➤ as a part of multiple endocrine neoplasia (MEN) syndrome.

de Quervain Thyroiditis

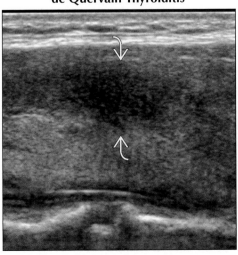

de Quervain Thyroiditis

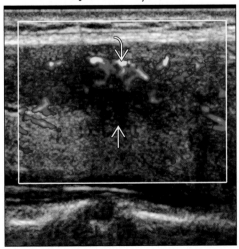

(Left) Longitudinal grayscale US shows an irregular, heterogeneously hypoechoic thyroid "nodule" ➤. The appearance is very similar to a malignant nodule; however, the patient had odynophagia and fever, suggesting de Quervain thyroiditis. The entire gland was involved after a few days. (Right) Corresponding longitudinal power Doppler US shows vascularity ➤ in the hypoechoic area/"nodule" ➡️, mimicking a malignant thyroid nodule.

HYPOECHOIC THYROID NODULE

Acute Suppurative Thyroiditis

(Left) Transverse US shows a large perithyroidal abscess ➡ with extension into the upper pole of the left lobe of the thyroid gland ➡. Note the CCA ➡ and areas of internal necrosis within the abscess ➡. (Right) Axial CECT in the same patient shows a large multiloculated perithyroidal abscess ➡ with intrathyroid extension ➡. Note the CCA ➡, trachea ➡, and necrotic areas of the abscess ➡.

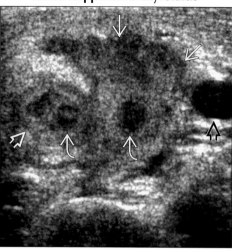

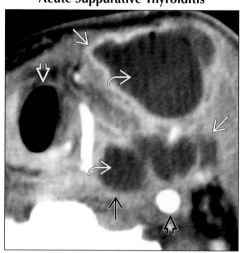

Acute Suppurative Thyroiditis

Anaplastic Carcinoma

(Left) Transverse US shows an anaplastic carcinoma. Note the ill-defined border ➡. Tissue plane between tumor and the trachea is lost, suspicious for tracheal invasion ➡. (Right) Transverse US shows an anaplastic carcinoma in the left lobe of the thyroid, seen as a large, ill-defined, hypoechoic mass ➡ with extracapsular spread ➡ invading the surrounding soft tissue. Note the CCA ➡ and anterior cortex of the vertebral body ➡.

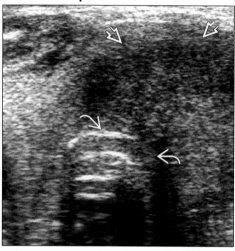

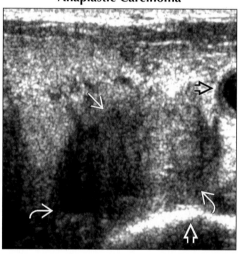

Anaplastic Carcinoma

Anaplastic Carcinoma

(Left) Axial CECT in the same patient shows extensive local infiltration by the tumor ➡ encasing the ipsilateral CCA ➡ and vertebral artery ➡, invading the ipsilateral prevertebral muscle, and crossing the midline ➡. (Right) Transverse T2WI MR with fat suppression in the same patient shows an irregular hyperintense area representing intratumoral necrosis ➡. Invasion of the prevertebral muscle and crossing of the midline ➡ are seen.

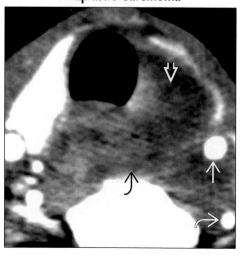

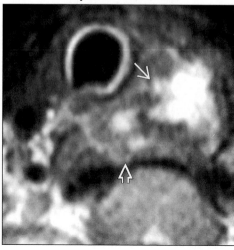

Anaplastic Carcinoma

HYPOECHOIC THYROID NODULE

Lymphoma

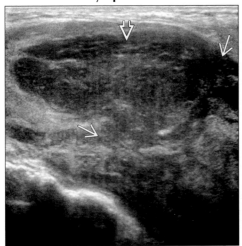

Lymphoma

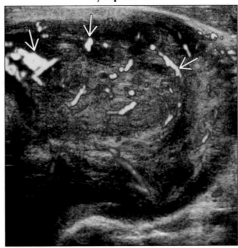

(Left) Longitudinal grayscale US shows an irregular, solid, hypoechoic mass infiltrating the lower pole of the thyroid ⇥, representing thyroid lymphoma. Note the ill-defined margins ⇥ and extracapsular spread. (Right) Corresponding transverse power Doppler US in the same patient shows marked disorganized internal vascularity ⇥ scattered throughout the lesion. The presence of associated lymphomatous nodes (not shown) was another clue to the diagnosis.

Metastasis

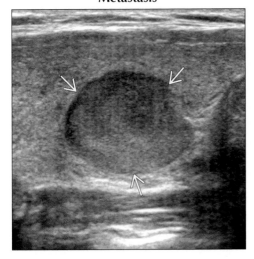

Metastasis

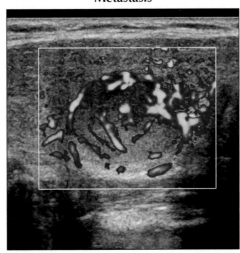

(Left) Longitudinal grayscale US in a patient with known cancer and disseminated disease shows a solid, heterogeneously hypoechoic, fairly well-defined, noncalcified nodule ⇥ in the thyroid, representing a solitary metastasis (in view of patient's history). (Right) Corresponding longitudinal power Doppler US shows profuse, disorganized, peripheral, and intranodular vascularity. Thyroid metastases are seen as part of disseminated disease, and the prognosis is usually grave.

Metastasis

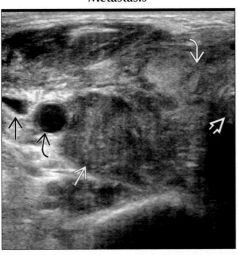

Metastasis

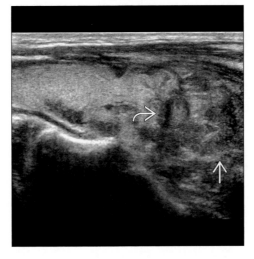

(Left) Transverse grayscale US shows metastatic cervical lymph node ⇥ from carcinoma of the lung invaded and infiltrated the thyroid gland, which shows multiple ill-defined, solid, hypoechoic nodules within ⇥. Note CCA ⇥, internal jugular vein ⇥, and trachea ⇥. (Right) Corresponding longitudinal US shows direct invasion of the lower pole of thyroid lobe ⇥ by metastatic cervical lymphadenopathy ⇥. Occasionally, thyroid lobes may be involved directly by esophageal or laryngeal primary.

CYSTIC THYROID NODULE

DIFFERENTIAL DIAGNOSIS

Common
- Colloid Cyst
- Hyperplastic Nodule
- Hemorrhagic Cyst

Less Common
- Papillary Carcinoma
- Acute Suppurative Thyroiditis

Rare but Important
- Follicular Carcinoma
- Congenital Cyst

ESSENTIAL INFORMATION

Key Differential Diagnosis Issues
- Thyroid cysts account for 15-25% of all thyroid nodules
- Most commonly seen in multinodular goiter (MNG) as combination of colloid cyst, hyperplastic nodule, and hemorrhagic cyst
- Most thyroid cysts are macronodules, which undergo degeneration with accumulation of serous fluid, colloid, or blood
  - "Solid" component of many cystic nodules is usually organized hemorrhage/blood clot
  - Presence/absence of vascularity helps to differentiate avascular hemorrhage from vascular tissue in thyroid carcinoma and hyperplastic nodule
- Thyroid carcinomas, particularly papillary carcinoma, may have prominent cystic component

Helpful Clues for Common Diagnoses
- **Colloid Cyst**
  - Well-defined, cystic, anechoic nodule with thick internal septa
  - Echogenic foci with "comet tail" artifacts may be adherent to septa/wall or dispersed in thick cystic content
  - "Comet tail" artifact due to reverberations from strong acoustic interface produced by inspissated colloid
    - When interrogating echogenic colloid foci, return to fundamental scanning mode to ensure "comet tails" are genuine artifacts and nonshadowing
    - Need to differentiate from punctate calcifications seen in papillary carcinoma
  - Internal debris may aggregate to form echogenic nodule, mimicking papillary carcinoma
    - Presence of punctate calcifications in solid component of papillary carcinoma
    - Use Doppler to differentiate from solid tissue
  - Sonographic appearance may be specific enough to avoid FNAC, which is often inadequate due to viscous content
  - Symptomatic nodules are due to internal hemorrhage or superimposed infection
    - Presence of fluid-sediment level suggests recent hemorrhage
    - US provides guidance for aspiration for symptomatic/cosmetic relief
    - May clinically present with sudden swelling at lower anterior neck or increase in size of known thyroid nodule
    - ± pressure symptoms (e.g., swallowing difficulty)
- **Hyperplastic Nodule**
  - Most commonly seen in background of hyperplasia in MNG
  - Focal hyperplasia of thyroid tissue forms nodule
  - Incompletely encapsulated/haloed vs. complete encapsulation in follicular adenoma
  - Cystic degeneration is common due to fluctuation in tissue response to thyroid-related hormone
    - Appearances range from multiple, dispersed, small cystic spaces to septate nodule to completely cystic nodule; frequently multiple
    - "Spongiform" appearance
    - May have adherent or dispersed "comet tail" artifact within
  - On Doppler, predominantly cystic nodule shows perinodular halo vascularity
    - However, marked intranodular vascularity is often seen in predominantly solid nodules
  - FNAC may be required to exclude neoplasm in nodules with equivocal US features
- **Hemorrhagic Cyst**
  - Hemorrhage into thyroid nodule, which may cause painful enlargement of thyroid nodule within hours or days
    - Rarely, may cause pressure symptoms, dysphagia, or dyspnea
  - Seen as diffuse, mobile, echogenic particulate material or fluid level ± echogenic blood clots in thyroid nodule
    - Echogenic blood clots are avascular on Doppler
  - Usually with background multinodular change
  - US-guided FNAC may be performed for symptomatic relief or cosmesis
  - Direct needle tip away from blood clots to facilitate aspiration of fluid

Helpful Clues for Less Common Diagnoses
- **Papillary Carcinoma**
  - Cystic change is not common in small tumors but often present in larger ones
  - Irregular, ill-defined nodule with cystic change; often seen against background of MNG
    - Eccentric solid portion may contain punctate calcification and is often hypervascular
    - May show local invasion of adjacent structures (e.g., strap muscles, trachea)
  - Metastatic nodes more likely to also show cystic change; appearance mimics primary tumor
    - Solid component of metastatic nodes from papillary thyroid carcinoma is hyperechoic
    - May contain punctate calcification within solid component
    - Chaotic vascularity within solid tumor portion
  - US-guided FNAC should direct needle tip to solid component (preferably calcified portion) for better yield
    - Aspirated fluid is high in thyroglobulin
- **Acute Suppurative Thyroiditis**
  - More common in children and adolescents
  - Left side involvement (95%) > > right side (5%)
  - Related to fistula tract extending from apex of pyriform sinus to lower anterior neck
  - Acutely present with fever, painful goiter, and odynophagia
    - History of recurrent episodes of left neck infection with incision and drainage
  - Perithyroidal abscess and soft tissue inflammation ± internal gas pockets

- Subsequently involves upper pole of thyroid
- Thyroiditis tends to be late occurrence due to inherent resistance of thyroid gland to infection (thick capsule, vascularity, and high iodine content)
  - CT/MR to exclude deep tissue and mediastinal involvement
  - Barium study after acute episode subsides to demonstrate pyriform fossa fistula

Helpful Clues for Rare Diagnoses

- **Follicular Carcinoma**
  - US-guided FNAC and core biopsy cannot differentiate follicular adenoma from carcinoma
  - Postoperative histology assesses capsular integrity and vascular invasion to establish diagnosis of follicular carcinoma
  - Therefore, on US, nodules are grouped as follicular lesions/neoplasms
    - Ovoid, solid, homogeneously iso-/hyperechoic
    - Hypoechoic nodule or hypoechoic portion in otherwise iso-/hyperechoic nodule raises possibility of malignancy
    - Border is well defined in less aggressive type and poorly defined in aggressive type
    - CT/MR help to evaluate extrathyroid extension of aggressive follicular carcinomas
    - Internal cystic area and coarse calcification are occasionally seen
    - Intranodular hypervascularity with "spoke-wheel" appearance on Doppler
- **Congenital Cyst**
  - True thyroid cysts lined with epithelium are rare
    - ≤ 1% of all thyroid nodules
  - Anechoic content ± fine cellular debris
  - Imperceptible walls and posterior acoustic enhancement

SELECTED REFERENCES

1. Frates MC et al: Subacute granulomatous (de Quervain) thyroiditis: grayscale and color Doppler sonographic characteristics. J Ultrasound Med. 32(3):505-11, 2013
2. Sofferman RA et al: Ultrasound of the Thyroid and Parathyroid Glands. New York: Springer. 61-150, 2012
3. Anil G et al: Thyroid nodules: risk stratification for malignancy with ultrasound and guided biopsy. Cancer Imaging. 11:209-23, 2011
4. Ito Y et al: Thyroid ultrasonography. World J Surg. 34(6):1171-80, 2010
5. Moon HJ et al: Can vascularity at power Doppler US help predict thyroid malignancy? Radiology. 255(1):260-9, 2010
6. Bonavita JA et al: Pattern recognition of benign nodules at ultrasound of the thyroid: which nodules can be left alone? AJR Am J Roentgenol. 193(1):207-13, 2009
7. Moon WJ et al: Are there any specific ultrasound findings of nodular hyperplasia ("leave me alone" lesion) to differentiate it from follicular adenoma? Acta Radiol. 50(4):383-8, 2009
8. Moon WJ et al: Benign and malignant thyroid nodules: US differentiation--multicenter retrospective study. Radiology. 247(3):762-70, 2008
9. Ahuja AT et al: Diagnostic Imaging: Ultrasound. 1st ed. Salt Lake City: Amirsys Publishing, Inc. 11-6-35, 2007
10. Hoang JK et al: US Features of thyroid malignancy: pearls and pitfalls. Radiographics. 27(3):847-60; discussion 861-5, 2007
11. Frates MC et al: Management of thyroid nodules detected at US: Society of Radiologists in Ultrasound consensus conference statement. Ultrasound Q. 22(4):231-8; discussion 239-40, 2006
12. Frates MC et al: Management of thyroid nodules detected at US: Society of Radiologists in Ultrasound consensus conference statement. Radiology. 237(3):794-800, 2005
13. Hegedüs L: Thyroid ultrasound. Endocrinol Metab Clin North Am. 30(2):339-60, viii-ix, 2001
14. Marqusee E et al: Usefulness of ultrasonography in the management of nodular thyroid disease. Ann Intern Med. 133(9):696-700, 2000

Colloid Cyst

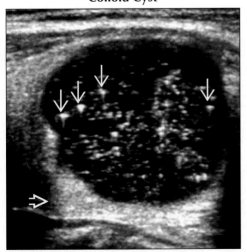

Longitudinal US shows the typical appearance of a colloid nodule with multiple "comet tail" artifacts ➡ scattered throughout the cyst. Note the thin walls and posterior acoustic enhancement ➡.

Colloid Cyst

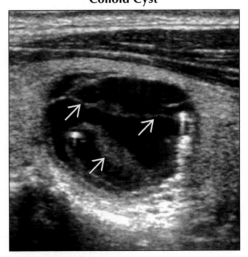

Longitudinal US shows a colloid nodule with "comet tail" artifacts. Note that the "comet tail" artifacts are adherent to the thick intranodular septa ➡, which are invariably avascular on Doppler.

CYSTIC THYROID NODULE

Hyperplastic Nodule

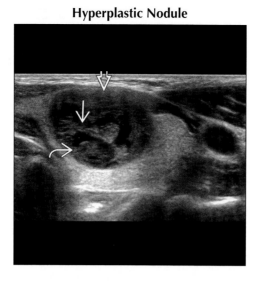

Hyperplastic Nodule

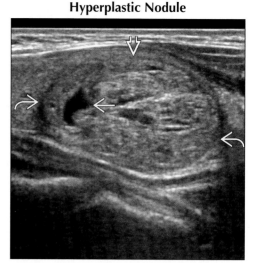

(Left) Transverse grayscale US shows a well-defined hyperplastic nodule ⇒ with cystic change, septa ➡, and internal debris ➡. Debris represents organized blood and is invariably avascular on Doppler. *(Right)* Longitudinal grayscale US shows a hyperplastic nodule ⇒ with cystic degeneration ➡ and complete halo ➡. On Doppler, such a halo is usually vascular (perinodular vascularity) and represents vessels in compressed thyroid tissue.

Hemorrhagic Cyst

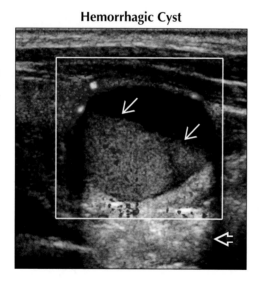

Hemorrhagic Cyst

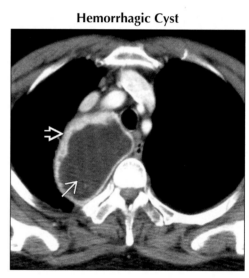

(Left) Longitudinal power Doppler US shows a thyroid nodule with fluid-debris level ➡ (mobile debris on real-time scan). The fluid-debris level, avascular nature, and posterior enhancement ➡ differentiate the hemorrhagic cyst from a solid nodule. *(Right)* Axial CECT shows cystic change ➡ within a thyroid nodule ➡ that extended into the mediastinum. CT better evaluates the inferior extent of large nodules. Aspiration yielded degraded blood products.

Papillary Carcinoma

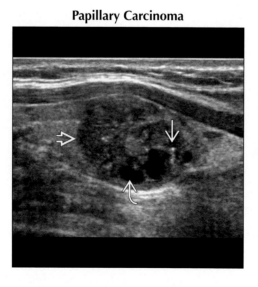

Papillary Carcinoma

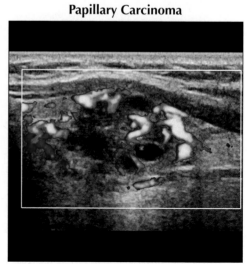

(Left) Longitudinal grayscale US shows a heterogeneous thyroid nodule ➡ with cystic change ➡ within. Multiple foci of punctate calcifications ➡ are seen scattered within the nodule, suggestive of papillary carcinoma. *(Right)* Corresponding longitudinal power Doppler US shows profuse chaotic intranodular vascularity, consistent with papillary thyroid carcinoma. US helps guide the needle towards the solid portion for diagnostic FNAC.

CYSTIC THYROID NODULE

Papillary Carcinoma

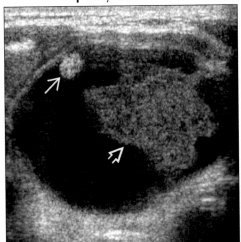

Papillary Carcinoma

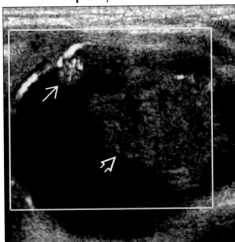

(Left) Transverse US shows a predominantly cystic nodule with 2 components of "solid" tissue: A small mural nodule ➡ and a large intranodular portion ➡. (Right) Transverse pulsed Doppler US in the same patient shows marked hypervascularity in the small solid portion ➡, but the larger portion is avascular ➡. Guided biopsy of the smaller nodule confirmed papillary carcinoma. The avascular component represents a blood clot.

Acute Suppurative Thyroiditis

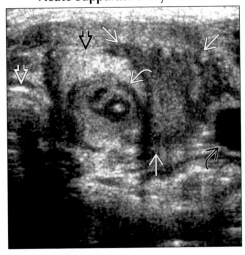

Acute Suppurative Thyroiditis

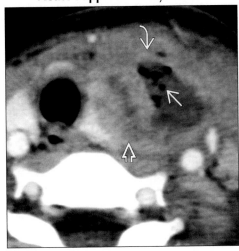

(Left) Transverse US shows a large perithyroidal abscess ➡ with intrathyroidal extension ➡ into the upper pole of the left lobe of the thyroid ➡. Note the trachea ➡ and common carotid artery (CCA) ➡. (Right) Axial CECT in the same patient shows a perithyroidal abscess ➡ with internal gas ➡ and an associated abscess in the left lobe of the thyroid ➡. CECT evaluates the extent of involvement and may show the sinus, seen as a track of air from the pyriform fossa.

Follicular Carcinoma

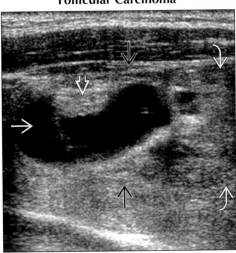

Follicular Carcinoma

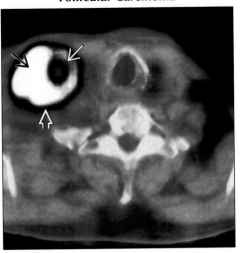

(Left) Transverse US shows an ill-defined thyroid nodule ➡ with an isoechoic solid component ➡ and cystic portion ➡. Note the ill-defined hypoechoic area ➡, which was hypervascular on Doppler (not shown). Surgery revealed follicular carcinoma. (Right) Axial FDG PET/CT fusion image shows a follicular carcinoma ➡ in the right lobe of the thyroid demonstrating avid FDG uptake ➡ except for a cystic component ➡ within the tumor.

CALCIFIED THYROID NODULE

DIFFERENTIAL DIAGNOSIS

Common
- Multinodular Goiter (MNG)

Less Common
- Papillary Carcinoma
- Anaplastic Carcinoma
- Follicular Carcinoma
- Medullary Carcinoma

ESSENTIAL INFORMATION

Key Differential Diagnosis Issues
- Calcification may be present in up to 30% of thyroid nodules
- Microcalcification: Tiny (< 2 mm) punctate echogenic foci ± posterior acoustic shadowing
  - One of the most specific features of malignancy; specificity of 85.8-95%, positive predictive value of 41.8-94.2%
  - Presence of microcalcifications in predominantly solid nodule increases cancer risk 3x compared with predominantly solid nodule without any calcification
  - May not be reliable predictor of malignancy in nodule size < 10 mm
- Macrocalcification: Calcification > 2 mm + posterior acoustic shadowing
  - More commonly seen in benign thyroid nodules and indicates longstanding disease
  - May be worrisome for malignancy if associated with microcalcifications or appearing in center of hypoechoic nodule
  - "Eggshell" calcification most often found in benign nodules; if calcified rim is interrupted, it is suspicious of malignancy
- US is more sensitive than CT and MR in detecting and characterizing punctate calcification
- Coarse shadowing calcification may obscure visualization of posterior part of lesion
  - Evaluating lesion from side or angling transducer may help
    - If this also fails, CT or MR may help
- When using machines with image optimization software, "comet tail" artifact may mimic echogenic foci from punctate calcifications
  - Scanning in fundamental mode may reveal thin shadowing from punctate calcification
  - Use grayscale image obtained during color/power Doppler
    - Automatically goes back to fundamental grayscale
  - Raising scanning frequency on fundamental scans may reveal fine shadowing from punctate calcification
    - As scanning frequency ↑, acoustic attenuation from calcification also ↑ and may show posterior shadowing
- For any lesion suspicious of malignancy, combine US with FNAC for definitive diagnosis
  - May be difficult to penetrate coarse dense calcification using fine needle

Helpful Clues for Common Diagnoses
- **Multinodular Goiter (MNG)**
  - Most common cause of calcified thyroid nodule

- Thyroid enlargement due to multiple cysts (simple, colloid, or hemorrhagic) and nodules (hyperplastic or degenerative)
- Nodules are well defined, haloed, and iso- to hypoechoic
- Early changes: Lower poles > > > upper poles
  - Background thyroid parenchymal echoes are heterogeneous
- Calcification develops with time; coarse, amorphous, or ring like
  - Most produce dense shadowing
- Always search for presence of malignant nodule against background of MNG (papillary, anaplastic carcinoma)

Helpful Clues for Less Common Diagnoses
- **Papillary Carcinoma**
  - Presents as painless thyroid nodule or neck mass (lymph node)
    - May be incidentally detected during US of neck for other causes
  - Solitary, multifocal (10-20%), or diffusely infiltrative
  - Ill-defined, hypoechoic (77-90%), solid nodule ± cystic change ± incomplete halo (15-30%)
  - Characteristic internal punctate calcification (psammoma bodies)
    - Fine discrete echogenic foci ± posterior acoustic shadowing
  - Metastatic lymph node
    - Ipsilateral > contralateral
    - May be very small (5 mm) but show characteristic appearance, such as round, hypoechoic/hyperechoic to muscle with punctate calcification
    - Large metastatic lymph nodes often show cystic change
  - Color Doppler US
    - Profuse disorganized intratumoral hypervascularity > > > hypovascularity
    - Disorganized intranodal vascularity in metastatic lymph node
- **Anaplastic Carcinoma**
  - Typically, rapidly enlarging goiter in elderly woman with long history of goiter
    - ± dysphagia, ± dyspnea
  - Grayscale US
    - Large, ill-defined, hypoechoic, necrotic (78%), heterogeneous mass against background of MNG
    - Internal calcification (58%), typically ring like, coarse, or amorphous, reflecting longstanding MNG
    - Often extracapsular spread with extensive local invasion
    - Internal jugular vein (IJV) thrombus: Due to compression or invasion
    - Nodal or distant metastases in 80% of patients
  - Color Doppler US
    - Necrotic tumor may be avascular/hypovascular (vascular infiltration/occlusion)
    - Vascularity in IJV thrombus suggests tumor thrombus and not bland thrombus
  - US is ideal to characterize tumor, identify extracapsular spread/local invasion, and guide FNAC for diagnosis
  - CT/MR to delineate entire tumor extent, tracheal, prevertebral, vertebral, and mediastinal invasion
- **Follicular Carcinoma**

- Differentiation of follicular adenoma and carcinoma cannot be made on imaging or biopsy
  - Therefore, called follicular lesion/neoplasm
- Definitive diagnosis relies on excision, as follicular carcinoma is defined by presence of vascular or capsular invasion
  - Majority of follicular carcinomas develop from preexisting follicular adenoma
- Sonographic features of follicular lesion
  - Well defined, oval, iso- to hyperechoic, homogeneous, solid, noncalcified
- Features more suggestive of carcinoma than benign adenoma
  - Hypoechoic, focally ill-defined border ± extrathyroid and vascular invasion
  - Hypoechoic, hypervascular change in otherwise iso- to hyperechoic nodule
  - Heterogeneous echo pattern, disorganized intratumoral hypervascularity
  - ± internal cystic change ± dense and coarse calcification
- **Medullary Carcinoma**
  - Middle-aged patient with lower neck mass or incidental finding in patient with family history of multiple endocrine neoplasia (MEN) syndrome
  - Uncommonly, may present with paraneoplastic syndromes: Cushing or carcinoid syndromes
  - Bilateral in 2/3 of sporadic cases; familial type almost always multifocal and bilateral
  - Hypoechoic, solid tumor; well defined > ill defined
  - Solitary, multiple, or diffuse (familial)
  - Echogenic foci (80-90%) = amyloid deposition + calcification
    - Calcifications typically dense and coarse with posterior acoustic shadowing (± central location)
  - 75% have lymphadenopathy at presentation
    - Involves mid and lower internal jugular chain and superior mediastinum
    - Appears as hypoechoic node ± calcification
  - Color Doppler US
    - Disorganized intratumoral and intranodal vascularity

- Nonfamilial form: Invariably mistaken for papillary carcinoma; diagnosis made by FNAC/biopsy
- CT/MR necessary to detect mediastinal and distant metastases

SELECTED REFERENCES

1. Kim BK et al: Relationship between patterns of calcification in thyroid nodules and histopathologic findings. Endocr J. 60(2):155-60, 2013
2. Lee J et al: Fine-needle aspiration of thyroid nodules with macrocalcification. Thyroid. 23(9):1106-12, 2013
3. Sofferman RA et al: Ultrasound of the Thyroid and Parathyroid Glands. New York: Springer. 61-150, 2012
4. Anil G et al: Thyroid nodules: risk stratification for malignancy with ultrasound and guided biopsy. Cancer Imaging. 11:209-23, 2011
5. Kwak JY et al: Thyroid imaging reporting and data system for US features of nodules: a step in establishing better stratification of cancer risk. Radiology. 260(3):892-9, 2011
6. Lu Z et al: Clinical value of using ultrasound to assess calcification patterns in thyroid nodules. World J Surg. 35(1):122-7, 2011
7. Lee SK et al: Follicular thyroid adenoma with eggshell calcification presenting as an intensely hypermetabolic lesion on 18F-FDG PET/CT. J Clin Ultrasound. 38(2):107-10, 2010
8. Moon HJ et al: Can vascularity at power Doppler US help predict thyroid malignancy? Radiology. 255(1):260-9, 2010
9. Bonavita JA et al: Pattern recognition of benign nodules at ultrasound of the thyroid: which nodules can be left alone? AJR Am J Roentgenol. 193(1):207-13, 2009
10. Lee SK et al: Follicular thyroid carcinoma with an eggshell calcification: report of 3 cases. J Ultrasound Med. 28(6):801-6, 2009
11. Park M et al: Sonography of thyroid nodules with peripheral calcifications. J Clin Ultrasound. 37(6):324-8, 2009
12. Kim BM et al: Sonographic differentiation of thyroid nodules with eggshell calcifications. J Ultrasound Med. 27(10):1425-30, 2008
13. Moon WJ et al: Benign and malignant thyroid nodules: US differentiation--multicenter retrospective study. Radiology. 247(3):762-70, 2008

Multinodular Goiter (MNG)

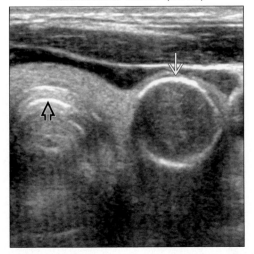

Transverse US shows a well-defined nodule in the left lobe of the thyroid with a complete ring of calcification ➡, which is consistent with a longstanding nodular goiter. Note the trachea ⮕.

Multinodular Goiter (MNG)

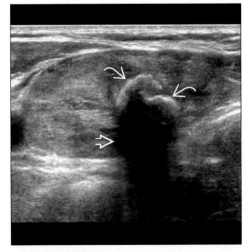

Transverse grayscale US shows multiple curvilinear calcifications ➡ with dense posterior acoustic shadowing ⮕ within a nodule in patient with MNG. The deep portion of the nodule is obscured by the shadowing.

CALCIFIED THYROID NODULE

Multinodular Goiter (MNG)

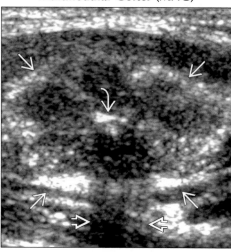

Multinodular Goiter (MNG)

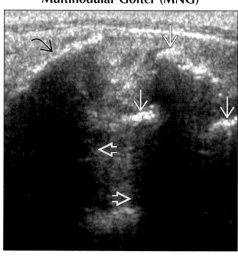

(Left) Longitudinal US shows a nodule in a patient with MNG with internal dense calcification ➡ and strong posterior acoustic shadowing ➡. Note the calcified echogenic rim ➡ of the nodule. *(Right)* Longitudinal US shows a thyroid nodule with both curvilinear peripheral calcification ➡ and central coarse calcification ➡. Note the posterior acoustic shadow ➡. Extensive calcification and shadowing obscure large parts of the nodule, making US suboptimal.

Papillary Carcinoma

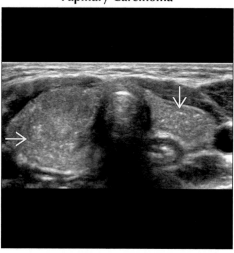

Papillary Carcinoma

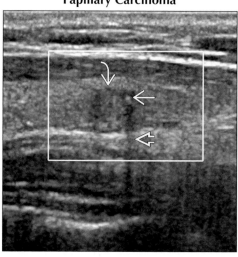

(Left) Transverse grayscale US shows multiple foci of punctate calcification ➡ diffusely scattered in both lobes of thyroid and subtle change in parenchymal echogenicity. Surgery confirmed diffuse sclerosing papillary thyroid carcinoma. *(Right)* Longitudinal power Doppler with color gain turned down (used as grayscale in fundamental mode) shows a small, ill-defined, hypoechoic thyroid nodule ➡ with fine internal punctate calcification ➡ and thin posterior acoustic shadow ➡.

Papillary Carcinoma

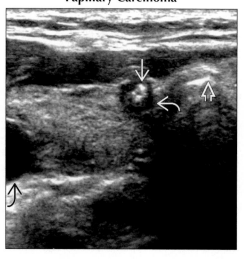

Papillary Carcinoma

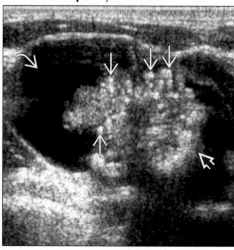

(Left) Transverse US shows a hypoechoic nodule ➡ with an indistinct border and characteristic internal punctate calcifications ➡. Note that small (5 mm) papillary carcinomas are frequently incidental findings. Note the trachea ➡ & common carotid artery (CCA) ➡. *(Right)* Longitudinal US shows a heterogeneous thyroid nodule with a large cystic area ➡ and an eccentric solid nodule ➡ with internal punctate calcifications ➡, typical findings of papillary carcinoma.

CALCIFIED THYROID NODULE

Anaplastic Carcinoma

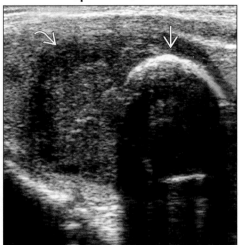

Anaplastic Carcinoma

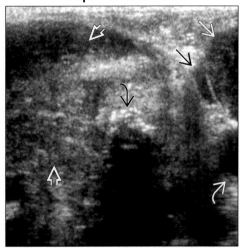

(Left) Longitudinal US shows a solid hypoechoic mass ⟹ with an ill-defined border around a calcified nodule ⟹ from an MNG. This appearance is typical for anaplastic carcinoma, which commonly develops in the setting of longstanding MNG. *(Right)* Transverse US shows a diffusely enlarged left lobe of the thyroid with a heterogeneous, infiltrating tumor ⟹ and eccentric coarse calcification ⟹. Note the associated malignant lymph node ⟹. Note the CCA ⟹ and internal jugular vein ⟹.

Follicular Carcinoma

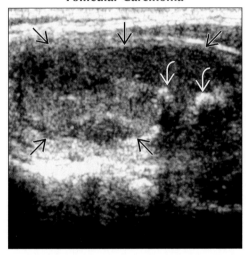

Follicular Carcinoma

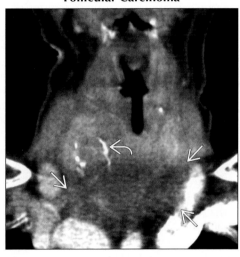

(Left) Longitudinal US shows an ill-defined, hypoechoic, heterogeneous thyroid nodule ⟹ that was confirmed as a follicular carcinoma on excision. Foci of coarse calcification ⟹ are occasionally seen in these tumors. *(Right)* Coronal reformatted CECT of the same patient shows extracapsular spread and extensive local invasion ⟹. Note the calcification ⟹, which was also seen on ultrasound.

Follicular Carcinoma

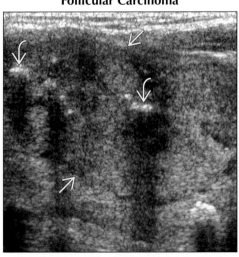

Medullary Carcinoma

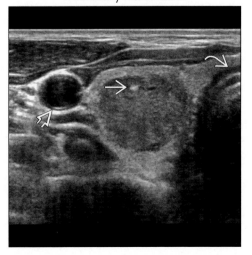

(Left) Longitudinal US shows an ill-defined, solid, hypoechoic nodule ⟹ with infiltrative borders and areas of dense shadowing calcification ⟹, confirmed as follicular carcinoma at surgery. *(Right)* Transverse US shows a well-defined, solid, hypoechoic nodule with a focus of calcification ⟹. This appearance is suspicious for thyroid carcinoma, usually papillary thyroid carcinoma. However, histology confirmed medullary thyroid carcinoma in this case. Note the trachea ⟹ and CCA ⟹.

ENLARGED PARATHYROID GLAND

DIFFERENTIAL DIAGNOSIS

Common
- Parathyroid Adenoma

Less Common
- Parathyroid Hyperplasia
- Parathyroid Cyst
- Parathyroid Carcinoma

ESSENTIAL INFORMATION

Key Differential Diagnosis Issues
- US accurately identifies parathyroid adenoma (PTA) in vicinity of thyroid gland
  - Scintigraphy best evaluates ectopic and intrathyroid parathyroid adenoma
- High-frequency transducer (9-12 MHz) is essential
- Color Doppler increases diagnostic yield
- Irrespective of nature of lesion, abnormal parathyroid glands are hypoechoic (compared with thyroid)
- Transverse scans quickly locate enlarged parathyroid, whereas longitudinal scans better evaluate internal architecture and vascularity
- Meticulous attention to technique and patient positioning yields better diagnostic results
  - Patient in supine position with extended neck to elevate low-lying PTA into neck
    - Neck extension is facilitated by putting small pillow/bolster under shoulder
    - Do not put patient in extended neck position for too long as it may exacerbate postural hypotension
- US has limited use in obese patients with short necks and following failed surgery
- Parathyroid lesion must be differentiated from thyroid nodule and paratracheal lymph node
  - Thyroid nodule is within confines of thyroid capsule
    - Pedunculated thyroid nodule may create diagnostic difficulty
    - US-guided aspiration of the nodule for parathyroid hormone (PTH) level helpful to confirm intrathyroidal parathyroid adenoma
  - Paratracheal lymph nodes, especially when small, are easily confused with normal/enlarged parathyroid gland
    - If enlarged, lymphadenopathy tends to be multiple and arranged in a chain
    - Lymph nodes have hilar architecture and vascularity
  - Normal longus colli muscle, blood vessels, and esophagus should not be mistaken for enlarged parathyroid
- US-guided FNAC easily performed for definitive diagnosis

Helpful Clues for Common Diagnoses
- **Parathyroid Adenoma**
  - Primary hyperparathyroidism occurs in 0.14% of adult population
    - Parathyroid adenoma accounts for 75-85% of cases; single > > multiple
    - Other less common causes include parathyroid hyperplasia (10-15%) and parathyroid carcinoma (< 1%)
  - Upper parathyroid glands
    - Deep to upper-mid pole of thyroid
    - Rarely located posterior to pharynx or esophagus

- Lower parathyroid glands
  - 65% inferior, lateral to lower pole of thyroid
  - 35% variably located along thymopharyngeal duct tract, extending from angle of mandible to lower anterior mediastinum
- Common ectopic locations
  - Near hyoid bone, within carotid sheath, intrathyroidal, intrathymic, and mediastinal
- Grayscale US
  - Well defined and hypoechoic with bright echogenic capsule, typically 1-3 cm
  - Deep to or in vicinity of thyroid glands, typically medial to common carotid artery (CCA)
  - Infrahyoid PTAs are usually spherical
  - Oval or flat if retrothyroid, as parathyroid glands in this position develop within longitudinally aligned fascial planes
  - "Arrowhead" appearance on longitudinal scan with "head" pointing superiorly
  - Bright echogenic line representing medulla may be seen in center
  - May show cystic change (multiple small cysts > solitary large cyst) or septa, representing cystic degeneration
  - Calcification is rare; more common in carcinoma or hyperplasia due to hyperparathyroidism
  - Hemorrhage may occur in larger lesions, causing cystic appearance with fluid level
- Color or power Doppler
  - PTAs are hypervascular with intraparenchymal/polar vascularity; 10% are avascular (lesions < 1 cm)
- Tc-99m sestamibi scan to confirm diagnosis
  - Focal increased radiotracer uptake on early and delayed images

Helpful Clues for Less Common Diagnoses
- **Parathyroid Hyperplasia**
  - Occurs as primary hyperparathyroidism or secondary/tertiary hyperparathyroidism in patient with chronic renal failure
  - Accounts for 10-15% of causes of primary hyperparathyroidism
    - Some are sporadic; others associated with MEN1, MEN2A, and familial hyperparathyroidism (autosomal dominant)
  - Diagnosis is based on biochemical and hormonal profile
  - Radiography shows typical bone changes
  - Main role of US is to identify glands when ethanol ablation is contemplated
  - Hyperplastic parathyroid glands are more spherical than with adenomas ± calcification
  - Scintigraphy employed in patients with clinical evidence of recurrence when previous surgery fails to identify all 4 glands
    - Probably due to ectopic parathyroid
- **Parathyroid Cyst**
  - Most are nonfunctional and asymptomatic
    - M < F, 40-60 years old
  - 20-30% functional
    - M > F, with hyperparathyroidism (may be subclinical)
  - US features
    - Solitary, unilocular, thin walled, and anechoic with posterior acoustic enhancement
    - Septation and loculation are uncommon

ENLARGED PARATHYROID GLAND

- Most are in lower neck near lower poles of thyroid gland but may be anywhere from angle of mandible to superior mediastinum
- 65% involve inferior parathyroid glands
- Cannot be definitely differentiated from branchial cleft cyst or thymic cyst
  - ○ US-guided FNAC may be performed for diagnostic and therapeutic purposes
    - Fluid is typically watery; PTH level is higher than in serum, even in nonfunctioning cyst
    - Helps differentiate from thymic cyst
- **Parathyroid Carcinoma**
  - ○ Most are hyperfunctioning
    - Constitute < 1% of patients with primary hyperparathyroidism
    - PTH level is exceptionally high compared with parathyroid adenoma
  - ○ In clinical setting of abnormally high PTH level and recurrent laryngeal nerve paralysis, parathyroid carcinoma must be suspected
  - ○ Final diagnosis usually made following surgery
  - ○ US features
    - Similar appearance to parathyroid adenoma
    - ± invasion of adjacent structures (thyroid, trachea, esophagus, longus colli muscle, recurrent laryngeal nerve)
    - ± calcification
    - ± immobility on swallowing
  - ○ 21-28% metastasize to cervical lymph nodes; less common than primary thyroid cancer
    - Solid, round, hypoechoic, ± intranodal necrosis
    - Color Doppler shows increased vascularity
    - Paratracheal or along jugular chain

SELECTED REFERENCES

1. Lee JH et al: Imaging of thyroid and parathyroid glands. Semin Roentgenol. 48(1):87-104, 2013
2. Vulpio C et al: Parathyroid-gland ultrasonography in clinical and therapeutic evaluation of renal secondary hyperparathyroidism. Radiol Med. 118(5):707-22, 2013
3. Phillips CD et al: Imaging of the parathyroid glands. Semin Ultrasound CT MR. 33(2):123-9, 2012
4. Sofferman RA: Parathyroid Ultrasound. In Sofferman RA et al: Ultrasound of the Thyroid and Parathyroid Glands. New York: Springer. 157-86, 2012
5. Wei CH et al: Parathyroid carcinoma: update and guidelines for management. Curr Treat Options Oncol. 13(1):11-23, 2012
6. Vazquez BJ et al: Imaging of the thyroid and parathyroid glands. Surg Clin North Am. 91(1):15-32, 2011
7. Dudney WC et al: Parathyroid carcinoma. Otolaryngol Clin North Am. 43(2):441-53, xi, 2010
8. Felger EA et al: Primary hyperparathyroidism. Otolaryngol Clin North Am. 43(2):417-32, x, 2010
9. Patel CN et al: Clinical utility of ultrasound and 99mTc sestamibi SPECT/CT for preoperative localization of parathyroid adenoma in patients with primary hyperparathyroidism. Clin Radiol. 65(4):278-87, 2010
10. Fakhran S et al: Parathyroid imaging. Neuroimaging Clin N Am. 18(3):537-49, ix, 2008
11. Fuster D et al: Localising imaging in secondary hyperparathyroidism. Minerva Endocrinol. 33(3):203-12, 2008
12. Shah S et al: Multimodality imaging of the parathyroid glands in primary hyperparathyroidism. Minerva Endocrinol. 33(3):193-202, 2008
13. Ahuja AT: Parathyroid Adenoma, Visceral Space. In Ahuja AT et al: Diagnostic Imaging: Ultrasound. 1st ed. Amirsys: Salt Lake City. 11-36-39, 2007
14. Huppert BJ et al: Parathyroid sonography: imaging and intervention. J Clin Ultrasound. 35(3):144-55, 2007
15. Kamaya A et al: Sonography of the abnormal parathyroid gland. Ultrasound Q. 22(4):253-62, 2006
16. Kettle AG et al: Parathyroid imaging: how good is it and how should it be done? Semin Nucl Med. 36(3):206-11, 2006
17. Uruno T et al: How to localize parathyroid tumors in primary hyperparathyroidism? J Endocrinol Invest. 29(9):840-7, 2006
18. Ahuja AT et al: Imaging for primary hyperparathyroidism--what beginners should know. Clin Radiol. 59(11):967-76, 2004
19. Meilstrup JW: Ultrasound examination of the parathyroid glands. Otolaryngol Clin North Am. 37(4):763-78, ix, 2004
20. Ihm PS et al: Parathyroid cysts: diagnosis and management. Laryngoscope. 111(9):1576-8, 2001

Parathyroid Adenoma

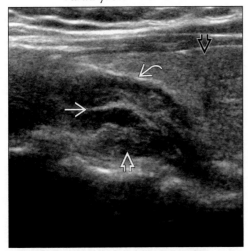

Longitudinal grayscale US shows a PTA ⬅ behind the thyroid gland ⬅. Note the echogenic center ➡ (medulla) with well-defined border and a sharp echogenic line ➡ separating the PTA from thyroid gland.

Parathyroid Adenoma

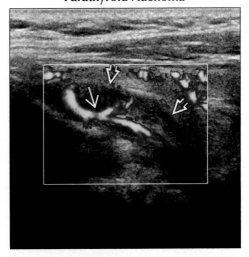

Corresponding longitudinal power Doppler US shows central vascularity ➡ in a PTA ⬅. Most PTAs are hypervascular with < 10% being avascular on Doppler.

ENLARGED PARATHYROID GLAND

Parathyroid Adenoma

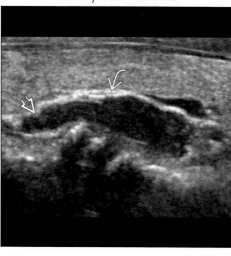

Parathyroid Adenoma

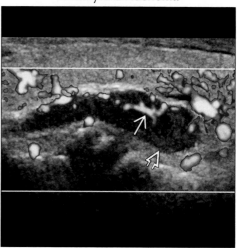

(Left) Longitudinal grayscale US shows an "arrowhead" appearance of a PTA, with the "head" ➡ pointing cranially. Note the bright echogenic capsule ➡ separating it from the thyroid gland anteriorly. *(Right)* Corresponding longitudinal power Doppler US shows central, linear, intraparenchymal hypervascularity ➡ in the PTA ➡, which is typical. Lesions that are deep-seated, < 1 cm, or have cystic necrosis may be avascular.

Parathyroid Adenoma

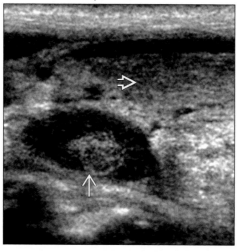

Parathyroid Adenoma

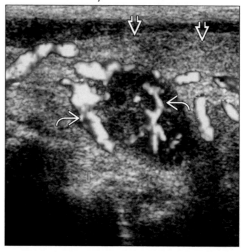

(Left) Longitudinal US shows a solid, well-defined, hypoechoic PTA ➡. Irrespective of the nature of the lesion, most PTAs are hypoechoic compared with the thyroid parenchyma ➡. This makes them conspicuous and readily visible when they are in the vicinity of the thyroid gland. *(Right)* Transverse power Doppler US in the same patient shows profuse parenchymal vascularity ➡ in the PTA. Note the thyroid ➡.

Parathyroid Adenoma

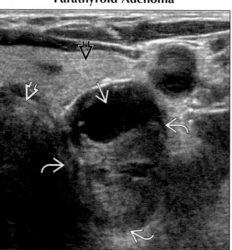

Parathyroid Adenoma

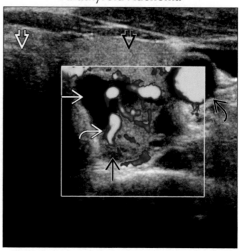

(Left) Transverse grayscale US shows a large PTA ➡ with a focal, well-defined, anechoic cystic area ➡ within. The appearance is consistent with cystic degeneration, which is often seen in large PTAs. Note the trachea ➡ and thyroid ➡. *(Right)* Transverse power Doppler US shows another PTA ➡ with cystic areas ➡ and intraparenchymal hypervascularity ➡. Multiple small cystic areas are more commonly seen rather than 1 large cystic area. Note the CCA ➡, trachea ➡, and thyroid ➡.

ENLARGED PARATHYROID GLAND

Parathyroid Adenoma

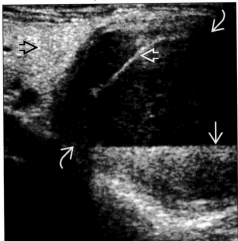

Parathyroid Adenoma

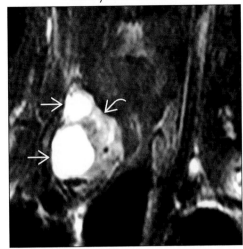

(Left) Transverse US shows a hemorrhagic PTA ➡. Note the internal fluid level ➡, septa ➡, and adjacent thyroid ➡. *(Right)* Coronal T2WI with fat suppression in the same patient shows the hemorrhagic PTA ➡. Note the cystic areas ➡ within. Such large lesions may compress the trachea, esophagus, and recurrent laryngeal nerve.

Parathyroid Adenoma

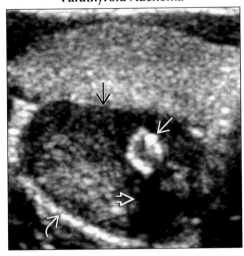

Parathyroid Hyperplasia

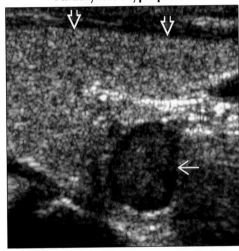

(Left) Transverse US shows a PTA ➡ behind the thyroid. Note calcification ➡ with acoustic shadowing ➡ and echogenic capsule ➡. Calcification is rare in a PTA and more commonly seen in hyperplasia due to hyperparathyroidism and parathyroid carcinoma. *(Right)* Longitudinal US shows an enlarged, well-defined, hypoechoic, noncalcified parathyroid gland ➡ in parathyroid hyperplasia. Note the thyroid ➡.

Parathyroid Cyst

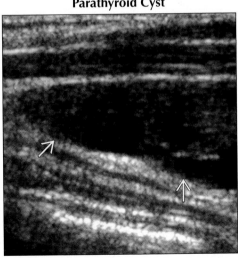

Parathyroid Cyst

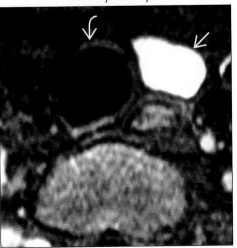

(Left) Longitudinal US shows a thin-walled parathyroid cyst ➡ inferior to the thyroid gland. *(Right)* Axial T2WI with fat suppression of the same patient shows the parathyroid cyst ➡, which is thin walled with homogeneous hyperintense fluid signal. Note the trachea ➡. Fluid aspirated from such cysts is usually clear and shows high parathyroid hormone levels compared with the serum.

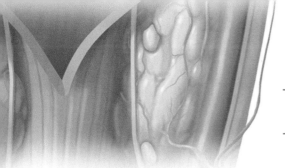

INDEX

INDEX

Index

ii

INDEX

INDEX

INDEX

INDEX

INDEX

INDEX

INDEX

INDEX

INDEX

INDEX

INDEX

INDEX